Communicating Clinical Decision-Making Through Documentation

Notice

Communicating Clinical Decision-Making Through Documentation

Coding, Payment, and Patient Categorization

Editors

Eric Shamus, PT, DPT, PhD, CEEAA
Professor, Chair Department of Rehabilitation Sciences
Florida Gulf Coast University
Fort Myers, Florida

Debra Stern, PT, DPT, MSM, DBA, CEEAA
Professor, Physical Therapy – Fort Lauderdale
Nova Southeastern University
Fort Lauderdale, Florida

William F. McGehee, PT, PhD, CEEAA
Associate Professor, School of Physical Therapy
Regis University
Denver, Colorado

Kara Gainer, JD
Director, Regulatory Affairs
American Physical Therapy Association
Alexandria, Virginia

Mc Graw Hill

New York Chicago San Francisco Athens London Madrid Mexico City
Milan New Delhi Singapore Sydney Toronto

Communicating Clinical Decision-Making Through Documentation: Coding, Payment, and Patient Categorization

Previously published as *Effective Documentation for Physical Therapy Professionals*, copyright © 2011, 2004 by the McGraw-Hill Companies, Inc.

1 2 3 4 5 6 7 8 9 DSS 26 25 24 23 22 21

ISBN 978-1-260-44066-9
MHID 1-260-44066-4

This book was set in Minion Pro by MPS Limited.
The editors were Michael Weitz and Peter J. Boyle.
The production supervisor was Catherine H. Saggese.
Project management was provided by Poonam Bisht and Jyoti Shaw.

This book is printed on acid-free paper.

Cataloging-in-publication data for this book is on file at the Library of Congress.

Contents

SECTION 4
Steps and Framework for Coding and Documentation

Contributors

Erika Albertini, PT, DPT
Activa Home Health
Boynton Beach, Florida

Nancy Campbell, PT
Orthonet
Fort Lauderdale, Florida

Matt Daugherty, MOT, DPT, DBA
Associate Professor
University of St. Augustine
St. Augustine, Florida

Helene H. Fearon, PT
Phoenix, Arizona

Claudia Senesac, PT, PhD, PCS
Clinical Professor
University of Florida
Gainesville, Florida

Jennifer Shamus, PT, DPT, PhD
Select Physical Therapy
Pembroke Pines, Florida

Rob Sillevis, PT, DPT, PhD
Assistant Professor
Florida Gulf Coast University
Fort Myers, Florida

Arie van Duijn, PT, EdD
Professor
Florida Gulf Coast University
Fort Myers, Florida

Tom Zeller, PT, DPT
Advanced Physical Therapy
Cape Coral, Florida

Contributors from Previous Editions

Martha Bloyer, PT, PCS
Miami, Florida

Barbara Deering, PT
Fort Lauderdale, Florida

Reuben Escorpizo, PT, DPT
Burlington, Vermont

Gerry Fluet, DPT
Newark, New Jersey

Scott Harp, PT, PhD
Orlando, Florida

Stephen M. Levine, PT, DPT
Fort Lauderdale, Florida

Rebecca S. Rosenthal, PT, MS, JD
Fort Lauderdale, Florida

Kathy Swanick, DPT
Fort Myers, Florida

Kay H. Tasso, PT, PCS, MA, PhD
Jacksonville, Florida

Preface

In a changing healthcare environment, physical therapists and physical therapist assistants need to be paid for services rendered. Therapists cannot afford third-party payer denial for services they provide. This textbook will help lay the foundation on what, how, and why to document. Clinical decision-making, evidence-based practice, legal issues, coding, and utilization review are just a few of the content areas covered.

Frequently asked Medicare billing and coding questions:

1. **Are Medicaid managed care organizations (MCOs) mandated by CMS to follow Medicare billing guidelines?**

A: No. MCOs must provide all benefits offered under the state plan, but can provide benefits additional to traditional Medicaid fee-for-service (FFS). MCOs are not mandated by the federal government (Centers for Medicare & Medicaid Services [CMS]) to follow federal Medicare billing and treatment guidelines, unless there is a state statute or regulation that mandates Medicaid MCOs in that state to follow Medicare guidelines. It is recommended that providers review their individual Medicaid MCO contractual agreements and meet with their prospective (and current) carriers to determine the details of the applicable billing and treatment polices applicable to physical therapist services.

2. **Can the physical therapist assistant complete the Medicare progress report?**

A: No. The physical therapist must write the entire progress report, but can use the information that was gathered by the physical therapist assistant and is in the physical therapist assistant's note. See Medicare Benefit Policy Manual Chapter 15, Section 220.3.

3. **Can I bill a re-evaluation (CPT 97164) every time a progress report is completed (at a minimum, every 10th treatment visit per Medicare coverage guidelines)?**

A: No. Continuous assessment of the patient's progress is a component of ongoing therapy services—it is not payable as a re-evaluation. Actual re-evaluations, however, are another matter—they are separately payable and should be conducted when indicated during an episode of care when the professional assessment of a physical therapist indicates significant improvement, decline, or change in the patient's condition or functional status that was not anticipated in the plan of care. Remember: A re-evaluation is not a routine, recurring service, but is focused on evaluating progress toward current goals, making a professional judgment about continued care, and modifying goals and/or treatment or terminating services. A formal re-evaluation is covered only if the documentation supports the need for further tests and measurements after the initial evaluation. According to CMS, indications for a re-evaluation include new clinical findings, a significant change in the patient's condition, or the patient's failure to respond to the therapeutic interventions outlined in the plan of care. Although some state regulations and state practice acts require re-evaluation at specific times, re-evaluations for Medicare beneficiaries also must meet Medicare coverage guidelines. The decision to provide a re-evaluation must be made by the physical therapist.

4. **Is direct care (1:1 rule) a Medicare rule?**

A: No. In fact, the language supporting the idea of "direct patient contact" appears in the American Medical Association's Current Procedural Terminology (CPT) book, in a section that accompanies the therapeutic procedure codes requiring that the "physician or qualified healthcare professional have direct (one-on-one) patient contact." The language is part of a resource aimed at providing a uniform language that will accurately describe medical, surgical, and diagnostic services—but it is not generated by CMS.

5. **Do I have to discharge patients from physical therapy when they reach the Medicare payment outpatient therapy threshold or targeted medical review threshold?**

A: As long as skilled physical therapy continues to be medically necessary, you should not discharge Medicare patients when they reach the outpatient therapy threshold or the targeted medical review threshold. What used to be the Medicare therapy caps now are annual thresholds that you can exceed when you append claims with the KX modifier for medically necessary services. This change from the earlier "hard" therapy caps is the result of the Bipartisan Budget Act of 2018 (BBA of 2018), which provides for Medicare payment for outpatient therapy services, including physical therapy, speech-language pathology, and occupational therapy services. If services exceed the annual threshold amounts, include the KX modifier as confirmation that services are medically necessary, as justified by appropriate documentation in the medical record. If you furnish medically necessary services over the targeted medical review threshold of $3,000, continue to affix the KX modifier and maintain the documentation to justify it. This medical review focuses on categories of providers deemed at higher risk for rejected claims.

Common reasons for denials by third-party payers include:

Technical errors such as:

- Identifier omission
- Incorrect form use
- Incorrect or inadequate information
- Missing physician's/nonphysician practitioner's (NPP's) signature and date of certification of the plan of care or progress note indicating the physician/NPP reviewed and approved the plan of care

Nontechnical errors such as:

- The medical documentation submitted did not show that the therapy services were reasonable and necessary and at a level of complexity that requires the skills of a therapist
  - Lack of detail for the level of severity
  - Illegibility
  - Good documentation in wrong place
  - Bad documentation anyplace
  - Billing information does not match documentation of care
  - Goals do not match problems or diagnosis
  - Outcomes or effectiveness of therapy services for patient's illness or injury (i.e., goals not achieved) are not documented
  - Patient achieved their restorative potential and was provided repetitive, nonskilled exercises
  - Documentation does not establish thorough objective measurements that the patient is making progress toward goals
  - Loss of function or functional limitation was not identified (problems were physiologically impairment based)
  - Potential for significant improvement not identified (goals were not significant enough to justify care, or patient was too high level or too low level)
  - Need for skilled therapist not identified (improvement would have been made without therapeutic intervention)
  - Skills of therapist are not required to actually carry out the maintenance program
  - Critical thinking not supported by evidence-based care

Incorporating all the general principles for documentation and health information management should help the therapist maintain records appropriately, organize the record, record appropriate information, and receive payment based on the documentation content. The therapist should seek to write only what is relevant and necessary and in an objective manner, using verbiage that indicates skill, but is universally understood based on all purposes of the medical record. By appreciating why payment for therapy services is denied, the therapist can reflect on documentation content guidelines and the importance of content adherence.

Acknowledgements

We would like to thank and acknowledge all the individuals who contributed to this book. Without their expertise and dedication, this book would not have been possible.

SECTION 1

How to Write Patient Care Notes

1 Introduction, Background, Purpose, and General Rules for Health Information Management

OBJECTIVES

Following completion of this chapter, the reader will be able to:

- Discuss the relationship between health information management and medical record keeping.
- Identify medical necessity for physical therapy.
- Define documentation according to the APTA Guide for Physical Therapist Practice.
- Understand the primary purposes of the medical record.
- Describe five secondary purposes of the medical record.
- Explain what is HIPAA and how is it relevant to health information management.

INTRODUCTION, BACKGROUND, AND PURPOSES OF THE RECORD

> *Clinical documentation is at the core of every patient encounter. In order to be meaningful, it must be accurate, timely, and reflect the scope of services provided. Successful clinical documentation improvement (CDI) programs facilitate the accurate representation of a patient's clinical status that translates into coded data. Coded data is then translated into quality reporting, physician report cards, reimbursement, public health data, and disease tracking and trending.*[1]

Although most purposes of physical therapy documentation have remained constant, in recent years and moving forward, the focus on value-based care is putting increasing emphasis on the need for value-based documentation. The elements of documentation need to imply value orientation.[2]

Documentation:

- *It is a tool for the planning and provision of physical therapist services and is a communication vehicle among providers.*
- *It is a record of care provided, including a report of the individual's status, physical therapist management, and outcome of physical therapist intervention.*
- *It may be used to demonstrate compliance with federal, state, payer, and local regulations.*
- *It provides a historical account of individual encounters that can be used as evidence in potential legal challenges.*
- *It may be used by third-party payers to assess appropriateness of service utilization that is required for payment.*
- *It may be used for policy or research purposes, including outcomes analysis.*[2]

As the complexity of healthcare has grown, so has the management of medical or health information, which is "the data related to a person's medical history, including symptoms, diagnoses, procedures and outcomes."[3] HealthIT.gov[4] defines an electronic health record (EHR) as a "digital version of a patient's paper chart, that are real time, patient-centered records that make information available instantly and securely to authorized users." Health information management (HIM) redefines the term medical record keeping as EHR or electronic medical records (EMR) which are now the norm, although some practices may still be using manual entry. The term EMR is a more focused, narrower record of patient health and care, such as that used in physical therapy practice, whereas the EHR is technically more comprehensive. However, the terms are often used interchangeably.

The American Health Information Management Association (AHIMA) is setting the standards for the overall science of HIM in an increasingly complex system.[3] A patient chart or record in any form is considered a legal document. As such, it is subject to state and federal laws, as well as medical record laws, HIM laws, state licensure laws for healthcare practitioners, and federal regulation and acts, especially the Health Information and Portability Accountability Act of 1996 (HIPAA). HIPAA set federal standards for accessing and handling medical information. Health information is also subject to regulations established by third-party payers, especially Centers for Medicare & Medicaid Services (CMS).

The American Physical Therapy Association board of directors approved the Guidelines: Physical Therapy Documentation of Patient/Client Management,[2] applicable to manual or electronic documentation, to provide "documentation guidance across all settings." The document provides an outline of the elements of physical therapist (PT) documentation with an outline of content expected in each, and is considered the professional standard.

For physical therapy professionals, documentation is a required practice by federal, state, facility, accreditation regulations, and guidelines. In some states, licensing laws include documentation content regulations and who is responsible for specific content: the PT or physical therapist assistant (PTA). In others, it is implied. However, it should be noted that any documentation laws are not dependent on who is paying the bill, but rather the physical therapy management of a patient itself.

According to the American Physical Therapy Association (APTA) *Guide to Physical Therapist Practice 3.0*,[5] documentation is any entry into the medical record and is required for all patient-related encounters. Although required in all settings with some differing requirements, effective, efficient, and appropriate documentation that complies with all purposes and regulations and reflects skilled care, including value, can be vexing to the practitioner. Documentation is not only required to justify if payment is indicated based on skilled care rendered but is being used to determine level of outcomes and potential bonus payment for the best outcomes. As requirements and guidelines are frequently updated by CMS, it is the individual responsibility of each PT or PTA to keep up with changing standards in all settings. Style and required content vary among facilities, organizations, agencies, and therapists, with electronic templates built into systems to facilitate minimum content. Some EHR/EMR systems allow more latitude in content than others. In reality, even with going electronic, practical application and entry are more challenging than theoretical application. However, many electronic systems now update their software automatically to facilitate practitioner compliance with changes and supply supplemental information about changing regulations to users.

Physical therapy became a billable service when the Medicare program was established with Title XVIII of the Social Security Act, implemented in 1966. According to the Social Security Act, when treating Medicare beneficiaries, all practitioners are required to document patient care and ascertain and establish the medical necessity of care. When Medicare was first implemented, most physical therapy was hospital based for both inpatient and outpatient treatment, and payment did not depend on, nor was it related to, record content. The scope and specificity for Medicare documentation in all settings, including outpatient, home health and inpatient rehabilitation, have been expanding since the 1970s. From an historical perspective, all delivered services initially required physician prescription or referral, ongoing physician visits, and justification of skilled care as evidenced by documentation. Depending on the setting—hospital, skilled nursing, outpatient, or home health—payment was on a fee-for-service or cost-based basis. In pure fee-for-service arrangements, increasingly rare in the twenty-first century, providers charged a fee and the third-party payer, including the designated Medicare intermediaries (now Medicare Administrative Contractors [MACs]), paid the bill. This system assumed the fees were reasonable and customary in a designated "community." Medicare's cost-based payment was derived from the costs incurred by the organization providing services to a Medicare beneficiary without regard for preset parameters, but rather categories that were acceptable for payment in skilled nursing facilities, rehabilitation agencies, and comprehensive outpatient rehabilitation facilities (CORF)s for physical therapy services. As healthcare costs began to and continued to escalate, fee-for-service has morphed on a continuous basis into more cost-effective payment systems for both the CMS Medicare program and the commercial insurance market, focusing on more prospective payment models and the resource-based relative value scale (RBRVS). Not all commercial payers tie their rates to the Medicare physician fee schedule, but many payers do follow the lead of Medicare in establishing their payment rates and policies and procedures.

The 1970s, which heralded both societal and healthcare changes, was a time of increasing medical malpractice claims, which continues even today. Malpractice suits remain more prevalent for physicians but occur in all types of settings and have affected physical therapy. Since the only evidence of care both during patient care and after patient discharge is the written record or EHR/EMR, the record content is critical in determining the validity of the claim and proving innocence or potential guilt of the healthcare provider. According to the Healthcare Providers Service Organization (HPSO)[6] that partners with the APTA to provide professional liability coverage for APTA members, the number of malpractice suits against PTs was and continues to be small. However, it continues to be the documentation coupled with appropriate standard of care that supports innocence and protects or potentially contributes to convicting the provider. In the 2016 HPSO claims report, there were approximately 3,000 claims over a 4-year period with a $10,000 or indemnity payment.[6] The cliché "if it wasn't written, it wasn't done" aptly described one aspect of the need for appropriate record content. Just having something written, however, is not the only defense, but rather having written information that is objective, complete, justifies, and describes the skilled care provided, with the value of the care included as determined by outcomes. With the APTA Vision 2020 of autonomous practice in an interprofessional environment and the change in the terminal PT educational degree to the doctor of physical therapy (DPT), there is an increasing need for thorough, accurate, complete, and skilled documentation demonstrating evidence-based care that provides the value needed for the level of severity of the patient.

As stated in the Medicare Benefit Policy Manual Chapter 15, Section 220.3:

> *Changes in objective and sometimes to subjective measures of improvement also help establish the need for rehabilitative services. The use of scientific evidence, obtained from professional literature, and sequential measurements of the patient's condition during treatment is encouraged to support the potential for continued improvement that may justify the patients' need for rehabilitative therapy or the patient's need for maintenance therapy.*

Before healthcare costs began escalating in the 1970s and 1980s, documentation content was not used to any extent to deny payment to the provider, as neither the federal government nor private industry had the technology to track claims in an efficient manner. However, with the advent of computerization in the 1980s, Medicare was able to track services for the first time. As this became possible, the Healthcare Finance Administration (HCFA), now CMS, embarked on a vigorous program to uncover fraud and abuse, as well as care that was not medically necessary for all Medicare-provided services, including physical therapy. In the early 1990s, commercial payers determined that they could also track services and determine if documentation supported the care rendered, making appropriate and skilled physical therapy documentation increasingly critical. Tracking resulted in the recovery of millions of dollars from fraudulent claims in the 1980s and 1990s and continues today with the expansion of Medicare and Medicaid fraud and incorrect payment initiatives throughout the country. According to the CMS.gov, "In the Tax Relief and Health Care Act of 2006, Congress required a permanent and national Recovery Audit Contractor (RAC) program to be in place by January 1, 2010" in all five Medicare regions.[7] The Medicare Fee for Service (FFS) recovery audit contractor (RAC) program instituted a 3-year pilot test to "identify and correct past improper Medicare payments, reduce future improper payments and improve its error rate (for all Medicare payments, not just physical therapy)."[7] The RACs were implemented in 2009. During its demonstration project alone, over $900 million in overpayments was identified based on audits of medical records/health information and billing records that did not support the care rendered, with minimal underpayment discovered. It is in the best interest of the RACS to discover overpayment, as they are paid based on discovery of overpayment and underpayment. Although this system is primarily Medicare based, all third-party payers conduct similar types of audits. In addition to the RACs, the federal General Accounting Office (GAO) through the Office of the Inspector General (OIG) has historically conducted audits for CMS and the Medicare and Medicaid programs. Physical therapy has regularly been identified as having documentation insufficient to support skilled care in a variety of domains.

There is an initiative in the private sector similar to the RACs, further emphasizing the need for physical therapy professionals to document skillfully in all venues. It should be noted that although CMS relative to Medicare does not include payment in its list of purposes of medical records, documentation and payment are integrally related, as evidenced by the practitioners ordered to "pay back" the federal government any payments not supported by appropriate documentation. As the healthcare industry continues to undergo reform, managed care—the initiative that seeks to deliver appropriate and cost-effective healthcare without sacrificing quality—demands an effective and efficient billing tracking process. Decreases in payment by third-party payers within a managed care environment, whether by decreased dollars per visit, visit limitation, or capitation, have forced physical therapy providers to ensure payment of all billable services, with justifiable care evidenced in documentation. The documentation must justify care that reflects the need for skilled services (medical necessity) along with the level of functional and medical severity, be concise and accurate (effective and efficient), and match all billing information with correct coding. The burden falls on the PT and PTA to justify the value of care delivered. In 2010, Congress passed the Affordable Care Act and created a national health plan initiative for individuals under age 65. Mandated purchase of healthcare coverage or paying a mandated "tax" was in effect until tax reform in 2018. Insurance coverage became available through federal or state marketplaces that sold plans ranging from the lowest or minimum required government laws to higher plans, named bronze, silver, gold, and platinum. As the value of the named metal increased, so did the amount of coverage purchased. All health insurance plans offered in the Affordable Care Act's Marketplace are required to cover a set of 10 categories of services. These include rhabilitative and habilitative services and devices (services and devices to help people with injuries, disabilities, or chronic conditions gain or recover mental and physical skills). Specific services may vary based on the state's requirements. Although content of documentation was not dictated by the plans, the expectation was and is consistent with that of other commercial insurance. Although there was and is debate about the success of this program, as the cost of plans continues to rise, it has resulted in an increase in coverage for millions of Americans. The 2018 tax reform, Tax Cuts and Jobs Act, signed in 2017, however, removed the requirement for Americans to purchase coverage and eliminated the tax penalty effective January 1, 2019. While not a documentation or value challenge for physical therapy, the future of the ACA is pending with the Supreme Court.

"CMS, an agency within U.S. Department of Health and Human Services (HHS)," is the single largest payer of healthcare in the United States, administering Medicare, Medicaid, and the State Children's Health Insurance Program (SCHIP or CHIP). CMS's Medicare program dictates basic content for documentation for rehabilitation professionals, including PTs. Data gathered by CMS is maintained in a national database, where it is stored and analyzed and used to "make decisions related to healthcare payment mechanisms, the effectiveness of healthcare services, and the general health of the Medicare population."[7] State governments that administer Medicaid (a shared federal and state program) and other third-party payers maintain similar data for decision-making purposes. However, since MACs contract with CMS to administer payment to the care provider, the regulations are open to interpretation by the payer as well as the care provider when there is no National Coverage Determination issued by CMS. Local coverage determinations (LCDs) are published by the MACs in each of 12 designated Medicare regions (as of June 2019) to clarify if a service is reasonable and necessary if there is no national coverage determination (NCD).[8] The one constant is that services must be skilled in nature and justified, as evidenced by documentation. This can result in coverage of a service or diagnosis in one or more regions, but not in others. The service provider must abide by the LCD in their jurisdiction.[8]

PTs need to make the connection in their documentation between the medical problem, the treatment or physical therapy-related functional problems, treatment diagnosis or physical therapy diagnosis, the PT's initial examination and evaluation, treatment/intervention, severity of the problem, and objective measures of beginning status and ultimately outcomes to indicate the value of care rendered. Goals should be established based on the World Health Organization's (WHO's) 2001 International Classification of Functioning, Disability and Health (ICF) model in consultation with the patient, how realistic the goals are based on prior level of function and presentation at the time of care, and length of stay (LOS) in a specific setting. With the introduction of alternative payment models, including bundled payment models, such as the Comprehensive Care for Joint Replacement Model (CJR), and a variety of prospective payment systems that use case-mix classification methodologies, including the Skilled Nursing Facility (SNF) Patient-Driven Payment Model (PDPM), which began on October 1, 2019, and the Home Health Patient Driven Groupings Model (PDGM), which began on January 1, 2020, documentation of patient status becomes increasingly important, as those who are responsible for covering patients throughout a continuum of care should be using the medical record to make decisions that are in the best interest of the patient.

PTs historically have been challenged in documenting the relationship between patient presentation, treatment/intervention, and goals to function and providing evidence that physical therapy is better than alternative patient management by other professionals or nonprofessionals. Lack of treatment diagnoses that are appropriate, that do not match interventions and goals, or that are not using standardized outcome measures that can be repeated to determine progress over time put payment success at risk as documentation is integrally related to payment for services as the only evidence of service provision.

Consistent terminology in both description and content is also a challenge for the PT and PTA. AHIMA[3] uses the general term health record to categorize what may be more commonly known, depending on setting, as the patient record (acute care), medical record (physician offices, physical therapy practices/departments), resident record (SNFs), or client record (ambulatory care, APTA). A health record contains all information about the patient, including the skilled documentation, and is most commonly electronic, although some elements may remain manual.[3] The *Guide to Physical Therapist Practice 3.0* refers to documentation as a role of the PT.[5] Documentation is defined in the *Guide to Physical Therapist Practice* as "any entry into the client record, such as consultation report, initial examination report, progress note, flow sheet/checklist that identifies the care/service provided, reexamination, or summation of care."[5] Colloquially, PTs are familiar with the term medical record, although non-APTA members may not be using the *Guide to Physical Therapist Practice*. Regardless of the terminology, the record is "the principal repository (storage place) for data and information about the healthcare services provided to an individual patient. It documents the who, what, when, where, what, and how of patient care."[5]

As the federal government mandates universal use of EHRs across all settings, regardless of whether a professional uses a pen, microphone or keyboard, narrative, SOAP format (subjective, objective, assessment, plan), or templates, the general principles, purposes, and content requirements remain the same.[9]

FUNCTIONS AND USERS OF THE HEALTH RECORD

According to AHIMA,[3] the basic purposes of documentation are to be used as a:

1. Basis for planning and treatment
2. Means of communication for attending health professionals
3. Legal entry describing the care the patient receives
4. Verification of services for payers
5. Database for health research and planning

This aligns with the Interprofessional Education Collaborative Core Competencies[10] that includes interprofessional communication practices, one of which is documentation.

The Institute of Medicine,[11] now called the National Academy of Medicine, divides the purposes into primary and secondary, where primary purposes directly relate to patient care (see Table 1-1) and secondary purposes indirectly relate to patient care (see Table 1-2).

Table 1-1 Primary Purposes of the Health Record

PATIENT CARE DELIVERY (PATIENT)
• To document services received • To constitute proof of identity • To self-manage care • To verify billing
PATIENT CARE DELIVERY (PROVIDER)
• To foster continuity of care (that is, to serve as a communication tool) • To describe diseases and causes (that is, to support diagnostic work) • To support decision-making about diagnosis and treatment of patients • To assess and manage risk for individual patients • To facilitate care in accordance with clinical practice guidelines • To document patient risk factors • To assess and document patient expectations and patient satisfaction • To generate care plans • To determine preventive advice or health maintenance information • To provide reminders to clinicians • To support nursing care • To document services provided

(continued)

Table 1-1 Primary Purposes of the Health Record (Continued)

PATIENT CARE MANAGEMENT
• To document case mix in institutions and practices • To analyze severity of illness • To formulate practice guidelines • To manage risk • To characterize the use of services • To provide the basis for utilization review • To perform quality assurance
PATIENT CARE SUPPORT
• To allocate resources • To analyze trends and develop forecasts • To assess workload • To communicate information among departments
BILLING AND REIMBURSEMENT
• To document services for payments • To bill for services • To submit insurance claims • To adjudicate insurance claims • To determine disabilities (for example, workers compensation) • To manage costs • To report costs • To perform actuarial analysis

SOURCE: Data from Dick, Steen, and Detmer.[11]

The primary purposes identified by the National Academy of Medicine are patient care delivery, patient care management, patient care support, and billing and payment.[11] Patient care delivery is the care provided by the professionals involved in a patient's care. This is used by providers to communicate what is being done and the outcome or patient response to treatment in order to ensure continuity of care, critical in an interprofessional practice environment. To this end, it is imperative that the record be available as needed to all providers and as appropriate, 24 hours a day. Patient care management refers to all of the activities related to a patient's management. Patient care support relates to facility management of resources, including trend identification for quality improvement and utilization review and management purposes. Billing and payment is the use of the record to provide justification for payment for the care rendered by describing the care in skilled terms.

The secondary purposes are education, regulation (compliance and accreditation), research, policy making (allocating resources and planning), and industry (research and development).

Table 1-2 Secondary Purposes of the Health Record

EDUCATION
• To document the experience of healthcare professionals • To prepare conferences and presentations • To teach healthcare students
REGULATION
• To serve as evidence in litigation • To foster post-marketing surveillance • To assess compliance with standards of care • To accredit professionals and hospitals • To compare healthcare organizations
RESEARCH
• To develop new products • To conduct clinical research • To assess technology • To study patient outcomes • To study effectiveness and cost-effectiveness of patient care • To identify populations at risk • To develop registries and databases • To assess the cost-effectiveness of record systems
POLICY MAKING
• To allocate resources • To conduct strategic planning • To monitor public health
INDUSTRY
• To conduct research and development • To plan marketing strategy

SOURCE: Data from Dick, Steen, and Detmer.[11]

Tables 1-3 and 1-4 list examples of the individual and institutional users of health records.[11] The patient identifiers are removed from all records used for purposes not directly related to patient care. In this way, the confidentiality of patient-identifiable information and the privacy of the individuals involved (both patients and providers) can be protected. However, HIPAA regulations require specific patient permission for any primary or secondary use of the medical record as of April 2003.

Based on the primary and secondary purposes of the record, it is evident that a wide variety of individuals may require and be legally entitled to access the medical record. With integrated EHRs, access through computers at convenient locations should facilitate optimal care through accessibility to all entries, legibility, and integrated information, with appropriate

Table 1-3 Representative Individual Users of Healthcare Records

PATIENT CARE DELIVERY (PROVIDERS)
Chaplains
Coders
Dental hygienists
Dentists dietitians
Family therapists
Laboratory technologists
Nurses (Nurse practitioners)
Occupational therapists (Occupational therapist assistants)
Optometrists
Pharmacists
Physical therapists (Physical therapist assistants)
Physicians (Physician assistants)
Podiatrists
Psychologists
Radiology technologists
Recreational therapists
Respiratory therapists
Social workers (Case managers)
PATIENT CARE DELIVERY (CONSUMERS)
Patients
Families
PATIENT CARE MANAGEMENT AND SUPPORT
Administrators
Financial managers and accountants
Quality managers
Records professionals
Risk managers
Unit clerks
Utilization review managers
PATIENT CARE REIMBURSEMENT
Benefit managers
Insurers (federal, state, and private)

(continued)

Table 1-3 Representative Individual Users of Healthcare Records (*Continued*)

OTHER
Accreditors
Government policy makers and legislators
Lawyers
Healthcare researchers and clinical investigators
Health sciences journalists and editors

SOURCE: Dick, Steen, and Detmer 1997, p. 76.[11]

Table 1-4 Representative Institutional Users of Health Records

HEALTHCARE DELIVERY (INPATIENT AND OUTPATIENT)
Alliances, associations, networks, and systems of providers
Ambulatory surgery centers
Donor banks (blood, tissue, organs)
Health maintenance organization (HMO) (or other third-party payers)
Home care agencies
Hospices
Hospitals (general and specialty)
Inpatient rehabilitation facilities (IRFs)
Nursing home (SNF)
Preferred provider organization (PPO)
Physicians' offices (large and small group practices, individual practitioners)
Psychiatric facilities
Public health departments
Substance abuse programs
MANAGEMENT AND REVIEW OF CARE
Medicare peer review organizations
Quality management companies
Recovery audit contractors (RACs)
Risk management companies
Utilization review and utilization management companies
REIMBURSEMENT OF CARE
Business healthcare coalitions
Employers
Insurers (federal, state, and private)

(*continued*)

Table 1-4 Representative Institutional Users of Health Records (*Continued*)

RESEARCH
Disease registries
Health data organizations
Healthcare technology developers and manufacturers (equipment and device firms, pharmaceutical firms, and computer hardware and software vendors for patient record systems)
Research centers
EDUCATION
Allied health/health science professional schools and programs
Schools of medicine: allopathic and osteopathic
Schools of nursing
Schools of public health
ACCREDITATION
Accreditation organizations
Institutional licensure agencies
Professional licensure agencies
POLICY MAKING
Federal government agencies
Local government agencies
State government agencies

Source: Data from Dick, Steen, Detmer 1997, p. 77.[11]

protection from public view. There may also be the ability for physicians to access records from a remote location directly to hospital systems, including all diagnostic testing, laboratory, and other reports through protected systems. Although terminology must be sophisticated and skilled enough to justify care, it must also be written in a manner that is clear and understood by other healthcare professionals, nonhealthcare professionals, and others. Other users can be divided into individual and institutional, needing the record for a variety of purposes. Each user may use and need the information from the record for a different purpose. A chaplain offering spiritual guidance and comfort uses information differently than a billing clerk, a third-party payer representative, PT, or surveyor/inspector (i.e., Joint Commission [JC], formerly the Joint Commission on Accreditation of Healthcare Organizations [JCAHO], or Commission on Accreditation of Rehabilitation Facilities [CARF]). It is also becoming more common for patients or patient representatives, such as family, legal guardian, or healthcare surrogate, to take a greater interest in the care provided. When harm comes to a patient, health professionals or the facility is suspected of harm, lawyers, or mediators may be readers of the record. With limited exceptions, the HIPAA Privacy Rule (the Privacy Rule) provides individuals with a legal, enforceable right to see and receive copies upon request of the information in their medical and other health records maintained by their health care providers and health plans. For more information on HIPAA, see Chap. 11 "Legal Issues" in the Medical Record. The regulations governing the standards for the security of electronic protected health information to be implemented by health plans, healthcare clearinghouses, and certain healthcare providers took effect in April 2003. The implications extend to not only current patients in any practice but the maintenance of records as well. AHIMA recommends 10 years for retention of records, JC is determined by state law, CARF requires policies but specifies no time limits, and the National Committee on Quality Assurance (NCQA) does not specify. State laws generally govern how long medical records are to be retained. However, HIPAA administrative simplification rules require a covered entity to retain required documentation for six years from the date of its creation or the date when it last was in effect, whichever is later. HIPAA requirements preempt State laws if they require shorter periods. Your State may require a longer retention period.[12]

The primary users of health records are patient care providers. However, many other individuals and organizations also use the information in health records. Managed care organizations, integrated healthcare delivery systems, regulatory and accreditation organizations, licensing bodies, educational organizations, utilization review screeners, providers in the continuum of care to determine qualifications for different discharge dispositions, third-party payers, and research facilities all use information that was originally collected to document patient care.

The National Academy of Medicine defines the users of health records as "those individuals who enter, verify, correct, analyze, or obtain information from the record, either directly or indirectly through an intermediary."[11] All users of health records influence clinical care in some way, but they use the information from health records for various reasons and in different ways. Some users (for example, nurses, physicians, and coding specialists) refer to the health records of specific patients as a part of their daily work. Many other users, however, never have direct access to the records of individual patients. Instead, they use clinical and demographic information.

As already noted, many individuals depend on the information in health records to perform their jobs. The individuals who provide direct patient care services include but are not limited to an interprofessional team of physicians, nurses, nurse practitioners, other allied health professionals, and other clinical service providers. Professions that are often listed as "allied health" include physician assistants (PAs), PTs, PTAs, registered nurses, respiratory therapists (RTs), nutritionists and dietitians, occupational therapists (OTs), occupational therapy assistants (OTAs), radiology technicians, sonographers, and medical laboratory technicians. Other medical professionals, such as pharmacists, social workers, psychologists, family therapists, podiatrists, and chiropractors, also provide clinical services.

The services directly administered by patient care providers are documented directly into the patient's health record. Other service providers (for example, medical laboratory technicians) submit separate written reports that become part of individual health records and are usually entered directly into the EMR. Although not physically tabbed as in manual records, different service sections are accessible in electronic records.

SUMMARY

"The convergence of clinical, documentation, and coding processes is vital to a healthy revenue cycle, and more important, to a healthy patient. To that end, CDI has a direct impact on patient care by providing information to all members of the care team, as well as those downstream who may be treating the patient at a later date."[3]

As stated by AHIMA,[3] the medical or client record, whether electronic or in rare cases manual, is a comprehensive set of information that chronicles an episode of medically related care rendered to an individual concurrently during patient care, retrospectively and for potential future patient care. The process of HIM is necessary in healthcare for a variety of reasons, with patient care being the most critical. It should include all information related to a patient expressed in terminology understood by all record users, both primary and secondary. Primary users of the record include those primarily involved in the care itself. Secondary users include most others. Regardless of the purpose the record serves, the content should be the same. By following general rules of medical record keeping and content, the PT should be able to create documentation or a complete record (depending on setting) that will be universally understood and withstand scrutiny by any reader, for any purpose.

REVIEW QUESTIONS

1. What is the relationship between health information management and medical record keeping?
2. Whose responsibility is it to determine medical necessity for physical therapy?
3. The advent of what technology facilitated the ability for Medicare and others to track services rendered to beneficiaries?
4. Relative to documentation, why has physical therapy not been considered an essential medical service?
5. What is documentation according to the APTA's *Guide for Physical Therapist Practice*?
6. Are the principles for documenting by manual entry different than for the electronic medical record? Defend your answer.
7. According to AHIMA, what are the primary purposes of the medical record?
8. Describe five secondary purposes of the medical record.
9. What does "user" mean in the context of the medical record? Give five examples and the purpose each would need to record for.
10. What is HIPAA and how is it relevant to HIM?

REFERENCES

1. *Clinical Documentation Improvement (CDI).* American Health Information Management Association. Available at www.ahima.org/topics/cdi. Accessed February 20, 2020.
2. *Guidelines: Physical Therapy Documentation of Patient/Client Management.* American Physical Therapy Association, Alexandria, VA. Available at https://www.apta.org/uploadedFiles/APTAorg/About_Us/Policies/BOD/Practice/DocumentationPatientClientMgmt.pdf. Published 2009. Accessed February 20, 2020.
3. *What Is Health Information?* American Health Information Management Association. Available at https://www.apta.org/apta-and-you/leadership-and-governance/policies/guidelines-documentation-patient-client-management. Published 2019. Accessed February 20, 2020.
4. *What Is an Electronic Health Record (EHR)?* HealthIT.gov. Available at https://www.healthit.gov/faq/what-electronic-health-record-ehr. Updated 2019. Accessed February 20, 2020.
5. *Guide to Physical Therapist Practice. 3.0.* Alexandria, VA: American Physical Therapy Association; 2016. Available at http://guidetoptpractice.apta.org/. Accessed February 20, 2020.
6. *Physical Therapy Professional Liability Exposure: 2016 Claim Report Update.* Healthcare Providers Service Organization. Available at http://www.hpso.com/Documents/pdfs/CNA_PT_CS_020116_CF_PROD_ASIZE_ONLINE_040417_SEC.pdf. Published January 2016. Accessed February 20, 2020.
7. *CMS Announces New Recovery Audit Contractors to Help Identify Improper Medicare Payments.* Centers for Medicare & Medicaid Services. Available at https://www.cms.gov/newsroom/fact-sheets/cms-announces-new-recovery-audit-contractors-help-identify-improper-medicare-payments. Published 2008. Accessed February 20, 2020.
8. *Local Coverage Determinations.* American Physical Therapy Association, Alexandria, VA. Available at https://www.apta.org/your-practice/payment/medicare-payment/coverage-issues/local-coverage-determinations-lcds. Published 2018. Accessed February 20, 2020.
9. Gnagey LT. Federal programs that paid hospitals to adopt electronic records delivers dramatic results. *Michigan News.* August 7, 2017. Available at http://ns.umich.edu/new/releases/24996-program-that-paid-hospitals-to-adopt-electronic-records-delivers-dramatic-results. Updated August 7, 2017. Accessed February 20, 2020.
10. Interprofessional Educational Collaborative. *Core Competencies for Interprofessional Practice.* Washington, DC: Interprofessional Educational Collaborative; 2016. Available at https://hsc.unm.edu/ipe/resources/ipec-2016-core-competencies.pdf. Accessed February 20, 2020.
11. Dick R, Steen E, Detmer D. *The Computer-Based Patient Record: An Essential Technology for Health Care, Revised Ed.* Washington, DC: National Academy of Sciences; 1997.
12. *Medical Record Retention and Media Formats for Medical Records. MLN Matters number. SE1022.* Centers for Medicare & Medicaid Services. Available at https://www.cms.gov/Outreach-and-Education/Medicare-Learning-Network-MLN/MLNMattersArticles/Downloads/SE1022.pdf. Accessed June 25, 2020.

2 Record Organization and General Principles

OBJECTIVES

Following completion of this chapter, the reader will be able to:

- Describe how manual records should be stored.
- Explain why legibility is imperative in the medical record.
- Describe the types of data found in the medical record.
- Explain how errors in the record should be corrected.
- Explain the risks involved if entries into the record are not timely.
- List why the use of abbreviations in the record is a potential problem for physical therapists.
- Explain the concept of accuracy in the record.
- Discuss objectivity in the medical record mean.
- Describe the relationship between payment and documentation.

GENERAL PRINCIPLES

The management of medical records, including content and organization, should be consistent throughout the organization or consistent within each discipline. General rules in organizational policies and procedures should be well defined for the professionals maintaining the record and ensure that all individuals abide by them. Additionally, the records should be organized so that individual pieces of information are easy to locate within the record as a whole. Therefore, all records in the same facility should be organized the same way whether they are hard copy or electronic. Problems can arise, for example, when physical therapy services in a skilled nursing facility are contracted out and the documentation systems do not interact with each other. There are legal cases where critical issues in terms of medical status, changes to medications, or patient complaints were not followed up on by the next practitioner due to a delay in the documentation systems.

REFERRAL INFORMATION

Referral information (self-referred, physician-referred or physician referred/prescribed, physician extender such as a nurse practitioner [NP] or physician assistant [PA], consultation, or other) should be included in the patient's medical record. Each state practice act provides who can refer to physical therapy and who can sign a plan of care. All states have some form of direct access to physical therapy services. If the patient comes with a written referral, that referral becomes part of the record. If referred by telephone or verbal order, the person who took the order must transcribe it, consistent with state law and facility policy. The transcription of the referral should also be followed up by a signed written referral, preferably an original rather than a fax. If the patient has direct access, that should be noted.

As defined by the Centers for Medicare & Medicaid Services (CMS) in the *Medicare Benefit Policy Manual* (MBPM), Chapter 15 Section 220:[1]

PHYSICIAN with respect to outpatient rehabilitation therapy services means a doctor of medicine, osteopathy (including an osteopathic practitioner), podiatric medicine, or optometry (for low vision rehabilitation only). Chiropractors and doctors of dental surgery or dental medicine are not considered physicians for therapy services and may neither refer patients for rehabilitation therapy services nor establish therapy plans of care for Medicare part B.[1]

VERBAL, TELEPHONE, OR E-MAIL/ELECTRONIC REFERRAL

The person taking the referral should transcribe the verbal orders. The entry itself should include what the referral is for, the time taken, how it was taken (i.e., phone, face to face, phone message, e-mail, fax, other), the prescribing individual's name, and the name of the person who entered it. Verbal, telephone, or e-mail electronic referrals require authentication, usually within 24 to 48 hours, by the prescribing professional, based on organizational or accreditation guidelines or requirements.

As stated in the CMS MBPM, Chapter 15, Section 220.1.1:[1]

***Although there is no Medicare requirement for an order**, [emphasis added] when documented in the medical record, an order provides evidence that the patient both needs therapy services and is under the care of a physician. The certification requirements are met when the physician certifies the plan of care. If the signed order includes a plan of care (see essential requirements of plan in §220.1.2), no further certification of the plan is required. Payment is dependent on the certification of the plan of care rather than the order, but the use of an order is prudent to determine that a physician is involved in care and available to certify the plan. The CORF services benefit does not recognize a non-physician practitioner (NPP) for orders and certification.*[1]

CERTIFICATION

According to CMS:[1]

Certification is the physician's/non-physician practitioner's (NPP) approval of the plan of care. Certification requires a dated signature on the plan of care or some other document that indicates approval of the plan of care.

220.1.3—Certification and Recertification of Need for Treatment and Therapy Plans of Care (Rev. 88, Issued: 05-07-08, Effective: 01-01-08, Implementation: 06-09-08) Reference: 42CFR424.24(c)

See specific certification rules in Pub. 100-01, Chapter 4, §20 for hospital services.

Method and Disposition of Certifications

Certification requires a dated signature on the plan of care or some other document that indicates approval of the plan of care. It is not appropriate for a physician/NPP to certify a plan of care if the patient was not under the care of some physician/NPP at the time of the treatment or if the patient did not need the treatment.

Since delayed certification is allowed, the date the certification is signed is important only to determine if it is timely or delayed. The certification must relate to treatment during the interval on the claim. Unless there is reason to believe the plan was not signed appropriately, or it is not timely, no further evidence that the patient was under the care of a physician/NPP and that the patient needed the care is required. The format of all certifications and recertifications and the method by which they are obtained is determined by the individual facility and/or practitioner.

Acceptable documentation of certification may be, for example, a physician's progress note, a physician/NPP order, or a plan of care that is signed and dated by a physician/NPP, and indicates the physician/NPP is aware that therapy service is or was in progress and the physician/NPP makes no record of disagreement with the plan when there is evidence that the plan was sent (e.g., to the office) or is available in the record (e.g., of the institution that employs the physician/NPP) for the physician/NPP to review.

For example, if during the course of treatment under a certified plan of care, a physician sends an order for continued treatment for 2 more weeks, contractors shall accept the order as certification of continued treatment for 2 weeks under the same plan of care. If the new certification is for less treatment than previously planned and certified, this new certification takes the place of any previous certification. At the end of the 2-week treatment (which might extend more than 2 calendar weeks from the date the order/certification was signed) another certification would be required if further treatment was documented as medically necessary. The certification should be retained in the clinical record and available if requested by the contractor.

Initial Certification of Plan

The physician's/NPP's certification of the plan (with or without an order) satisfies all of the certification requirements noted above in §220.1 for the duration of the plan of care, or 90 calendar days from the date of the initial treatment, whichever is less. The initial treatment includes the evaluation that resulted in the plan.

Timing of Initial Certification

The provider or supplier (e.g., facility, physician/NPP, or therapist) should obtain certification as soon as possible after the plan of care is established, unless the requirements of delayed certification are met. "As soon as possible" means that the physician/NPP shall certify the initial plan as soon as it is obtained, or within 30 days of the initial therapy treatment. Since payment may be denied if a physician does not certify the plan, the therapist should forward the plan to the physician as soon as it is established.

The Medicare contractor may consider evidence of diligence in providing the plan to the physician during review in the event of a delayed certification. Timely certification of the initial plan is met when physician/NPP certification of the plan is documented by signature or verbal order, and dated in the 30 days following the first day of treatment (including evaluation). If the order to certify is verbal, it must be followed within 14 days by a signature to be done timely. A dated notation of the order to certify the plan should be made in the patient's medical record.

Recertification is not required if the duration of the initially certified plan of care is more than the duration (length) of the entire episode of treatment.

Review of Plan and Recertification

Reference: 42CFR424.24(c), 1861(r), 42CFR 410.61(e).

The timing of recertification changed on January 1, 2008. Certifications signed on or after January 1, 2008, follow the rules in this section. Certifications signed on or prior to December 31, 2007, follow the rule in effect at that time, which required recertification every 30 calendar days. Payment and coverage conditions require that the plan must be reviewed, as often as necessary but at least whenever it is certified or recertified to complete the certification requirements. It is not required that the same physician/NPP who participated initially in recommending or planning the patient's care certifies and/or recertifies the plans.

Recertifications that document the need for continued or modified therapy should be signed whenever the need for a significant modification of the plan becomes evident, or at least every 90 days after initiation of treatment under that plan, unless they are delayed.

Physician/NPP Options for Certification

A physician/NPP may certify or recertify a plan for whatever duration of treatment the physician/NPP determines is appropriate, up to a maximum of 90 calendar days. Many episodes of therapy treatment last less than 30 calendar days.

Therefore, it is expected that the physician/NPP should certify a plan that appropriately estimates the duration of care for the individual, even if it is less than 90 days. If the therapist writes a plan of care for a duration that is more or less than the duration approved by the physician/NPP, then the physician/NPP would document a change to the duration of the plan and certify it for the duration the physician/NPP finds appropriate (up to 90 days). Treatment beyond the duration certified by the physician/NPP requires that a plan be recertified for the extended duration of treatment. It is possible that the therapist will discharge patients before the end of the estimated treatment duration because some will improve faster than estimated and/or some successfully progressed to an independent home program.

Physicians/NPPs may require that the patient make a physician/NPP visit for an examination if, in the professional's judgment, the visit is needed prior to certifying the plan, or during the planned treatment. Physicians/NPPs should indicate their requirement for visits, preferably on an order preceding the treatment, or on the plan of care that is certified. If the physician wishes to restrict the patient's treatment beyond a certain date when a visit is required, the physician should certify a plan only until the date of the visit. After that date, services will not be considered reasonable and necessary due to lack of a certified plan. Physicians/NPPs should not sign a certification if they require a visit and a visit was not made. However, Medicare does not require a visit unless the National Coverage Determination (NCD) for a particular treatment requires it (e.g., see Pub. 100-03, §270.1—Electrical Stimulation (ES) and Electromagnetic Therapy for the Treatment of Wounds).

Restrictions on Certification

Certifications and recertifications by doctors of podiatric medicine must be consistent with the scope of the professional services provided by a doctor of podiatric medicine as authorized by applicable state law. Optometrists may order and certify only low vision services. Chiropractors may not certify or recertify plans of care for therapy services unless state laws, such as Florida, permit chiropractic referral. This does not however, align with Medicare regulations.

Delayed Certification

References: Medicare Benefit Policy Manual Chapter 15 Section 220.1.3(D)[1] and §1835(a) of the Social Security Act 42CFR424.11(d)(3)

Certifications are required for each interval of treatment based on the patient's needs, not to exceed 90-calendar days from the initial therapy treatment. Certifications are timely when the initial certification (or certification of a significantly modified plan of care) is dated within 30-calendar days of the initial treatment under that plan. Recertification is timely when dated during the duration of the initial plan of care or within 90-calendar days of the initial treatment under that plan, whichever is less. Delayed certification and recertification requirements shall be deemed satisfied where, at any later date, a physician/NPP makes a certification accompanied by a reason for the delay.

Certifications are acceptable without justification for 30 days after they are due. Delayed certification should include one or more certifications or recertifications on a single signed and dated document. Delayed certifications should include any evidence the provider or supplier considers necessary to justify the delay. For example, a certification may be delayed because the physician did not sign it, or the original was lost. In the case of a long delayed certification (over 6 months), the provider or supplier may choose to submit with the delayed certification some other documentation (e.g., an order, progress notes, telephone contact, requests for certification or signed statement of a physician/NPP) indicating need for care and that the patient was under the care of a physician at the time of the treatment.

Such documentation may be requested by the contractor for delayed certifications if it is required for review. It is not intended that needed therapy be stopped or denied when certification is delayed. The delayed certification of otherwise covered services should be accepted unless the contractor has reason to believe that there was no physician involved in the patient's care, or treatment did not meet the patient's need (and therefore, the certification was signed inappropriately).

See Examples below for where payment should and should not be denied based on a delay of certification.

Example

Payment should be denied if there is a certification signed 2 years after treatment by a physician/NPP who has or had no knowledge of the patient when the medical record also shows, for example, no order, note, physician/NPP-attended meeting, correspondence with a physician/NPP, documentation of discussion of the plan with a physician/NPP, documentation of sending the plan to any physician/NPP, or other indication that a physician/NPP was involved in the case.

Example

Payment should not be denied, even when certified 2 years after treatment, when there is evidence that a physician approved needed treatment, such as an order, documentation of therapist/physician/NPP discussion of the plan, chart notes, meeting notes, requests for certification, certifications for intervals before or after the service in question, or physician/NPP services during which the medical record or the patient's history would, in good practice, be reviewed and would indicate therapy treatment is in progress.

Example

Subsequent certifications of plans for continued treatment for the same condition in the same patient may indicate physician certification of treatment that occurred between certification dates, even if the signature for one of the plans in the episode is delayed. If a certified plan of care ends on March 30 and a new plan of care for continued treatment after March 30 is developed or signed by a therapist on April 15 and that plan is subsequently certified, that certification may be considered delayed and acceptable effective from the first treatment date after March 30 for the frequency and duration as described in the plan. Of course, documentation should continue to indicate that therapy during the delay is medically necessary, as it would for any treatment. The certification of the physician/NPP is interpreted as involvement and approval of the ongoing episode of treatment, including the treatment that preceded the date of the certification unless the physician/NPP indicates otherwise.

Denials Due to Certification

As discussed in Medicare Benefit Policy Manual Chapter 15 Section 220.1.3(E):

Denial for payment that is based on absence of certification is a technical denial, which means a statutory requirement has not been met. Certification is a statutory requirement in Social Security Act 1835(a)(2) ("periodic review" of the plan).

For example, if a patient is treated and the provider or supplier cannot produce (on contractor request) a plan of care (timely or delayed) for the billed treatment dates certified by a physician/NPP, then that service might be denied for lack of the required certification. If an appropriate certification is later produced, the denial shall be overturned. In the case of a service furnished under a provider agreement, as described in 42CFR489.21, the provider is precluded from charging the beneficiary for services denied as a result of missing certification.

However, if the service is provided by a supplier (in the office of the physician/NPP or therapist), a technical denial due to absence of a certification results in beneficiary liability. For that reason, it is recommended that the patient be made aware of the need for certification and the consequences of its absence. A technical denial decision may be reopened by the contractor or reversed on appeal, as appropriate, if delayed certification is later produced.

CLINICIAN

From the CMS MBPM Chapter 15, Section 220:[1]

The clinician is a term used by CMS and in Pub 100-04, Chapter 5, Section 10 or Section 20, to refer to only a physician, non-physician practitioner or a therapist (but not to an assistant, aide, or any other personnel) providing a service within their scope of practice and consistent with state and local law. Clinicians make clinical judgments and are responsible for all services they are permitted to supervise.

Services that require the skills of a therapist, may be appropriately furnished by clinicians, that is, by or under the supervision of qualified physicians/NPPs when their scope of practice, state, and local laws allow it and their personal professional training is judged by Medicare contractors as sufficient to provide to the beneficiary skills equivalent to a therapist for that service.[1]

STORAGE

Records must be kept in locked, fireproof storage and accessible only to those directly involved with the patient. Electronic records must be password coded, and screens must be shielded from public view. Security measures, such as firewalls, should also be in place. Clinic notes should not be taken home.

INDIVIDUAL CHARTS AND FOLDERS

In facilities that are not billing and are using manual entry, there should be a single, hard copy "chart." If manila file folders are used, it is a best practice to use a new folder for each new patient. If it is the policy of the facility to reuse folders, all references on and in the folder to the prior patients should be obliterated for privacy purposes.

LEGIBILITY

All entries must be legible, not only to the writer but to anyone who may need or is entitled to record access. Illegibility may give the impression of carelessness and rushed efforts. For electronic records, consistent font style and size should be used with manual entry. In these systems, entries must be legible if an electric pen is allowed for manual notes or signatures. As most signatures are not legible, it is critical that all licensed professionals use their state license numbers following their names so they can be identified. In the case of students, following their designation of student physical therapist (SPT) or student physical therapist assistant

(SPTA), they should also print their names for future identification. All individuals working with the patient should be identified for future reference.

DATA TYPES

Although not applicable to individual entries, the record as whole, regardless of the setting, consists of four types of data, whether manual or electronic:

1. Personal
2. Financial
3. Social
4. Medical

ERRORS IN THE RECORD

Entries cannot be physically removed, completely covered, or otherwise made illegible. In legal cases, it is assumed the facility or therapist is hiding something when this occurs. If items that should have been entered are recalled at any time following the documentation for a specific encounter, an addendum can be added. It must be placed in the next available space in the record and should include the time and date of entry. It should then state "Addendum to entry of ________." In the electronic record all notes should be time-stamped. If an entry is placed in an incorrect area or incorrect chart, a single line through the content and date identified needs to be included and information maintained.

If an error in spelling, location, or other minor error is made, a single line should be put through the incorrect entry. The correction should be made above the incorrect entry, with the date and initials of the person correcting beside it. Neither correction fluid (White Out) nor correction tape should be used in a hard-copy medical record. See below Example for an entry with an error correction.

Example

8/26/20 ES

18 y.o. male adm ~~8/25/20~~ with R femur fx.

Alterations to the medical record are considered fraudulent. Therefore, even if an incorrect entry is made on a new page and discovered, technically, it should not be removed. Although this is current practice now, the privacy and confidentiality components of the Health Insurance Portability and Accountability Act of 1996 (HIPAA) may eventually require a change in this practice

Additionally, do not leave blanks or skip lines and always enter information chronologically. Blanks may give the impression that information was forgotten and may leave opportunity for record alteration. Single lines can be drawn through or across multiple blank lines or spaces. However in a system in which there are running chronological entries, the space that follows the final signature on an entry is not considered blank space and should not be lined out.

In electronic records, corrections must be made consistent with laws and acceptable practice.

In electronic records, errors should not just be deleted. It should be noted in an addendum that an entry is incorrect, and the addendum should then include the correction. Facilities using electronic records should have internal policies regarding entry error correction

TIMELINESS OF ENTRY AND TIME OF SESSION

Whether entries are dictated, manually written, or electronically computer generated, either typed in or voice transcribed, they should be composed as close to the time of service delivery as possible, preferably at the time the treatment is being rendered or immediately following. Timeliness of entry input saves time and ensures accuracy, as the physical therapist (PT) does not have to "remember" what they did later. Additionally, if harm comes to the patient between physical therapy visits, immediate documentation of patient status following treatment can protect the provider. Discharge entries and summaries should also be completed in a timely manner for accuracy. Although good practice is to complete this within 24 hours of discharge, it is up to the therapist to follow facility policies and procedures. Regulations are in place for some settings that do not require documentation for each visit; however, even if a full note is not required, the date and record of interventions performed should, at a minimum, be entered in some format. According to the American Physical Therapy Association (APTA), there should be an entry for every visit or encounter between the patient and provider. Absence of an entry for any visit or encounter may result in denial of payment, since there is no proof of the visit. Documentation for all patients treated or who did not receive treatment but were scheduled should be completed before a therapist or assistant leaves the facility for the day.

Dictated Documentation. For Medicare purposes, dictated therapy documentation is considered completed on the day it was dictated. The qualified professional may edit and electronically sign the documentation at a later date.[1]

Dates for Documentation. The date the documentation was made is important only to establish the date of the initial plan of care because therapy cannot begin until the plan is established unless treatment is performed or supervised by the same clinician who establishes the plan. However, contractors may require that treatment notes and progress reports be entered into the record within 1 week of the last date to which the progress report or treatment note refers. For example, if treatment began on the first of the month at a frequency of twice a week, a progress report would be required at the end of the month. Contractors may require that the progress report that describes that month of treatment be dated not more than 1 week after the end of the month described in the report.[1]

SPELLING AND GRAMMAR

Although correct spelling and grammar would seem a given, carelessness does occur. The provider must correctly spell all words and write in a logical, coherent manner, as there are multiple uses for the record and multiple people who will be using it. Incorrect spelling and grammar may lead the reader to believe inadequate care has been rendered. Professionals are expected to be able to spell. For electronic entry, some systems may have spelling checks and grammar checks. If your system has these capabilities, it is recommended that they be used before finalizing entries. Spelling can also be checked easily with cell phones with internal dictionaries. Many words are spelled correctly that a spelling check will change. It is critical to review all changes that the spelling check recommends. The spelling check will check to see if a word is spelled wrong, but not if the incorrect word is spelled correctly. For example, in the phrase "the 50-year-old mature woman," if *manure* was used instead of *mature*, it would not be caught. Other examples include "the person is *egotistical* versus *ego testicle*" and "the medication the person is taking is *antidepressants* versus *auntie depressants*." The homonyms there, their, and there or your and you're will not be caught by the spelling check. The spelling check will not correct words in all caps or abbreviations in capital letters.

ABBREVIATIONS

Only standard abbreviations and acronyms should be used. The dilemma in physical therapy is standardization. Refer to Appendix A for a list of some standard abbreviations. However, PTs who work in organizations, facilities, or solo/independent practice often have specific policies and procedures on using abbreviations. Individuals should not use self-developed abbreviations that are not universally understood. Abbreviations for specific physical therapy treatments or interventions should only be used in conjunction with universally accepted Current Procedural Terminology (CPT) codes, which are universally required for billing, to ensure categorical understanding. For example, other PTs or rehabilitation professionals may understand PNF for "proprioceptive neuromuscular facilitation," but nonrehabilitation professionals would not know it is a form of therapeutic exercise. Additionally, if abbreviations have multiple meanings, such as WFL: "within functional limits" or "within full limits," the PT should provide a key on the form being used. These specific terms however, are better expressed by numeric representation versus general statements. The latest Joint Commission regulations recommend elimination of the use of all abbreviations to minimize medical error and maximize effective interprofessional communication.

ACCURACY

All documentation entries and intervention content should match billing dates, attendance grids, and appointment book entries. In the content itself, the medical diagnosis should be the one established by the referring medical professional as appropriate. The physical therapy diagnosis or treatment diagnosis should be established by the PT by description, matching International Classification of Disease codes (ICD 10 version), and must match the patient complaints, problems identified during the assessment, the goals established (functionally oriented), the intervention selected, and the frequency and duration of care. Each entry should match the appropriate billing date. The codes entered for billing purposes should match the codes and/or verbiage indicated in the record. CPT coding terminology should describe the interventions categorically. The physical therapy diagnosis may be functionally oriented and therefore may either differ from or correspond with the medical diagnosis. The onset date of the physical therapy problem should be clearly indicated and should be "recent," even if the medical problem is chronic in nature. Throughout the record, all information should match.

A physical therapy diagnosis is not the same as a medical diagnosis, and is actually a determination of the primary problem for which the patient is receiving skilled care. For states in which PTs are not legally authorized to diagnose, the description would be the physical therapy problem. The Medicare forms specifically require differentiation between the medical diagnosis and the physical therapy or treatment problem or diagnosis (see Appendix C).

Author Note

As stated in the Medicare Claims Processing Manual, Chapter 5, Section 10.3.2:

Bill the most relevant diagnosis. As always, when billing for therapy services, the diagnosis code that best relates to the reason for the treatment shall be on the claim, unless there is a compelling reason to report another diagnosis code. For example, when a patient with diabetes is being treated with therapy for gait training due to amputation, the preferred diagnosis is abnormality of gait (which characterizes the treatment). Where it is possible in accordance with State and local laws and the contractors' local coverage determinations, avoid using vague or general diagnoses. When a claim includes several types of services, or where the physician/NPP must supply the diagnosis, it may not be possible to use the most relevant therapy diagnosis code in the primary position. In that case, the relevant diagnosis code should, if possible, be on the claim in another position.

Careful attention should be paid to homonyms, words that sound the same but are spelled differently and have different meanings, such as gait and gate and their and there. Care should also be taken to avoid any other commonly confused terms or concepts, such as left and right.

Information should be presented in an organized manner and indicate functional goals attained by the patient/client in a linear progression. The appropriate forms, as determined by policy and procedure or external requirements such as third-party payers, should always be used.

AUTHENTICATION AND COMPLETION

To ensure authenticity and as a means of illustrating completion, the medical record entry should be signed by the PT or PTA who writes it. An electronic signature has been deemed legally acceptable in electronic records. Signature stamps, however, are not acceptable.

Signature means a legible identifier of any type acceptable according to policies in Pub. 100-08, Medicare Program Integrity Manual, Chapter 3, §3.3.2.4 concerning signatures.[1]

A legible signature should appear with every entry. If the entry spans multiple pages, it should appear on each page, with continuation indicated. The signature should be the provider's full name and appropriate professional designation (i.e., PT or PTA) and should be signed the same way each time. The individual's medical license number should accompany the signature to ensure identification and authentication of the provider of service. See below Examples for Counter Signatures.

Example

Susan Smith, PT # 0001977

Depending on state, national, and local laws or accreditation requirements, SPTs and recent graduates with temporary licenses may require countersignature or co-signature for authentication by the supervising licensed PT. According to Roach, "The purpose of countersignatures is to require a professional to review, and if appropriate, indicate approval of action taken by another practitioner. Usually, the person countersigning a record entry is more experienced or has received a higher level of training than the person who made the original entry. In any case, the person required to countersign should be the individual who has the authority to evaluate the entry."[2]

Example

Kevin Johnson, SPT

Susan Smith, PT # 0001977

DATE

From the CMS MBPM, Chapter 15, Section 220:[1]

A DATE may be in any form (written, stamped, or electronic). The date may be added to the record in any manner and at any time, as long as the dates are accurate. If they are different, refer to both the date a service was performed and the date the entry to the record was made. For example, if a physician certifies a plan and fails to date it, staff may add "Received Date" in writing or with a stamp. The received date is valid for certification/re-certification purposes. Also, if the physician faxes the referral, certification, or re-certification and forgets to date it, the date that prints out on the fax is valid. If services provided on one date are documented on another date, both dates should be documented.[1]

NATIONAL PROVIDER IDENTIFIER NUMBER

Conditions of coverage and payment for outpatient physical therapy (PT), occupational therapy (OT) or speech-language pathology (SLP) services rely on the certification of the plan of care (POC). The National Provider Identifier (NPI) of the certifying physician or non-physician practitioner (NPP) must be included on the therapy claim. See Pub. 100-04, Medicare Claims Processing Manual, Section 10.3.5. https://www.cms.gov/Regulations-and-Guidance/Guidance/Manuals/downloads/clm104c05.pdf. The NPI is a required 10-digit free registration of a unique number for covered healthcare providers including physical therapists.[1]

COURTESY

The record is not the place for complaints, criticism, blame, anger, arguments, or expressions of frustration with other healthcare team members. The tone of the entries should be as neutral as possible. If multiple attempts have been made by the therapist to contact a physician or another professional and he or she has not responded, simply record the date and time the call was made. Let others pass judgment. Avoid underlining for emphasizing negatively toned entries, do not change from cursive to print or vice versa, and do not write larger in some parts of the entry than others or in capital letters in hard-copy entries. In electronic records, or if manually printing, avoid using all capital letters, as capitals indicate anger, bolding components, or underlining.

CONTENT INCLUSION

Document all telephone calls, missed appointments, instructions given to the patient or caregiver, discussion with families, verbal or telephone orders from physicians (followed by signed written orders in as close to 24 hours as possible), instructions to other health professionals, all communication about the patient, and all relevant session or encounter information, including identification of anyone who may have observed the therapy session.

All entries should be brief, meaningful, and as objective as possible, including primarily facts. Do not write just for the sake of writing. Avoid phrases and words that are meaningless or have multiple meanings. If tempted to use the adjective "confused," for example, it is better to describe the behaviors that led you to use the word. See Example below for a content inclusion for a patient that is confused.

Example

Instead, if the patient is confused, write:

Although patient could not identify the therapist nor where he was, he was able to actively participate in the therapy session.

Avoid phrases such as "tolerated treatment well," as it does not objectively describe any behavior or response to treatment. Describe instead what the patient or client accomplished in terms of time and aerobic capacity or endurance, or use another choice of objective descriptions. For example:

Patient was able to complete 60 minutes of active therapeutic exercise and gait, with only brief rest periods in between and stabilizing of blood pressure after 2 minutes of rest. This has improved, as patient required up to 5 minutes for vital signs to return to normal previously.

Avoid physical therapy jargon or terms and phrases only understood by PTs. What is written will influence the reader's impression of your care. Anyone that needs access to the record for any reason must be able to understand what is written. In the case of payment, lack of understanding by the third-party payer representative may result in initial denial of a claim.

Terminology should be descriptive so that treatment can be duplicated or a clear picture of the patient is painted. Descriptive documentation should include impairments and functional limitations, justifying care based on functional improvement.

HEADINGS OR TITLES

Preprinted forms or electronic templates usually include section headings or titles. In addition to section titles or headings, the whole entry itself should be titled (i.e., Physical Therapy Evaluation, Physical Therapy Notes, Physical Therapy Progress Report, etc.). In sections where narrative, paragraph, or "freeform" entries may be included, it is better to categorize information—for example, Interventions: gait training. Even when using the SOAP (subjective, objective, analysis/assessment, plan) format, subheadings can be used to clarify and better organize data. If categories extend to more than one page, either the back of a page or a new page, there should be an indication that it is a continuation. All pages should be numbered, and the total number should be clear (i.e., 1/4, 2/4, 3/4, 4/4).

ILLUSTRATIONS OR PICTURES

Pictures or illustrations can be effective tools for entering information into the record. They can be drawn with ink and must be clearly labeled, dated, and signed. Preprinted pictures must be clearly labeled as well (see Figure 2-1 for an example of a body diagram that can be utilized for documentation purposes). Photographs or video, CD, and digital recordings may also be included, but there must be signed permission and protection consistent with the HIPAA.

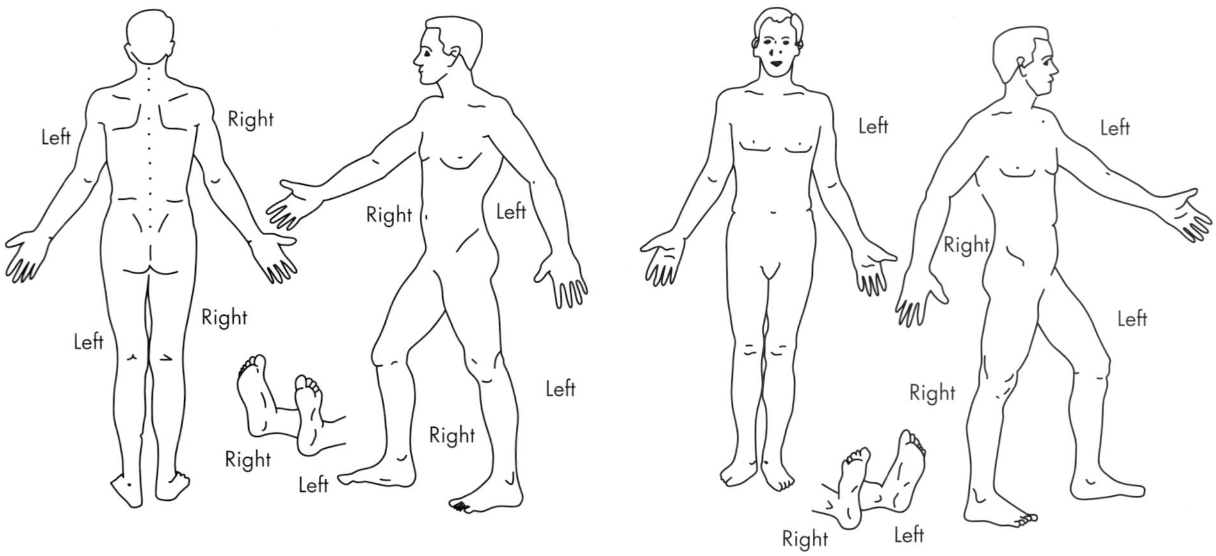

Figure 2-1. The pain chart.[3] Instructions: Please use all of the figures to show exactly where all your pains are, and where they radiate to. Please be as precise and detailed as possible. Shade or draw with blue marker for pain. Use yellow marker for numbness and tingling; red marker for burning or hot areas; and green marker for cramping. Only the patient is to fill out this sheet. *(Reproduced, with permission, from Melzack R. Pain Measurement and Assessment. New York, NY: Raven Press; 1983. Copyright ©1970 by Dr, Ronald Melzack.)*

TREATMENT DAY

From the CMS MBPM Chapter 15, Section 220:[1]

Treatment day means a single calendar day on which treatment, evaluation and/or reevaluation is provided. There could be multiple visits, treatment sessions/encounters on a treatment day.[1]

TREATMENT SESSION

From the CMS MBPM Chapter 15, Section 220:[1]

Visits or treatment sessions begin at the time the patient enters the treatment area (of a building, office, or clinic) and continue until all services (e.g., activities, procedures, services) have been completed for that session and the patient leaves that area to participate in a non-therapy activity. It is likely that not all minutes in the visits/treatment sessions are billable (e.g., rest periods). There may be two treatment sessions in a day, for example, in the morning and afternoon. When there are two visits/treatment sessions in a day, plans of care indicate treatment amount of twice a day.[1]

OBJECTIVITY

All entries should be as objective as possible, avoiding subjectivity and including facts. Personal opinion should be avoided. If a patient comes in smelling of alcohol, yelling obscenities, and staggering, avoid documenting that they are drunk; rather, document your observations of their behavior. Drunkenness can only be established legally by blood alcohol levels. Indeed, other medical conditions such as ketoacidosis may mimic drunkenness or alcohol breath.

Provide only the behaviors or signs that you have observed or assessed. When entering statements made by the patient, use quotation marks. When entering quotes, be careful when taking statements out of context.

ECONOMY OF VERBIAGE

All notes should be as efficient as possible, using only those words that are absolutely necessary. Nonessential words, such as pronouns and other modifiers, can be omitted. The reader will know, once the patient is identified, that entries are about the patient, unless otherwise stated. When selecting words, if there are short alternatives, utilizes them as long as the demonstration of skilled physical therapy is still implied. The use of commonly used or facility-approved symbols is also acceptable as a means of economizing on words. Bulleting or numbering can be used to present items in a series. Electronic entries may have a selection of phrases based on function or diagnosis (see Appendix A for abbreviations). For patient goals, "Patient will be able to…:" is written once—it does not need to be repeated for every goal. It would only be necessary to clarify if a goal was for someone other than the patient. For example, "the husband will be able to demonstrate safe and effective transfers with patient from the wheelchair (WC) to and from the bed."

PATIENT

From the CMS MBPM, Chapter 15, Section 220:[1]

Patient, client, resident, and beneficiary are terms used interchangeably to indicate enrolled recipients of Medicare covered services.[1]

CLAIM DENIAL ISSUES AND DOCUMENTATION

Although communicating the care of the patient is probably the most important purpose of documentation, the record is also used for payment purposes. There are APTA guidelines regarding pro bono care and wellness care. It is the responsibility of the professional providing care to ensure that the content of any entries in the patient record justify the intervention provided. The entries must therefore contain the information necessary to communicate with other practitioners involved in the care and ensure payment (as well as serve the other purposes of the medical record and documentation). When considering general principles of documentation and those specific to physical therapy, discussion of the Office of the Inspector General (OIG) reports and identification of reasons for physical therapy denials in the Medicare system is warranted. These reports are accessible to the public and are available on the OIG website (http://www.oig.dol.gov/).[4] The reasons include both technical errors and content errors that did not justify skilled PT intervention. Attention to the general principles of documentation can prevent denial for most of the elements cited and help the practitioner ensure appropriate content. The problems identified in the OIG audits, although performed on Medicare records, are universally applicable.

Common reasons for denials include the following:

- Documentation did not support certification of the plan of care for physical therapy services
- The physician's or NPP's signature and date of certification of the plan of care or progress note indicating the physician/NPP reviewed and approved the plan of care is required
- Identifier omission
- Incorrect form use
- Incorrect information
- Inadequate/imprecise
- Illegibility
- Good documentation in wrong place
- Bad documentation in any place
- Billing information did not match documentation of care
- Goals did not match problems or diagnosis
- Effectiveness of therapy services for patient's illness or injury (i.e., goals not achieved) not documented
- Patient had achieved their restorative potential and was provided repetitive, nonskilled exercises (care exceeded date of goal achievement)
- Patient did not require the care of a skilled therapist (either care was not skilled, maintenance was too general, or the documentation did not indicate skill)
- Loss of function or functional limitation not identified (problems were physiological impairment based)
- Potential for significant improvement not identified (goals were not significant enough to justify care, or patient was too high level or too low level)
- Need for skilled therapist not identified (improvement would have been made without therapeutic intervention)
- No indication of medical necessity
- Maintenance-type therapies being provided (rote, repetitive treatment to maintain same level of function)

There are other common reasons for denial that will be described by the OIG for the general knowledge of the therapist. Since authorization is frequently required in a managed care system for physical therapy services, the following reasons for denial deserve attention. Although not considered documentation of care, they are part of the client's medical record. Authorization or preauthorization is the permission of the third-party payer or managed care organization (MCO) to provide a specified number of physical therapy visits to a beneficiary. It usually includes total number of visits to an approved provider, based on a specific diagnosis, with treatment authorized for a specific diagnosis for a specific body area or body part.

As large third-party payers such as Blue Cross Blue Shield (BCBS) provide multiple insurance products, having provider status with one type or division does not automatically mean the therapist has provider status with another. For example, if a PT has a Medicare provider number through BCBS, it does not give the individual provider status with the health maintenance organization (HMO) or point-of-service (POS) plan, unless the contract specifically stipulates otherwise. Preauthorization or authorization does not necessarily ensure payment. Documentation still has to support the necessity of skilled therapy services. For PTs providing Medicare Part B services, they must apply for individual Medicare identification numbers by enrolling in Medicare.

Reasons for denials based on authorization include the following:

- Unauthorized treatment (where preauthorization is required)
- Unapproved provider (practice is not an approved provider for the payer)
- Exceeded approval limit (exceeded preauthorized number of visits in total, or goals were achieved in fewer than approved visits and treatment continued)
- Treatment for other than “authorized” body area
- Part of care justified by documentation, but not all (partial denial, either patient reached goals and there was continued care, or only some of the documentation was skilled in nature)
- Documentation did not support the need for skilled physical therapy (not medically necessary)

NONCOVERED CONDITIONS AND SERVICES

It is also the service provider’s responsibility to be aware of medical conditions and services not covered by the third-party payer. Regardless of the documentation, noncovered services will not be paid regardless of therapist efforts or goals. See Chap. 13 “Coding,” for examples of Medicare noncovered services and conditions. Some payers may not pay for services rendered unless provided by a PT only. This is also the responsibility of the PT to know.

ACTIVE PARTICIPATION

From the CMS MBPM, Chapter 15, Section 220:[1]

ACTIVE PARTICIPATION of the clinician in treatment means that the clinician personally furnishes in its entirety at least 1 billable service on at least 1 day of treatment.[1]

SUMMARY

Millions of dollars in Medicare overpayments are identified annually. More than a third were due to lack of medical necessity identifiable in the documentation, such as payments for skilled physical therapy for patients with *no functional* diagnosis requiring physical therapy. Incorrect coding was at the root of another percentage of the overpayments. Auditors check codes by comparing the code with the documentation in the medical record to support that level of code. Results such as these have led to increasingly aggressive efforts by CMS to identify fraud and abuse in the Medicare system. All fiscal intermediaries and third-party payers are making the same efforts. With the advent of technology, audits and reviews can easily be performed to identify discrepancies.

Incorporating all of the general principles for documentation should help organize the record, record appropriate information, and get services paid based on the documentation. The therapist or assistant should seek to write only what is relevant and necessary, in an objective manner, using verbiage that indicates skill but is universally understood by all potential users of the medical record. Appreciating why payment for physical therapy services is denied and why services are paid to the therapy team can reflect on documentation content guidelines and the importance of content adherence.

REVIEW QUESTIONS

1. How should manual and electronic records be stored?
2. Why is legibility imperative in the medical record?
3. Describe the types of data found in the medical record.
4. Explain how errors in the record should be corrected. Give two examples in different domains.
5. Explain the risks involved if entries into the record are not timely.
6. Why is the use of abbreviations in the record a potential problem for a PT?
7. Explain the concept of accuracy in the record.
8. What is a co-signature? Provide an example of application in physical therapy documentation.
9. What does objectivity in the medical record mean?
10. What is the relationship between payment and documentation? Give six examples of denial based on the documentation.
11. What type of follow-up should there be for verbal, telephone, or electronic referrals or orders?
12. A physical therapy entry includes the statement "patient was uncooperative." Rewrite this statement using appropriate verbiage.

REFERENCES

1. Covered Medical and Other Health Services. In: *Medicare Benefit Policy Manual*. Baltimore, MD: Centers for Medicare & Medicaid Services. Available at https://www.cms.gov/Regulations-and-Guidance/Guidance/Manuals/Downloads/bp102c15.pdf. Accessed August 15, 2020.
2. William RH Jr, Hoban RG, Broccolo BM, Roth AB, Blanchard TP. *Medical Records and the Law*. 4th ed. Sudbury, MA: Jones and Bartlett Publishers; 2006.
3. Melzack R. *Pain Measurement and Assessment*. New York, NY: Raven Press; 1983.
4. *Office of Inspector General,* OIG. Available at http://www.oig.dol.gov/. Accessed August 15, 2020.

3 Application of Models for Organization and Guidelines for Content

OBJECTIVES

Following completion of this chapter, the reader will be able to:

- Compare and contrast the basic types of medical record organization.
- Explain what goes in each section of the SOAP formatted note.
- Give examples of three types of individual entry formats.
- List what needs to be included in a checklist or flow sheet.
- Explain what a disablement model is.
- Understand the different components of the ICF.
- Compare and contrast the medical diagnosis and the physical therapy diagnosis (physical therapy problem).
- Describe the difference between the initial examination and the evaluation.

RECORD FORMATS

A variety of record formats are used by physical therapists (PTs). Categorically, they include source-oriented, problem-oriented, and integrated systems.

The *source-oriented medical record keeping (SOMR)* system has been commonly used in hospitals and skilled nursing facilities for decades. Each record, or "chart," is divided into sections by profession or service given (i.e., physical therapy, nursing, medical, physician orders, laboratory, etc.). Patient problems are not separated and notes between caregivers are not integrated because they are "parallel" in nature. Entries in each section are usually in chronological order. It may be time consuming for the PT to glean patient information from the SOMR because of this structure. Additionally, within each section, the methodology for recording information may be different for each discipline, but each discipline should be consistent with itself. This record keeping allows for easy access by a service group provider, but makes it difficult for overall assessment of the patient.

A component of the *problem-oriented medical record (POMR)* system, the SOAP (subjective, objective, assessment/analysis, plan) or SOAPIER (SOAP implementation of plan, evaluation of the implemented plan, and revision of the plan if necessary) note, has been commonly used by PTs, but less so with the advent of electronic medical records (EMRs). Common use, however, should not be misunderstood to translate to the best or most effective or efficient method for every situation. In an effort to improve patient record keeping, in 1958 Dr. Lawrence Weed of the University of Vermont began exploring alternative types of record entries. The POMR, developed in 1969, focuses on a patient's specific problems in an integrated and coordinated manner between professionals.[1,2] Weed's system includes the initial assessment, problem list, initial plan, progress notes, and discharge summary. All patient problems are included and numbered, active (current) and past, and all professionals involved in the patient's care contribute to the list. In the "pure" system, only one problem can be addressed on a SOAP progress note. Physician orders, not included in the initial plan, are cross-coded for relevance by number to the problems identified. Notes in the POMR are recorded in the SOAP or SOAPIER format. Dr. Weed offered categories to assist professionals in clarifying information.[1,2]

Author's Note

Beware of statements that are irrelevant to care or out of context that may be misunderstood and result in denial of services.

S Subjective data (what the patient, family member, or significant other says the patient feels or is doing, *only as relevant to the specific episode of care and problem*)

O Objective data (what the professional performs, observes, or inspects in a reproducible manner as relevant to function as possible and clearly presented)

A Assessment or Analytical (summary of S and O with interpretation and professional judgment in order to justify care, including progress toward goals, if using SOAP only vs. SOAPIER)

P Plan (intervention plan)

I Implementation of plan

E Evaluation of the implemented plan

R Revision of the plan if necessary

The SOAP or SOAPIER entries may be supplemented by flow sheets for ongoing and frequent interventions. For the discharge summary or summation of care, each problem identified needs a separate SOAP note by each professional providing intervention for the problem in the Weed format.

In order to adapt the SOAP note format to record-keeping regulations, an additional P for the patient problem, may be added before the S: PSOAP. In a hospital setting or skilled nursing facility (SNF), the record may be source oriented but the physical entry may be in POMR format, SOAP or PSOAP, or SOAPIER. Another change in SOAP-type entries in the past decade is the introduction of functional outcomes reporting (FOR). *Documenting Functional Outcomes*[3] furthered the concept of FOR introduced by Swanson. This type of documenting stresses function and goals related to the same problem and can be presented in SOAP format, the FOR format, or narrative format.

Dr. Weed's contribution to health or medical record keeping has, to date, passed the test of time. He envisioned "a future in which every patient will have a birth to death problem list on record for use by any hospital. This list, available through a central computer bank, would provide healthcare professionals with a patient's complete data base, anytime, anywhere."[12] Although Dr. Weed's vision has been a long time in coming, it is interesting to note that his vision is being realized. The recent experimental advent of implantable data chips is the realization of Dr. Weed's vision.

The third category of record keeping is the *integrated health record format*. All entries and forms by each discipline are arranged in chronological order without separation.

INDIVIDUAL ENTRY FORMATS

There are a variety of formats for individual entries in addition to SOAP, including problem, status, and plan (PSP); problem, status, plan, and functional goals (PSPG); data, evaluation, and performance goals (DEP); FOR; narrative; patient client management format; use of clinical tools; flow sheets/checklists; and illustrations. The latter three should be used more as supplements to the others than as stand-alone entries. In the past decade, documentation by exception and critical pathway documentation have also been introduced.

Problem, Status, and Plan

P Patient problems and/or medical diagnosis

S Patient/family/caretaker input as relevant and objective data

P Treatment plan/treatment rendered

Problem, Status, Plan, and Functional Goals

P Patient problems and/or medical diagnosis

S Patient/family/caretaker input as relevant and objective data

P Treatment plan/treatment rendered

G Functional goals/progress toward goals

Data, Evaluation, and Performance Goals

D Patient/family/caretaker input as relevant and objective data

E Identification of patient problems, interpretation of data, treatment plan/treatment rendered

P Functional goals/progress toward goals

Functional Outcome Report

The FOR includes the reason for referral, functional limitations (these differ some from the American Physical Therapy Association [APTA] ICF Model), physical therapy assessment, physical therapy problems, functional outcome goals/progress toward goals, treatment plan/treatment rendered, and rationale.

Narrative

Entries are made by category of intervention, but should be consistent with terminology from Current Procedural Terminology (CPT) coding, in that prior to listing individual interventions, they should be preceded by the CPT code verbiage (i.e., gait training, therapeutic exercise, therapeutic activities) in paragraph-style format, objective intervention and patient response, progress toward goals, and plan or modifications to plan. There may be conclusions or assessments drawn, depending on the purpose of the entry (i.e., treatment vs. progress over time). Headings should be differentiated so that information can be readily identified.

PATIENT MANAGEMENT

This method is related to the patient management process purported in the *Guide to Physical Therapist* practice. In it, appropriate categories are used as headings in which information can be included, consistent with the guide categories of the systems and subcategories such as aerobic capacity, assistive and adaptive devices, sensory integrity, etc.

CLINICAL TOOLS

A variety of scales, indexes, tests, and measures are commonly used in physical therapy. However, the use of tools must be coordinated with the diagnosis (if there is a disease-specific tool), interventions, and results external to the assessments or data gathered and entered onto the tool form. The information contained in the tool should always be summarized in supporting entries in a functional, objective manner in order to be meaningful to other professionals involved in care and any reader. Examples of clinical tools are the Berg Balance, Timed Up and Go, and the Folstein Mini Mental. If physical therapy intervention is addressing the deficits identified by the tools, the tools should be repeated at a minimum at discharge. The OPTIMAL,[4] developed in coordination with the APTA, is an example of a survey-style tool that can be used at both initial exam and evaluation and focuses on function. The OPTIMAL is one of the tools recommended by the Centers for Medicare & Medicaid (CMS) for Medicare Part B outpatients.[4]

APTA'S OPTIMAL DATA COLLECTION INSTRUMENT[4]

APTA's OPTIMAL remains the copyrighted intellectual property of *Physical Therapy* (PTJ). OPTIMAL is used for Functional Limitation Reporting for therapy services. The OPTIMAL assessment tool can be used to quantify beneficiary function. OPTIMAL can assist with reporting functional limitations as follows:

- Scoring of OPTIMAL asks the patient to identify his or her primary goal of physical therapy. This will help with patient-centered care and provide additional information for the PT to determine the primary goal.[4]
- OPTIMAL's scoring of the patient's perceived difficulty and confidence in performing a specific activity can help the PT make a clinical judgment on the severity of the impairment limitation restriction.[4]
- APTA does not require entities to request permission for using OPTIMAL. This applies to (1) clinicians within their facilities for patient care; (2) education institutions using material for in-classroom use; (3) entities conducting research; and (4) entities wishing to use it in commercial products or services, including other publications, courses, or software programs. (Copyright © 2012, 2006, 2005 American Physical Therapy Association. All rights reserved.)

FUNCTIONAL INDEPENDENCE MEASURE

The Functional Independence Measure (FIM) (Guide for the Uniform Data Set for Medical Rehabilitation, 1996) is used to determine the severity of disability on a scale of 1 to 7 and indicates how much assistance the individual needs to perform activities of daily living. Developed by the University of Buffalo (Dr. Carl V. Granger), the FIM scores are used to measure progress as a result of intervention and are commonly used for inpatient rehabilitation. The Uniform Data Set administers the system.[5] Fees are charged for participation in the system and analysis of the data for one organization compared to similar organizations in the system. FIM is functionally oriented, using variables such as transfer, toileting, and gait. It is an 18-item ordinal scale. The WeeFIM is the version of FIM used for pediatric application. All professionals using the FIM are specially FIM trained and certified for consistency with scoring.

FOCUS ON THERAPEUTIC OUTCOMES

The Focus on Therapeutic Outcomes (FOTO) system is designed to measure outcomes of care in the outpatient setting. Like the FIM system, fees are charged for participation in the system and analysis of the data for your organization compared to similar organizations in the system.[6]

FLOWSHEETS AND CHECKLISTS

Flowsheets and checklists may contain dates, treatments, attendance, or a variety of other activities. Generally, a check mark is used to mark a specific box for the care provided. Initials of the person who provided the care are preferable to discourage others from entering on the record. Flowsheet or checklist entries should be accompanied by notes to clarify entries and "skill" or rate the effectiveness of the intervention. Although functional, they should not be used as stand-alone forms. See Table 3-1 for a flowsheet example. The downside of using these types of entries is that treatment sessions may appear unskilled if there are no clarifying entries addressing the skill needed.

CRITICAL PATHWAYS/CLINICAL PATHWAYS

Within each patient's therapy plan, target processes and sequences of care, known as critical or clinical pathways, are determined upon the initial visit or diagnosis and generally follow a precise timeline. The pathways are generally experientially or evidence based and may be used to replace traditional forms of documentation, since they require only a signature and date when a goal is achieved on a preprinted pathway form. The term "critical pathway" relates to the original pathways developed in acute care for "critically ill" patients. Clinical pathways are more applicable in rehabilitation for patients not "critically" ill. See Table 3-2 for a clinical pathway example.

DOCUMENTATION BY EXCEPTION

The documentation by exception style of record keeping consists of using anticipated or typical treatments and goals that are pre-established and available on preprinted forms in manual entry systems. The only entries required would be variations from the established "norms." In electronic or computerized systems, the user enters the initial diagnosis, and the treatment information appears in a retrievable file in a data bank. This method is not recommended because it does not allow for entry of specific patient information and is often too generalized.

PRINCIPLES SPECIFIC TO PHYSICAL THERAPY

Documentation content can be organized and simplified with the use of conceptual models or frameworks. Models are frequently used in industry and theoretical sciences to make categorization of information easier to study, organize, apply, and discuss. The APTA provides models in the *Guide to Physical Therapist Practice.*[7] The information in the guide is presented using a clinical decision-making model (CDMM) (see Figure 3-1). Using the CDMM can help therapists organize their examination (tests and measures), evaluation, interventions, and all record-keeping documentation.

In May 2001, the advent of the International Classification of Functioning, Disability and Health (ICF) begun with its approval by the 191 member states of the World Health Organization (WHO)[8] during the 54th World Health Assembly (WHA). The ICF is a conceptual framework and classification system that provides a universal understanding of health using a broad consideration of functioning-related factors and contextual factors to include personal and environmental factors. The ICF was intended for use in research, surveillance,

Table 3-1 Flowsheet Example

Flowsheet Example 1

TX:	8/26/20	8/27/20	8/28/20
Ther ex	*JLS*		
Gait Training	*JLS*		
Therapeutic Activities		*JLS*	
Self-Management		*JLS*	*JLS*

Supplemental entries by date:

8/27/20 "Pain at 3/10 during activity after last session." Able to inc. resistance from 5 to 8#'s for quad ext/flex, 30 reps. Demonstrated ability to ascend and descend 5 steps without use of handrails, no knee buckling. Requires tactile facilitation during LE ther ex to fully engage the L quadriceps and control contractions. Steady improvement noted toward goals *Jon L. Smith, PT*, #1234

Flowsheet Example 2

Patient: Grant Shamus

Please indicate # of units as applicable for each procedure (or a check ✓if units are nonbillable) and initials of individual treating

Procedure	11/07/20
Gait training 97116	1 unit *LR*
Ther ex 97110	1 unit *LR*
Neuromuscular re-ed 97112	1 unit *LR*
Cold pack (CP) 97010	1 unit *LR*
Home Instruction	✓ *LR*

Supplemental entries by date:

11/07/20:

Progressed from FWRW to axillary crutches: CG & VC: ascend and descend 5 steps, grass, carpet, even surface 50′, × 3 reps each. Ther ex, active in standing L hip: in all planes, 10 reps, single leg stance R, 10 sees with balance loss to L. CP L hip in sidelying at end of session × 15 mins. Pain▾from 6/10 to 3/10 following CP. Add 2# resistance next visit, cont 3x/week. *Lynn Robert,* PT 1234

Flowsheet Example 3

Pt: Grant Shamus

Please indicate # of units as applicable for each procedure and initials of individual treating

Procedure	11/07/20
Gait Training	1
97116	*LR*

crutches	✓
carpet	✓
stairs	✓
curbs	
grass	✓
Therapeutic Exercise	1
97110	*LR*
Active	✓
Standing	✓
Supine	
Sidelying	
Prone	
Resistive	
Standing	
Supine	
Sidelying	
Prone	
Neuro-muscular Re-ed	1
	LR
97112	
Balance	✓
Cold Pack	1
97010	*LR*
Home	✓
Instruction	*LR*

Supplemental entries by date:

11/07/20:

Progressed from FWRW to axillary crutches: CG & VC: ascend and descend 5 steps, grass, carpet, even surface 50′ × 3 reps each. Ther ex, active in standing L hip: in all planes, 10 reps, single leg stance R, 10 secs with balance loss to L. CP L hip in sidelying at end of session × 15 mins. Pain decreased from 6/10 to 3/10 following CP. Add 2# resistance next visit, cont 3x/week. *Lynn Robert*, PT 1234

and reporting per WHA resolution. The World Confederation for Physical Therapy endorsed the ICF in June 2003, and the APTA followed with its endorsement of the ICF in June 2008.

Exclusive of the models, guidelines for documentation were first established for Medicare by the Healthcare Finance Administration (HCFA, now CMS). Initially the guidelines were used by the Medicare fiscal intermediaries (FIs), or carriers, now referred to as Medicare Administrative Contractors (MACS), to verify provision of services to beneficiaries by physicians. The guidelines were not, however, used extensively until the 1970s. By the 1970s, computers could track adherence and costs to the system, which began to grow exponentially. When third-party payers (also known as carriers) gained access to technology and the revelation that they, too, could track provision of care, documentation for non-Medicare beneficiaries had to undergo the same scrutiny. Though somewhat general in nature, there is standard information required by Medicare. Many of the guidelines were

Table 3-2 Clinical Pathway Examples

Clinical Pathway Example 1

Medical Diagnosis: ______________________________

PT Diagnosis: ______________________________

Weight-Bearing Status: __________RLE__________LLE

PT Name: Print: __________ Signature: __________ Initials: __________

PT Name: Print: __________ Signature: __________ Initials: __________

PT Name: Print: __________ Signature: __________ Initials: __________

Post-op day achieved	IEP: Quad sets, ankle pumps	Able to recall precautions	LTD Asst bed mob	I bed mobility	I sit <>supine	Min Asst sit <> stand	Min Asst Gait with walker, 25′	Sup standing with device	Pain level with movement
1	*JLS*	*JLS*							10/10
2			*JLS*						9/10
3				*JLS*	*JLS*	*JLS*			7/10
4							*JLS*	*JLS*	6/10
5	Discharge status:								

Indicate if status different from that above:

Supplemental entries as indicated:

Clinical Pathway Example 2

Medical Diagnosis:

S72.002A Fracture of unspecified part of neck of left femur, initial encounter for closed fracture

PT Diagnosis:

R26.9 Unspecified abnormalities of gait and mobility

Weight-bearing status: FWB RLE **PWB** 50% LLE

PT: Name: Print Jennifer Allan DPT **Signature**: *Jennifer Allan* **Initials:**

PT: Name: Print: Lynn Robert PT **Signature**: *Lynn Robert* **Initials:** *LR*

PT: Name: Print:__________ **Signature**__________ **Initials:** __________

	Gait training 97116	Gait training	Gait training	Gait training	Ther ex 97110	Ther ex	Ther ex	Instructions
Date	**1 crutches even surface**	**1 crutches carpet**	**1 crutches grass/ outdoor**	**1 crutches stairs**	**3/5 strength L hip: ✓ abd**	**3+/5 strength L hip: ✓ abd**	**4-/5 strength L hip: ✓ abd**	**I HEP**
11/02/20					✓ *get*			✓ *get*
11/06/20	✓ *LR*					✓ *LR*		✓ *LR*

Discharge status:

Interim supplemental entries as indicated:

11/02/20:

Progressed from FWRW to axillary crutches 4 point gait: CG & VC: even surface 50′, × 3 reps. Ther ex, active on mat in antigravity positions: L hip: in all planes, 10 reps, single leg stance R, 5 secs with balance loss to L. Able to sleep 4 hours uninterrupted by pain. Progress to ther ex in standing next visit, cont 3x/week. *Jennifer Allan,* DPT 2234

11/06/20:

Progressed from FWRW to axillary crutches: CG & VC: ascend and descend 5 steps, grass, carpet, even surface 50′, × 3 reps each. Ther ex, active in standing L hip: in all planes, 10 reps, single leg stance R, 10 secs with balance loss to L. CP L hip in sidelying at end of session × 15 mins. Pain ↓from 6/10 to 3/10 following CP. Able to sleep up to 6 hours now. Add 2# resistance next visit, cont 3x/week. *Lynn Robert,* PT 1234

written into Medicare manuals in the 1970s and 1980s, but it was not until a decade later that Medicare attempted to standardize forms or formats for payment.

It should be noted that the information required in Medicare documentation is very similar to that recommended in the APTA *Guidelines for Physical Therapy Documentation*. The Medicare documentation guidelines can be obtained on the Internet by accessing Medicare provider manuals at https://www.cms.gov/Regulations-and-Guidance/Guidance/Manuals/Internet-Only-Manuals-IOMs.

THE DISABLEMENT MODEL

As early as the 1970s, disablement models were developed with the help of sociologist Saad Nagi to categorize the impact of medical conditions on function for the WHO.[8] The WHO, part of a component organization of the United Nations, which also developed the International Statistics Classification of Diseases and Related Health Problems, more commonly known as ICD (i.e., ICD-10), developed an alternative model in 1980: the International Classification of Diseases, Impairments, Disabilities, and Handicaps (ICDIDH). The National Center for Rehabilitation and Research developed a similar model in 1992. See Table 3-3 for the disablement models.

In its current version, the *Guide to Physical Therapist Practice*[7] uses the ICF framework as the theoretical basis for its terminology. Familiarity with the model should help the PT in conceptualizing and actualizing documentation of care, as all components should be addressed in the medical or client record. There are four categories in the model: pathology or pathophysiology, impairment, functional limitation, and disability. Pathology or pathophysiology is a situation in which an injury is caused by a disorder, condition, or disease. Impairment is the physiologic or system problem itself (i.e., integument, cardiopulmonary or neuromuscular, psychological, or anatomic problem). Functional limitation is activity limitation that occurs as a result of the impact of the impairments on a physical "action, task, or activity in an efficient, typically expected, or competent manner."[7] Disability is the inability to perform expected self-care, leisure, work, community, and social roles.

With the endorsement of the ICF by the APTA, the ICF is integrated in the *Guide to Physical Therapist Practice*. This development makes the awareness and understanding

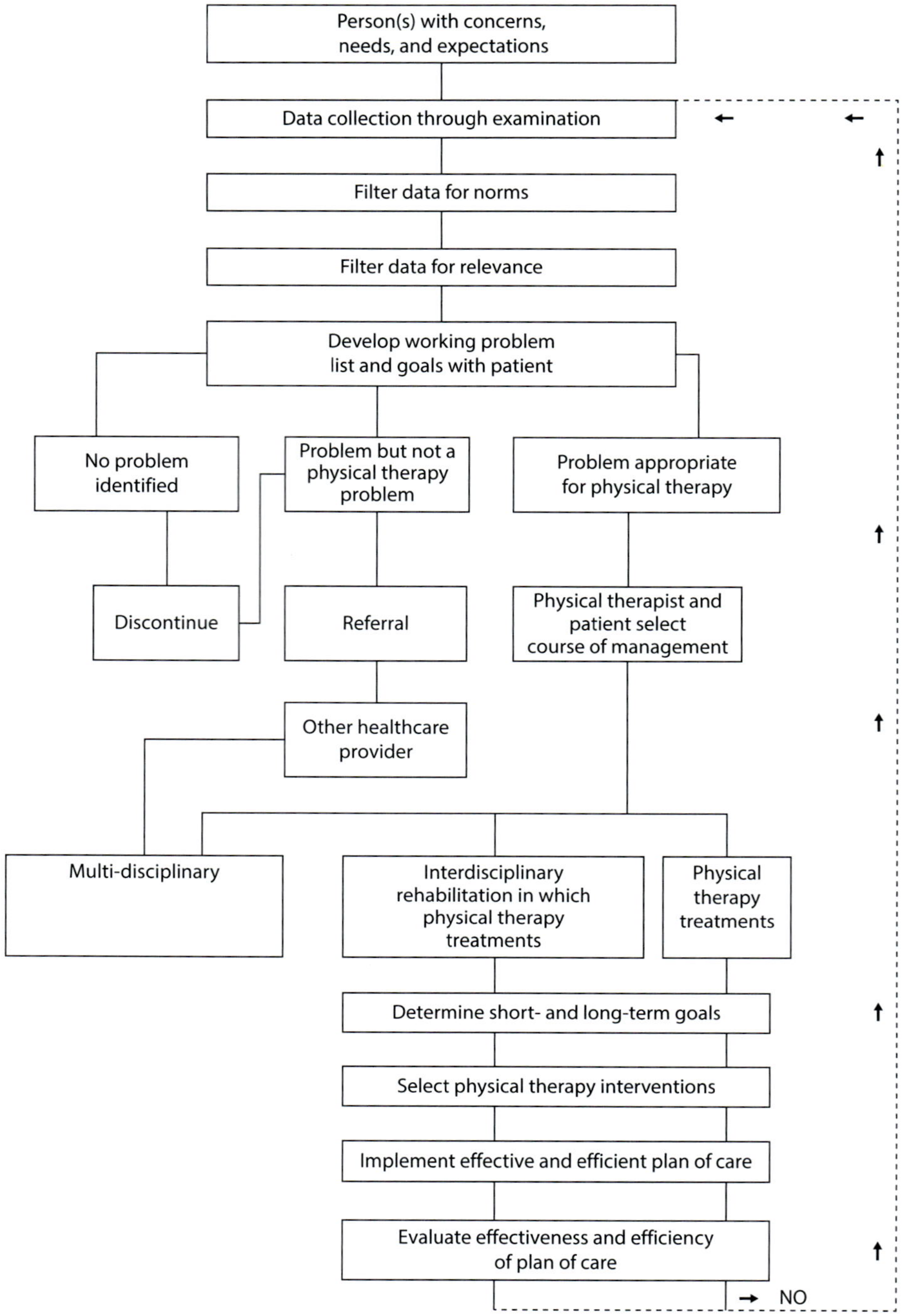

Figure 3-1. Clinical decision-making model (CDMM).

of PTs of the ICF a necessary tool in order to document a comprehensive picture of their patients' health, functioning, and disability. The ICF (see Figure 3-2) is made up of different interactive components: health condition, functioning variables (body functions and body structures, activity, and participation), and contextual factors (environmental and personal). Within the ICF, functioning (or disability) as it relates to the patient's health condition provides information not only at the individual (intrinsic) level but also at the societal (extrinsic) level. This makes the ICF framework essential in the whole process of documentation because of its inclusiveness. See Figure 3-3 for the definition of the different components included within the ICF.

Table 3-3 Disablement Models

	NAGI	WHO	NATIONAL CENTER FOR REHABILITATION AND RESEARCH	ICF
Categorization of condition	Active pathology: Interruption or interference with normal processes and efforts of the organism to regain normal state	Disease: The intrinsic pathology or disorder	Pathophysiology: Interruption with normal physiologic developmental processes or structures	Health condition: Diseases, disorders, and injuries
Impairment	Anatomic, physiologic, mental, emotional abnormalities, or loss	Loss or abnormality of psychological, physiologic, or anatomic structure or function at organ level	Loss or abnormality of cognitive, emotional, physiological, or anatomic structure or function	Impairments are problems in body function or body structure, such as a significant deviation or loss.
Activities	Functional limitation: Limitation in performance at the level of the whole person	Disability: Restriction or lack of ability to perform an activity in a normal manner	Functional limitation: Restriction or lack of ability to perform in action in the manner or range consistent with the purpose of an organ system	Activity limitations or difficulties an individual may have in executing activities
End state	Disability: Limitation in performance of socially defined roles and tasks within a social, cultural, and physical environment	Handicap: Disadvantage as a result of impairment or disability that limits or prevents fulfilment of a normal role depending on age, gender, or sociocultural factors for the person	Societal limitation: Restriction attributable to social policy or barriers that limit fulfilment of roles	Participation restrictions or problems an individual may experience in involvement in life situations
Other factors				Environmental factors as facilitators or barriers to functioning Personal factors as positive or negative influences at the individual level

The ICF is a system that is part of the Family of International Classifications (FIC) by the WHO. The ICF classification complements the WHO's ICD-10, which contains information on diagnosis and health condition, but not on functional status. In some cases, both could also overlap (i.e., impairment of body parts and/or body function). Both the ICF and ICD-10 are under the auspice of the WHO Collaborating Centres for the FIC. In the ICD-10, the integration of the ICF enables the complementary role of each system. In physical therapy practice, comprehensive description of functioning, regardless of the etiology, is vital in addressing problems of the patient that are common to more than one health condition.

Other related roadmap developments in the implementation of the ICF include the following:

- Consolidated Health Informatics (CHI) recommended the use of ICF as the "vocabulary" (November 2006)

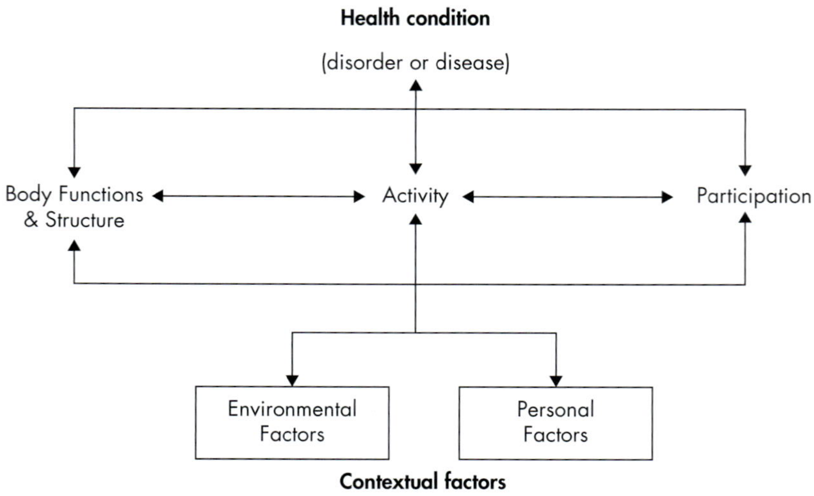

Figure 3-2. The ICF model.

Health Condition: diseases, disorders, and injuries

Functioning Components:

(1) Body Structures: anatomical parts of the body such as organs, limbs and their components
(2) Body Functions: physiological functions of body systems (including psychological functions)
(3) Activity: execution of a task or action by an individual
(4) Participation: involvement in a life situation

Contextual Factors:

(5) Environmental Factors: make up the physical, social and attitudinal environment in which people live and conduct their lives.

(6) Personal Factors: include gender, age, coping styles, social background, education, profession, past and current experience, overall behaviorpattern, character and other factors that influence how disability isexperienced by the individual.

Figure 3-3. Definition of the ICF components.

- National Committee on Vital and Health Statics, an advisory to the Secretary of Department of Health and Human Services in the United States, agreed with the recommendation of CHI regarding the use of the ICF Initiative 2006 Recommendations on the Functioning and Disability Domain (accepted by DHHS secretary in 2007)
- Integration of the ICF in the Unified Medical Language Systems (UMLS)

The prevailing trend in the evolution of disablement (or enablement) models is toward functioning-based rather than the pure medical/diagnostic model. This trend reflects consideration of the society and the environment (macro level) in addition to capturing information at the individual level (micro level). As we go further into the realm of an ICF-based system of healthcare documentation, PTs must reflect the ICF model components for payment.

The ICF is structured around the following broad components:

- Body functions and structure
- Activities (related to tasks and actions by an individual) and participation (involvement in a life situation)
- Additional information on severity and environmental factors

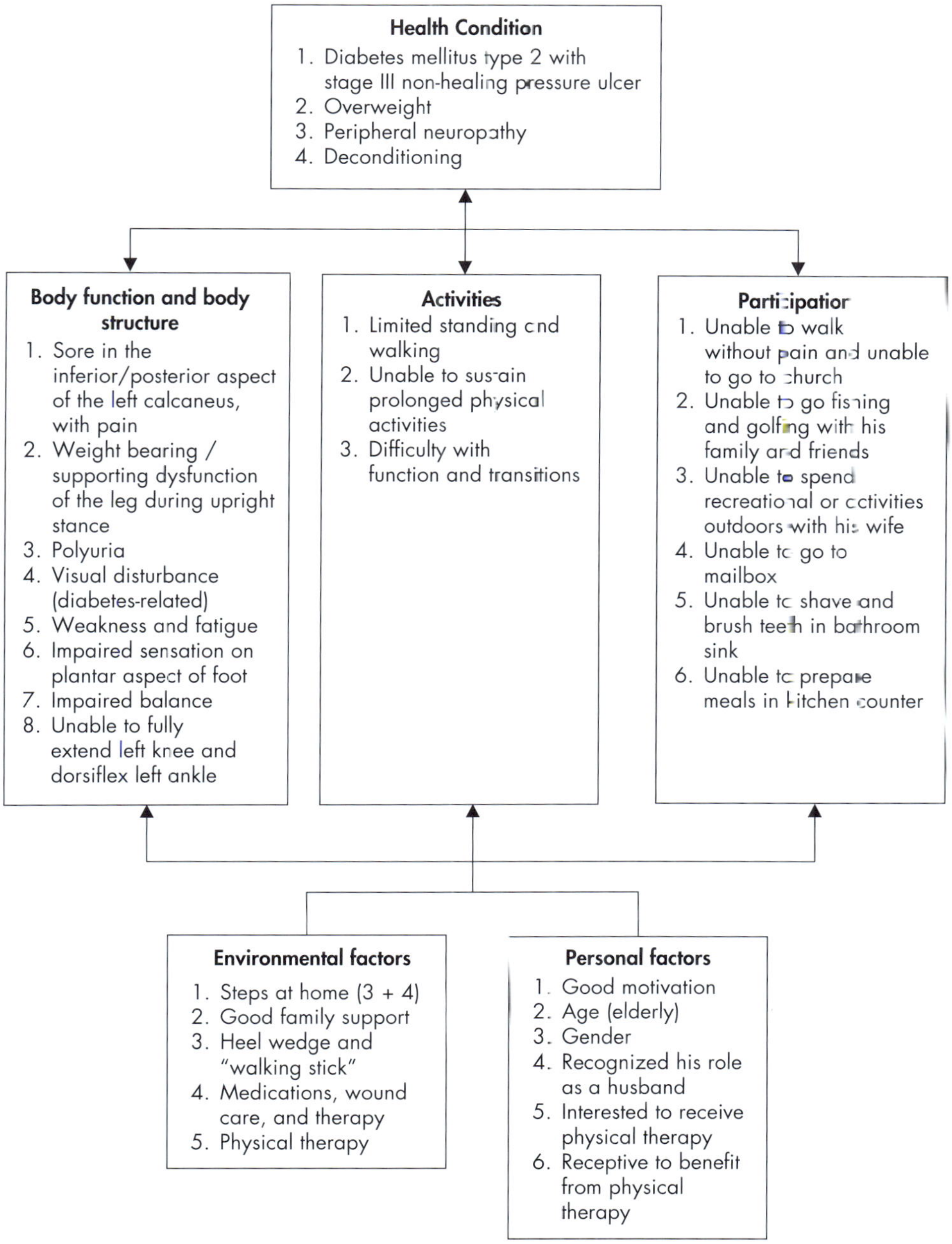

Figure 3-4. Case illustration based on the ICF components.

Figure 3-4 illustrates the application of the ICF in a case format. The main purpose of this figure is simply to convey to the documenting clinician a framework by which the ICF can operate to define "what" needs to be documented in order to generate informed clinical management. Having said that, the clinician can modify "how" the ICF could be applied depending on the documentation and payment requirement of the payer. Because the ICF is universal on the basis of the WHO,[8] specific adaptations made should not be a major problem, but would rather create a great impression to the payers of the clinician's effort to document their patient's level of functioning.

By addressing all four elements of the disablement model, the PT should be able to appropriately address patient needs and problems, regardless of the format the PT selects to enter the information (i.e., SOAP or narrative). The functional goals of the episode of care should be based on resolution or management of the impairments as they relate to function, decrease or eliminate functional limitations, and decrease or eliminate disabilities. The record should not, however, ever reflect concentration on physiologic impairment or resolution of impairments, unless a clear relationship is established between the impairment and its impact on functional improvement. Patient problems can be summarized in the initial examination or evaluation by using the classification headings, which better articulate the treatment goal. *If specifics have already been stated in the body of the document,* deficits can be summarized as presented in below Example.

Example

Impairments	Functional limitations	Disabilities
• Limited bilateral knee flexion 30°/135°	• Unable to climb stairs in home • Unable to sit at table or desk • Unable to squat	• Unable to work as a truck driver

This is characteristic of the functional reporting model. With an appropriate form of development and organization, goals and anticipated dates can be added as columns to clearly relate impairments to functional limitations and disabilities, as well as to specific categories of interventions.

Another application of the disablement model as a tool to facilitate critical thinking and organization of record content is the CDMM (see Chapter 10). The CDMM helps the therapist organize the patient management process from initial visit through discharge, using the same documentation process throughout. Recording of the information gained by history and interview and various tests and measures should assist in filtering the data for relevance to physical therapy management. Clearly documenting problem summaries and setting realistic functional goals should result in a well-constructed initial evaluation document.

The *Guide to Physical Therapist Practice*[7] suggests six components for patient management that lead to "optimal outcomes":

Diagnosis
↕
Evaluation
↕
Examination
↕
Prognosis
↕
Intervention
↕
Outcomes

The specific elements in the six components can be correlated to the categories of information that should be included in the written record, as follows.

Diagnosis

Based on the examination results and clinical judgment, the therapist determines the physical therapy diagnosis or problem and correlates it with the appropriate functional ICD-10 code. The initial examination or evaluation should also include the physician's referring diagnosis. However, the therapist should be aware of medical diagnoses that absolutely do not match actual treatment diagnoses, as they will interfere with payment, as shown in below Example.

Example

Medical diagnosis: Fractured humerus	ICD-10: S42.296B Diagnosis Code – Other non-displaced fracture of upper end of unspecified humerus, initial encounter for open fracture

This may be sufficient if the referral was for treatment of the healing humerus or the individual had become dependent in terms of self-care. However, if the referral was because the patient had lost gait functionality because of prior walker use, then the physical therapy diagnosis or problem should be different, as given in below Example.

Example

PT diagnosis: Gait abnormality	ICD-10: R26.1 Diagnosis Code – Paralytic gait

A diagnosis that does not match the problems, interventions, or goals identified will result in denial of the claim.

Generally, an acute medical event, such as the onset of a cerebrovascular accident (CVA), fracture, multiple trauma or multisystem illness, or presence of comorbidities or complex medical condition will justify, with appropriate documentation, skilled physical therapy. However, the addition of functionally oriented diagnoses such as hemiplegia, cerebral ataxia, gait abnormality (Paralytic or ataxic) will better support the need for therapy intervention.

Examination

Information and data obtained during the examination process (tests and measures) lead the therapist to clinical judgments, including appropriate systems, screening, and more specific tests and measures to determine the patient needs. The specific tests and measures are usually categorized on a "form" entitled "PT Evaluation" with varying formats.

Evaluation

Based on information and data collected in the initial examination, the PT makes clinical judgments regarding patient care, including identification of the physical therapy problems or diagnosis(es) and potential need for consultation or referral. According to the APTA *Guidelines for Documentation,* this stage is called the initial examination and evaluation/consultation. In total, this entry should answer the following questions:

1. Who is the patient?

   Demographics, medical history, social history, prior or concurrent services (avoid duplication), onset
2. Where is the patient functionally?

   Causative impairments, functional limitations, disabilities
3. What is/are the primary problems the patient has?

System tests and measures, impairments, medical/social/psychological problems that may affect care

4. What is the applicable physical therapy diagnosis?

   The primary problem that will be addressed correlated to the appropriate ICD-10 code

5. Can the problems be affected by physical therapy intervention?

   Identification of effective and efficient intervention for the problem(s) as determined by the PT and consistent with patient's and family's perceptions and needs

6. If yes, which will be addressed during this episode of care?

   Identification of the problem(s) that will be addressed in the plan of care

7. If no, what will the disposition be?

   If not accepting the individual for care, identify reason: lack of expertise in area of problem, has other problems that need referral in addition to those for physical therapy, problems identified are not within scope of physical therapy

8. What is the level of severity of this case?

9. Is evidence-based care provided? (Medicare and other payers may have slightly different requirements. Please always check payer policy.)

According to to the Medicare Benefit Policy Manual Chapter 15 Section 220.3, the PT must document the following elements of patient care:

- Medical diagnosis
- Treatment impairment or dysfunction
- Subjective observation
- Objective observation (e.g., identified impairments, severity or complexity of patient , results from a measurement functional instrument (If instrument not included, documentation is required to indicate objective, measurable beneficiary physical function))
- Assessment (includes rehabilitation potential)
- Plan (information pertinent to the plan of care)

Prognosis

According to the *Guide to Physical Therapy Practice,*[7] the prognosis is included in the initial examination/evaluation document, including the plan of care (interventions), goals or level of function anticipated as a result of the therapeutic intervention, and frequency and duration of treatment. Contents for the plan of care are outlined by CMS for Medicare beneficiaries. However, they can be applied to all settings and carriers. The prognosis also includes the individual's rehabilitation potential, which is relevant to the physical therapy goals and prior level of function. If an individual is accepted for care, the rehabilitation potential should be at a minimum good, as it is based on the goals established. "Excellent" may appear to indicate to the reader that the individual may not need services. If the PT chooses "fair," it may be acceptable, assuming the patient is too ill to make any other determination at the time.

Intervention

These are the specific skilled physical therapy treatments and methods used to affect the patient's problems. Treatments should be described with terminology that matches the Current Procedural Terminology (CPT) system, developed by the American Medical Association (AMA) or Healthcare Common Procedure Coding System (HCPCS). All of these achieve goals established by the PT in conjunction with the patient. The interventions must match specific problems identified in the initial exam or re-exam (with goals modified as indicated) and specific goals.

Outcomes Assessment

This phase of treatment occurs when the results of the interventions or treatments are evaluated. The *Guide to Physical Therapy Practice*[7] includes the re-examination of the patient to determine if changes or modifications are needed in the interventions. If the patient is not demonstrating progress toward the desired outcomes or achieving the anticipated results from the interventions or treatment at any point in time, re-evaluation of treatment options is necessary. Possible adjustments in treatment include changing the intervention and determining a change in medical status necessitating referral back to the physician or initial referral in states with direct access. The outcome or progress level during care must be clearly indicated in the documentation. If some or all of the goals are not achieved, the reasons for lack of accomplishment must be included. These outcomes must also reflect back to the initial goals and modifications during the episode of care.

The *APTA Physical Therapy Outcomes Registry*[10] is a qualified clinical data registry (QCDR). This *Physical Therapy Outcomes Registry* allows for:

- Benchmark outcomes—without additional data entry
- Optimize your practice with insights from easy-to-use dashboards
- Empower PTs to provide the most effective patient care
- Market your practice to referring physicians, payers, patients, and employers
- Maximize payment from private payers with outcomes data

With healthcare moving to outcomes-based payment, PTs need to understand how they perform, identify areas to improve quality, and manage patient populations.[10]

SUMMARY

There are three basic formats for client record organization: the SOMR, POMR, and integrated systems. Of the three, the SOMR—the system that divides the record by service or discipline—is the most common. Each service, however, may choose within the SOMR to make their entries in the "model" of their choice. The most common entry formats for physical therapy are a SOAP and narrative for ongoing entries, with flowsheets and checklists for intervention parameters. A variety of customized formats, often self-designed, are used for initial examination/evaluation and discharge summaries and disposition.

In the *Guide to Physical Therapist Practice,*[7] the APTA used to support the Nagi disablement model to help organize patient care and the documentation. In the model, information is divided into pathology, impairment, functional limitation, and disability. The *Guide to Physical Therapist Practice*[7] identifies six elements that must be included in the record: the physical therapy diagnosis or problem (as well as the medical diagnosis, as applicable), examination, evaluation, prognosis, intervention (continuation of care), and outcomes assessment (summation of episode of care). Application of the concepts presented in the *Guide to Physical Therapist Practice*[7] and the CDMM can assist the PT in completing appropriate documentation.

With the APTA's endorsement of the ICF/WHO, the *Guide to Physical Therapist Practice,*[7] along with other documentation efforts in physical therapy practice, now reflect the ICF. The ICF shares a common interface with the *Guide to Physical Therapist Practice*[7] and the CDMM, and hence the ICF was meant to be complementary. Whereas the ICF defines "what" to measure, the *Guide to Physical Therapist Practice*[7] can provide ways and means on "how" to operationalize the ICF components in practice.

The recognition and understanding of enablement models, particularly the ICF, would be helpful in daily documentation within the context of CMS guidelines and private insurers in terms of guidance toward standard formats for documentation and payment. Another importance of enablement models is in the standardization of the contents of documentation, enhancing the ability of the clinician to track treatment outcomes. Electronic Medical Records (EMRs) used for documentation may be custom designed or have standardized formats. They may include drop down built in menus or items or allow original narrative. All however, must facilitate inclusion of common elements and skilled content.

REVIEW QUESTIONS

1. What are the basic types of medical record organization? Compare and contrast these types.
2. Explain what goes in each section of the SOAP formatted note. What is the difference between the SOAP and SOAPIER?

3. Give examples of three types of individual entry formats. Compare and contrast each format.
4. What is your opinion regarding the popularity of the SOAP format?
5. What is a clinical tool and its relevance to documentation? Give two examples.
6. Why is it not prudent to use a checklist or flowsheet without additional narrative or written entries?
7. What are the different models being used in physical therapy practice?
8. Explain what a disablement model is. Which model is used by the APTA in the *Guide to Physical Therapist Practice?*
9. What is the ICF? What are the different components of the ICF?
10. Give your own example entry for each of the ICF components.
11. Explain the categories in the disablement model employed in the *Guide to Physical Therapist Practice.* Include examples for each category.
12. Give an example of an impairment, the resulting functional problem, and possible disability.
13. Compare and contrast the medical diagnosis and the physical therapy diagnosis (physical therapy problem).
14. What is the difference between the initial examination and the evaluation?
15. How can the ICF help in patient evaluation and tracking patient progress?
16. How do you determine the level of severity for the patient?

REFERENCES

1. Weed LL. Medical records that guide and teach. *N Engl J Med.* 1968; 278:11, 593-600, 652-657. doi:10.1056/NEJM196803142781105.
2. Weed LL. *Medical Records, Medical Education, and Patient Core: The Problem Oriented Medical Record as a Basic Tool.* Cleveland, OH: Case Western Reserve Press; 1969.
3. Abeln S, Stewart D. *Documenting Functional Outcomes in Physical Therapy.* St. Louis, MO: Mosby-Year Book; 1993. ISBN-10:0801663598.
4. *APTA's Outpatient Physical Therapy Improvement in Movement Assessment Log* (OPTIMAL1.1). Alexandria, VA: American Physical Therapy Association. Available at https://www.sralab.org/sites/default/files/2017-07/OPTIMAL_BaselineForm.pdf. Accessed August 10, 2020.
5. *Uniform Data System for Medical Rehabilitation,* 270 Northpointe Parkway, Suite3 00, Amherst, NY 14228. email: info@udsmr.org. Available at http://www.udsmr.org. Accessed August 10, 2020.
6. *Focus on Therapeutic Outcomes,* Inc. Available at www.foto-inc.com. Accessed August 10, 2020.
7. *Guide to Physical Therapist Practice*, 3.0. Alexandria, VA: American Physical Therapy Association. Available at http://guidetoptpractice.apta.org/. Accessed August 10, 2020.
8. World Health Organization. Available at www.who.int/en. Accessed August 10, 2020.
9. *Medicare Benefit Policy Manual Chapter 15 – Covered Medical and Other Health Services.* Centers for Medicare & Medicaid Services. Available at https://www.cms.gov/Regulations-and-Guidance/Guidance/Manuals/downloads/bp102c15.pdf. Accessed August 15, 2020.
10. *APTA Physical Therapy Outcomes Registry.* Alexandria,VA: American Physical Therapy Association. Available at http://www.ptoutcomes.com/home.aspx. Accessed August 10, 2020.

ADDITIONAL REFERENCE

International Classification of Functioning, Disability and Health (ICF). National Centers for Health Statistics. Centers for Disease Control and Prevention. Available at https://www.cdc.gov/nchs/icd/icf.htm. Accessed August 10, 2020.

4 The Electronic Medical Record*

Stephen M. Levine† and Helene M. Fearon

OBJECTIVES

Following completion of this chapter, the reader will be able to:

- Explain the history of electronic medical record (EMR) development leading up to the current mandate for transitioning to an EMR.
- Explain the concept of "meaningful use" in regards to EMR adoption.
- Explain the difference between an electronic medical record and electronic health record.
- Compare and contrast the benefits of point of care use of EMR versus workstations or documenting outside the patient visit.
- Discuss the three primary considerations when considering software for the electronic medical record.
- Analyze the relationship between an EMR system and evidence-based practice.

Author's Note

The terms electronic health record (EHR) and electronic medical record (EMR) are often used interchangeably, although they are different. While the EMR is used by clinicians and staff within one healthcare organization, the EHR conforms to nationally recognized interoperability standards and can be created, managed, and consulted by authorized clinicians and staff across more than one healthcare organization. For purposes of this chapter, the term EMR will be used, but should be recognized to include EHR as well.

Edited by Eric Shamus, PT, DPT, PhD, for new edition.

†*This chapter is dedicated to the memory of Stephen M. Levine.*

The implementation and use of electronic medical records (EMR) is one of the highest priorities for healthcare providers, organizations, and government agencies in the United States. An EMR can provide many benefits for providers and their patients and can improve care by enabling functions that paper medical records cannot deliver:

- ***Complete and accurate information.*** An EMR allows the healthcare professional to have the information they need in a timely fashion in order to provide the best possible care, at the best possible time. The ability to access the patient's complete health history before beginning the evaluation and treatment processes affords additional support for the provider's clinical decision-making process, as well as facilitating the patient's involvement in their own healthcare. Use of an EMR has the impact of bringing an individual's complete health information picture into the process of getting appropriate care earlier rather than later. The result of use of this technology is better healthcare decision-making and more coordinated care.
- ***Better access to information.*** EMRs facilitate greater access to the information healthcare providers need to support high-quality and efficient care and improve the health outcomes of their patients. EMRs also allow information to be shared more easily among physician, therapist, and other healthcare provider offices; hospitals; and across health systems, leading to better coordination of care. There are many integrated outcome programs. Physical therapists (PTs) need to be able to use quality measures to articulate the value they bring to the healthcare system, given that in the near future payment for services will depend on quality measure performance.[1]
- ***Patient empowerment.*** Use of EMRs empowers individuals to take a more active role in their health and in the health of others for whom they have responsibility. Patients can receive electronic copies of their medical records and share their health information securely over the Internet with whomever they choose. EMRs can support better follow-up information for patients—for example, after a clinical visit or hospital stay, instructions and information for the patient can be effortlessly provided and reminders for other follow-up care can be sent easily or even automatically to the patient.

DEFINING KEY TERMS

The National Alliance for Health Information Technology (NAHIT) was hired by the Office of National Coordinator of Health Information Technology (ONC) to create key health information technology (IT) definitions. The executive summary of the report explains why defined terms are needed:

> *The ambiguity of meaning created by not having a shared understanding of what these key terms signify becomes an obstacle to progress in health IT adoption when questions about a term's definition and application complicate important policy expectations or directives, contractual matters, and product features. Differences in how a term is used can cause confusion and misunderstanding about what is being purchased, considered in proposed legislation, or included in current applicable policies and regulations.*[2]

The following list is not exhaustive, but meant to provide short definitions of key terms that healthcare providers should understand as health information technology (HIT) literacy is enhanced:

- **Electronic medical record (EMR):** An electronic record of health-related information on an individual that can be created, gathered, managed, and consulted by authorized clinicians and staff *within one healthcare organization.*
- **Electronic health record (EHR):** An electronic record of health-related information on an individual that conforms to nationally recognized interoperability standards and that can be created, managed, and consulted by authorized clinicians and staff *across more than one healthcare organization.*

> *An EMR aligns with the prevailing state of electronic records today (whether the record is branded an EMR or an EHR). However, the movement of the industry is toward electronic records that are capable of using nationally recognized interoperability standards, which is a key defining component of an EHR. With the passage of time, electronic records not capable of exchanging information interoperably will lose their relevance. Thus the term EMR is on course for eventual retirement.*[2]

As noted by ONC in a May 1, 2019, blog, EMRs are "a digital version of the paper charts in the clinician's office.... But the information in EMRs does not travel easily out of the practice." Whereas "EHRs focus on the total health of the patient ... EHRs are designed to reach out beyond the health organization that originally collects and compiles the information."[3]

- **Personal health record (PHR):** An electronic record of health-related information on an individual that conforms to nationally recognized interoperability standards and that can be drawn from multiple sources while being managed, shared, and controlled by the individual.
- **Health information exchange (HIE):** The electronic movement of health-related information among organizations according to nationally recognized standards.
- **Health information organization (HIO):** An organization that oversees and governs the exchange of health-related information among organizations according to nationally recognized standards.
- **Regional health information organization (RHIO):** A health information organization that brings together healthcare stakeholders within a defined geographic area and governs HIE among them for the purpose of improving health and care in that community.
- **Clinical decision support (CDS):** Consists of programs designed to assist health professionals with decision-making tasks, linking health observations (signs and symptoms) with health knowledge (best practices and current research) to influence choices made by clinicians to improve care (see the section "Determining the Right EMR: Criteria for Consideration" for additional information).
- **Client/server application:** EMRs reside on a hard drive or a server. The client/server application describes the relationship between two computer programs in which one program, the client, makes a service request from another program, the server which fulfills the request. In this environment, a facility will view and document in a medical record while it resides on the hard drive or server located within that facility or a facility-owned network (see "Determining the Right EMR: Criteria for Consideration" for additional information).
- **Application service provider (ASP):** An ASP is a business that deploys, hosts, and manages access to software applications for multiple parties from a central location that is cloud based. The information is encrypted for privacy and complies with HIPAA. The ASP charges a subscription fee to users of the applications, which are delivered over the Internet or other public or private network. The application software resides on the vendor's system and is accessed by users through a Web browser or by special-purpose client software provided by the vendor (see "Determining the Right EMR: Criteria for Consideration" for additional information).
- **Integrated (end-to-end) EMR:** An integrated practice management and EMR system (often heard discussed as an "end-to-end" system) refers to applications that are developed by the same vendor, share a single database or development platform, and are designed to share complex data between applications.
- **Interoperability:** Provides the ability of software and hardware on multiple pieces of equipment made by different companies or manufacturers to communicate and work together. This need is essential for the sharing of health-related information. An established system must obtain standards to enable systems to exchange information reliably and securely. It also requires critical mass of health IT adoption within the delivery system to create and share health-related information electronically.

THE PUSH TOWARD ELECTRONIC MEDICAL RECORDS:

Understanding the Current Environment

Health Information Technology (HIT) is changing rapidly in the United States. The goal at the federal level is to have EMR systems in use across the country in all provider settings. A 2008 study published in the *New England Journal of Medicine* found that only 4% of doctors nationwide used a fully functioning EMR system, while only an additional 13% said they had a basic system.[4] As of 2017, nearly 9 in 10 (86%) of office-based physicians had adopted any EHR. Nearly 4 in 5 (80%) had adopted a certified EHR (see Figure 4.1).[5]

In 2015 more than 4 in 5 of all nonfederal acute care hospitals had adopted a basic EHR with clinician notes. Ninety-six percent of nonfederal acute care hospitals have possession of an EHR certified by the U.S. Department of Health and Human Services (HHS). This percentage is consistent through 2017 (see Figure 4.2).[6]

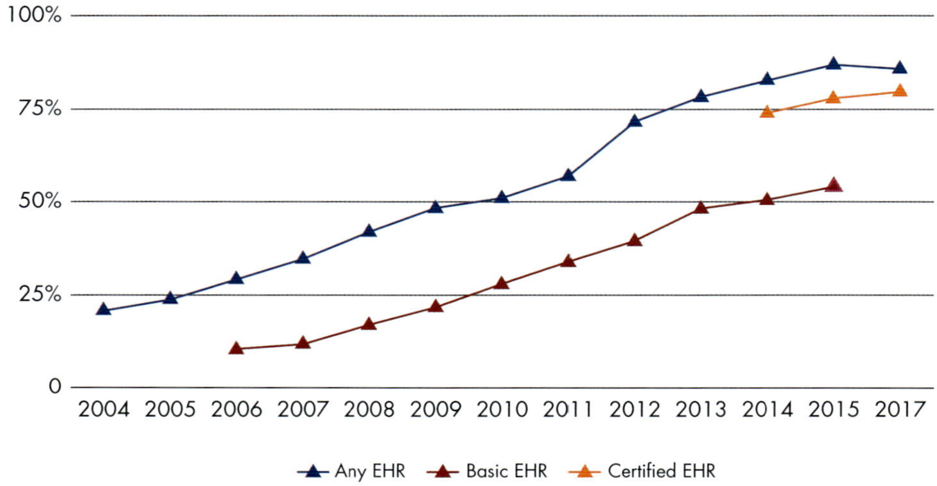

Figure 4-1. Percentage of office-based physicians using any electronic health record (EHR)/electronic medical record (EMR) system and physicians that have a certified EHR/EMR system, by U.S. state: National Electronic Health Records Survey, 2017.[5]

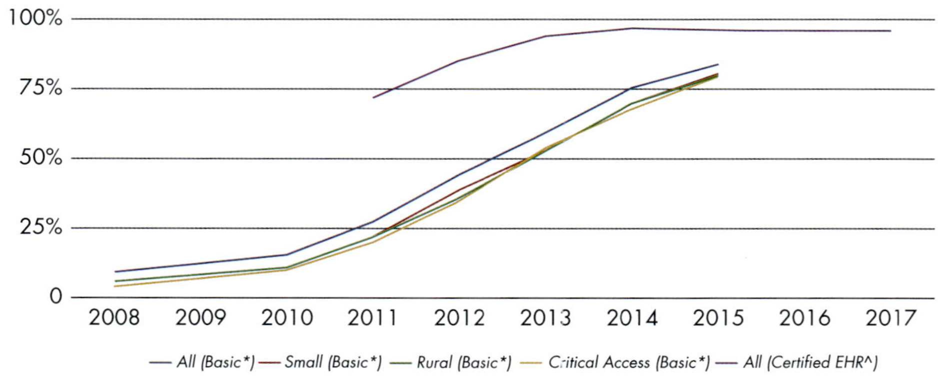

Figure 4-2. 2017 Nonfederal acute care hospital electronic health record adoption. (Reproduced from the Office of the National Coordinator for Health Information Technology. Non-federal Acute Care Hospital Electronic Health Record Adoption, Health IT Quick-Stat #47.[6])

At the current rate of adoption, it is predicted that EMR systems will reach maximum penetration by 2024, 10 years beyond the federal goal.[7] Reasons for lack of adoption are not fully understood, but published studies and articles related to the use of EMRs are increasing significantly.

The idea of an EMR is not new. In 1991, the Institute of Medicine, rebranded as the National Academy of Medicine in 2015, organized a task force that examined issues of medical record systems. In the conclusion of the examination, the IOM reported the computer-based record was an "essential technology for healthcare."[8] In 1997, IOM conducted a follow-up report that identified steady progress toward developing computerized health systems, but noted no system supported all the features of a comprehensive system.

By 2003, the DHHS began promoting widespread use of modern IT. DHHS asked IOM to identify core health delivery–related functionalities, including an EHR functional model. Following the proposal in 2004, the Bush administration made HIT one of the nation's top priorities. DHHS launched the "Decade of Health Information Technology," with goals for EHRs for most Americans in 10 years. An initiative of the DHHS's National Health Information Infrastructure is to "enable regional information sharing throughout the continuum of care by establishing healthcare policies and promoting effective use of data and vocabulary standards."[8]

As the country slowly but steadily has become more aware and accepting of EMRs over the past 20 years, the time was right for the next major step in this initiative. That step occurred when President Obama signed into law the American Recovery and Reinvestment Act of 2009 (ARRA) on February 17, 2009. This law provides for ONC to promote the development of a nationwide interoperable HIT infrastructure:

> *The Office of the National Coordinator for Health Information Technology (ONC) is at the forefront of the administration's health IT efforts and is a resource to the entire health system to support the adoption of health information technology and the promotion of nationwide health information exchange to improve healthcare. ONC is organizationally located within the Office of the Secretary for the U.S. Department of Health and Human Services (HHS).*[9]
>
> *ONC is the principal federal entity charged with coordination of nationwide efforts to implement and use the most advanced health information technology and the electronic exchange of health information. The position of National Coordinator was created in 2004, through an Executive Order, and legislatively mandated in the Health Information Technology for Economic and Clinical Health Act (HITECH Act) of 2009.*[9]

The HIT Policy and Standards Committee, with input from public and private stakeholders (e.g. physicians), established and created recommendations on the HIT policy framework, standards, implementation specifications, and certification criteria for electronic exchange and use of health information. The DHHS goal was to adopt an initial set of standards, implementation specifications, and certification criteria by December 31, 2009.[9]

The ARRA provides financial incentives through the Medicare program to encourage physicians and hospitals to adopt and use *qualified EMRs* in a *meaningful way* (as defined by the Secretary of Health and Human Services). As defined in the legislation, a qualified EMR system is one that "includes patient demographic and clinical health information, such as medical history and problem lists; and has the capacity to:

(i) provide clinical decision support;
(ii) support physician order entry;
(iii) capture and query information relevant to healthcare quality;
(iv) exchange electronic health information with, and integrate such information from other sources."[9]

ONC was authorized to provide competitive grants to states for providers who become early adopters of qualified EMRs. Medicare incentive payments were designed based on an amount equal to 75% of the secretary's estimate of allowable charges. Incentive payments made to users of the qualified EMR are intended to be reduced in subsequent years through 2015.

WHAT IS "MEANINGFUL USE"?

In the context of the EMR incentive programs, demonstrating meaningful use is the key to receiving the incentive payments from the government to assist with the costs associated with transitioning to an EMR. Adopting an EMR means more than using a simple electronic documentation program as a depository of data in a word processor. "Meaningful use" is defined as meeting a series of objectives that make use of EMRs' potential to have an impact on the improvement of quality, efficiency, and patient safety in the healthcare system through the use of certified EHR technology (CEHRT).

Author's Note

According to CMS, "CEHRT gives assurance to purchasers and other users that an EHR system or module offers the necessary technological capability, functionality, and security to help them meet the meaningful use criteria. Certification also helps healthcare providers and patients be confident that the electronic health IT products and systems they use are secure, can maintain data confidentially, and can work with other systems to share information."[10]

On July 13, 2010, Centers for Medicare & Medicaid Services (CMS) published the final rule on "meaningful use" of CEHRT that specified the objectives providers must have achieved in payment years 2011 and 2012 to quality for incentive payments. The final rule:

- Specified initial criteria that eligible professionals, eligible hospitals, and critical access hospitals (CAHs) must meet to demonstrate meaningful use and qualify for incentive payments.
- Included "core" criteria that all providers must meet to qualify for payments, while also allowing provider choice among a "menu set" of additional criteria.
- Outlined a phased approach to implement the requirements for demonstrating meaningful use. This approach initially establishes criteria for meaningful use based on currently available technological capabilities and providers' practice experience. CMS will establish graduated criteria for demonstrating meaningful use through future rulemaking.

At the same time, ONC published a final rule specifying the technical capabilities that EHR technology must have to be certified and to support providers in achieving the "meaningful use" objectives. Specifically, the rule:

- Set initial standards, implementation specifications, and certification criteria for EHR technology under the incentive program.
- Coordinated the standards required of EHR systems with the meaningful use requirements for eligible professionals and hospitals.[11]

With these standards in place, providers could be assured that the CEHRT they adopt is capable of performing the required functions to comply with CMS's meaningful use requirements and other administrative requirements of the Medicare and Medicaid EHR incentive programs.

By focusing on the effective use of EHRs with certain capabilities (note the ONC regulations were focused on aspects of HIT that relate more to an EHR than an EMR), the Health Information Technology for Economic and Clinical Health (HITECH) Act made clear that the adoption of records is not a goal in itself: it is the use of EHRs to achieve health and efficiency goals that matters. HITECH's incentives and assistance programs seek to improve the health of Americans and the performance of their healthcare system through "meaningful use" of EHRs to achieve five healthcare goals:

- to improve the quality, safety, and efficiency of care while reducing disparities;
- to engage patients and families in their care;
- to promote public and population health;
- to improve care coordination;
- to promote the privacy and security of EMRs.

Beginning in 2011, the Medicare and Medicaid EHR Incentive Programs were developed to encourage eligible professionals (EPs) and eligible hospitals and CAHs to adopt, implement, upgrade (AIU), and demonstrate meaningful use of CEHRT. In subsequent years' rulemaking, CMS continued its advancement of CEHRT utilization, focusing on burden reduction and improving interoperability and patient access to health information.

On October 16, 2015, CMS issued a final rule specifying the requirements that EPs, eligible hospitals, and CAHs must meet in order to qualify for Medicare and Medicaid EHR incentive payments and avoid downward payment adjustments under the Medicare EHR Incentive Program. In addition, it changed the Medicare and Medicaid EHR Incentive Programs reporting period in 2015 to a 90-day period aligned with the calendar year. This final rule with comment period also removed reporting requirements on measures that had become redundant, duplicative, or topped out from the Medicare and Medicaid EHR Incentive Programs. In addition, this final rule with comment period established the requirements for Stage 3 of the program as optional in 2017 and required for all participants beginning in 2018. The final rule with comment period continues to encourage the electronic submission of clinical quality measure (CQM) data, establishes requirements to transition the program to a single stage, and aligns reporting for providers in the Medicare and Medicaid EHR Incentive Programs.

Also on October 16, 2015, ONC, through a final rule, finalized a new edition of certification criteria (the 2015 edition health IT certification criteria, or "2015 Edition") and a new 2015 Edition Base EHR definition, while also modifying the ONC Health IT Certification Program to make it open and accessible to more types of HIT and HIT that supports various care and practice settings. The 2015 edition establishes the capabilities and specifies the related standards and implementation specifications that CEHRT would need to include to, at a minimum, support the achievement of meaningful use by EPs, eligible hospitals, and CAHs under the Medicare and Medicaid EHR Incentive Programs when such addition is required for use under these programs.[10]

As required by the Medicare Access and CHIP Reauthorization Act of 2015 (MACRA), the Quality Payment Program (QPP) includes a Merit-based Incentive Payment System (MIPS) performance category that focuses on meaningful use of CEHRT, previously referred to in the CY 2017 and CY 2018 QPP final rules as the "advancing care information" performance category. CMS subsequently changed the name of the performance category to the "Promoting Interoperability" performance category in QPP Year 2.[12] MACRA created the QPP that rewards value and outcomes in one of two ways: MIPS, which is divided into four performance categories (quality, clinical practice improvement activities, meaningful use of CEHRT, and resource use or cost) and Advanced Alternative Payment Models (APMs).

Author's Note

To learn more about the Quality Payment Program, visit www.qpp.cms.gov.[12] APTA also has numerous resources about MIPS and Advanced Alternative Payment Models on its Website.

It is all but inevitable that "meaningful use of CEHRT" will continue to evolve within the boundaries of what is reasonably possible using technology available today. Achieving meaningful use with CEHRT is not an easy task for PTs and other provider types who were ineligible for the financial and technical assistance that was afforded to physicians and hospitals. However, it is something that needs to happen if improvement in patient care is the overriding objective of healthcare reform. The onus will be on the vendors of EMR products to ensure that their products can be "meaningfully used" by the users in line with what is included by CMS in its regulations governing the QPP, as well as any other regulatory requirements.

It is critical for PTs and other nonphysician healthcare professionals, as well as long-term care and post-acute care facilities, to understand the need to effectively implement EMRs that will be consistent with current and government standards and allow for the achievement of the goals of EMR and, ultimately, EHR adoption.

Unfortunately, there are numerous barriers preventing PTs and other nonphysicians from adopting CEHRT for purposes of participation in the Medicare QPP. The ONC certification process has established standards and other criteria for structured data that providers' EHRs must use in order to achieve CEHRT under the QPP. However, CEHRT requirements are designed for prescribing professionals and do not capture tasks performed by nonphysician professionals using different types of EHRs. Consequently, the vast majority of EHR technology developed for use by PTs and other nonphysician providers cannot fully satisfy the technology requirements outlined in 42 CFR 414.1305, therefore hindering these providers' capability to participate in the Promoting Interoperability category of MIPS (and eventually MIPS Value Pathways [MVPs]) or APMs.

To move to a more standardized and interoperable environment; facilitate PTs' and other nonphysicians' participation in MIPS, MVPs, and APMs in the future; and promote increased interoperability and care coordination, the American Physical Therapy Association (APTA) is aggressively advocating to the federal government that it help nonphysician providers, including PTs, adopt and implement CEHRT.

Healthcare providers who are in the process of selecting and implementing EMR software would be advised to include in their contracts that not only the vendor's product would be qualified, but the vendor would incorporate features that will make it possible for them to demonstrate meaningful use of CEHRT. The burden of demonstrating that the system is being put to "meaningful use" is on the provider. However, the vendor for nonphysician healthcare professionals, such as PTs, must make that process easier.

Professional organizations have also weighed in on the adoption of EMRs/EHRs. The American Medical Association (AMA) is committed to EHR adoption that streamlines the clinical and business functions of a physician's office and helps physicians provide high-quality care to patients. The APTA's position with regard to the use of electronic records is favorable: APTA "supports meaningful and standardized data collection by physical therapists through the adoption of interoperable electronic health record (EHR) systems in all practice settings that can advance patient services, improve quality, and demonstrate the value of physical therapist services to patients and clients, payers, policy makers, and the provider community."[13]

Clearly, the current healthcare environment has created a road map to HIT adoption, and APTA, through its highest policy-making body, the House of Delegates, has focused the profession on this goal. However, before making the transition to an EMR, PTs must have a clear understanding of the terminology used in the HIT environment, the benefits, barriers, and pitfalls of adopting EMRs; be aware of the cultural evolution required for successful implementation; understand how best to prepare for this transition; and know what features and criteria should be reviewed before making a decision on what system is right, both for immediately identified needs and for long-term successful implementation and use.

ELECTRONIC DOCUMENTATION: BENEFITS AND BARRIERS

Benefits of Electronic Medical Records

EMRs and HIE can help clinicians provide higher-quality and safer care for their patients. By adopting EMRs in a meaningful way, clinicians can:

- **Know more about their patients**. Information in EMRs can be used to coordinate and improve the quality of patient care.
- **Make better clinical decisions.** With more comprehensive information readily and securely available, clinicians will have the information they need about treatments and conditions—even best practices for patient populations—when making treatment decisions.
- **Save money.** EMRs require an initial investment of time and money. But clinicians who have implemented them have reported reductions in the amount of time spent locating paper files, transcribing, and spending time on the phone with labs or pharmacies; more accurate coding; and reductions in reporting burden.[14,15]

There are many benefits to utilizing an EMR. The most critical reason is the availability and improved access to clinical information. By having one point of entry for patient information in an organization, clinicians have access to all patient information as necessary, including patient demographics, and accurate and complete payment sources. Having complete and reliable patient information immediately available improves communication with the patient concerning their care and allows for better case management, team communication, and decision-making. By improving the quality and readability of documentation, there is also great potential for improved payment. An EMR also provides the ability to streamline business processes by reducing redundant front-office activities by eliminating use of forms and paper in general. Hard-copy medical records take up large amounts of space and have the potential of being misfiled or lost. The storage of discharged EMRs is simpler, cheaper, easier to retrieve, and can be backed up or saved in duplicate on networks or disks.

EMRs have the ability to provide a practical delivery mechanism for clinical practice guidelines, which assist with clinical decision-making. It also allows for a clinician to evaluate and assess valuable sources of data providing new information about quality outcomes and practice styles. EMRs have the ability to track and report consistent, positive, and effective outcomes by entering coded data that facilitates advanced computer-based decision support. This will aid in identifying inconsistencies in utilization of care that compromise quality and will also assist in standardizing care and minimizing quality disparities. The ability to easily identify and report outcomes serves to empower research feedback loops that can help turn American healthcare into a self-improving system, leading to a significant potential to lower overall healthcare costs. The coordination of care that results from effective use of an interoperable EMR improves the availability, timeliness, and accuracy of data. Sharing of patient information among authorized professionals improves as well continuity of care and timeliness of diagnosis and treatment.

An EMR will not only assist with clinical aspects of the practice setting but also provide an enormous benefit to the clerical aspect of a practice. An integrated or end-to-end EMR system has several positive impacts that are detailed in the following section:

Scheduling Component

Assists in decreasing patient and administrative staff time spent in managing appointments, while providing important practice management reports reflecting data related to patient visits (i.e., new patients, returning patients, cancellations, no shows, referral sources, and patterns).

Documentation and Billing Component

Patient demographic data, both administrative and clinical in nature, collected prior to or at the start of care and merged with the clinical documentation completed by the clinician or other appropriate staff provides for more accurate billing of services and fewer opportunities for clinical errors as a result of improved legibility, accuracy, and accessibility of treatment and progress notes, which can reduce the possibilities for insurance denials or misinterpretations of data and may help decrease provider cost per visit and improve revenues. Electronic data will also improve interdepartmental and interprovider communication and increase the ability to have remote access to patient information. In addition, effective EMRs will increase full integration and documentation of clinical information; increase timeliness of patient tracking and follow-up; reduce the time frame of administrative filing, finding, and pulling records; and eliminate lost or damaged paper records.

Data Management Component

Electronic documentation has demonstrated increases in operational efficiency, clinical productivity, and office workflow. Improving workflow has been identified to be a primary motivation for implementing EMR systems.[14] Productivity is a key success factor in any business, including physical therapy, and clinicians who may be required to see a specific number of patients per day and complete all necessary documentation within the framework of their working day will find that after successful transition, EMRs will assist in tracking key indicators that can facilitate identification of trends that would require a call to action to facilitate the effective management of the clinical practice.

A fully implemented EMR may increase revenue due to allowing for a more complete charge capture of services that are provided and efficiently and correctly documented. EMRs assist in decreasing undercoding or up-coding of services, thus avoiding audit paybacks, and will reduce billing errors and turn-around time, as well as staff time spent on data entry. EMRs facilitate claims submission and third-party payment, and importantly, effective systems will assist providers in meeting the compliance requirements of CMS and other third-party payers, thereby reducing the risk of payment denial and reducing duplication of services. Revenue can be enhanced further with an EMR that has the ability to monitor the payment patterns of the payers. This becomes critical, since some third-party payment rates are better than others, and if a facility knows which physicians are referring patients with better insurance payment rates, that facility could improve their net profits without having an effect on productivity by focusing their marketing on those physicians. If a facility knows which insurance companies do not pay well for treatment, marketing of those physicians that refer those patients could be reduced.

Barriers to Adoption of Electronic Medical Records

Given the benefits to implementation and use of an EMR, there are also significant barriers that should be considered and addressed in order to be best prepared for this opportunity. Understanding these barriers, and potential solutions to them, will greatly assist PTs in the successful transition from paper documentation to an EMR. Implementation of an EMR has been demonstrated to follow the 80/20 rule, where 80% of the work of implementation is spent on issues of change management and 20% is spent on technical issues related to the technology itself. The various barriers to EMR implementation can be categorized into four main types: financial barriers, technological barriers, attitudinal and behavioral barriers, and organizational change barriers.[16] Each area also presents with potential solutions for addressing these barriers that should assist the PT in easing the transition process.

Financial Barriers

Typically, the most significant barrier to the adoption of an EMR is the high initial "up-front" costs related to the purchase of hardware and software, installation, interfacing with existing programs, administrative and clinical training, and having adequate and appropriate space to house necessary hardware, such as servers. After the initial cost, there are also ongoing costs associated with technical support, hardware updates, and ongoing maintenance , monthly cloud subscriptions and potential individual user access costs. There is also often an underdeveloped business case made to support transition, meaning there may be an uncertain return on investment (ROI) and slow financial benefits to the outlay of initial costs. Finally, high initial time costs are also of concern, meaning the time spent with EMR installation, training, and motivating and cheerleading staff can be a drain on staff resources that could otherwise be focused on patient care and other revenue-generating activities.

One of the potential solutions to the financial burden may include considering a modular system that allows for obtaining an EMR system incrementally with smaller up-front investment. This "building" of a full-scale EMR system over time may work if there is no intention to purchase an integrated product. A company or practice may also use a phased implementation approach, purchasing or renting more complex EMR components in a planned manner for a later implementation process or adding hardware (laptop computers, workstations, etc.)

as the number of users or utilization of the software increases. If initial financial outlay is a concern, it is advisable to strongly consider an ASP, which is discussed in more detail later in this chapter. The ASP model reduces specific costs associated with EMRs, specifically software upgrades, server, and other hardware costs, to decrease the initial costs in the areas of hardware and maintenance. It is important to recognize that ROI cost is not instant, since cost savings are realized in the medium to long term and are also associated with elimination of paper charts, encounter forms, integration of referrals, decrease in data entry and transcription, and improvement in claim capture. EMRs also have the potential to increase the "bottom-line" annual financial ROI through increasing billing revenue with more complete capture of services provided. An EMR should facilitate a decrease in coding and billing errors and improve the turn-around time of a claim's eventual payment.

Another impact of successful adoption should be reduced staff time performing data entry, decreased patient and administrative staff time making appointments and filing activities related to paper charts, and a decrease in staff turnover due to efficiency gains with an EMR that are not present with handwritten processes. Research also shows that EMRs have the potential to save provider time in the long run by enhancing clinical processes and workflow practice efficiency; improving the clinicians' ability to make sound clinical decisions in a timely manner; decreasing provider documentation and dictation time by using templates with documentation prompts; increasing timeliness of patient tracking and follow-up; increasing full integration and documentation of clinical records; and improving the legibility, accuracy, and accessibility of documentation, leading to reduced denials on medical review. Clear data exists that demonstrate net financial benefits from successful implementation of EMRs, with some studies citing between $20,000 and $86,400 per physician/healthcare provider over a 5-year period, and others recovering up to 11.9% of net patient service revenue attributed to excessive administrative complexity costs, which are typically eliminated after successful EMR adoption.[14,15]

Technological Barriers

Technological barriers include inadequate technical support, inadequate data exchange and fragmentation, inadequate Internet connectivity, issues of customization, security and privacy issues, usability issues, and the current lack of interoperability standards incorporated into EMR programs. Regarding technical support, often there is considerable time spent obtaining support from various software, hardware, networking, backup, and service vendors and limited clinician knowledge of technical troubleshooting. Insufficient equipment or equipment inadequacy may cause a problem due to limited access to workstations, older hardware, and lack of adequate backup and storage limitations. Internet connectivity that is inadequate or inconsistent can slow down and/or decrease the efficiency of the system. The lack of ability to customize EMR systems to fit specific office needs, including diagnosis-specific forms and documentation shortcuts, can also present barriers. Concerns for privacy, confidentiality, and security of EMR and Internet-based communication can also pose barriers to the implementation and use of an EMR. A system may have inadequate data exchange or data fragmentation and lack interoperability. EMR systems require standards to be met in areas related to content, information capture and representation, quality assurance, and clinical decision support. Any deficit in these standards produces a risk for a technological barrier. "Usability," or the ease with which healthcare providers can employ the EMR technology in order to achieve the goal related to this transition, is one of the major factors hindering widespread adoption of EMRs.[16] Usability has a strong, often direct, relationship with clinical productivity, error rate, user fatigue, and user satisfaction—critical factors for EMR adoption. Clinicians lose productivity during the training days and potentially for months afterward as they adapt to the new tools and workflow.

In order to limit some of the technological barriers, it is important to arrange for comprehensive technical and process support. Technical support is a critical component of successful EMR implementation, and comprehensive technical support from vendors needs to be included in contract negotiations (see "Training and Support"). This is often overlooked or eliminated from contracts by the provider due to cost concerns; however, doing so is generally short sighted. Major EMR advocacy groups such as the Healthcare Information and Management Systems Society (HIMSS) (www.himss.org), professional organizations, vendors, and major healthcare organizations are developing IT systems that adequately communicate and exchange healthcare data. Data-producing organizations are increasingly using data standards such as HL7, which is an abbreviation for **Health Level Seven**, a standard for exchanging information between medical applications that defines a format for the transmission of health-related information. With regard to customization concerns, when purchasing or renting an EMR system, make sure the contract has adequate terms for the provision of complementary changes and adequate support to customize the EMR system to meet the needs, including the management of data, of your particular practice (see "Customization Ability").

Privacy, confidentiality, and security concerns are mitigated by the fact that all data exchanged between EMR servers must be encrypted to protect confidentiality and must comply with the privacy and security requirements promulgated within the Health Insurance Portability and Accountably Act (HIPAA). It is critical that vendors implement administrative, physical, and technical safeguards to maintain data confidentiality, integrity, and availability. Typically, vendors are well aware of these requirements, and these safeguards are built into systems. Providers should verify this compliance with any EMR vendor with whom they are considering contracting. However, often providers, in an attempt to develop shortcuts in practice, may not use these protection systems and therefore even though the EMR offers these protections, confidentiality and privacy can be breached easily. One such shortcut is not logging out of the program after each use so that anyone can access the data from the same computer, or providers that use the same login information for each provider or employee (often the login of the practice owner or department manager). Both of these situations should be avoided!

Attitudinal and Behavioral Barriers

Resistance to change is cited repeatedly in the literature as the primary barrier to successful implementation of an EMR. This and other attitudinal and behavioral barriers of office staff and clinicians generally focus on the concern about how IT systems will change the delivery of care and relationships between and among providers and patients. Staff may have an aversion to clinical applications of technology and a belief that use of EMRs will decrease clinical productivity and affect financial payment. Attaining technical competency can develop into a barrier if the providers are uncomfortable with computers or use of technology in necessary communications. Also, electronically inputting information may initially take practitioners more time than writing or dictating, especially if current handwritten notes are substandard.

The lack of clear leadership in transitioning to an EMR is also a major behavioral barrier. The lack of leadership may cause staff to build a resistance to change, and even have an underlying fear of job loss. Some clinicians, due to a lack of understanding of the technology, may see the clinical decision support tools provided in more sophisticated EMR solutions as a "cookbook" approach to treatment, causing a perception that the healthcare provider will lose individuality or choice. There are also varying ranges of acceptance, technological access, and computer literacy among patients and healthcare consumers, who may also have concerns about access, content, and dissemination of private information.

The initial disruption of a facility's or practice's administrative and clinical services workflow associated with the introduction of new IT systems and how to align these systems into this workflow often is met with significant resistance, as there is clearly an initial disruption in some financial, clinical, and organizational processes in moving to a paperless system. And finally, the lack of financial incentives available to PTs for implementation of EMR systems from the government may cause therapists to avoid "biting the bullet" and planning now for such a transition.

The appropriate use and implementation of an EMR system can overcome these attitudinal and behavioral barriers and create solutions for moving forward with efficiency and effectiveness. An effective EMR system can increase provider–patient communication abilities and improve patient satisfaction and patient self-care abilities, according to several studies.[8]

Examples of these communications that could save time and enhance provider effectiveness are the use of e-mail messaging rather than phone calls, allowing for a better identification of patient needs. Interoffice electronic communication can increase communication and coordination between healthcare providers and support staff. Coordination of care is affected by improving the availability, timeliness, and accuracy of messages among healthcare providers; the sharing of patient information among authorized professionals; and the continuity of care and timeliness of diagnosis and treatment.

Additionally, concerns about technical competency are in decline, further reducing attitudinal barriers. Provider and consumer attitudes toward the use of technology and EMRs have progressed in a positive direction dramatically over the years, keeping pace with legislative initiatives and advances in the area.

In 2014, Rutten et al. researched patient perceptions of use of EMRs and ratings of care quality.[17] Rutten et al. found that EMR use was significantly more frequent by females; younger age groups; non-Hispanic whites; and those with higher education, higher incomes, health insurance, and a usual source of healthcare.[17] Rutten et al. also found that physician use of the EMR had significantly higher ratings of quality of care.[17]

The Pew Research Center examined technology use among seniors (age 65 and up).[18] In 2016, 67% of seniors use the Internet and 4 in 10 seniors were smart phone owners. This is in comparison to 2013 when 2 in 10 seniors were smart phone users. Smart phone ownership was highly correlated with household income and education.[18]

It is important to identify an "EMR champion," or a practice should not attempt to implement a transition at all. One of the best predictors of success in the transition of using an EMR is leadership by a designated individual in the user community.[19] EMR implementation requires the commitment of an individual who effectively creates and communicates a shared vision, empowers staff to act on the vision, plans short-term "wins," and embraces an IT culture for continuous quality improvement. Simply put, it is essential to identify a person to be the EMR advocate in the practice or facility, and it is important to know that it is often not the practice owner who best meets this responsibility!

Organizational Change Barriers

The final barriers to adopting an EMR are those related to organizational change. The concern that technology may interfere with the therapist–patient communication and relationship is often cited as a primary concern. Migration from paper to a paperless system can be difficult if the process is not appropriately planned. Workflow redesign can be difficult, particularly in gaining consensus in regard to the various aspects of the workflow in the facility or practice. Customization and standardization can be challenging and take time in order to be effective. Resource allocations and responsibilities are likely to change, and process issues are exposed, which can cause hard feelings among staff. There will also be, without a doubt, temporary reductions in productivity due to training in new tools and an uncertainty about the types of training and skills needed to adopt IT systems for healthcare quality.

In attempting to mitigate these barriers, understand that the use of therapist–patient e-mail communications may optimize face-to-face interactions and has the potential to increase patient satisfaction and patient self-care and compliance. It is important to avoid parallel paper and electronic data entry, as doing so will likely cause frustration, as well as increase the time commitment necessary to effectively transition to a paperless system. To facilitate the transition away from paper, administrative staff can enter information in advance from paper to paperless systems and scan recent reports and transfer past information from paper charts into the new EMR system. If the technology choice does not include adopting an integrated solution, it is important to set up efficient data exchange systems between your practice's scheduling, documentation, and billing software. Efficiencies are maximized when information is entered only once electronically and passed automatically through to the necessary interfaces and processed seamlessly. Organizational change barriers are minimized when there is a well-planned work process redesign to eliminate paper-based clinical processes. And because EMR implementation in a provider's office changes how the practice does almost everything, staff needs adequate training in order to maximize success. These areas will be discussed more fully in the section "Preparing for the Transition to an EMR: Strategic Recommendations for Successful Implementation."

PHYSICAL THERAPIST PRACTICE AND THE EMR: PITFALLS AND KEY POINTS TO CONSIDER

PTs should be aware of the various pitfalls that exist in the current EMR marketplace. The pitfalls described in this section represent some of the most common issues that may inhibit successful implementation of an EMR within a physical therapy clinic or facility, and if understood and addressed in context of the setting, can be avoided.

- **System selected or implemented without understanding documentation requirements**: Documentation is the bane of most therapists' existence, and unfortunately, it is a skill that most therapists have not taken adequate time to develop. In looking for an EMR, therapists tend to search for programs that will allow them to complete a note in a matter of seconds or minutes, and to be sure, there are some programs that allow this to occur. However, choosing a system before understanding the documentation requirements that are consistent with the Standards of Practice, state licensing laws, third-party requirements, and other regulations could result in significant time and money spent on a system that might be fast, but that will not assist the therapist in providing effective, efficient, and compliant documentation consistent with medical necessity or regulatory requirements. Staying current on the documentation requirements for physical therapy practice will ensure that any EMR selected is consistent with those requirements. Shortcuts are nice, but if a therapist ends up having to pay back all of the third-party payment received because the product of their electronic documentation does not pass muster, then the therapist has not done themselves or their patients any good!
- **System developed without adequate clinician input**: Many EMR systems are developed without the knowledgeable input of clinicians who understand best practice and who can provide the necessary information, requirements, and regulatory nuance to the programmers who drive the content into the EMR system. Be sure to look for an EMR program that has had the involvement of PTs, but also be sure those therapists have appropriate credentials and expertise in the rules, regulations, standards, and clinical guidelines governing the practice of physical therapy.
- **Limited practice management options built into system:** Providers have to decide if they will invest in an integrated (or end-to-end) system, which includes scheduling, documentation, billing, and practice management, or focus only on a documentation system in hopes of integrating with the scheduling or billing software already in use (see "Determining the Right EMR: Criteria for Consideration"). The greatest efficiencies are gained with a system that allows for robust practice management capabilities, providing data that will assist in growing and maintaining a healthy business, provide outcomes, and allow for efficient and effective practice management over the entire process of the patient interface.
- **Equating an electronic documentation system (i.e., word processing-based system) to a true EMR/EHR:** If providers do not understand the true benefits of an EMR, they are likely to equate a simple word processing system or a depository of data with the power of an EMR. While word processing systems will assist in creating legible documents and may allow the flexibility of designing or customizing a system to meet specific needs, they typically do not integrate evidence-based practice or assist in improving quality of care by incorporating clinical decision support systems. It is worth the investment in time to understand the development of the system and its ability to incorporate the elements of a true EMR system.
- **Software is not compliant with current rules and regulations:** Providers often believe that an EMR system inherently incorporates third-party rules and regulations into its programming and that using these systems will protect the therapist from deficiencies and

paybacks in the event of an audit. The rules and regulations governing therapy services are complex, and remaining compliant with them takes a considerable effort. Many EMR systems profess to incorporate compliance rules related to documentation, coding, and billing, but the provider needs to ensure that due diligence is performed on these systems to identify and understand the process in which this occurs. Client/server-based systems can have difficulty maintaining compliance due to the significant lag time in providing updated versions of software, whereas ASP products should be able to maintain such compliance much more easily (see "Determining the Right EMR: Criteria for Consideration").

- **Software that was originally designed for different market:** Many EMR products being marketed to physical therapy professionals have actually been designed for the physician or other healthcare provider marketplace, and either therapists customize these EMR products to meet their individual needs or the vendor may retrofit its product for the therapy marketplace. This approach makes compliance with professional standards and rules and regulations pertaining to physical therapy services difficult and often creates significant barriers to successful EMR adoption.
- **Lack of due diligence in evaluating systems and vendors:** Making the decision to purchase an EMR based on word-of-mouth recommendations, the amount of users, or aggressive sales techniques without performing adequate due diligence will likely lead to a difficult transition and possibly even a mismatch between expectations and what is delivered as an outcome of using the program. Take the time to have staff use the program with real patients in order to make the most appropriate decision. A large majority of vendors recognize that allowing a practice, facility, or therapist to try the system before committing to purchasing or leasing the system can only assist in the successful outcome. Finally, be sure to check references of those who have been using the software!
- **Lack of inclusion of key staff in decision-making process:** Obtaining "buy-in" from the key staff is critical in contributing to a successful transition to an EMR. Staff will be the ones using the system and learning how to incorporate it into their daily routine. Make sure to include them in the marketplace assessment, if not for each product reviewed, at least for the two to three that are identified as top choices. Bringing the staff into the process early on, so that they are part of the decision-making process, has been shown to be important in a successful transition.[20]
- **Having tunnel vision during the process:** Many choices will need to be made in selecting the right EMR, and often choices are made based on biases before even beginning to explore the potential options available. For example, some clinicians feel strongly that they want to use a client/server system so that they maintain their data on a local hard drive and will not even entertain the idea of an ASP model for fear of not having access to their data when and where they want it. In actuality, ASP systems can offer more security than a typical server-based system, in that backup and redundancy systems are in place to ensure secure access to your data from any Internet-compatible computer, and they generally can meet many other needs that client/server systems can not. The key is to recognize any biases that may exist and set them aside while analyzing various products.
- **Focusing only on immediate needs:** It is all too common for clinicians to focus on their most immediate need in adopting a system—usually this means trying to gain efficiencies so that you can spend less time on documentation and related activities and more time treating patients. While this is certainly an important reason for adopting an EMR, focusing only on this aspect, without also ensuring that professional standards, compliance, audit protection, evidence-based practice guidelines, and clinical decision support systems are also integrated, will likely result in short-term feelings of success. That is until your coding, documentation, medical necessity, or outcomes are questioned by third-party payers, review organizations, or licensing boards.
- **Lack of adequate system training before, during, and after implementation:** Lack of adequate training is one of the biggest obstacles to successful implementation of an EMR. See the section "Training and Support," and ensure that adequate resources are dedicated to this critical area.

- **Lack of anticipation of reduced productivity during initial implementation:** An understandable (and valid) concern regarding EMR adoption is related to decreased practitioner productivity during implementation and its impact on day-to-day operations. It is typical to have productivity decrease during the early stages of implementation, and it is critical to anticipate and plan for this reduction. One study identified that a manager in a large paper-based practice said he expected "2–3 weeks of disastrous inefficiency followed by 4–6 months of relative inefficiency."[2] While implementation of an EMR system typically does not result in this reality, not anticipating and planning for a reduction in productivity can result in a less-than-successful attempt at EMR adoption. Modifying therapist schedules, phasing in implementation, and appropriate scheduling of implementation processes in less busy times will all help to mitigate these productivity losses and allow for an easier transition and achievement of a more productive clinic. The desired result is less time spent on administrative tasks and more on the clinical management of patients.
- **Lack of an understanding of the true purpose and value of an EMR:** If you have gotten this far, you should be recognizing that the value of an effective EMR system is far greater than simply the use of electronic documentation. By understanding and embracing this paradigm change as a health professional in the U.S. healthcare system, along with the evolution of evidence-based care, providers will recognize that a transition to an effective EMR system will change almost everything about a practice. While this process can be stressful, the outcome of taking this step will be demonstrated in the use of an efficient EMR that will not only improve documentation skills, capture clinical services with correct coding, and enhance revenue but will result in an improved quality of care, enhanced outcomes, and greater patient satisfaction.

COMPUTERS AT THE POINT OF CARE: INTRODUCING HEALTH INFORMATION TECHNOLOGY INTO THE THERAPIST–PATIENT RELATIONSHIP

The gains in operational efficiency and use of clinical decision support to affect patient management and outcomes are best recognized when an EMR is used while the therapist is actually interacting with the patient, or at the "point of care." While detrimental effects on provider–patient rapport are often cited as a barrier to implementation of a point-of-care (PoC) EMR system in a busy practice, research has demonstrated that patients did not indicate a sense of loss of rapport with their healthcare providers when an EMR was used during their outpatient visit, and in fact in-room computing appeared to have positive effects on provider–patient interactions and care experience.[21-23]

Author's Note

It is important to focus on the patient and not the computer screen. Depending on the patient's culture, eye contact may or may not be desired.

Communication skills and information processing are the cornerstones of achieving quality in healthcare. Computers play a pivotal role in information management for many industries, in that their ability to store, correlate, and retrieve enormous quantities of information quickly and accurately makes them ideally suited to manage voluminous amounts of information.[22] However, computers potentially alter the traditional manner that therapists, physicians, and other healthcare providers use to communicate with patients. Treatment-room computers can add complexity to the organization and flow of the visit by increasing the amount of clinical information (mental tasks) or introducing additional physical tasks, which has the potential to shift the clinician's attention and involvement away from the patient to the keyboard and monitor. Effective use of computers in the outpatient treatment room are often dependent upon clinicians' baseline skills that are carried forward and are amplified, positively or negatively, in their effects on clinician–patient communications.[23] For those with greater visit organization skills, the presence of a computer provides a new tool to help organize relevant clinical data as well as visit tasks. For those with poorer organization skills, the presence of computers can multiply the sense of disorganization of the visit and can extend its length. Frankel et al.[23] demonstrated that clinicians who integrated data gathering (interview) and data recording (written chart entry) activities into their conversations with patients prior to implementation of an EMR were able to seamlessly integrate the computer into their visits, both initially and at 6 months following implementation of an EMR.[23]

Clinicians' comfort with, and ability to navigate an electronic device influences whether its use during a visit facilitates or impedes communication. Typing abilities and organization of information efficiently affect overall communication with the patient. The ability to use an EMR to effectively recall and share data or information on patient status or progress (often using visually appealing graphs or charts) will typically enhance clinician–patient communication. Effective use of computers should appear seamless and natural.

Some factors and barriers to communication include nonverbal behavior, computer navigation, mastery of skills, and spatial organization. The visual and cognitive attention required for a clinician to enter and retrieve data while maintaining the flow of the visit can be complex. There are three key ways by which clinicians can maintain communication with patients during computer use. The first is verbally, by maintaining a conversation when looking at a computer screen or typing. The second is visually, by making eye contact with the patient intermittently during computer use. The literature demonstrates that maintaining or re-establishing eye contact at least every 15 seconds or when talking to a patient provides the necessary connection with the patient.[23] The third key way is postural, where the clinician positions his or her head or torso toward the patient rather than having their back to the patient during computer use. Studies show that clinicians who are able to use frequent eye contact, proper bodily orientation, and vocalization are able to stay connected to their patients as they use a computer.[23]

Physical configuration of the computer, the monitor, treatment table, and clinician's chair can make communication more or less challenging. Computer location should easily permit the clinician to alternate attention between the computer monitor while simultaneously entering information and positioning the monitor in such a way that allows sharing of the information on the monitor with patients, which will enhance communication and understanding by the patient.[21,23]

Longitudinal studies have been published on the impact of treatment room computing on physician–patient interactions. Gadd and Penrod reviewed overall visit satisfaction, satisfaction with the physician's level of familiarity, and communication about medical issues and degree of comprehension with decisions made during the visit, which all increased with PoC EMR use.[24] Gadd and Penrod showed a significant increase in the level of overall patient satisfaction during the visit after introduction of the computer into the treatment room in the seventh month after introduction as compared to baseline. Moreover, there was no significant drop in overall satisfaction immediately after computer introduction.[24]

The use of computers resulted in the patients' perceptions that physicians were more familiar with them as persons and with their medical history.[21] There was an increased satisfaction with a level of communication about their medical care, including the explanation of diagnosis and treatment, the patient's participation in the decision-making process, and focus on prevention of illness and promoting good health. Further, patient satisfaction is not significantly different after introduction of the computer in the areas of the personal manner of interaction with the physician, the perception of physician's concern for their emotional and physical well-being, and how carefully their physician listened to them. Garrison et al. revealed that a majority of patients in family medicine clinics believe that computer use has a positive effect on the overall quality of care at the visit.[22] All areas of review demonstrated that patient satisfaction improved significantly over baseline levels by 7 months after implementation of an EMR. Few studies have found that introducing computers into treatment rooms had an adverse effect on physician–patient communications. However, it is important to understand that there are differences between the effects of providers learning to use computers and EMRs in treatment rooms while they are also trying to engage with patients versus the experienced computer user, who is able to more easily integrate the familiar use of computers into treatment rooms during outpatient visits.

Incorporating PoC documentation requires an understanding of the differences in hardware requirements necessary for efficient and effective practice. Applying an EMR at PoC requires a computer be taken into the treatment area with the patient. As a result, the most effective and efficient alternative for electronic documentation that can facilitate PoC documentation includes laptops, personal digital assistants (PDAs), netbooks, iPads, and the like. Some laptops and other devices have touch screen and electronic signature capture capabilities that can improve the speed of documentation and overall productivity. The technology available for PoC EMR use will only continue to improve and as healthcare professionals become more and more comfortable with incorporating technology into the therapist–patient relationship.

Workstations, although still in widespread use, may make the transition to an efficient and effective PoC paradigm more difficult. A workstation is usually a desktop computer that may have a printer attached. Based on the number of users, a kiosk can be set up in a central location where clinicians can document information as time allows. Because the computer is in a central location, clinicians typically have to document their clinical findings, interventions, and other notes on paper while they are with the patient and then enter the information into the computer or wait for access to the kiosk. If a paper record is created before electronic entry, it actually increases documentation time and decreases efficiency. All created papers records; for example, handwritten notes; should be destroyed or stored in accordance with other hard copy records.

Although workstations do not provide for the most efficient use of the clinician's time and may limit productivity, some clinics or facilities may feel more comfortable by "dipping their toe in the water," so to speak, and not investing in hardware for each clinician. Some have installed individual workstations at predetermined "desk" areas. Although this may provide each therapist a station, the lack of portability of the hardware may result in these being located away from the treatment area, which decreases the efficiency because the therapist must be at the station to document. There may also be competition for the work stations, delaying entries.

PREPARING FOR THE TRANSITION TO AN EMR: STRATEGIC RECOMMENDATIONS FOR SUCCESSFUL IMPLEMENTATION

An effective implementation of an EMR changes almost every aspect of a PT's practice. It is therefore critical to recognize that a successful EMR implementation process starts long before the physical deployment of the application on-site. The implementation plan needs to be thought out well before selecting a vendor. Each year, EMR systems are deployed in many healthcare provider practices throughout the country, typically with clear clinical and financial objectives. However, some of these systems are later uninstalled by practices after they have found them to be too costly in terms of lost time, productivity, and revenue. So how does a practice become one of the success stories instead of one of the casualties? The answer does not necessarily lie in choosing the right EMR system, although that is certainly important. Instead, the answer lies in making sure the practice has the kind of culture that is compatible with an EMR initiative—and in laying the groundwork for a successful implementation long before the EMR system is up and running.[25]

Although the shift to an EMR system may be mandated, its primary success or failure will depend upon the readiness of the practice's employees to embrace change, because as process changes go, this will likely be one of the biggest they have ever encountered! Planning strategically to go through this process will provide the best potential for successful transition to an EMR. The following 10 steps provide a basic framework for moving from a paper to a paperless system.

1. **Identify an EMR "champion."**

   One of the best predictors of success in an EMR implementation is clinician leadership. EMR implementation requires the commitment of a therapist leader, a sort of "EMR champion," who creates and communicates a shared vision, empowers staff to act on the vision, plans short-term wins, and embraces an IT culture for quality improvement.[19] Identification of this "champion" is one of the most important decisions that will affect the success of the implementation process, and should typically be a clinician who has the respect of the rest of the staff, and, if it is not the owner of the practice or manager of the rehabilitation department, has a direct line of communication to that person.

2. **Perform a workflow analysis.**

   There is almost always an initial disruption of office workflow associated with the introduction of new IT systems, and knowing how to align these systems into the practitioner workflow is critical for a successful implementation. In addition, there is an initial disruption in some financial, clinical, and organizational processes in moving to a paperless system as well.

   It is important for a practice to conduct a thorough assessment of its current workflow prior to initiating an EMR transition. Not only does this provide the practice with an excellent baseline for assessing its EMR needs, but it also will help to identify and reduce or eliminate any potential bottlenecks that could impede the EMR progress once it is installed or adopted. Just as important, the practice can begin to establish some reasonable expectations for the EMR system. For example, planning to initiate the use of an EMR on a Monday with an expectation that things will run smoothly at 100% productivity by that Friday is not realistic.

   It is prudent to prepare to incorporate an EMR system in your daily office workflow by knowing your patient demographics, staff roles, practice environment, and office processes and work patterns. Begin to analyze the workflow of your office by reviewing current workflow from intake to discharge, taking special care to perform a forensic review of your current processes related to coding, billing, and documentation. This process includes a review of the current roles and functions related to administrative operations as well, identifying who is currently doing what tasks. The greatest efficiency and effectiveness will be gained by matching the required tasks to the talent of specific staff, providing the training necessary to maximize success, and involving your staff in this redesign process. This initial process will allow you to identify areas of deficiency and develop a plan to correct those deficiencies. It is generally best to diagram the workflow process by using flow maps and flowcharts to make it easier to identify waste, bottlenecks, and inefficiencies. Once these have been identified, use small tests of change to find solutions to patient flow problems. This will then allow you to promote implementation of an EMR into an efficient process, rather than incorporating historical inefficiencies into your new workflow.

3. **Determine what data is desired as an output from your EMR system.**

   The workflow analysis should help you to understand the relationship between data collection and information that is produced and utilized. In order to do this, it is important to determine the purpose of data collection and information sharing, such as diagnosis classification, outcomes identification, justification for skilled care, marketing, and adherence to third-party requirements. A clinician must determine what information is important to their practice from a clinical and administrative perspective. It is necessary to determine the target audiences (such as other therapists, physicians, case managers, and third-party payers) and their likely use of information, since each of these stakeholders will want or require different things from the output of your EMR.

   By understanding compliance requirements, it is easier to determine the data to be collected and the method of input of that data in your EMR system. Therapists will often complain that documenting in an EMR system takes much longer than handwriting their documentation, without the understanding that their current documentation skills may not be sufficient, or that their current documentation does not meet professional standards or regulatory requirements. One of the biggest benefits of adopting an EMR system should be the assistance it provides in adhering to compliance requirements, so it is important to recognize current areas of deficiency and use the transition to an EMR to assist in improving compliance literacy. It will also be necessary to determine the most effective interface to efficiently input data into system for your staff and establish what application hardware (workstations, laptops, or handhelds) will be used for documentation.

Vendors will often identify the myriad of reports available in their systems as a reason to consider their product, when in truth there are a handful of reports that will provide you the most valuable data for the successful management of your practice. Be careful not to find yourself buried under piles of data that do not help you to manage your practice at a high level, sometimes referred to as "analysis paralysis." Ensure your EMR system can seamlessly translate your practice's key data elements into meaningful and usable information that will assist you in efficiently understanding the profile of your practice.

4. **Include clinical input into development and decision-making process.**

   Implementing an EMR will likely challenge your current paradigm, and therefore it is important to assess the impact of the pending adoption of an EMR system on the organization itself. This is often best initiated by including the perspectives of therapists who will be using the system in the end. Including key staff in the marketplace analysis and in the review of any system that may potentially be adopted will go a long way in helping staff "buy in" into EMR implementation. However, it is important to remember that gaining consensus from everyone on the final product to adopt may take time, and agreement on any customization and standardization may be a difficult process. This is time well spent as long as the expectations for an outcome from this process are clear to all involved. In some cases, it assists to discuss timelines for decision-making regarding choices related to EMR choices.

5. **Understand the concepts of documentation, medical necessity, and regulatory requirements prior to the decision-making process.**

   Becoming aware of and staying current in professional standards, third-party payment policy, regulatory requirements, and coding and documentation guidelines and requirements are critical, but often-overlooked, components of patient management. Understanding these aspects of a practice will likely help avoid system choices that may not provide the necessary data capture to provide essential alerts related to compliance in these areas. An EMR that takes these areas into consideration should better ensure the efficient support the clinician requires to meet medical necessity requirements as defined by various third-party payers, allowing for a greater focus on patient care with less frustration, or a faulty sense of security related to compliance issues. Unfortunately, there are too many EMR products that do not accurately incorporate appropriate compliance requirements into the coding and documentation software. As a result, the therapist who is unaware of these requirements and has not taken the time to remain current in this critical area may end up submitting false claims to third-party payers.

   Although a thorough discussion of what constitutes a false claim and the potential penalties associated with this is beyond the scope of this chapter, awareness of compliance requirements allows a critical analysis of potential systems prior to purchase commitment. It is strongly recommended that a practice undergo a documentation and coding audit both pre- and post-implementation to establish baseline adherence to professional requirements and ensure a successful transition and implementation to a compliant paperless system.

6. **Determine desired system characteristics.**

   There are many different ways and types of documenting both on paper and in an EMR. On paper, blank sheets may be used to document the various components of the record. Templates as well as fill-in-the-blank forms for specific types of evaluations and treatments and assorted flow sheets and checklists are also used. EMR systems also offer similar characteristics and formats. There are template-driven systems that allow a clinician to fill in the blanks, and there are knowledge-base-driven systems that allow a clinician to document in any way they deem necessary. Knowledge-based systems that integrate clinical decision support will provide a huge advantage in incorporating evidence-based practice, compliance standards, and outcomes ability into a practice, and while data entry may be a bit more structured, the benefits usually far outweigh any downside. And as with paper or manual entry, once an EMR format is adopted, there should be consistency in the utilization and content capture among therapists and within a practice or facility.

7. **Test system performance and usability.**

   Clinicians can easily become frustrated with a poorly performing system. An EMR must meet or exceed user expectations. It is best to plan your implementation in advance and test the product carefully (preferably before making that final purchase) to ensure adequate software and hardware system performance. It is also important to select a system that will support future growth and functionality. Rules and regulations are always changing, and it is important to ensure that these changes can be incorporated into an EMR system timely and completely. Usability is a key factor in a successful implementation, so spend some time testing the system to make sure it is intuitive, makes sense to the clinicians and administrative personnel who will be using it, and matches the flow of patient examination. One of the best ways to do this is by participating in any opportunity for beta testing of a new or developing program. Doing so not only provides the ability to "test drive" the system, but participating in a beta opportunity is an excellent way to contribute to the development of a system and incorporate individual practice processes into a system that may be selected for adoption.

8. **Do not "work around" standards.**

   It is crucial not to "work around" standards that are incorporated into EMR systems. Coded observations and quantitative results are necessary for incorporation of automatic clinical guidelines, driving clinical decision-support systems, and other high-level functions. Ensuring data quality is paramount to achieving the full functionality of an EMR and for providing credible clinical outcomes. If users find themselves creating "work arounds" to meet payer or other stakeholder requirements, the system is not working for you. Adoption of an EMR should also include an acknowledgement that these standards exist and are important and result in a commitment to necessary data capture and adherence to future data standards.

9. **Avoid duplicate processes.**

   It is critical to understand that regardless of the system identified, efficiencies and productivity increases will only be gained if providers avoid parallel paper and electronic data entry. For clinicians, utilizing a PoC process where data is entered directly into the system while the therapist is with the patient is the most efficient system. In addition, during any transition, having administration staff enter information in advance from paper to paperless systems is helpful, so that demographic and health history information is entered in advance of the visit and key reports are scanned into the EMR so that they are easily accessible to the clinician when needed. Ultimately, maximal efficiencies are gained when work processes are redesigned to eliminate paper-based clinical processes and move to an effective paperless system. By setting deadlines for specific paper processes to transition to electronic interfaces, staff can keep track of their own progress in avoiding inefficient duplication of efforts.

10. **Do not skimp on training.**

    Training of staff is often minimized or underestimated. Training is critical to successful software implementation and use. If a facility does not know how to use a software application or what it is capable of doing, they will not receive the full benefits of it. This can lead to eventual dissatisfaction with the application. Levels of training can vary from having to travel for training, on-site training, Web-based training and tutorials, to manuals for self-paced education and training. But regardless, training should be multidimensional, including system navigation, training in new roles and workflows, and training methods to ensure data integrity. Therapists should take full advantage of training available as part of any EMR choice. The next section will provide greater insight into this most important aspect of EMR implementation.

TRAINING AND SUPPORT

The key to successful implementation and use of hardware or software is the type of training and support a facility receives as it transitions to an EMR. Software programs touted as being the most efficient and effective will quickly become ineffective if the end user does not know how to use the application. Typically, software companies usually provide some customer service and technical support for an agreed upon period. Most vendors will offer higher levels or extended coverage for an additional cost, and these costs can be on a per usage, monthly, or annual basis. The skill level of the end users will dictate the level of customer service and support a facility requires. Product and technical support and services should not be neglected or negotiated out of a contract to save money. Most importantly, all training should be reinforced by the facility itself by making sure they utilize a "train the trainer" method with their staff in order to ensure that in the event of staff turnover, remaining staff could train new staff or that system training is procured.

The method of training should be carefully considered and planned to effectively and efficiently meet the needs of the clinic or facility. On-site training is useful because a trainer can see how a facility operates and provide suggestions of how their system can be best implemented into the facility's workflow. However, on-site training can be expensive, even cost prohibitive, if a facility must bring in a trainer every time a facility needs additional training or has a new employee. Self-paced manuals are typically included with the software, but for some providers can also be the least effective method of training. The manuals will always be available as a refresher or for new employees, but will not necessarily provide a facility with helpful hints of how an application can be best implemented in a facility.

Web-based technology has improved dramatically in the last few years, making training through the Internet both informative and extremely useful. There are several options for Web-based training, including self-paced tutorials, recorded Web training, and live Web-based training. Self-paced tutorials and videos are similar to viewing a slide or PowerPoint presentation, guiding you through the application. Recorded Web-based training often provides the user with more useful information, with helpful tips and tricks not always available in a self-paced tutorial. Live Web-based training is a real-time session with a trainer via the Web with the added ability to share computer screens, making training specific to the issues identified. This method provides the end user with live training without the expense and inconvenience of traveling.

As an added benefit, staff training on EMR implementation and office redesign has the potential to increase individual skills, confidence, and familiarity with IT systems. Preparation for actual EMR training can be broken down into three basic steps:[26]

1. **Identify current skill levels of staff:** Employee baseline skill levels and comfort with computers will vary depending upon the age and background of employees. Younger employees most likely have grown up using cell phones, texting, and e-mailing and are extremely comfortable with technology as a part of their daily routines; these are the people you probably need to worry about least! Other employees may come from a generation that is less "tech-savvy," making it imperative that their baseline computer skill level be determined before rolling out an EMR. Many EMR "failures" are really failures of planning on the part of practice owners and administration. No matter what training method or schedule you choose, make sure that those with less computer literacy have learned the basics of PC or Mac applications and Web browsing (for ASP users) before scheduling your training sessions.
2. **Bring everyone up to the necessary skill level:** Determine the core skills that will be needed with the new EMR system. These core skills will be based, in part, on whether an ASP-based system or a client/server one is selected. ASP systems are Web-based, and

more and more people are becoming comfortable with using the Internet. But there are certain basic skills that should not be taken for granted: turning a computer on and off, setting a default printer, following password protocols, and logging on and off properly are small things that can frustrate users if they are not comfortable with these and other basic actions.

3. **Design a training plan for the new EMR:** Whatever method you choose, a training plan will need to be developed based on the skills of particular staff. Start with the basics of the system, then use a building block approach, adding on common tasks that all employees need to use (such as scheduling) followed by increasingly complex functions depending on an employee's particular job tasks. Basic EMR training should incorporate basic terminology, workflow, security, usability, and communications. After a general orientation, it is best to identify some "super users" who will become very proficient with the system and will help train additional staff, particularly new staff that may come on after the initial implementation. These "super users" usually consist of clinicians who championed the new system, but could also include office managers, practice owners, or other key administrative staff. The "train the trainer" strategy has many benefits, including developing in-house "experts" who know the program well enough to problem-solve issues that may develop because of unique practice styles, culture, and workflows.

Although it is advisable to plan to minimize business interruption and monitor organizational progress while training, it is best to aim for training that is distraction-free. With phones ringing and patients walking through the door, therapists and support staff can find themselves learning the system in 15-minute snatches—a formula for frustration. Careful planning will create longer blocks of uninterrupted learning. Ideally, shutting down the office completely allows for the most focus, but may not be practical. If this is not an option, open the office late one morning or close early in the afternoon to dedicate the time necessary. If possible, schedule fewer patients than usual on training days, or plan for training on light patient days. This will ensure that patient care is not negatively affected. While it is usually prudent to accept the vendor's recommendation on training hours and schedule, it is not reasonable to try to learn everything all at once—this may just create "glazed-over" expressions and frustrations by trying to master new technology quickly.

It is important to instill the right culture through the right messaging as you embark on the training process. Getting therapists and other clinicians and staff mentally prepared for EMR training is another key to a successful launch.[27] Even in the most progressive offices, some therapists need a bit of a nudge (or a more forceful shove!) to embrace the new technology. This "encouragement" can typically occur by using a combination of selling the benefits of the new system and firmly announcing that the EMR train is leaving the station, whether they are on it or not. But be mindful—although encouragement and incentives often work better than threats, one resistant employee who may resent the added technology because they see it as a threat to their job security may, if allowed to spread this anxiety unchecked, derail the entire atmosphere and training process.

Finally, ongoing technical and professional support of an application after the initial training is crucial to the overall success of the software. If the software application is not working correctly, it will have a significant negative impact on the efficiency and effectiveness of the staff and facility. Therapists need to understand how a particular vendor will provide ongoing training both in instances when new therapists need to learn the program and when enhancements to the software and new features have been incorporated. Levels of support can vary from continuous live support, to limited hours of support, to e-mail communication. Within these types of support, the level of expertise can vary significantly. Some companies will provide support strictly for technical difficulties associated with their software. Others will support the software and the hardware that their system runs on, while still others will have clinicians on staff that can assist a facility with more legal, ethical, and clinical decision-making issues. But the key here is simple: Understand what support is available from the vendor, what the cost of that support is, and when that support is available to you. Negotiate any needed enhancements in this area prior to the purchase of the software. A live support line that is available 6 AM to 6 PM Eastern time would not do you much good if you have a problem at 4 PM Pacific time!

EMR AND THIRD-PARTY PAYMENT: MINIMIZING RISK AND IMPROVING COMMUNICATION FOR PAYMENT OF PHYSICAL THERAPY SERVICES

Documentation shapes the process of clinical reasoning and provides justification for payment of physical therapy services. Regulatory changes continually push even the best-prepared practitioner to work overtime to maintain the training, policies, and standards related to documentation and coding for clinical services. The issue of medical necessity has become a primary focus of payer and regulatory agency audits. Billing for services that are not adequately justified in medical records can become an issue related to the potential fraud or abuse, carrying a significant risk to the provider. The adoption of EMRs has been identified as one potential tool for reducing negative audit experiences, as well as improving quality of care.

In the current healthcare payment climate, it is common for third-party payers to request medical records for the purposes of determining whether payment for services already rendered will be provided or whether a refund for payments already made is required. Over the past few years, these incidents have become more frequent, driven in large part by third-party payers who recognize the lack of awareness and compliance by many therapy providers in the areas of documentation, coding, and billing practices.

The third-party focus on the payment for rehabilitation services is instructive, in that it provides an opportunity for therapists to examine their clinical programs to better demonstrate that what they do and how they do it and that it is valuable and worthy of appropriate payment. Yet in many cases, physical therapy is perceived as unskilled or unnecessary and therefore undervalued by the third party's payment methodology. The PT has the opportunity to change the third-party perception of physical therapy by doing a better job of reflecting the use of current evidence; demonstrating clinical reasoning in their approaches to patient care; and demonstrating successful outcomes of their clinical approaches through more accurate documentation, coding, and billing practices. An effective EMR can greatly assist in this process.

Audit flags are identifiers on claim forms or in documentation that alert auditors or reviewers to potential fraud, abuse, or overutilization and indicate further investigation is necessary in order for the payer to justify payment of that particular claim. There are several common audit flags that providers should be aware of when evaluating potential EMR programs or self-auditing their own system. While some of these audit flags are not specific to electronic documentation and exist in handwritten documentation formats as well, EMR systems can increase the likelihood of some audit flags more than others (if for no other reason than the improved legibility of the record!). Awareness of these flags and ensuring that the EMR you choose minimizes the risk of them will greatly assist in reducing the potential of negative audits by third-party payers.

The following audit flags are seen commonly in many existing EMR systems:

- ***Evaluation notes reduced to one page, without necessary information to justify medical necessity.*** Too often, the desire to have reports printed to only one page to either save paper or provide physicians with summary reports because of fear that they do not want to (or would not) read this clinical information causes therapists to minimize information they collect or that they enter into their EMR system. It is important to remember that there are a variety of stakeholders for whom therapy documentation is important: referral sources, third-party payers, colleagues, attorneys, etc. It is important to collect and report the data that will support medical necessity, as well as minimize the risk in the event of any legal action. Many EMRs allow for various formats to be printed once the initial evaluation is complete and documented in the system. It is best to understand all the options available for reporting to third parties.
- ***Canned and generalized "assessment" statements that do not give a proper representation of the patient's progress or justification of the need for therapy services.*** The adoption of an EMR does provide significant efficiencies, one of which may be a menu of phrases that can be populated into various sections of documentation. Using these phrases repeatedly,

without the ability to edit them or individualize them to the specific patient, may lead third-party payers to question the legitimacy or credibility of the documentation.

- ***Generalized statements often leading to standardized notes that go unchanged by clinicians from visit to visit.*** Often, the review of documentation from EMR systems by third-party payers will identify notes that are essentially duplicated visit after visit, with only the date or some other small nuance modified. Although there may be great similarities between visits over a short period, typically, no two physical therapy visits will be identical, particularly if the patient is making progress toward established goals. The documentation of each visit should reflect the differences in provider interaction, progression of treatment, and patient response to treatment at each visit.
- ***The signature area for the physician on the Medicare Pan of Care (POC) is printed on a separate page than the required POC elements.*** Medicare requires that the physician or nonphysician provider (NPP) (per Medicare qualification requirements) certify a POC. That POC must include, at a minimum, the patient's diagnoses; long-term treatment goals; and the type, amount, frequency, and duration of treatment. Often, a signature box prints out on a separate sheet of paper than these items, and in fact, often the signature box is the only item on the last page of the POC. In these circumstances, the Medicare contractor may have difficulty identifying if the required certification was related to the required elements, and further, there is no guarantee that those elements can not be modified without the knowledge of the physician or other referring practitioner such as a Nurse Practitioner (NPP) or a Physician Assistant (PA). Page numbers on the POC document may be useful to indicate a signature as being linked to information found on a previous page of the document.
- ***Programs will often carry over previously measured objectives, which are repeated each visit as if they are being obtained, but are actually just being repopulated from prior visits.*** Documentation on each visit should pertain to data that is collected at each visit. Historical measures are appropriate to add to a visit if they are being compared to new data or referenced in regard to modifications in the POC. When these measures are simply included in a visit note and only reference historical data, this causes confusion and may be perceived as a lack of progress, since the values are not changing.
- ***Minutes for each procedure identified in the EMR populate a unit charge for a Current Procedural Terminology (CPT) code, regardless of the amount of time spent with the patient on that procedure.*** This may be especially challenging if an intervention for a Medicare beneficiary is less than 8 minutes and may not, therefore, align with the 8-minute rule. One of the largest areas for audits is related to the accurate reporting of the time spent with a patient. The CPT codes that describe direct contact should be reported based on the time spent with the patient; however, the number of units of these codes submitted for payment on each visit cannot exceed the total time spent with the patient. Most programs populate units for any number of minutes identified (4, 8, 10, etc.) without aggregating the minutes, resulting in therapists submitting claims for payment that reflect more time spent than actually occurred. This type of billing could constitute a false claim and subject the provider to severe penalties. An effective EMR will assist the PT in establishing this relationship and minimizing audit risk in this area, aligning with the ICF model.
- ***Documentation of nonspecific subjective comments, functional status, or tests and measures on initial examination or follow-up visits.*** Many EMR systems provide standardized measurements that reflect findings that are overly general and do not provide sufficient information from which to objectively measure progress throughout the rehabilitation program. One of the benefits of an EMR is the ability to collect specific data and use that data to measure objective progress throughout the episode of care. The absence of this level of specificity or objectivity will likely cause third-party payers to question the legitimacy of the care or medical necessity of the treatment provided.
- ***Objective data populated in the medical record relates to impairments only, without relationship to objective measures identifying limitations in functional activity.*** Although not specific to an EMR, therapists have historically focused their data collection on

impairments, such as pain, strength, and range of motion. While limitations in these areas are important, limitations in impairments are only considered a basis for skilled therapy if they are affecting functional performance. An effective EMR will assist the PT in establishing this relationship and minimizing audit risk in this area.

- ***Goals that are nonspecific, not related to functional activity limitations, or not related to findings on examination.*** An area of significant problem in therapy documentation is in goal development. Medical necessity and compliance adherence require therapy goals to be specific, objective, and functionally related. While not an audit flag specific to EMR, computerized documentation may cause these inadequacies to be more easily identified, thus increasing the likelihood of problems on audit. An effective EMR should provide the tools to enhance appropriate functional goal development using the data gathered and input during the examination process.
- ***Focus of documented interventions is on activities the patient is performing, rather than the therapist interaction with the patient to justify the need for skilled care.*** Historically, PTs have focused their documentation on lists of exercises and activities that the patient is performing, without providing any indication of how therapist involvement is necessary to meet the established goals. EMRs often provide significant detail on sets and repetitions of exercises, but offer no indication as to why the patient could not be performing those exercises at home or in a community health club. EMRs should assist the therapist in identifying their interactions with the patient to assist in justifying the need for skilled care.
- ***The initial POC does not change or is too general and does not provide specific detail necessary to drive interventions.*** Compliance requirements and documentation standards require the parameters of specific interventions to be identified within the documentation. If these parameters are not identified in the initial POC, then they must be identified on each visit that they are provided. Further, when additions, deletions, or modifications to the established POC are made, the POC should be modified. EMRs often identify overly general elements in the POC (therapeutic exercise, manual therapy, etc.), or the POC is not modified in the documentation as it occurs.
- ***Discharge notes do not summarize treatment, progress, or provide for recommendations for follow-up.*** The absence of discharge summaries as a routine component of therapy documentation has been identified as a significant issue among third-party payers and review agencies. When they are documented, they often do not include the necessary components of a discharge note. EMRs, given their ability to collect, collate, and retrieve data, should provide significant value in complying with this aspect of professional responsibility. However, therapists must understand the required components of a discharge summary and ensure that the EMR system they adopt will trigger them to efficiently document this information.

While no EMR can assure that you will never be audited, an effective EMR, designed specifically with the rehabilitation professional in mind, can be a significant asset in ensuring compliance with third-party payment rules, practice act regulations, and Standards of Practice. This improved compliance can assist dramatically in reducing the risk of negative audit consequences and increasing the likelihood of enhanced revenue capture based on documented justification for billed services.

DETERMINING THE RIGHT EMR: CRITERIA FOR CONSIDERATION

When evaluating EMR systems, the application should fit into the workflow of the practice and assist in improving productivity. Any system that adds work to the practice's processes without adding efficiencies or disrupts the workflow of the end users without significant benefits will not be accepted and will eventually have a negative impact on productivity levels. The EMR system should be intuitive to users, support them in documenting appropriate information, and assist with case management. If a system can provide these things, it will improve the clinician's efficiency and productivity, allowing them to spend more quality time with their patients. There are a multitude of criteria and features that PTs should review prior to purchasing a system.

There are many benefits to using an EMR. However, there are multiple aspects to consider before implementing any system. There are three primary considerations in evaluating any software application:

- First, is it going to improve the workflow and functionality of the practice?
- Second, is the application going to improve productivity, case management, and payment?
- Third, is the application going to improve compliance and practice management?

Once an application meets a facility's basic criteria, the next steps to evaluate are training and customer support. As was discussed in the previous section, training and support are key to user acceptance and obtaining maximum benefit from the system. After a system is implemented, there will be a learning curve before complete user acceptance and improved productivity. With practice and dedication to the system, the rewards of effective and efficient documentation, increased productivity, and increased revenues can be realized.

Key Features to Consider

There are many features provided in today's EMR systems, and the ability to identify key groups of these when evaluating the right system for a particular clinic or facility is critical as a component of the due diligence necessary for successful implementation. The following is a noncomprehensive list of program features, grouped by category, which should assist the rehabilitation provider in this process, recognizing that many other sources of criteria analysis and feature recommendations are available in the marketplace.

The first three features—ASP versus client/server, integrated systems versus best of breed, and the integration of clinical decision support systems—are among the most important, and as a result are discussed in more detail.

ASP versus Client/Server

With the growth in technology and the need for timely enhancements to EMR systems as well as the desire for providers to access medical records where and when it is convenient to them, the trend has been to shift from what is known as a client/server model to an ASP cloud based platform for EMR systems. This is one of the most significant decisions to be made in choosing an EMR.

In the client/server option, providers (or clients) host the EMR software on their internal computer responsible for running the software (called a server) and purchase the EMR licenses outright. This requires substantial capital as well as an internal IT staffing that can constantly stay on top of maintaining the server. Servers are typically out of date within 3 to 4 years, so this model is only for those clients that can afford to update and repair the internal network. Also, software is a "fluid" product, and after purchasing, it is important to recognize that the vendor typically is continuing to modify and program new enhancements and features. With this model, it will be necessary to not only ensure the vendor is making timely changes, particularly related to compliance and regulatory elements, but that a clinic is equipped to update and maintain a dedicated server with the new software on a regular basis.

In contrast, an ASP is a remotely hosted (cloud based) software system accessed via an Internet Web browser, where the EMR application, database (where all the patient data is stored), and server all reside in a central location outside the therapist's office and are maintained by the EMR vendor or other third party. The server is secure and HIPAA compliant and clinicians and staff use a secure login to access the EMR, in the same way they would access a secure banking site. The ASP allows clinicians to access the program and associated patient information at any time, from any place with Internet access.

Although ASP systems do not eliminate all hardware requirements (printers, scanners, and laptops or workstations are still necessary), they do allow for outsourcing the maintenance and repair of the critical server to outside IT professionals. This can be a significant time and money saver, and is one reason for the sharp increase in ASP system development over the past few years. EMR software updates (which can be challenging and time-consuming for a client/server system to keep up with) are done by the ASP vendor and are included as part of the monthly service charge. The ASP vendor also is responsible for performing regular backups of patient data and providing redundant systems that are crucial functions that can jeopardize a practice if done poorly (or not at all) by practices maintaining their own systems. And with an ASP system, the cost and hassle of replacing the server (typically the most expensive piece of hardware) every 3 to 4 years is eliminated.

From a cost perspective, in a client/server option, a practice purchases a perpetual license for the software. After the EMR is paid for (often in installment payments), the remaining financial obligation to the vendor is an annual support payment, which typically covers new updates and technical support. Annual support fees typically range from 18% to 20% of the retail cost of the software.[28]

In contrast, with an ASP option there is no up-front cost for the software. Users may pay a monthly fee for as long as the service is used, or another subscription-type payment model may be chosen. Fees can range from $250 to $1,000 per provider, per month, plus the cost of a reliable, high-bandwidth connection to the Internet. The ASP fee is typically inclusive, covering technical support, software upgrades, daily database backups, and any server maintenance. Training and implementation costs may or may not be included in the monthly fee for an ASP.

Often the ASP versus client/server decision primarily revolves around how much IT support, server maintenance, and data management a practice is willing to absorb. For practices that have the staff, ability, and resources to maintain a server, perform the backups religiously, attend to the details of technical troubleshooting, and manage complex software upgrades, a client/server model may be a good choice and sometimes can be less expensive in the long run. But if the tasks described earlier are daunting or terrifying, then ASP is a better choice for a practice. Experts will usually recommend the ASP model based on the ability to assess the past and see where large software companies (such as Microsoft) are heading, because even if a provider has the wherewithal to handle the upgrades, maintenance, etc., it still does not prove to be financially advantageous to do so. In the long run, the ASP model has projected savings of up to 30% based on reduced labor costs related to maintenance and support and reduced ownership costs related to hardware expenses over client/server programs.

Best-of-Breed versus Integrated (End-to-End) Systems

Most practices in the market for their first EMR already have computerized practice management (or billing) systems. In deciding on an EMR, they will need to make an important decision, which is whether or not to keep the existing practice management system and interface it with a new EMR (if possible), known as the "best-of-breed" approach, or purchase an integrated system that combines a new EMR with new practice management software, sometimes known as implementing an end-to-end solution.

With the best-of-breed approach, each software application is selected based on its inherent qualities. If the practice management and EMR systems selected come from different vendors and need to exchange data, it will be necessary to build an interface that allows this exchange. When combining EMR and practice management systems from different vendors, registration interfaces are the most common. This allows front-desk staff to automatically send data for new patients entering a practice to the new EMR. Without a registration interface, staff must separately enter patient data into the practice management and EMR systems.

In contrast, integrated (or end-to-end) systems share the same database. This means that when front-desk staff enters patient data into an integrated system, the information becomes instantly available to everyone in the office, using the scheduling, billing, or EMR portion of the system. With integrated systems, a single vendor provides the convenience of a single point of contact for support and technical concerns. In addition, the requirement to manage the technical aspects of building and maintaining an interface between the EMR and practice management systems is eliminated. Most importantly, there will be significant efficiency gains from the systems' shared applications. Because truly integrated systems share a common database, they allow sophisticated interactions between the EMR and practice management systems.[29] One such example of this is the development of clinical decision support systems, which function most effectively in a fully integrated EMR. Another example is the integration of documentation with billing.

In a fully integrated system, documentation during a visit populates the appropriate CPT codes, which are then sent electronically to the practice's billing department. This process will typically ensure that documentation supports the CPT codes billed to a third party. The billing staff then reviews the charges for proper coding and can quickly and efficiently post the claim. This type of seamless data exchange is difficult (and generally expensive) to achieve when interfacing between two separate systems.

Many tasks within therapy practices require different staff members to share data quickly and accurately. Integrated systems are built with this data sharing in mind; best-of-breed systems are not.

Clinical Decision Support System

Computerized clinical decision support systems (CDSSs) are information systems (software) designed to improve clinical decision-making about individual patients. In a CDSS, characteristics of individual patients are matched to a computerized knowledge base, and software algorithms generate patient-specific recommendations.[30] An EMR that integrates a CDSS provides a powerful tool to capture coded clinical information that can be linked to knowledge of evidence-based treatment to provide tailored recommendations *at the point of care*. So, by utilizing an EMR with an integrated CDSS, while the therapist is actually examining or treating the patient, the clinician improves the ability to make sound clinical decisions in a timely manner and decrease documentation and dictation time by using evidence-based recommendations and other aspects of decision support. Appropriate systems *seamlessly* integrate into the current workflow of busy clinicians by suggesting actions at a time when a clinician is still in the process of clinical documentation. Such integrated clinical decision support should assist in closing the large and well-documented gap between best evidence and actual practice.

CDSSs are designed to facilitate clinical management. A provider can save time in the long run and improve the quality of care by enhancing clinical practices and workflow practice efficiency. Typical components suggested for inclusion in a CDSS related to rehabilitation care include:

- Actions and recommendations based on specific examinations/evaluation findings
- Clinical guidelines
- Electronic alerts
- Documentation prompts
- Reference materials
- Reports related to captured patient data

An additional critical element of CDSS is computerized *clinical reminders*, or computer-generated suggestions about clinical care for individual patients that are informed by data stored in the EMR. These suggestions are based on programs that operationalize evidence-based practice as computable rules that are integrated into the clinical application. In addition to clinical reminders, more comprehensive CDSSs include administrative and compliance reminders.

Although there are barriers to the implementation of a CDSS, which include the failure of practitioners to use the CDSS, poor usability or integration into practitioner workflow, or practitioner nonacceptance of computer recommendations, compared with manual initiation, the automatic prompting of a CDSS has been demonstrated to improve integration into practitioner workflow, as well as provide better opportunities to correct inadvertent deficiencies in care.[30] Although some providers have voiced concern about increased practitioner dependence on CDSSs, with eroded capacity for independent decision-making, others advocate strongly that the use of CDSSs actually confirms the decision-making process while improving the efficiency and quality of care. CDSSs are considered so important to the future of quality healthcare that the Office of the National Coordinator for Health Information Technology (ONCHIT) included this criterion in the final rule establishing the initial set of standards, implementation specifications, and certification criteria for EHRs.

Additional Features for Consideration

Customization Ability

Many providers get caught up in the concept of "my workflow" versus the "EMR workflow." Some providers are looking for an EMR vendor to customize the system based on their current paper and clinical workflow, whether or not that workflow is efficient or based on evidence. EMRs have the ability to standardize the approach to physical therapy evaluation and intervention and reduce the unwarranted variation in PT practice.

Unwarranted variation in practice has been identified as a root cause of excessive and inappropriate healthcare utilization, resulting in less-than-optimal quality and efficiency. This unwarranted variation is typically caused by the "unique approach" to the evaluation and treatment of patients that are maintained by individual healthcare providers, and may be a result of such things as working for an organization that dictates practice styles, following the teachings of the latest, greatest "guru," or simply the result of habit—"It's always been done this way." Such variation may be further perpetuated by practice "philosophies" that PTs often tout as marketing or differentiating strategies for their practices or facilities.

Individual practitioner approaches, when not informed by the best current evidence, have become one of the root causes of what the third-party payer sees as excessive and potentially inappropriate utilization—the result of which may be demonstrated in less-than-optimal quality and efficiency of care. Physical therapy, as seen from the third-party perspective, is notorious for demonstrating unexplained variations in practice patterns. This is typically the result of efforts to put into place various clinical protocols or policies that may not be based in current best evidence, but instead use information gained in seminars or publications that are not consistently reflective of current evidence and out of context with other clinical programs and approaches. The PT has the opportunity to change the third-party perception of physical therapy by doing a better job of reflecting the use of current evidence; demonstrating clinical reasoning in their approaches to patient care; and demonstrating successful outcomes of their clinical approaches through more accurate documentation, coding, and billing practices.

While it is important to ensure adequate provisions for customization, this customization should occur within the structure of a necessary standardization of approach, using best available evidence whenever possible. And while some customization is necessary, customization that eliminates necessary documentation requirements simply to reduce the time it takes to document or eliminate evidence-based clinical decision support can add to the unwarranted variation in PT practice, resulting in decreased quality and effectiveness, increased cost, increasing audits, and demand for return of identified overpayments.

Compliance Adherence

Generally, compliance in the larger context means adherence to laws and regulations of the land, and when specifically applied to the medical world, a focus is on maintaining regulatory compliance in all activities of documentation, coding, and billing for professional services. A compliant process and environment are an absolute necessity when considering the manner in which regulatory organizations are closely monitoring all aspects of healthcare activities, including those related to patient quality of care, documentation of services to support charges, and other financial transactions between the provider and the beneficiary. How will a therapy practice ensure that what ends up in the chart accurately reflects the care that was provided to the patient, as well as the services that were billed? An effective EMR system should include the incorporation of compliance requirements and programming of payer/regulatory changes seamlessly and in a timely manner. Through utilizing an integrated EMR, the burden of assessing compliance is lessened dramatically. A well-designed system that incorporates these requirements and changes will greatly assist the clinical staff in performing their documentation, and it is this documentation that then automatically determines the services to be coded and billed, a process that is easily performed once reviewed by the responsible staff. Typically, ASP systems are significantly more timely and complete with compliance updates.

Focus on Functional Activities

Professional standards and third-party payer requirements focus on the attainment of measurable functional goals based on activities and impairments that are identified on the initial evaluation. When evaluating an EMR system for documentation abilities, a facility should look at its ability to generate previous and current levels of function; identify measurable impairments and functional limitations; facilitate outcomes data collection; integrate the International Classification of Functioning, Disability, and Health (ICF); and develop and track measurable functional goals that identify the impact of noted impairments on activity performance.

Clinical Reporting Flexibility

Documentation is performed for various reasons, and documentation is read and utilized by many who are involved in the delivery and payment of our services. Physicians and third-party payers utilize documentation of therapy services for determining appropriateness of patients' responses and medical necessity, while state practice acts, compliance requirements, and medical/legal and risk management focus on specifics in documentation that could assist in malpractice or regulatory challenges. One report written in an ineffective and/or inefficient manner, while meeting the criteria for one set of eyes, will undoubtedly have another glaze over by the time they get to the third page of your initial evaluation report! The ability to generate multiple report formats as needed by the various entities that are the recipients of the documentation will simplify and reduce administrative work.

In choosing an EMR, look for a system that allows for documentation to be produced in a timely manner, is easy to review, and provides each intended recipient with the information they need (and want). Some applications generate template forms that may give a referral source the kind of information they need to make appropriate decisions concerning their patient's care, but may not include the information necessary to comply with your state practice act or third-party payment requirements. Other applications may provide too much information or be too "busy," making it difficult for the referral source to extract the information they are looking for. The ideal application would allow a clinician to document everything that is important and necessary to their clinical practice and patient/client management and be able to report this information in both a detailed evaluation or follow-up note that becomes part of the medical record, and also provide a summary report that could be provided to the referral source with only the information they want and need. Providing the physician with the appropriate information to make him or her effective and productive may have a positive impact on the amount of referrals that physician sends, while still allowing the therapist to be compliant with necessary standards, rules, and regulations.

Tracking and Alert Systems

One of the greatest strengths of EMR systems, particularly those that integrate clinical decision support systems, is the ability to track various actions or statistics and notify the user based on predetermined parameters that are established by either the vendor or the end user. A few of the tracking and alert parameters to look for include the following.

Authorization and Resource Management. It is important that interventions and services that are medically necessary be paid appropriately by either the third-party payer or the patient. Awareness of coverage limitations prior to treatment will allow clinicians to best manage patients within the limits of the patient's financial abilities. When evaluating EMR systems, a facility should seek features that assist with case management, tools to ensure optimal charge capture for documented services, and alerts to inform the clinicians before their patient's authorization expires. Knowing the status of patients allows the therapist to make better clinical decisions and provide extended care for the patients who need it. With such alerts, the clinician can educate the patient as to their coverage and take appropriate action to seek additional authorization, obtain payment for additional services directly from the patient, or discharge the patient.

Additionally, one of the keys to managing a successful practice is the ability to manage the available resources related to payment for services. Payers manage their resources by limiting the number of covered visits or length of treatment under an insurance plan, by limiting the dollar amount paid per visit, or by limiting the duration of the benefit. If a patient is treated outside of the parameters established by the payer, the payer may refuse to pay for the treatment delivered. Having the ability to monitor the resource status of each patient will enable the clinician to develop an appropriate plan of care, manage the patient's care efficiently, maximize therapist productivity, and improve payment by informing patients prior to exceeding third-party payment limits and informing patients of their financial responsibility at the appropriate time.

Ability to Identify and Track Functional Improvement. Medicare and many workers' compensation providers are requiring that clinicians have functional documentation to support continued care. Professional resources, including APTA's *Guide to Physical Therapist Practice 3.0*[31] and *Defensible Documentation*,[32] identify recommended examination, tests and measures, and interventions, as well as proper documentation of these. There has been a greater demand for functional outcome-oriented documentation and the incorporation of evidence-based practice through research to justify therapy services. When a facility evaluates EMR systems, the system should be evaluated on its incorporation of these and other professional guidelines. The system should have the ability to generate the treating or PT diagnosis in addition to the medical diagnosis and track outcomes data related to interventions provided and functional status achieved at discharge. Being familiar with these resources and others that are available will assist in the review and decisions related to making an EMR choice.

Utilization and Attendance Tracking. It can be difficult to keep track of every active case in a facility. If a patient goes on vacation for a week or cancels appointments as a result of illness, this patient entry can become lost and therefore be missing in the system. Certainly lost or missing patients mean lost revenue in the short run, but trends like this can also affect patient satisfaction or be reflected in more significant practice concerns. An effective EMR system should be able to track patients that have not been seen in a facility for an established period of time and alert the therapist when a patient has not been seen in a set time without a discharge, thus allowing the clinician to be able to take appropriate action in a timely fashion. By responding to these alerts, a clinician may be able to recapture lost visits, improve facility revenues, and better assist their patients in returning to a previous level of function. Besides attendance tracking, the ability to track utilization of services based on diagnosis code, insurance category, therapist, etc., will provide significant information to allow for practice growth through more efficient and effective management.

Dashboard Availability

Dashboards are one of the most intuitive and interactive ways to display data so that clinicians and managers can make intelligent, data-driven decisions about their practice on a daily basis. The best dashboards should allow for the flexibility to view both high-level reports and detailed listings down to the patient account level. One of the benefits of having an EMR is the ability to report captured key data in an efficient manner to allow for efficient and effective practice management. There are several key areas that can be reported on dashboards within an EMR. For example, a patient dashboard will display a summary of all appropriate patient information stored in the EMR and is updated in real time, without the need for manually updating the information. Data such as patient demographics, problems/diagnoses, notes, and other helpful information to make necessary clinical decisions are typical components of the patient dashboard. Financial dashboards will provide real-time data on dimensions of a practice, such as collection ratios, adjustment ratios, and extensive accounts receivable reporting. Practice management dashboards include such statistics as number of new patients, visits, and procedures, with the ability to identify each based on CPT code, diagnosis code, insurance type, and various other statistics.

These calculations can provide quick and useful information when monitoring the health and stability of a practice or facility. Used as a management tool, these dashboard ratios and statistics paint a picture of fluctuations in payer patterns, practice billing operations, patient statistics, or other influencing factors that can help efficiently focus a practice's efforts in the overall management of clinical and administrative operations.

Financial/Revenue Report Availability

One area of responsibility for most office staff is the ability to report on the quantity of patients treated, revenue generated, and money collected from co-pays (and durable medical equipment if the facility is a provider). By having this information readily available, a facility is able to quickly assess whether they are making or losing money. When choosing an EMR, a facility should be able to generate these reports quickly and easily, without having to do additional data entry.

Outcomes Reporting

Outcomes measurements, the ability to compare the results of an action or process over time, are part of the next wave of EMR applications. Certain outcomes, such as time from injury to release to partial or full employment, are easy to calculate and track if they are entered as dates. They can be recalled for specific procedures, clinicians, diagnoses, and payers. More advanced outcome measurements, such as improvement in the Disabilities of the Arm, Shoulder and Hand (DASH) scale or other scales can be integrated into existing EMRs. Maintaining outcomes in an integrated EMR will allow practices to monitor their outcomes, benchmark them against published standards, and participate in new pay-for-performance or value-based purchasing initiatives as they are created. When evaluating various EMR systems, remember that this is likely going to provide you with an opportunity to track and report data that previously took hours, if not days, to identify and embrace new methods to continue to provide better care

The Physical Therapy Outcomes Registry is a platform that allows all PTs and practices to leverage EHR data to improve patient outcomes. APTA has partnered with FIGmd, a leading IT company that specializes in EHR-integrated registries, to power the Physical Therapy Outcomes Registry.[33]

Incorporation of Third-Party Payment Policy

Collecting payment for services provided is often a challenge. There is a plethora of reasons why a payer may deny or refuse to pay a claim, and moreover, payers also aim to ensure that there is documentation to support the bills submitted for payment. Several different types of edits can be applied to charges. The most common types of edits are known as the National Correct Coding Initiative (NCCI or CCI).[34] Additionally, local medical review policies (LMRPs) or local coverage decisions (LCDs) often have crosswalks that identify diagnoses for which a particular CPT code will be considered for payment. There are also billing rules, such as cascading or multiple procedure payment reductions, that may have an impact on how a facility submits a bill for payment.

As described on the Medicaid.gov Website, "CMS' NCCI promotes national correct coding methodologies and reduces improper coding which may result in inappropriate payments of Medicare Part B claims and Medicaid claims."[34] NCCI Procedure-to-Procedure (PTP) code pair edits are automated prepayment edits that prevent improper payment when certain codes are submitted together for Part B–covered services.

In addition to PTP code pair edits, the NCCI includes a set of edits known as Medically Unlikely Edits (MUEs). An MUE is a maximum number of units of service (UOS) allowable under most circumstances for a single Healthcare Common Procedure Coding System/Current Procedural Terminology (HCPCS/CPT) code billed by a provider on a date of service for a single beneficiary. For more information about NCCI edits, refer to *How to Use the Medicare National Correct Coding Initiative (NCCI) Tools*.[34]

> **Author's Note**
>
> The majority of commercial payers load the CCI edits into their systems. The workers' compensation programs and self-insured plans could create their own edits.

Medicare Part A and Part B local medical review policies are used to assist therapists in submitting correct claims for payment.

In choosing an EMR, a facility should ensure the application takes any billing and coding edits into account to ensure efficient submission of claims and timely payment. Further, payers generally have contract-specific fee schedules, so any EMR you select should be able to support many different contractual fee schedules, as well as provide alerts if a particular insurance company does not cover a particular service or there is a need to submit charges with CPT codes that are different than would typically be associated with an intervention.

Legal Adherence and Risk Mitigation

With regard to the incorporation of HIPAA and other legal elements, there are many legal aspects in the day-to-day operations of a physical therapy business. When evaluating an EMR system for a facility, one should make sure that the application follows professional standards and Medicare guidelines for documentation and is compliant with HIPAA regulations. There are also federal and state guidelines that need to be monitored. By implementing an EMR system that keeps current with the legal aspects of documentation, a facility can improve overall productivity and minimize risk of noncompliance.

In the past, making certain errors was a mistake, but in an environment that has ratcheted up the scrutiny, making certain errors may be considered fraud. Examples include overbilling and billing for treatment that was not actually rendered. It is a continual challenge to keep track of all the regulatory requirements, so your EMR system should assist you with this. All data exchange must be encrypted to protect confidentiality, and it is essential to avoid access to patient data by unauthorized individuals in or associated with the practice. EMR systems typically implement safeguards to maintain data confidentiality, integrity, and availability. From an administrative perspective, these include access management and workforce security; from a physical perspective, such things include facility controls and workstation access; and from a technical focus, these include audit control, system integrity, and user authentication. When evaluating EMR systems, it is critical to ensure that the system will reduce exposure to fraud and risk, rather than making day-to-day activities more challenging to monitor and control.

Automation of Administrative Functions

An effective EMR system should have the ability to automate current administrative office functions such as appointment reminders, insurance eligibility, and patient follow-up. The inclusion of PoC documentation, coding, and billing alerts related to missing or incorrect information will greatly enhance administrative efficiency.

Individuals' Perceptions of the Privacy and Security of Medical Records and Health Information Exchange

A majority of individuals are confident that their medical records are safe from unauthorized viewing but have concerns when health information is electronically exchanged. (see Figure 4.3)[35]

A majority of individuals (74%) are confident that their medical records are safe from unauthorized viewing but have concerns (66%) when health information is electronically exchanged. These perceptions are unchanged since 2011. Ten percent of individuals reported withholding information from their healthcare provider due to privacy and security concerns regarding their medical record. This is down from 15% of individuals in 2014.[35]

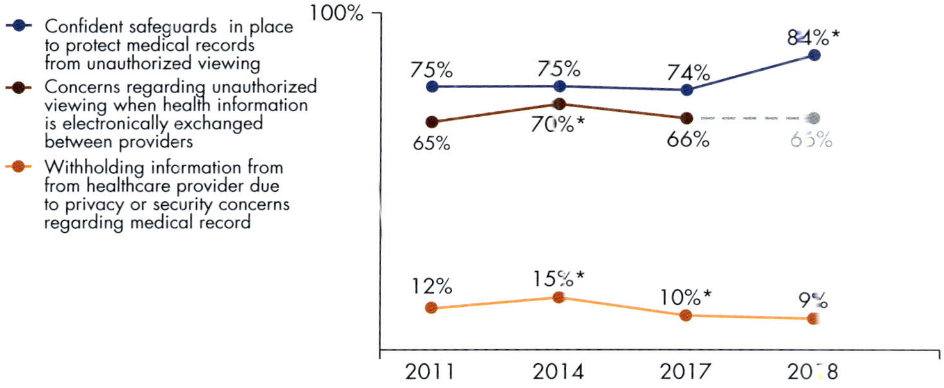

Figure 4-3. Individuals' perceptions of the privacy and security of medical records and health information exchange.[35]

*Notes: *Significantly different from previous year ($p < 0.05$). Denominator represents all individuals; weighted percentages reflect national estimates.*

Breaches of Unsecured Protected Health Information[36]

Based upon data collected by the HHS Office for Civil Rights, as of February 1, 2016, protected health information breaches affected over 113 million individuals in 2015. In 2015, hacking incidents comprised nearly 99% of all individuals affected by breaches, and the number of reported hacking incidents, 57, comprised over 20% of all reported breaches. From 2010 to 2014, 97 hacking incidents affected fewer than 4 million individuals, less than 10% of all reported breaches and affected individuals during this time.

However, despite the rise in breaches related to hacking incidents, reported breaches related to other incidents and the number of individuals affected by these breaches are down in 2015. Through February 1, 2016, theft, loss, improper disposal, and unauthorized access or disclosure of protected health information comprised 208 of all reported breaches (N=265), down from 216 (N=285) in 2014 and 211 (N=262) in 2013. These four types of breach incidents affected 1.4 million individuals in 2015, compared to 10.7 million in 2014 and 6.7 million in 2013.

In 2015, 4 of the 51 hacking incidents involved an EMR. One hacking incident affected 3.9 million individuals' health information—nearly all the individuals affected by an EMR hacking incident in 2015.[36]

Notes:

[1] The HIPAA Breach Notification Rule: http://www.hhs.gov/ocr/privacy/hipaa/understanding/coveredentities/breachnotificationifr.html, requires healthcare providers, health plans, and other HIPAA-covered entities to notify affected individuals when their health information is breached, as well as the HHS secretary and the media where a breach affects more than 500 individuals. As required by Section 13402(e)(4) of the HITECH Act, the secretary of HHS must post a list of breaches of unsecured protected health information affecting 500 or more individuals.

[2] A breach may involve any of the following types of incidents: theft, loss, hacking/IT incident, improper disposal, unauthorized access/disclosure, other, or unknown (not reported or data missing).

[3] Breach incidents may involve any of the following information, information technology, or devices: paper/films, network server, laptop, desktop computer, e-mail, electronic medical record, other portable electronic device, or other.

See Table 4.1 for the CMS Electronic Record Incident report template.

ADAPTABILITY TO FUTURE CHANGES

Thanks to legislation that implemented meaningful use and MIPS, EHR adoption is near 100%. Future policies will further promote greater interoperability and improved patient

Table 4-1 CMS Electronic Record Incident Report Template[37]

Date/Time:					
INCIDENT TRACKING NUMBER					
CMS	**HHS**	**US CERT**		**NCISS Risk Rating**	
				**** = Required information***	
REPORTING INDIVIDUAL CONTACT INFORMATION					
Name*			**Email***		
Office Number*	**Cell Number**		**Dept/OPDIV***	**User ID**	
Name(s) of Dept/OPDIV or individual notified of security incident:					
Dept/OPDIV		**Name/Title**		**Date/Time Notified**	
IMPACTED USER CONTACT INFORMATION					
Name*			**E-mail***		
Office Number*	**Cell Number**		**Dept/OPDIV***	**User ID**	
INCIDENT INFORMATION					
Date and Time Activity First Detected					
Date:				Time:	
Number of Systems Impacted		Number of Records Impacted		Number of Users Impacted	

Impact Categories

Functional Impact

- ☐ No Impact
- ☐ No Impact to Services
- ☐ Minimal Impact to Noncritical Services
- ☐ Minimal Impact to Critical Services
- ☐ Significant Impact to Noncritical Services
- ☐ Denial of Noncritical Services
- ☐ Significant Impact to Critical Services
- ☐ Denial of Critical Services/Loss of Control

Information Impact

- ☐ No Impact
- ☐ Suspected But Not Identified
- ☐ Privacy Data Breach
- ☐ Proprietary Information Breach
- ☐ Destruction of Noncritical Systems
- ☐ Critical Systems Data Breach
- ☐ Core Credential Compromise
- ☐ Destruction of Critical System

Recoverability

- ☐ Regular
- ☐ Supplemented
- ☐ Extended
- ☐ Not Recoverable

Attack Vectors Taxonomy

Attack Vector

- ☐ Unknown
- ☐ Attrition
- ☐ Web
- ☐ E-mail/Phishing
- ☐ External/Removable Media
- ☐ Impersonation/Spoofing
- ☐ Improper Usage
- ☐ Loss or Theft of Equipment
- ☐ Other

Incident Attributes

Location of Observed Activity

- ☐ Level 1 – Business Demilitarized Zone (DMZ)
- ☐ Level 2 – Business Network
- ☐ Level 3 – Business Network Management
- ☐ Level 4 – Critical System DMZ
- ☐ Critical System Management
- ☐ Critical Systems
- ☐ Safety Systems
- ☐ Unknown

Incident Category*

- ☐ Lost/Stolen Asset (*Section A*)
- ☐ PII Breach (*Section B mandatory*)
- ☐ Malicious Code (*Section C*) (Cat 3)
- ☐ Unauthorized Access (*Section D*) (Cat 1)
- ☐ Improper Usage (*Section E*) (Cat 4)
- ☐ Exercise/Network Defense Testing (*Sect F*)
- ☐ Denial of Service (*Section G*) (Cat 2)
- ☐ Scans/Probes/Attempted Access (*Sect G*)
- ☐ Investigations (*Section G*) (Cat 6)

Type of Device Involved in Incident* Check below			
			Operating System
☐ Tablet ☐ Cell Phone ☐ Computer (Nonspecific) ☐ Computer Files ☐ Desktop Computer	☐ Domain Controller ☐ E-mail ☐ Hard Drive (External) ☐ Hard Drive (Internal) ☐ Laptop ☐ Paper Documents	☐ CD/DVD ☐ PDA ☐ Server ☐ Tape/DLT/DASD ☐ USB Thumb Drive ☐ Other________	☐ Windows ☐ Linux ☐ Unix ☐ Mac

Source IP/Network (*Attacker*)		**Destination IP/Network** (*Victim*)
Source Computer Name (*if known*)		**Destination Computer Name** (*if known*)
Antivirus Vendor		**Antivirus Signature Version Number**
Encryption		**Encryption Type/Vendor**
☐ YES	☐ NO	N/A

Section A: Lost/Stolen Asset	
PII Involved? (if so, complete Section B) ☐ YES ☐ NO	**Brief Description** Include actions taken, asset brand/model, date and time, location of theft/damage and whether or not PII was exposed
Actions Taken: (Please state if no further action is needed.)	

Section B: PII Breach		
Breach Category Check below		
☐ Document Theft ☐ Hardware/Media Theft ☐ Document Loss ☐ Hardware/Media Loss	☐ Document Lost in Transit ☐ Hardware/Media Lost in Transit ☐ Improper Usage ☐ Unintended Manual Disclosure	☐ Unintended Electronic Disclosure ☐ Unauthorized Access ☐ Hacking or IT Incident ☐ Document Sent to Wrong Address

Number of PII Lost or Compromised List Number below	
Exact number of PII:	Otherwise, check: ☐ Unknown

Brief Description:
Ensure to include the format of the PII (i.e., e-mail, web, database, etc.), population affected, lost/stolen, summary timestamp, and the actions taken if any.
Actions Taken: (Please state if no further action is needed.)

Section C: Malicious Code

Malware Type (Check One)		Operating System?
☐ Worm	☐ Denial of Service (DoS)	☐ Windows
☐ Virus	☐ Other	☐ Linux
☐ Trojan	____________	☐ Unix
☐ Buffer Overflow	____________	☐ Mac
	____________	

Name of Malware If Known
N/A

Action Taken Regarding Malware?			Prior to Event, Was Affected Node Properly Patched?
☐ Quarantined	☐ Cleaned	☐ Left Alone	☐ Yes ☐ No

Description of Current Actions Taken (if any):

Section D: Unauthorized Access

Describe Violation
Actions Taken (if any)
(Please state if no further action is needed.)

Section E: Improper Usage/Policy Violation

Type of Violation					
(P2P) File Sharing	*Instant Messenger*	*Inappropriate Websites*	*Remote Access*	*Unapproved Software*	Other (Describe)
☐	☐	☐	☐	☐	☐

Describe Violation: (i.e., software name and version, URL address if applicable)
N/A
Describe Incident
Actions Taken (if any)
(Please state if no further action is needed.)

Section F: Exercise/Network Defense Testing

Testing Approval Provided By	**Contact Number**	**Testing Time Period**

Brief Description: Include reason for testing and the networks and systems tested.
Actions Taken: (Please state if no further action is needed.)

Section G: Denial of Service, Scans/Probes/Attempted Access, and Investigations

Describe Violation
There is no evidence that this information has been further used or disclosed inappropriately.
Actions Taken (if any)
(Please state if no further action is needed.)

Section H: Additional Information

Indicators of Compromise
Provide any indicators of compromise developed or used to identify the activity (if available).
Signatures
Provide any signatures triggered or developed to identify the activity (if available).
Detection Measures
Provide any detection measures developed in relation to the incident (if available).

access to their medical record information. It is most important when shopping for a system to consider those things that are not yet known in the industry or about your specific utilization of a system and consider the standards related to specific aspects of the EMR that, while it may not be required today, will be required for physical therapy professionals in the future. After all, the purchase of an EMR is a long-term investment in your practice and your profession.

CURRENT STATE OF EMRs

The current state of EMRs specific to rehabilitation has seen some consolidation in the market, and there has been some change in what the most used systems include and offer to their customers, including integrated outcomes programs.

> *The Physical Therapy Outcomes Registry is an approved Qualified Clinical Data Registry (QCDR) by the Centers for Medicare and Medicaid Services (CMS) for the 2019 Merit-Based Incentive Payment System (MIPS). Twenty-seven PT-specific quality measures are supported within the Registry for the 2019 MIPS reporting year. APTA's Registry is the only physical therapy–specific QCDR that has experience reporting MIPS data since 2017. After enrollment is complete, FIGmd's patented read-only software, Registry Practice Connector, can run in the background of an EHR system, pulling pertinent data into the Physical Therapy Outcomes Registry on a scheduled basis. The Physical Therapy Outcomes Registry empowers you to:*[33]

- Benchmark outcomes—*without* additional data entry
- Easily participate in MIPS and maximize your payment incentive
- Optimize your practice with insights from easy-to-use dashboards
- Empower PTs to provide the most effective patient care
- Market your practice to referring physicians, payers, patients, and employers
- Maximize payment from private payers with outcomes data

FINAL THOUGHTS

Most PTs recognize the importance, and value, of appropriate coding and documentation of clinical services, yet the process of learning and implementing all of the necessary information to adequately document the clinical care provided to patients, not to mention the time it can take to do so, can be overwhelming. But if an appropriate and effective EMR system is implemented, the process of documentation can not only efficiently meet the clinical, legal, regulatory, and payment requirements that currently exist, it can also serve to enhance the patient encounter, facilitate improved functional outcomes, and increase a company's bottom line while at the same time reducing the risk of punitive audits. To achieve these goals, it is critical for therapists to increase their "compliance IQ" as well as improve their "documentation hygiene" and then to embrace, after appropriate education and due diligence, the transition to an EMR. For in that transition, a computerized documentation system will not only assist PTs to meet new legislative requirements and become a significant administrative and compliance asset, it will become a most valuable partner in the provision of efficient, effective, and evidence-based physical therapy care.

REVIEW QUESTIONS

1. What constitutes fraud in the medical record?
2. Explain the history of EMR development leading up to the current mandate for transitioning to an EMR.
3. Explain the concept of "meaningful use" with regard to EMR adoption.
4. Explain the difference between an electronic medical record and electronic health record.

5. Compare and contrast ASP versus client/server EMR platforms.
6. Compare and contrast the benefits of point-of-care use of EMR versus workstations or documenting outside the patient visit.
7. What is the key to user acceptance and obtaining maximum system benefit? Defend your answer.
8. What are the three primary considerations when considering software?
9. What is the relationship between an EMR system and evidence-based practice?

REFERENCES

1. *Value Based Payment Models.* American Physical Therapy Association, Alexandria, VA. Available at https://www.apta.org/your-practice/payment/medicare-payment/alternative-payment-models/apms-an-introduction. Accessed July 20, 2020.
2. *Defining Key Health Information Technology Terms.* Department of Health and Human Services. Available at https://www.healthitanswers.net/health-it-terminology/. Published April 28, 2008. Accessed August 10, 2020.
3. Garrett P, Seidman J. EMR vs HER - what is the difference? *Health IT Buzz.* Available at https://www.healthit.gov/buzz-blog/electronic-health-and-medical-records/emr-vs-ehr-difference. Published January 4, 2011. Accessed February 20, 2020.
4. DesRoches CM, Campbell EG, Rao SR, et al. Electronic health records in ambulatory care—a national survey of physicians. *N Engl J Med.* 2008;359(1):50-60.
5. *Office-based Physician Electronic Health Record Adoption.* The Office of the National Coordinator for Health Information Technology. Available at https://dashboard.healthit.gov/quickstats/pages/physician-ehr-adoption-trends.php. Published January 2019. Accessed February 20, 2020.
6. *Non-federal Acute Care Hospital Electronic Health Record Adoption.* The Office of the National Coordinator for Health Information Technology. Available at https://dashboard.healthit.gov/quickstats/pages/FIG-Hospital-EHR-Adoption.php. Accessed February 20, 2020.
7. Zandieh SO, Yoon-Flannery K, Kuperman GJ, Langsam DJ, Hyman D, Kaushal R. Challenges to EHR implementation in electronic-versus paper-based office practices. *J Gen Intern Med.* 2008;23(6):755-61.
8. Vreeman DJ, Taggard SL, Rhine MD, Worrell TW. Evidence for electronic health record systems in physical therapy. *Phys Ther.* 2006;86(3):434-46, discussion 446-9.
9. *About the ONC.* The Office of the National Coordinator for Health Information Technology (ONC). Available at https://www.healthit.gov/topic/about-onc. Reviewed February 2019. Accessed February 20, 2020.
10. *Certified HER Technology.* Centers for Medicare & Medicaid Services. Available at https://www.cms.gov/Regulations-and-Guidance/Legislation/EHRIncentivePrograms/Certification. Accessed August 10, 2020.
11. *HER incentive programs 2015 through 2017 (modified stage 2) overview.* Centers for Medicare & Medicaid Services. Available at https://www.cms.gov/Regulations-and-Guidance/Legislation/EHRIncentivePrograms/Downloads/2015_EHR2015_2017.pdf. Accessed February 20, 2020.
12. *Quality Payment Program.* Centers for Medicare & Medicaid Services. Available at www.qpp.cms.gov. Accessed August 10, 2020.
13. *Delivery of Value Based Physical Therapy Services.* HOD P06-19-20-47. American Physical Therapy Association, Alexandria, VA. Available at https://www.apta.org/apta-and-you/leadership-and-governance/policies/delivery-value-based-pt-services. Published June 2008. Accessed February 20, 2020.
14. Blanchfield BB, Heffernan JL, Osgood B, Sheehan RR, Meyer GS. Saving billions of dollars-and physicians' time-by streamlining billing practices. *Health Aff.* 2010 Jun;29(6):1248-1254.
15. Menachemi N, Collum TH. Benefits and drawbacks of electronic health record systems. *Risk Manag Healthc Policy.* 2011;4:47-55.
16. Wang SJ, Middleton B, Prosser LA, et al. A cost-benefit analysis of electronic medical records in primary care. *Am J Med.* 2003 Apr;114(5):397-403.
17. Rutten LJ, Vieux SN, St Sauver JL, et al. Patient perceptions of electronic medical records use and ratings of care quality. *Patient Relat Outcome Meas.* 2014;5:17-23.
18. Anderson M, Perrin A. *Technology use Among Seniors. Internet & Technology.* Pew Research Center. Available at https://www.pewresearch.org/internet/2017/05/17/technology-use-among-seniors/. Published May 17, 2017. Accessed February 20, 2020.
19. Miller RH, Sim I. Physicians' use of electronic medical records: barriers and solutions. *Health Aff.* 2004;23(2):116-26.
20. Garavand A, Mohseni M, Asadi H, Etemadi M, Moradi-Joo M, Moosavi A. Factors influencing the adoption of health information technologies: a systematic review. *Electron Physician.* 2016 Aug;8(8):2713-2718.
21. Hsu J, Huang J, Fung V, Robertson N, Jimison H, Frankel R. Health information technology and physician-patient interactions: impact of computers on communication during outpatient primary care visits. *J Am Med Inform Assoc.* 2005;12(4):474-80.

22. Garrison GM, Bernard ME, Rasmussen NH. 21st-century health care: the effect of computer use by physicians on patient satisfaction at a family medicine clinic. *Fam Med.* 2002;34(5):362-8.
23. Frankel R, Altschuler A, George S, et al. Effects of exam-room computing on clinician-patient communication. *J Gen Intern Med.* 2005 Aug;20(8):677-82.
24. Gadd CS, Penrod LE. Dichotomy between physicians' and patients' attitudes regarding EMR use during outpatient encounters. *Proc AMIA Symp.* 2000;275-279. Available at http://www.ncbi.nlm.nih.gov/pmc/articles/PMC2243826/. Accessed February 20, 2020.
25. Koo CC. Getting Ready for EMR. Physician practices should consider several key factors before selecting an electronic medical record system. *Health Manag Technol.* 2004;25(8):26,28. Available at http://www.providersedge.com/ehdocs/ehr_articles/Getting_Ready_for_an_EMR.pdf. Accessed February 20, 2020.
26. Polack P. Training your staff for EMR. *Med Pract Trends.* October 29, 2008.
27. Lowes R. EMR Success: training is the key. *Med Econ.* 2004;81(9):TCP 11-4.
28. Kane LR. Best EMRs for small practices. *Medscape Business Medicine.* May 21, 2009. Available at https://www.medscape.com/viewarticle/702950_2. Accessed February 20, 2020.
29. Kleaveland B. The tech doctor: best-of-breed or integrated systems? *Physicians Practice.* 2007 June 17:17(9). Available at https://www.physicianspractice.com/health-it/tech-doctor-best-breed-or-integrated-systems. Accessed February 20, 2020.
30. Garg AX, Adhikari NKJ, McDonald H, et al. Effects of computerized clinical decision support systems on practitioner performance and patient outcomes. *JAMA.* 2005;293(10);1223-1238.
31. *Guide to Physical Therapist Practice, 3.0.* American Physical Therapy Association, Alexandria, VA. Available at http://guidetoptpractice.apta.org/. Accessed August 10, 2020.
32. *APTA's Defensible Documentation for Patient/Client Management.* American Physical Therapy Association, Alexandria, VA. Available at https://www.apta.org/your-practice/documentation. Accessed July 22, 2020.
33. *Physical Therapy Outcomes Registry.* American Physical Therapy Association, Alexandria, VA. Available at http://www.ptoutcomes.com/HowItWorks/. Accessed February 20, 2020.
34. *How to Use the National Correct Coding Initiative.* Centers for Medicare & Medicaid Services. Available at https://www.cms.gov/Medicare/Coding/NationalCorrectCodInitEd. Published January 2020. Accessed February 20, 2020.
35. *Individuals' Perceptions of the Privacy and Security of Medical Records and Health Information Exchange.* Health IT Quick-Stat #58. Office of the National Coordinator for Health Information Technology. Available at https://dashboard.healthit.gov/quickstats/pages/consumers-privacy-security-medical-record-information-exchange.php. Published June 2019. Accessed February 20, 2020.
36. *Breaches affecting 500 or more individuals.* U.S. Department of Health and Human Services (HHS) Office for Civil Rights. Available at https://ocrportal.hhs.gov/ocr/breach/breach_report.jsf. Published February 1, 2016. Accessed February 20, 2020.
37. *CMS electronic record incident report template.* Centers for Medicare & Medicaid Services. Available at https://www.cms.gov/Research-Statistics-Data-and-Systems/CMS-Information-Technology/InformationSecurity/Info-Security-Library-Items/RMH-Chapter-08-Incident-Response-Appendix-K-Incident-Report-Template. Accessed February 20, 2020.

ADDITIONAL RESOURCES

APTA HIPAA Resource Webpage

The Health Insurance Portability and Accountability Act (HIPAA) imposes numerous requirements on patient privacy and security issues. The APTA offers informational resources and links for providers to learn about compliance with HIPAA regulations. Available at https://www.apta.org/your-practice/compliance/hipaa.

Health Information Technology (HIT)

Updates on HIT program development and legislation, as well as APTA's related advocacy efforts. New guidelines on de-identification of protected health information. Available at http://www.apta.org/FederalIssues/HIT/

How to Implement EHRs

HealthIT.gov has developed a resource for providers and professionals to help with implementing EHRs. This is a six-step process with many useful resources. Available at https://www.healthit.gov/playbook/

ONC Guidance on EHR Vendor Contract Negotiations

This document explains a few key EHR contract terms and what you need to know about them. Understanding these terms may help you select an appropriate EHR system and protect your practice or organization from business and patient safety risks that may arise when you rely upon EHRs for critical aspects of your operations. Available at https://www.healthit.gov/sites/default/files/ehr_contracting_terms_final_508_compliant.pdf

APTA CONNECT

Created through a partnership between APTA and Cedaron Medical, Inc., APTA CONNECT is a point-of-care, computerized patient record system designed specifically for physical therapists. APTA CONNECT offers useful reports to track patient progress, practice management trends, referral, and resource utilization. Any data, be it initial patient registration or follow-up appointment, needs to be entered only once, regardless of the number of users. With APTA CONNECT, you can compare your performance from different time periods or benchmark your clinicians with each other. If you want an administrative report that is not currently available in APTA CONNECT, you can create it on-site and save it to meet your exact needs. Available at https://www.apta.org/your-practice/documentation/connect.

The Agency for Healthcare Research and Quality (AHRQ)

AHRQ and its community of contractors and grantees have developed tools to help healthcare organizations plan for, implement, and evaluate health information technology (IT). These tools describe and recommend strategies for addressing some of the common challenges organizations encounter when working with health IT systems. Available at http://healthit.ahrq.gov/portal/server.pt?open=512&objID=919&parentname=CommunityPage&parentid=8&mode=2&in_hi_userid=3882&cached=true

Office of the National Coordinator for Health Information Technology (ONC)

The Office of the National Coordinator for Health Information Technology (ONC) is the principal federal entity charged with coordination of nationwide efforts to implement and use the most advanced health information technology and the electronic exchange of health information. The position of national coordinator was created in 2004 through an executive order and legislatively mandated in the Health Information Technology for Economic and Clinical Health Act (HITECH Act) of 2009. Available at https://www.healthit.gov/topic/about-onc

HealthIT.gov

HealthIT.gov is a product of the joint efforts of the Office of the National Coordinator for Health Information Technology (ONC) and the Agency for Healthcare Research and Quality (AHRQ). It is intended that this site will eventually include content from other agencies within the Department of Health and Human Services (DHHS), as well as other federal agencies in health IT such as The Department of Defense/Health Affairs (DoD/HA), the Department of Veterans Affairs/Veterans Health Administration (VA/VHA), and others. Available at https://www.healthit.gov/

5 Content Standardization and Component Requirements

OBJECTIVES

Following completion of this chapter, the reader will be able to:

- Discuss the basic requirements for Medicare documentation.
- Identify ten content elements required in the initial examination and evaluation.
- Analyze the relationship between the patient/client's prior level of function and physical therapy.
- Describe the basic content requirements for a plan of care.
- Discuss the recommended frequency of documentation.
- List examples of terms that should be avoided in documentation.
- Compare and contrast certification and recertification in the Medicare context.
- Discuss under what circumstances is gait training skilled versus unskilled.

GENERAL DOCUMENTATION REQUIREMENTS

There are basic requirements for all physical therapy services: initial examination/evaluation, plan of care (POC), ongoing documentation of care/continuum of care, re-evaluation, and discharge summary or summation of care. The Centers for Medicare & Medicaid Services (CMS) was the first to delineate documentation requirements for physical therapists (PTs) by a payer source. Although there are some differences depending on the setting and the type of organization, the basic requirements are always included. Documentation is also guided by insurance mandates and language in a state's practice act. Florida, for instance, has documentation requirements that each therapist has to follow, although they are similar to those required by CMS for Medicare. The American Physical Therapy Association (APTA) has developed guidelines for documentation that are similar to the Medicare guidelines (see Table 5-1). The APTA guidelines represent best practice standards.

The use of standardized formats or templates for documentation and billing purposes aids in maintaining consistency within an organization or facility, as well as between therapy

Table 5–1 Medicare (CMS) and APTA Guidelines For Documentation

Medicare (requires some forms or similar format and content)	**APTA: Guide for Documentation** (provider choice of format)
Physician's/NPP's approval/signature on initial Plan of Care (POC)	Referral or referral mechanism (prescription)
Developed by PT	
Evaluation	Initial examination/evaluation
	History
Identification of objective losses by system	Systems review
	Tests and measures
	Evaluation: judgment
	Physical therapy diagnosis
	Level of severity
Prognosis	Prognosis
	Patient involvement in goals
	Measurable goals related to impairment, functional
POC	Limitations, disabilities
	Plan of care
	Authentication
Ongoing documentation of interventions	Progress report at least every 10 days
	Continuation of care
	Every visit or encounter
Re-evaluation/recertification of POC	Re-examination
Discharge	Summation of episode of care

personnel. Blank forms or pages lead to inconsistency and omission of information that may be crucial in supporting medical necessity for skilled physical therapy services. Although predesigned or keyed forms (or formats in the electronic medical record) do not guarantee the quality of content, if keys or legends are provided in each category, the information is more likely to be included. The APTA's *Guide to Documentation* includes sample forms (see Appendix E).[1] The forms in the guide are not detailed (with the exception of the history) and therefore should be used only as a guide to develop forms that best suit a facility's or organization's needs. This is applicable to manual entry forms as well as electronically generated formats.

Because these documentation elements are generic and widely used, therapists should attempt to use them consistently, regardless of the third-party payer or payment system. Durable medical equipment, such as orthotics or wheelchairs, may require not only the standard documentation to identify need but additional supporting letters from the therapist and/or physician, or state-specific forms, such as for Florida Medicaid wheelchairs.

The third-party payer will determine some of the documentation requirements that therapists will have to consider. There are varieties of forms or formats required or strongly recommended for billing of services. Examples include the CMS form number 1450 (also sometimes referred to as the UB-04 and, prior to that, the UB-92), the standard claim form used by institutional providers to bill Medicare Administrative Contractors (MACs) when a paper claim is allowed, which has been revised to include the National Provider Identification (NPI) number,[2] and the CMS Form Number 1500 (see Appendix C),[3] which providers sending professional and supplier claims to Medicare on paper must use.

Example

Coding for billing and documentation content

The treating PT or PTA documents the treatment preceding all descriptions with CPT verbiage.

Therapeutic exercise: passive stretching; 5 reps x 15 seconds of the hamstrings, reciprocal inhibition quadriceps/hamstrings to facilitate hamstring lengthening, manual resistive exercise with progressive resistance knee extension/flexion.

Since this is a timed code, either the billing department or the treating PT/PTA would need to ensure that the time was included.

1 unit 97110 /15 minutes: Therapeutic exercise: passive stretching; 10 reps x 30 seconds of the hamstrings, reciprocal inhibition quadriceps/hamstrings to facilitate hamstring lengthening, manual resistive exercise with progressive resistance knee extension/flexion.

As stated in the CMS Publication 100-04 Internet Only Manual Medicare Claims Processing Manual Chapter 26 Section 1:[4]

The Administrative Simplification Compliance Act (ASCA) requires that Medicare claims be sent electronically unless certain exceptions are met. Providers meeting an ASCA exception may send their claims to Medicare on a paper claim form. Providers sending professional and supplier claims to Medicare on paper must use Form CMS-1500 (see Appendix C) in a valid version. This form is maintained by the National Uniform Claim Committee (NUCC), an industry organization in which CMS participates. Any new version of the form must be approved by the White House Office of Management and Budget (OMB) before it can be used for submitting Medicare claims. When the NUCC changes the form, CMS coordinates its review, any changes, and approval with the OMB.

Author's Note

Medicare A/B MACS (B), durable medical equipment (DME) MACs, physicians, and suppliers are responsible for purchasing their own CMS-1500 claim forms. Forms can be obtained from printers or printed in-house as long as they follow the specifications developed by the NUCC. The only acceptable claim forms are those printed in Flint OCR Red, J6983 (or exact match) ink. Although a copy of the CMS-1500 form can be downloaded, copies of the form cannot be used for submission of claims, since your copy may not accurately replicate the scale and Optical Character Recognition (OCR) color of the form. The majority of paper claims sent to carriers and durable medical equipment regional carriers (DMERCs) are scanned using OCR technology. This scanning technology allows for the data contents contained on the form to be read while the actual form fields, headings, and lines remain invisible to the scanner. Photocopies cannot be scanned and therefore are not accepted by all carriers and DMERCs.

You can find Medicare CMS-1500 completion and coding instructions, as well as the print specifications, in Chapter 26 of the Medicare Claims Processing Manual (Pub.100-04). In order to purchase claim forms, you should contact the U.S. Government Printing Office at 1-866-512-1800, local printing companies in your area, and/or office supply stores. Medicare will accept any type (i.e., single sheet, snap-out, continuous feed, etc.) of the CMS-1500 claim form for processing. Each of these vendors sells the CMS-1500 claim form in its various configurations (single part, multipart, continuous feed, laser, etc.).[5]

As discussed in CMS Publication 100-04, Medicare Claims Processing Manual, chapter 5, rehabilitation agencies, when permissible, submit their claims to Medicare contractors using the ASC X12 837 institutional claim format (frequently referred to as CMS-1450 or UB-04 claim form). PTs in private practice, meanwhile, submit their claims using the ASC X 12 837 professional claim format (frequently referred to as CMS-1500 claim form). Check each commercial payer and Medicaid program policy to ensure understanding of the payer's coverage, coding, and billing requirements.[5]

Regardless of the form used for the documentation, the goal of the provider should be to submit a clean, error-free claim that matches the information both in the initial forms and reports and subsequent forms. If information is requested to support the bill, it should be self-explanatory and reinforce the information and charges on the claim form. It is essential that the instructions that come with each form be followed. In some cases, as in the use of the CMS-1500 form, modifiers are used to further specify a certain service or explain a service. For instance, Modifier 59[6] may be reported if the two procedures are performed in distinctly different 15-minute time blocks. Modifier 59 should not be used if the two procedures are performed during the same time block.[6]

The majority of non-Medicare payers follow the same coding and documentation initiatives as Medicare, including the National Correct Coding Initiative Procedure-to-Procedure Edits (CCI Edits).[7]

Author's Note

As stated on the APTA website, CMS developed the National Correct Coding Initiative (NCCI) to promote national correct coding methodologies and to control improper coding that leads to inappropriate payment in Part B claims. CMS developed its coding policies based on coding conventions defined in the American Medical Association's Current Procedural Terminology (CPT) manual, national and local policies and edits, coding guidelines developed by national societies, analysis of standard medical and surgical practices, and a review of current coding practices. For an explanation of the rationale for NCCI edits and as a general reference, carriers and fiscal intermediaries can use the *National Correct Coding Initiative Coding Policy Manual for Medicare Services*, which is updated annually.

NCCI includes three types of edits: NCCI procedure-to-procedure (PTP) edits, Medically Unlikely Edits (MUEs), and add-on code edits. PTP edits and MUEs are contained in a single table that includes the PTP code pairs that should not be reported together for a number of reasons, as explained in the *NCCI Coding Policy Manual*.

- **NCCI PTP edits** prevent inappropriate payment of services that should not be reported together. Each edit has a Column One and Column Two

HCPCS/CPT code, called a "pair." If a provider reports the two codes of an edit pair for the same beneficiary on the same date of service, the Column One code is eligible for payment, but the Column Two code is denied unless a clinically appropriate NCCI-associated modifier is permitted and reported. The NCCI PTP edits are divided into two provider types:

Practitioner—Applied to claims submitted by PTs in private practice, as well as by other nonphysician practitioners (NPPs) and physicians and by ambulatory surgery centers.

Hospital—Applied to claims submitted for services that are paid under the outpatient prospective payment system; for example, outpatient hospital services, Part B skilled nursing facilities, comprehensive outpatient rehabilitation facilities, outpatient physical therapy and speech-language pathology providers, and certain claims for home health agencies billing under types of claims identified as 22X, 23X, 75X, 74X, and 34X.

- **MUEs** prevent improper payment for an inappropriate number or quantity of the same service on a single day. An MUE for a Healthcare Common Procedure Coding System (HCPCS)/CPT code is the maximum number of units of service under most circumstances able to be reported by the same provider for the same beneficiary on the same date of service. MUEs are divided into three provider types:

  Practitioner MUEs are applied to all claims submitted by PTs, physicians, and other practitioners.

  DME Supplier MUEs are applied to claims submitted to DME MACs.

  Facility Outpatient MUEs are applied to all claims for types of bills identified as 13X, 14X, and 85X (critical-access hospitals).

- **Add-on code edits** consist of a listing of HCPCS and CPT add-on codes with their respective primary codes. An add-on code is eligible for payment only if one of its primary codes is also eligible for payment.[7]

Author's Note

Always check the CCI edits list to determine whether a modifier, such as Modifier 59,[6] can be used for a code pair. Frequently, when CPT 97140—manual therapy is billed with another code, such as 97530—therapeutic activities, the 59 modifier must be used to override the edit. If the appropriate modifier is not used, the insurer will likely reject the claim, stating that the services cannot be billed separately unless using the modifier. Documentation would also have to delineate this in the treatment. The CCI edits are updated on a quarterly basis and can be found on CMS's website. For additional information, see CMS's Modifier 59 Article[6] and APTA's web page on NCCI.[7]

It is the responsibility of the treating PT or physical therapy assistant (PTA) to know for the sake of documentation and billing if a payer has adopted the CCI edits.[7]

In addition to the use of forms, the terminology used in the documentation must be universally understood by all possible record "readers," yet sophisticated enough to justify the skilled care rendered. In this context, there are terms that can and should be used and terms that should be avoided. Terms that may be used by the therapist in conversation should not necessarily appear in the documentation. According to Baetan et al.[8] "Functional phrase alternatives are terms or phrases that convey to the reviewer the skilled nature of the service provided . . . the concept of using functional phrase alternatives can be expanded to all practice settings."[8]

CATEGORIES AND APPROPRIATE TERMINOLOGY

What to Avoid

There are words and verbiage that are considered "red flags" in professional documentation and may result in an automatic denial from some payers, but not necessarily others.

- Avoid using the terms "walking" when referring to gait training and "maintain" (unless used in the context of balance ability). The word walking should only be used in the context of quoting a patient, as in: Patient stated, "he wants to walk."
- Avoid repeated statements that indicate a patient is not progressing, is noncompliant or uncooperative, or is still unable, unless the intention is to discontinue the physical therapy. If any nonspecific words such as these are used, they should be clarified.
- Avoid using nondescriptive terms such as patient is "the same," "not improving," or "still not compliant." It is better to identify some aspect of the treatment that the patient is able to perform and demonstrate progress in, such as "The patient is now able to…"

Example

Patient is demonstrating noncompliance with this home exercise regime; stated: "I hate doing those exercises, so I'm not."

Patient was uncooperative during therapy today; he shouted to therapist "Go to hell," then picked up the walker and threw it toward the therapist.

This should also be avoided when describing the training or education a caregiver is receiving. For most skills that involve caregivers, a reasonable time must be established, similar to that for a specific patient goal.

Example

An initial established goal on a POC is:

Husband will be able to safely and consistently transfer patient (his wife) from the WC to and from the bed by ____________(indicate date or number of sessions)

Avoid in treatment or progress reports comments such as "husband is still unable to safely transfer wife" in spite of multiple training sessions.

Instead: Husband is now able to transfer his wife from the WC to the bed with minimal verbal instructions.

If it appears that the husband will not be able to execute a stand pivot or sliding board transfer, the goal needs to be terminated or modified (e.g., Husband will be able to safely and consistently transfer patient from the WC to bed using a mechanical lift.).

- Avoid terms without clear meaning, such as "uncooperative," confused," and "agitated," unless the plan is to discharge or unless specific clarification follows.
- Use of the word "maintain" should be used with caution. Other terms without clear meaning include tolerated well; general increase in; general improvement, strengthening, or supervision; poor carry through; declined in function; not responding to treatment; improved (unless objective data follows); and increased or decreased pain without reference to a scale that can be measured and related to function.

What to Include

Descriptive, objective terminology and data and measures should be included in your documentation. Examples include functionally oriented goals, distances, deficits with progress toward goals, and functional limitations and disabilities that can be affected during the episode of care by resolving impairments.

- Include documentation of essential function. Essential functions are those that an individual has to do versus wants to do. Any type of leisure activity, for example, is not an essential function. The ability to achieve in one's home to functionally move room to room, self-care, or get to the bathroom for toileting in functional times is essential.
- Once a patient has progressed to outpatient status, community safety and function must also be addressed. Use comparisons that illustrate progress and provide instruction in precautions, independent exercise, and caregiver training.
- Use skilled terminology that matches CPT code verbiage for interventions (i.e., therapeutic exercise, gait training) so that documentation content truly matches the billing codes. Terminology as indicated in the *Guide to Physical Therapist Practice 3.0*[9] is also acceptable and should include application of practice patterns for goals, interventions, and progress.
- Whenever possible, numbers—assuming they are universally understood or a key is provided—should be used to communicate in the medical record. Range of motion (ROM) should be expressed as fractions, indicating total "normal" range based on a standard (i.e., 120°/130° for shoulder flexion/extension, 45°/135° for knee flexion, and so on). ROM should be written to indicate the goal and the reason it is necessary, or the "in order to…" component.

Example

Increase AROM L shoulder flexion from 95°/180° to 180°/180° in order to maximally flex L shoulder and return to job as a house painter.

- Muscle performance or strength should be expressed in fractions based on a standardized scale, such as the 0/5 to 5/5 scale (using + or – as indicated). Strength goals should be written to indicate the goal strength and the reason it is necessary. Stating in a goal that "muscle strength will be increased by 1 grade" does not include a frame of reference for anyone reading the record.

Example

Increase strength of L shoulder flexion from 3/5 to 5/5 in order to return to job as a house painter, and sustain full flexion of the shoulder up to 6 hours/day.

If a patient, however, such as a geriatric client, can only perform maximal resistance with a single repetition or only early in the day, caution should be used when using a standard strength scale to describe muscle performance. In this case, the therapist may prefer to use verbiage that more accurately describes the reality of what the patient can do or describe strength relative to functional activities performed. Instead of writing quadriceps strength 5/5, it is better to identify the patient can only perform sit to stand out of the chair one time.

- Records should also include numeric expression of assistance with the component for which help is needed (i.e., minimal or limited assistance of 25%, moderate or extensive assistance of 50%, maximal or extensive assistance of 75%, or total assistance 100%), applied for transfers, transitional movements, gait, wheelchair mobility, balance, or other objective measures of gait with use of consistent terminology.

- Since the CPT code is gait training, consistently use "gait". Also included should be the components of the activity for which the percentage (%) assistance is needed. The entry, avoiding introduction of the term "ambulation" (although CMS accepts the use of the term). Walking is not a skilled term. It should also be noted that when using percentages to describe patient ability or dependence, the part of the activity that the patient needs assistance with should be included in the daily or weekly documentation, although it is not needed in the initial goal setting.

Example

Gait Training: fixed front wheeled rolling walker, even surface, no directional changes, 3-point discontinuous pattern; PWB LLE, minimal assist of 25% to keep walker from veering L/R, verbal instructions for consistent pattern, and for intermittent facilitation of PWB on LLE.

The initial examination is presented again as an overview because its importance cannot be stressed enough. If the appropriate content is in the initial examination or evaluation, including objective measures, reliable and valid tests and measures that are functionally oriented or disease specific, identified physical therapy problems, and clear delineation of the patient's deficits or problems that can be affected in a reasonable amount of time (frequency and duration), with appropriate goals and interventions, the appropriate baseline will be established for the total episode of care.

INITIAL EXAMINATION OR EVALUATION

The APTA includes four main documentation elements: initial examination and evaluation, visit, reexamination, and conclusion of episode of care summary. Practitioners may be more familiar with the colloquial terms of initial evaluation, daily/weekly notes, progress notes/reports, and discharge reports or summaries. (See Chapter 12 for more detailed specific information.)

What is important for each, regardless of the name, is the content. The initial report sets the tone for the record and should clearly establish the need for skilled therapy and the level of severity. Many of the elements included should be repeated in the discharge summary to determine if indeed the care rendered matched the initial problems and plan—especially standardized tests and measures. All data should be communicated as objectively as possible to allow for objective goal setting and justification of care. The categories from "Referral through Precautions" to "Reason for Skill through Authentication" should be included in all records. The PT will have to make decisions regarding which baseline tests and measures should be included based on the patient's primary complaint(s) and if disease-specific measurement tools are indicated.

Initial Visit

Author's Note

According to the *Guide to Physical Therapist Practice 3.0*[9] there are five elements of patient care: examination, evaluation, diagnosis, prognosis, and intervention.

Evaluation. The initial examination and evaluation is an integral component of physical therapy services. It is the clinical judgment of the PT based on the synthesis of data, information, and findings to establish the diagnosis, prognosis, and plan of care. It establishes the baseline data (including identified functional problems and related impairments that can be affected by skilled PT intervention) necessary for assessing the level of severity, expected rehabilitation potential, setting realistic (functionally oriented) goals, and measuring progress. The evaluation of the patient's condition must be the basis for the PT's treatment goals.

Author's Note

Evaluations only, without justification for intervention, may not be paid. The examination component of the evaluation should be psychomotor, observational and objective. The complete evaluation includes the cognitive clinical decision making based on the findings and realistic goals based on prognosis, medical status and other relevant information.

For record authenticity purposes, it is preferable to include as much information as possible in the record at the initial visit so an initial plan can be developed. In some situations, some of the tests and measures may have to be completed on subsequent visits. All initial patient visits should also include self or caretaker completion of an intake form with demographic information, payer/insurance information, reason for physical therapy, other treatment for current condition, and medical history form that has information that can be easily checked off. Medications, including prescription, over the counter, and supplements, should also be included for the PT to review.

Content of Initial Visit Documentation

1. ***Referral Information.*** The three types of referrals in physical therapy are self-referred, physician, and NPP referral. The ability to accept referrals may depend on state law and from whom a payer will accept referrals. If the patient is referred, the diagnoses and treatment requested must be included on the referral. The referral process may also include specific authorization if the patient is a member of a managed care plan. There are no standard referral requirements. If there are specific referral requirements, they would be based on the state practice act or payer specific.

   Although a Medicare beneficiary can start an episode of care through self-referral, the established treatment POC will have to be approved by a physician within 30 days of the first date of treatment. By signing the POC, the physician certifies that the beneficiary needs skilled rehabilitation services. However, the physician who approves the POC need not have seen the patient immediately preceding the referral. Nor does it have to be the same physician who approves and signs subsequent POC for recertification. He or she must advise the PT of the beneficiary's medical history, current diagnosis, and medical findings. This should include any precautions or contraindications to specific activities or indicate intensity of rehabilitation services.
2. ***Health Insurance Portability and Accountability Act (HIPAA) acknowledgement.*** A signed acknowledgement of the organization's HIPAA policies is required for all patients.[10]
3. ***Signed Consent.*** Consent to treat by the patient, legal guardian, or parent is required. There should also be signed or verbal consent to treat once treatment and effects are explained. In the case of verbal consent, the therapist should state in the documentation that treatment was discussed and that the patient or appropriate representative has agreed to treatment.
4. ***Patient Identification Information.*** Full name, gender, date of birth, and language spoken, including primary and secondary.

5. ***Start of Care Date (SOC).*** Date of the initial examination/evaluation to indicate the initiation of the episode of care.
6. ***Medical Diagnosis.*** Document the patient's primary and secondary diagnoses using the International Classification of Diseases, Tenth Revision, Clinical Modification (ICD-10-CM).[11]
7. ***Physical Therapy Diagnosis.*** The PT, based on the initial examination, establishes the physical therapy diagnosis or primary physical therapy problem. While the PT can list a physical therapy diagnosis, which is more functionally oriented, it is preferred to use a medical diagnosis, as this is what payers recognize, assuming the medical diagnosis (es) aligns specifically to the physical therapy.
8. ***Onset Date.*** *Should be recent.* If a chronic condition, list date of acute or recent exacerbation. Recent is usually no more than 3 to 6 months prior to the SOC, as this date will help the PT identify that skilled service is necessary.
9. ***Medical History.*** Include comorbidities (may be summarized if on separate intake form completed by patient with only relevant information summarized in the evaluation) and medications, as they may affect physical therapy, recent hospitalizations, circumstances regarding onset, general medical history including surgeries, and any prior treatment for the same problem by PTs or other practitioners. Information should also be obtained to ensure the patient is not receiving any simultaneous services that could be considered duplicative and will result in payment denial.
10. ***Related Medical Testing Results.*** As available to the PT.
11. ***Level of Severity.*** APTA and its collaborators developed a three-tiered system of CPT evaluation codes that went into effect beginning in 2017.[1] The evaluation codes reflect three levels of patient presentation: low complexity (97161), moderate complexity (97162), and high complexity (97163), and replace the current 97001 code. The new re-evaluation code (97164) replaces the current 97002. (See Chapter 12 for more detailed information.)
12. ***Patient/Family Therapy Goals.*** Goals are determined based on examination results and needs of the patient and family that are relevant and appropriate for the episode of care. This is a critical component consistent with the World Health Organization's (WHO) International Classification of Functioning, Disability, and Health (ICF).[12]

    Appropriate identification of patient problems with relevant goals is another key to successful documentation. Although goals should be functionally oriented, impairment-based goals should be included as they relate to function. The goals of the patient or caregiver(s) need to be addressed in the documentation. However, they must be achievable and appropriate for the episode of care. The therapist should provide goals for only the episode in which they are providing care. If a continuum is expected (i.e., acute care, to inpatient rehabilitation, to home health, to outpatient), each therapist establishes the goals for the setting and time period for which the patient is under their care. A therapist in one setting should never establish goals for therapy rendered in another setting.
13. ***Prior Functional Level.*** This should include mobility (home and community); work, school, leisure, and self-care (ADL [activities of daily living], IADL [instrumental activities of daily living]); and family care responsibilities/child care/elder care.
14. ***Social History/Support.*** Handedness: right/left; employment income source, school, leisure; family status; living arrangements (type of dwelling, presence or absence of stairs, location of bedrooms and bath); and support system.
15. ***Precautions/Contraindications/Barriers.*** Precautions may relate to medical conditions, as with cardiac precautions; surgical, as in total hip precautions for a posterolateral approach, weight bearing, or other. This should include the therapist's evolution and documentation of yellow flags. Contraindications would indicate that some procedure should not be performed for a specific reason (i.e., electrical stimulation to a body area close to a nonshielded pacemaker, or ultrasound use over a nonhealed fracture site). Barriers may include such things as physical barriers in a living environment, illiteracy, language, financial limitations, or lack of regular transportation. There could be a situation (red flag)

that physical therapy is contraindicated, and the patient will be referred to the appropriate healthcare provider.

16. ***Baseline Data from Tests and Measures***
    - ADLs (instrumental and functional; compare to prior level of function)
    - Aerobic capacity; activity tolerance/endurance
    - Balance
    - Cardiovascular/pulmonary
    - Cognition
    - Coordination
    - Gait ability or nongait mobility
    - General integrity
    - Hearing
    - Joint integrity
    - Mobility (bed, wheelchair)
    - Motor control/movement patterns (gross and fine motor skills)
    - Muscle performance/strength
    - Musculoskeletal status/findings
    - Neuromuscular/neuromotor development
    - Pain (measurable scale of 0/10 to 10/10, specifying body part and pain at rest and activity)
    - Posture
    - ROM: active versus passive versus active assistive; joint contracture
    - Reflexes
    - Sensory/proprioception
    - Systems review (as relevant to problem for specific episode of care)
    - Tone
    - Transfers/transitional movement
    - Vascular: capillary refill, skin temperature/condition, edema, extremity hair patterns, nails
    - Vision
    - Vital signs: radial pulse (other peripheral as applicable, blood pressure, respiration rate, breathing pattern) before, during, and after
    - Anthropometrics
    - Integument integrity: Wounds/ulcerations/any abnormalities or potential areas of concern
    - Functional deficits/abilities

    Whenever possible, standardized tests and measures that are functionally based or disease specific should be used. These can then be repeated throughout the patient's episode of care and at discharge to measure the patient's progress. Medicare Part B requires that standard tests and measures be used at initial examination or evaluation. The APTA OPTIMAL is one of the recommended measures.[13] However, the clinician can determine which test or measure is most appropriate.
17. ***Device Use.*** Protective or adaptive; orthotics (including splints and supports); prosthetics; assistive gait devices; communication devices (i.e., augmentative communication devices, communication boards, speech, hearing aids, glasses, electrolarynx [external]).

    Note: Passy-Muir valves have replaced the need for an electrolarynx in some cases in recent years.
18. ***Results of Any Special Tests.*** When possible, include language supporting the validity, sensitivity, or specificity of the test you use. Using this kind of language builds the case that there is a certain probability that a condition is present and that skilled service is indicated.
19. ***Architectural/Safety Considerations.*** The physical considerations of the home, work, school, and other environments/buildings, including access, presence of stairs, elevators,

ramps, bathrooms, door widths, bathroom accessibility, and so on. Safety relates to the patient's ability to function safely in an environment based on their abilities.

20. ***Prior Level of Function (PLOF).*** This is a general description of what the patient was able to do functionally prior to the "current episode" of illness, pathology, surgery, etc.

Example

PLOF

Patient was independent in gait without an assistive device, able to drive, perform all self-care, work, and participate in leisure activities.

21. ***Reason for Skilled Care, Referral or Need for Therapy Services, Assessment/Professional Judgment***

Example

Patient is now dependent for gait, transfers, bed mobility, and self-care.

22. ***Problem Summary.*** The physical therapy medical record should also include a summary of deficits identified in baseline data, preferably delineating the relationship between impairments and the functional limitations and disabilities but avoiding physiological impairment focus. This is where you justify in summary form the need for physical skilled services.

The current ICF model[12] includes a "list of body functions and structure, and a list of domains of activity and participation. Since an individual's functioning and disability occurs in a context, the ICF also includes a list of environmental factors." There is a difference in functional outcome reporting versus the *Guide to Physical Therapist Practice 3.0*[9] regarding impairment and functional limitation. In the Nagi disablement model, which is used in the second edition of the *Guide*, gait is considered an impairment. Gait in different environments and levels of quality, speed, and functional purposes are considered functional limitations. For Medicare purposes, concentration should be on essential functional activities (EFAs) as much as possible, based on the setting in which the patient is being treated. For example, home health would concentrate on EFA in the home. Once the progression is made to outpatient status, essential activities would expand into the environment outside the home and appropriate safe function.

23. ***Plan of Care.*** The physical therapy POC should include specific planned interventions using CPT or HCPCS terminology, including patient/caregiver instruction and a statement regarding patient and family involvement in goal setting. The POC should list the frequency and duration of the treatment and include all short- and long-term goals (time defined, functionally oriented). Rehabilitation potential for achievement of goals and prognosis should also be included, along with a statement of the medical necessity or need for skilled physical therapy (see Chapter 7 for more information on the definition of skilled services). Medicare requires the plan of care include diagnoses; long-term treatment goals; and type, amount, duration, and frequency of therapy services.

Author's Note

Medicare providers may have a separate document entitled POC since a physician/NPP signature is required.

- ***Authentication.*** Authentication consists of the signature of the both the PT and the certifying physician/NPP (for a Medicare POC) with attestation of the need for skilled physical therapy and agreement with the POC.

The POC must be kept on file and available for the MAC's review if requested. A physical therapy POC must include the type, amount, frequency, and duration of the services that are to be furnished and indicate the treatment diagnosis and anticipated goals.

24. ***Physical Therapist of Record***. The physical therapist who performs the initial evaluation of a patient shall be the physical therapist of record for that patient with ultimate responsibility. The physical therapist of record shall remain as such until a reassignment of that patient to another physical therapist of record has occurred.

It's the concept of hand off in the record.

With current staffing patterns in different venues in which physical therapy is performed, the evaluating PT may not be the PT responsible for the physical therapy management of the patient if he or she works per diem, part-time, occasionally or rotates to different units or sites. In these cases, the evaluating PT should indicate to whom the oversite should be shifted and as of when.

CMS guidelines for Medicare coverage of outpatient physical therapy, encompassed within the Medicare Benefit Policy Manual Chapter 15, states the following:[14]

The services must relate directly and specifically to a written treatment plan as described in this chapter. The plan, (also known as a POC or plan of treatment) must be established before treatment is begun. The plan is established when it is developed (e.g., written or dictated). The signature and professional identity (e.g., MD, DPT, OT) of the person who established the plan, and the date it was established must be recorded with the plan. After the plan has been created, it still needs to be certified within 30 days by the referring physician/NPP (consultation with the treating PT is recommended). Only a physician may establish a plan of care in a CORF.

Treatment under a plan. The evaluation and treatment may occur, and are both billable either on the same day or at subsequent visits. It is appropriate that treatment begins when a plan is established. Therapy may be initiated by qualified professionals or qualified personnel based on a dictated plan. Treatment may begin before the plan is committed to writing only if the treatment is performed or supervised by the same clinician who establishes the plan. Payment for services provided before a plan is established may be denied.

Two plans. It is acceptable to treat under two separate POCs when different physicians/NPPs refer a patient for different conditions and the payment is by two separate entities. It is also acceptable to combine the POCs into one plan covering both conditions if one or the other referring physician/NPP is willing to certify the plan for both conditions and payment is from the same entity. The treatment notes continue to require timed code treatment minutes and total treatment time and need not be separated by plan. Progress reports should be combined if it is possible to make clear that the goals for each plan are addressed. Separate progress reports referencing each POC may also be written at the discretion of the treating clinician or at the request of the certifying physician/NPP, but shall not be required by contractors.

There shall be different POCs for each type of therapy discipline. When more than one discipline is treating a patient, each must establish a diagnosis, goals, etc., independently. However, the form of the plan and the number of plans incorporated into one document are not limited as long as the required information is present and related to each discipline separately. For example, a PT may not provide services under an occupational therapist POC. However, both may be treating the patient for the same condition at different times in the same day for goals consistent with their own scope of practice. The amount of treatment refers to the number of times in a day the type of treatment will be provided. Where amount is not specified, one treatment session a day is assumed.

- ***Goals****. Long-term treatment goals should be developed for the entire episode of care in the current setting. When the episode is anticipated to be long enough to require more than one* *certification, the long-term goals may be specific to the part of the episode that is being certified. Goals should be measurable and pertain to identified functional impairments. Therapists typically also establish short-term goals, such as goals for a week or month of therapy, to help track progress toward the goal for the episode of care. If the expected episode of care is short—for example, therapy is expected to be completed in 4 to 6 treatment days—the long-term and short-term goals may be the same. In other instances, measurable goals may not be achievable, such as when treatment in a particular setting is unexpectedly cut short (such as when care is transferred to another therapy provider) or when the beneficiary suffers an exacerbation of his or her existing condition terminating the current episode; documentation should state the clinical reasons progress cannot be shown.*

- ***Frequency and Duration****. The frequency and duration must be specific, especially for Medicare, and not given in ranges. Physical therapy services are to be furnished in accordance with the plan of care established by the PT and approved by the physician responsible for the patient's care and may not be altered in type, amount, or duration by the therapist (except in the case of an adverse reaction to a specific treatment). The frequency refers to the number of times in a week the type of treatment is provided. Where frequency is not specified, one treatment is assumed. If a scheduled holiday occurs on a treatment day that is part of the plan, it is appropriate to omit that treatment day unless the clinician who is responsible for writing progress reports determines that a brief, temporary pause in the delivery of therapy services would adversely affect the patient's condition.*

The duration is the number of weeks, or the number of treatment sessions, for this POC. If the episode of care is anticipated to extend beyond the 90-calendar-day limit for certification of a plan, it is desirable, although not required, that the clinician also estimate the duration of the entire episode of care in this setting. The frequency or duration of the treatment may not be used alone to determine medical necessity, but these factors should be considered with other factors such as condition, progress, and treatment type to provide the most effective and efficient means to achieve the patient's goals. For example, it may be clinically appropriate, medically necessary, most efficient, and effective to provide short-term intensive treatment or longer-term and less frequent treatment depending on the individual's needs. It may be appropriate for therapists to taper the frequency of visits as the patient progresses toward an independent or caregiver-assisted self-management program with the intent of improving outcomes and limiting treatment time.

Example

Frequency and duration: 5x/week for 2 weeks, then 3x/week for 2 weeks 2x/week for 6 weeks

- Medical record documentation maintained by the PT with the certifying physician/NPP signature and must clearly indicate the medical necessity of each physical therapy modality covered by the Medicare program.
- The physician/NPP or PT *must document the patient's functional limitations in terms that are objective and measurable.* Documentation must show objective loss of joint motion, strength, or mobility (i.e., degrees of motion, strength grades, levels of assistance.) related to function.
- All claims submitted with an unlisted service or procedure must be accompanied by documentation that describes the service, supports medical necessity, and the rationale for using the treatment modality.

This previous section describes the minimum requirements for documentation. It is anticipated that clinicians may choose to make their plans more specific in accordance with good practice. For example, they may include these optional elements: specific treatment interventions, procedures, modalities or techniques, and the amount of each. Also, notations in the medical record of the beginning date for the plan are recommended, but not required, to assist Medicare contractors in determining the dates of services for which the plan was effective.

- **Changes to Therapy Plan (Medicare's requirements under 220.1.2).** *Changes are made in writing in the patient's record and signed by one of the following professionals responsible for the patient's care:*
  - *Physician/NPP*
  - *PT*
  - *Registered professional nurse or physician/NPP on the staff of the facility pursuant to the oral orders of the physician/NPP or therapist*

While the physician/NPP may change a plan of treatment established by the therapist providing such services, the therapist may not significantly alter a plan of treatment established or certified by a physician/NPP without their documented written or verbal approval. Physician/NPP certification of the significantly modified POC shall be obtained within 30 days of the initial therapy treatment under the revised plan. An insignificant alteration in the plan would be a change in the frequency or duration due to the patient's illness, or a modification of short-term goals to adjust for improvements made toward the same long-term goals. If a patient has achieved a goal or has had no response to a treatment that is part of the plan, the therapist may delete a specific intervention from the POC prior to physician/NPP approval. This shall be reported to the physician/NPP responsible for the patient's treatment prior to the next certification.

CERTIFICATION OF PLAN OF CARE

All providers billing for physical therapy services are required to maintain an established plan of treatment as a permanent part of the patient's clinical record. The plan must be established as soon as possible relative to the start of care.

METHOD AND DISPOSITION OF CERTIFICATION

Per the Medicare Benefit Policy Manual Chapter 15 Section 220.1.3:[14]

Certification requires a dated signature on the plan of care or some other document that indicates approval of the plan of care. It is not appropriate for a physician/NPP to certify a plan of care if the patient was not under the care of some physician/NPP at the time of the treatment or if the patient did not need the treatment. Since delayed certification is allowed, the date the certification is signed is important only to determine if it is timely or delayed. The certification must relate to treatment during the interval on the claim. Unless there is reason to believe the plan was not signed appropriately, or it is not timely, no further evidence that the patient was under the care of a physician/NPP and that the patient needed the care is required. The format of all certifications and recertifications and the method by which they are obtained is determined by the individual facility and/or practitioner. Acceptable documentation of certification may be, for example, a physician's progress note, a physician/NPP order, or a plan of care that is signed and dated by a physician/NPP, and indicates the physician/NPP is aware that therapy service is or was in progress and the physician/NPP makes no record of disagreement with the plan when there is evidence the plan was sent (e.g., to the office) or is available in the record (e.g., of the institution that employs the physician/NPP) for the physician/NPP to review. For example, if during the course of treatment under a certified plan of care a physician sends an order for continued treatment for 2 more weeks, contractors shall accept the order as certification of continued treatment for 2 weeks under the same plan of care. If the new certification is for less treatment than previously planned and certified, this new certification takes the place of any previous certification. At the end of the 2 weeks of treatment (which might extend more than 2 calendar weeks from the date the order/certification was signed) another certification would be required if further treatment was documented as medically necessary.

TIMING OF INITIAL CERTIFICATION

According to Medicare Benefit Policy Manual Chapter 15 Section 220.1.3:[14]

The provider or supplier (e.g., facility, physician/NPP, or therapist) should obtain certification as soon as possible after the plan of care is established, unless the requirements of delayed certification are met. "As soon as possible" means that the physician/NPP shall certify the initial plan as soon as it is obtained, or within 30 days of the initial therapy treatment. Since payment may be denied if a physician does not certify the plan, the therapist should forward the plan to the physician as soon as it is established. Evidence of diligence in providing the plan to the physician may be considered by the Medicare contractor during review in the event of a delayed certification.

Timely certification of the initial plan is met when physician/NPP certification of the plan is documented, by signature or verbal order, and dated in the 30 days following the first day of treatment (including evaluation). If the order to certify is verbal, it must be followed within 14 days by a signature to be timely. A dated notation of the order to certify the plan should be made in the patient's medical record.

Recertification is not required if the duration of the initially certified plan of care is more than the duration (length) of the entire episode of treatment.

Author's Note

For specific certification rules for hospital services, please see Publication 100-01 Internet Only Manual Medicare General Information, Eligibility, and Entitlement, Chapter 4, Section 20: https://www.cms.gov/Regulations-and-Guidance/Guidance/Manuals/Downloads/ge101c04pdf.pdf

Recertification of Plan of Care (Plan of Treatment)

Per Medicare Benefit Policy Manual Chapter 15 Section 220.1.3:[14]

Payment and coverage conditions require that the plan must be reviewed, as often as necessary but at least whenever it is certified or recertified to complete the certification requirements. ***It is not required that the same physician/NPP who participated initially in recommending or planning the patient's care certify and/or recertify the plans****. Recertifications that document the need for continued or modified therapy should be signed whenever the need for a significant modification of the plan becomes evident, or* ***at least every 90*** *days after initiation of treatment under that plan, unless they are delayed.*

Author's Note

CORF requirement, MBPM Chapter 12 Section 30:

"The CORF physician or the referring physician for physical therapy, occupational therapy and speech-language pathology services, must review the plan of treatment at least once every 90 days certifying that the patient needs or continues to need skilled rehabilitation services, the rehabilitation plan of treatment is being followed and that the patient is making progress in attaining the established rehabilitation goals. The 90-day period begins with the first day of rehabilitation therapy. (For survey and certification the plan of treatment review must meet the requirements at 42CFR 485.58(b)). When the patient has reached a point where no further progress is being made toward one or more of the rehabilitation goals, or the skills of a therapist are no longer required, Medicare coverage ends with respect to that aspect of the rehabilitation plan of treatment." https://www.cms.gov/Regulations-and-Guidance/Guidance/Manuals/Downloads/bp102c12.pdf.

Author's Note

Sending recertifications out a few days prior to the due date with a note of explanation and a return addressed envelope with an arrow "sticky" indicating where the signature goes or faxing and then sending it out to be signed may prevent undue delay.

Each facility should have a policy regarding how to obtain an original signature on orders or referrals taken verbally, by fax, or through other means if not in writing by the physician/NPP.

Author's Note

The patient's plan normally need not be forwarded with the claim but is retained in the provider's file. The provider must certify on the billing form that the plan is on file. The plan and other documentation must be submitted upon request.

Make sure the plan is established or reduced to writing either by the person who established the plan or by the PT when the PT makes a written record of that person's verbal/oral, electronic, e-mail or faxed orders before treatment begins. The plan must be promptly signed by the ordering physician and therapist and incorporated into the patient's clinical record.

DELAYED CERTIFICATION

Per Medicare Benefit Policy Manual Chapter 15 Section 220.1.3:[14]

Certifications are required for each interval of treatment based on the patient's needs, not to exceed 90 calendar days from the initial therapy treatment. Certifications are timely when the initial certification (or certification of a significantly modified plan of care) is dated within 30 calendar days of the initial treatment under that plan. Recertification is timely when dated during the duration of the initial plan of care or within 90 calendar days of the initial treatment under that plan, whichever is less. Delayed certification and recertification requirements shall be deemed satisfied where, at any later date, a physician/NPP makes a certification accompanied by a reason for the delay. Certifications are acceptable without justification for 30 days after they are due. Delayed certification should include one or more certifications or recertifications on a single signed and dated document.

Delayed certifications should include any evidence the provider or supplier considers necessary to justify the delay. For example, a certification may be delayed because the physician did not sign it, or the original was lost. In the case of a long delayed certification (over 6 months), the provider or supplier may choose to submit with the delayed certification some other documentation (e.g., an order, progress notes, telephone contact, requests for certification or signed statement of a physician/NPP) indicating need for care and that the patient was under the care of a physician at the time of the treatment. Such documentation may be requested by the contractor for delayed certifications if it is required for review.

It is not intended that needed therapy be stopped or denied when certification is delayed. The delayed certification of otherwise covered services should be accepted unless the contractor has reason to believe that there was no physician involved in the patient's care, or treatment did not meet the patient's need (and therefore, the certification was signed inappropriately).

Daily Treatment Notes or Progress Notes:
APTA: Continuum of Care. Daily Note/Treatment Note (format of choice)
Content of subsequent visit documentation

1. **Title of entry if not provided on form** (e.g., PT Treatment Note, PT Progress Note)
2. **Date.** Indicate the date of service.
3. **Patient's legal name.** First and last.
4. **Number of units for each intervention or time.** Timed codes are in 15-minute intervals. However, Medicare has an "8-minute" billing rule. When only one service is provided in a day, providers should not bill for services performed for less than 8 minutes. For any single timed CPT code in the same day measured in 15-minute units, providers bill a single 15-minute unit for treatment greater than or equal to 8 minutes, through and including 22 minutes. If the duration of a single modality or procedure in a day is greater than or equal to 23 minutes, through and including 37 minutes, then two units should be billed.
5. **Where treatment was rendered.** This may include how the patient got to the location (if it's not standard for all patients).
6. **Specific interventions**. Indicate what treatment interventions were used and where applied (i.e., lower extremity) with parameters including patient position.
7. **Equipment issued**, if any.
8. **Response/assessment of improvement**. Document the response to the intervention at visit (+ or −) or episode of care that you are describing. Include objectives measures when appropriate.
9. **Patient-related instructions**. Any patient-related instructions given or communication and if the patient was accompanied by someone else. (Indicate who this person was and the relationship to the patient. Document the instructions that were given to this person if indicated).
10. **Plan for follow-up visit**. Documentation identifying the plan for the subsequent visit or continued care.
11. **Authentication** (signature of PT, PTA, or both).

NOTE: *According to the Medicare Benefit Policy Manual Chapter 15 Section 220.3(E): Treatment Note:*[14]

The purpose of these notes is simply to create a record of all treatments and skilled interventions that are provided and to record the time of the services in order to justify the use of billing codes on the claim. Documentation is required for every treatment day, and every therapy service. The format shall not be dictated by contractors and may vary depending on the practice of the responsible clinician and/or the clinical setting. The treatment note is not required to document the medical necessity or appropriateness of the ongoing therapy services. Descriptions of skilled interventions should be included in the plan or the progress reports and are allowed, but not required daily. Non-skilled interventions need not be recorded in the treatment notes as they are not billable. However, notation of non-skilled treatment or report of activities performed by the patient or non-skilled staff may be reported voluntarily as additional information if they are relevant and not billed. Specifics such as number of repetitions of an exercise and other details included in the plan of care need not be repeated in the treatment notes unless they are changed from the plan.

Documentation of each treatment shall include the following required elements:

- Date of treatment.
- Identification of each specific intervention/modality provided and billed, for both timed and untimed codes, in language that can be compared with the billing on the claim to verify correct coding. Record each service provided that is represented by a timed code, regardless of whether or not it is billed, because the unbilled timed services may affect the billing.
- Total timed code treatment in minutes and total treatment time in minutes. Total treatment time includes the minutes for timed code treatment and untimed code treatment. Total treatment time does not include time for services that are not billable (e.g., rest periods). For Medicare purposes, it is not required that unbilled services that are not part of the total treatment minutes be recorded, although they may be included voluntarily to provide an accurate description of the treatment, show consistency with the plan, or comply with state or local policies. The amount of time for each specific intervention/modality provided to the patient may also be recorded voluntarily, but contractors shall not require it, as it is indicated in the billing. The billing and the total timed code treatment minutes must be consistent. See Pub. 100-04, chapter 5, section 20.2 for a description of billing timed codes.
- Signature and professional identification of the qualified professional who furnished or supervised the services and a list of each person who contributed to that treatment (i.e., the signature of Colin Brooks, PTA, with notation of phone consultation with Grant Shamus, PT, supervisor) when permitted by state and local law). The signature and identification of the supervisor need not be on each treatment note, unless the supervisor actively participated in the treatment. Since a clinician must be identified on the POC and the progress report, the name and professional identification of the supervisor responsible for the treatment is assumed to be the clinician who wrote the plan or report. When the treatment is supervised without active participation by the supervisor, the supervisor is not required to co-sign the treatment note written by a qualified professional. When the responsible supervisor is absent, the presence of a similarly qualified supervisor on the clinic roster for that day is sufficient documentation, and it is not required that the substitute supervisor sign or be identified in the documentation.

APTA Re-examination and Progress Notes or Reports: Periodic entries—weekly, biweekly, or monthly—are compiled based on the daily entries. According to Baetan et al., "The focus of the progress report is on the problems identified in the initial evaluation or any new problems that have developed since the last formal re-evaluation [*or initial examination/evaluation*]. Documentation describing the skilled intervention provided, complicating factors that may have affected the duration of skilled care, and comparative data."[8]

Significant progress toward functional goals, modification of goals, and completion of goals should be evident. If progress is not demonstrated, justification of this lack of progress, as well as justification for continued care with modified goals and plans as indicated, must be included. Authentication of any change in care is required.

If the entry is a progress note (narrative or SOAP format), the following is also needed:

1. **Brief statement of overall functional progress**, not necessarily addressing all goals (as in progress reports) In a SOAP format, this would be the "A," or assessment/analysis section.
2. **Additions/deletions of treatments**

Author's Note

A progress note would include the same information as a treatment note, in addition to a statement of progress relative to the initial or interim goals established. It is usually longer, as it relates to a longer period of time (i.e., a week, multiple weeks).

DOCUMENTATION OF CONTINUATION OF CARE

According to the Medicare guidelines, "The office/progress note must contain necessary and sufficient information, which indicates the services were actually provided and were reasonable and necessary to treat the patient's condition." The categories described in the APTA's *Defensible Documentation* include "Documentation of intervention or services provided and current patient/client status, and Documentation of Reexamination."[1] It is the therapist's or organization's responsibility to determine the format in which the information should be included.

NOTE: *According to the Medicare Benefit Policy Manual Chapter 15 Section 220.3(D): Progress Report:*[14]

The Progress Report provides justification for the medical necessity of treatment. ***For Medicare payment purposes, the minimum progress report period must be at least once every 10 treatment days.*** *For Medicare payment purposes, information required in progress reports shall be written by a clinician that is, either the physician/NPP who provides or supervises the services, or by the therapist who provides the services and supervises an assistant. It is not required that the referring or supervising physician/NPP sign the progress reports written by the therapist.*

Note: Although PTAs may write elements of the progress report dated between the therapist's report, reports written by PTAs are not complete progress reports. *The PT must write a progress report during each progress report period, regardless of whether the physical therapist assistant writes other reports.* The elements of a progress report are discussed in the following sections.

Note: A re-evaluation should not be completed before every progress report routinely, but may be appropriate when assessment suggests changes not anticipated in the original POC.

Author's Note

According to the Medicare Benefit Policy Manual Chapter 15 Section 220:[14]

Re-evaluation is separately payable and is periodically indicated during an episode of care when the professional assessment of a clinician indicates a significant improvement, or decline, or change in the patient's condition or functional status that was not anticipated in the plan of care. Although some state regulations and state practice acts require re-evaluation at specific times, for Medicare payment, re-evaluations must also meet Medicare coverage guidelines. The decision to provide a re-evaluation shall be made by a clinician.

DISCHARGE SUMMARY

APTA Summation of Episode of Care and Discharge Report or Discharge Evaluation:

At the end of the episode of care, the patient status, summarized from initial examination and evaluation through the final visit, is required. This summary should address all initial or modified goals and progress or achievement of them. If goals were not achieved, indicate why.

The summation should also include:

- A description of interventions rendered during care, including total number of sessions and the duration (dates) and frequency of the sessions. If specific tests and measures were administered at the initial visit, they should be repeated to show objective change and improvement.
- The patient's discharge disposition, plan for next level of care with recommendations as applicable (including home with instructions), and any other instructions or training, equipment dispensed, and safety concerns. Authentication is required.

Author's Note

In circumstances where timely discharge reports are not completed, a summary may be the best way to close out a record based on the information included in the daily entries. If a patient self-terminates care, a discharge summary indicating such with a summary of care determined by the daily entries should be completed when it has been established that the patient is not returning. A discharge report or evaluation that includes analysis and plans for further care requires completion by a PT. According to the APTA, all summations of care should be completed by the PT. Medicare requires that a PT see a Medicare patient pre-discharge and complete the discharge summary.

In practice settings that use outcome assessment measures, such as the APTA Physical Therapy Outcomes Registry[15] or Focus on Therapeutic Outcomes (FOTO), used in outpatient settings, values at initial examination and final re-examination should be included.

Author's Note

APTA launched the Physical Therapy Outcomes Registry in 2017 to provide a user-friendly system for collecting uniform data on patient and client outcomes. Data will help guide best practices, help providers meet regulatory reporting requirements, generate benchmarking reports, and help shape payment policy.[15]

NOTE: *According to the Medicare Benefit Policy Manual Chapter 15 Section 220.3(D): Discharge Note (or Discharge Summary):*[14]

Medicare requires a Discharge Note for each episode of outpatient treatment. *In provider settings where the physician/NPP writes a discharge summary and the discharge documentation meets the requirements of the provider setting, a separate discharge note written by a therapist is not required. The discharge note shall be a progress report written by a clinician and shall cover the reporting period from the last progress report to the date of discharge. In the case of a discharge unanticipated in the plan or previous progress report, the clinician may base any judgments required to write the report on the treatment notes and verbal reports of the assistant or qualified personnel. In the case of a discharge anticipated within 3 treatment days of the progress report, the clinician may provide objective goals which, when met, will authorize the assistant or qualified personnel to discharge the patient. In that case, the clinician should verify that the services provided prior to discharge continued to require the skills of a therapist, and services were provided or supervised by a clinician. The discharge note shall include all treatment provided since the last progress report and indicate that the therapist reviewed the notes and agrees to the discharge. At the discretion of the clinician, the discharge note may include additional information; for example, it may summarize the entire episode of treatment, or justify services that may have extended beyond those usually expected for the patient's condition. Clinicians should consider the discharge note the last opportunity to justify the medical necessity of the entire treatment episode in case the record is reviewed. The record should be reviewed and organized so that the required documentation is ready for presentation to the contractor if requested.*

Medicare: Reasonable and Necessary Outpatient Physical Therapy Services

To be covered under Medicare, physical therapy services must relate directly and specifically to the plan of treatment described in the Medicare Benefit Policy Manual, Chapter 15,

Section 220,[14] and be reasonable and necessary to the treatment of the individual's illness or injury. Services related to activities for the general well-being and welfare of patients (i.e., general exercises to promote overall fitness and flexibility and activities to provide diversion or general motivation) do not constitute physical therapy services for Medicare purposes.

A physical therapy initial evaluation (excluding routine screening) is covered when it is reasonable and necessary for the qualified PT to determine if there is an expectation that either rehabilitative or maintenance services are appropriate for the patient's condition. When a patient exhibits a demonstrable change in physical functional ability, re-evaluations are covered to re-establish appropriate treatment goals (re-evaluations are also covered for ongoing assessment of the patient's rehabilitation needs). Initial evaluations or re-evaluations that are determined reasonable and necessary are covered even though the expectations are not realized or when the evaluation determines that skilled rehabilitation is not needed.

Author's Note

Evaluations only, without justification for intervention, may not be paid.

- ***Reasonable and necessary.*** In order for services to be considered reasonable and necessary, the services must be considered under accepted standards of medical practice to be a specific and effective treatment for the patient's condition.

The services must be of such a level of complexity and sophistication or the condition of the patient must be such that the services required can be safely and effectively performed only by or under the supervision of a qualified PT. Services that do not require the performance or supervision of a PT are not considered reasonable or necessary physical therapy services even if they are performed or supervised by a PT.

There must be an expectation that the condition will improve significantly in a reasonable (and generally predictable) period of time based on the assessment made by the physician of the patient's restoration potential after any needed consultation with the qualified PT. Alternatively, the services must be necessary to establish a safe and effective maintenance program required in connection with a specific disease state. The amount, frequency, and duration of the services must be reasonable.

Author's Note

When the MAC determines the services furnished were of a type that could have been safely or effectively performed only by or under the supervision of a qualified PT, it presumes that such services were properly supervised. However, this assumption may be rebutted. If, in the course of a medical review, the MAC finds that physical therapy services are not being furnished under proper supervision, the MAC denies the claim.

Medicare will not pay for physical therapy student–rendered care. However, the student may assist the PT if the PT is directly supervising and not engaged in treating other patients at the same time.

Claims for physical therapy services denied because the services are not considered reasonable and necessary are excluded from coverage and are thus subject to consideration under the waiver of liability provision in §1879 of the Social Security Act.

Types of Therapy

Rehabilitative Therapy

To constitute physical therapy, a service must be reasonable and necessary to the treatment of the individual's illness. If an individual's expected restoration potential is insignificant in relation to the extent and duration of physical therapy services required to achieve such potential, the services are not considered reasonable and necessary. In addition, there must be an expectation that the patient's condition will improve significantly in a reasonable (and generally predictable) period of time. If at any point in the treatment of an illness it is determined that the expectations will not materialize, the services are no longer considered reasonable and necessary and are excluded from coverage. All therapy provided consists of skilled and medically necessary services and is appropriate to each patient's POC.[16]

Author's Note

According to Medicare Benefit Policy Manual Chapter 15, Section 220.2:[14]

Rehabilitative therapy includes services designed to address recovery or improvement in function and, when possible, restoration to a previous level of health and well-being. Therefore, evaluation, re-evaluation and assessment documented in the Progress Report should describe objective measurements which, when compared, show improvements in function, decrease in severity or rationalization for an optimistic outlook to justify continued treatment. Improvement is evidenced by successive objective measurements whenever possible (see objective measurement and other instruments for evaluation in the §220.3.C of this chapter). If an individual's expected rehabilitation potential is insignificant in relation to the extent and duration of therapy services required to achieve such potential, rehabilitative therapy is not reasonable and necessary.

Maintenance Therapy

Skilled therapy services that do not meet the criteria for rehabilitative therapy may be covered by Medicare in certain circumstances as maintenance therapy under a maintenance program.

The goals of a maintenance program would be, for example, to maintain functional status or to prevent or slow further deterioration in function. Coverage for skilled therapy services related to a reasonable and necessary maintenance program is available in the following circumstances:

- Establishment or design of maintenance programs: If the specialized skill, knowledge, and judgment of a qualified therapist are required to establish or design a maintenance program to maintain the patient's current condition or to prevent or slow further deterioration, the establishment or design of a maintenance program by a qualified therapist is covered.
- If skilled therapy services by a qualified therapist are needed to instruct the patient or appropriate caregiver regarding the maintenance program, such instruction is covered. If skilled therapy services are needed for periodic re-evaluations or re-assessments of the maintenance program, such periodic re-evaluations or re-assessments are covered.

According to CMS, "The deciding factors are always whether the services are considered reasonable, effective treatments for the patient's condition and require the skills of a therapist, or whether they can be safely and effectively carried out by nonskilled personnel or caregivers."[14]

Co-Treatment/Team Therapy

There may be instances where two or more disciplines are providing therapy services to the same patient. There may also be occasions where these services are duplicative. Your MAC uses your documentation to determine if duplication exists.

For guidance on appropriate Medicare billing in the outpatient setting, please refer to CMS's 11 Part B Billing Scenarios for PTs and OTs:[16]

> *Therapists, or therapy assistants, working together as a "team" to treat one or more patients cannot each bill separately for the same or different service provided at the same time to the same patient. CPT codes are used for billing the services of one therapist or therapy assistant. The therapist cannot bill for his/her services and those of another therapist or a therapy assistant, when both provide the same or different services, at the same time, to the same patient(s). Where a physical and occupational therapist both provide services to one patient at the same time, only one therapist can bill for the entire service or the PT and OT can divide the service units. For example, a PT and an OT work together for 30 minutes with one patient on transfer activities. The PT and OT could each bill one unit of 97530. Alternatively, the 2 units of 97530 could be billed by either the PT or the OT, but not both. Similarly, if two therapy assistants provide services to the same patient at the same time, only the service of one therapy assistant can be billed by the supervising therapist or the service units can be split between the two therapy assistants and billed by the supervising therapist(s).*

For guidance on appropriate Medicare billing in the inpatient setting, please refer to CMS's regulations and policies for the applicable setting.

Author's Note

Please also refer to the Joint Guidelines for Therapy Co-treatment under Medicare produced by the APTA, American Speech-Language-Hearing Association (ASHA), and American Occupational Therapy Association (AOTA).

The following are some examples where there is not a duplication of services:

1. ***Transfers.*** Physical therapy instructs the patient in transfers to ascertain the level of safety with the techniques. Occupational therapy instructs and utilizes transfers as they relate to the performance of daily living skills (e.g., transfer from wheelchair to bathtub for bathing).
2. ***Pulmonary.*** Physical therapy teaches the patient an adapted breathing program. Occupational therapy carries the breathing retraining program into ADL training.
3. ***Hip Fractures/Arthroplasties***. Physical therapy instructs the patient in hip precautions and gait training. Occupational therapy carries out and reinforces the precautions when training the patient in ADLs (e.g., lower extremity dressing, toileting, and bathing).
4. ***Stroke.*** Physical therapy utilizes upper extremity neurodevelopmental treatment (NDT) techniques to assist the patient in positioning the upper extremities on a walker and in gait training. Occupational therapy utilizes upper extremity NDT techniques to increase the functional use of upper extremities for dressing, bathing, grooming, and so on.

   As with all rehabilitation services, your documentation must indicate a reasonable expectation that the patient will make material improvement within a reasonable period of time.
5. ***Professional Services.*** Services are sometimes performed by speech-language pathologists, occupational therapists, and PTs in concert with other health professionals. Services may be documented as performed by a team, with each member performing unique roles. Do not document duplicate services. Clearly delineate roles. Services may include but are not limited to the following example:

Example

One professional is assisting with positioning, adaptive self-help devices, inhibiting abnormal oromotor, and/or postural reflexes while another professional is addressing specific exercises to improve oromotor control, determining appropriate food consistency form, assisting the patient in difficulty with muscular movements necessary to close the buccal cavity, or shaping food in the mouth in preparation for swallowing. Another professional might address a different role, such as increasing muscle strength, sitting balance, and head control.

Relate the documentation to either loss of function or potential for change. As with other conditions and disorders, the reasonableness and necessity of services must be evident in your documentation.

Include:

- Changes in condition or functional status
- History and outcome of previous treatment for the same condition
- Other information that would justify the start of care

Even where a patient's full or partial recovery is not possible, a skilled service still could be needed to prevent deterioration or to maintain current capabilities.

Author's Note

If there are complicating comorbidities or the potential for decline, skilled services may be indicated on an inpatient, home health, or outpatient basis.

Example

A primary need of a nonambulatory patient may be frequent changes of position in order to avoid development of decubitus ulcers. However, since such changing of position does not ordinarily require skilled nursing or skilled rehabilitation personnel, it would not constitute a skilled service, even though such services are obviously necessary. However, if instruction to caretakers is needed for positioning and transfer training, the short-term skilled instruction, with appropriate documentation, should be covered.

Example

A patient has undergone peripheral vascular disease treatment, including revascularization procedures (bypass), with open or necrotic areas of skin on the involved extremity. Skilled observation and monitoring of the vascular supply of the legs is required.

Example

A patient has undergone hip surgery and has been transferred to an SNF. Skilled observation and monitoring of the patient for possible adverse reaction to the operative procedure, development of phlebitis, skin breakdown, or need for the administration of subcutaneous heparin is both reasonable and necessary, as well as rehabilitation services to regain function.

Example

A patient has been hospitalized following a heart attack and, following treatment but before mobilization, is transferred to the SNF. Because it is unknown whether exertion will exacerbate the heart disease, skilled observation is reasonable and necessary, as skilled mobilization and rehabilitation is initiated until the patient's treatment regimen is essentially stabilized.

Example

A frail 85-year-old man was hospitalized for pneumonia. The infection was resolved, but the patient, who had previously maintained adequate nutrition, will not eat or eats poorly. The patient is transferred to an SNF for monitoring of fluid and nutrient intake, assessment of the need for tube feeding, and forced feeding if required. Observation and monitoring by skilled nursing personnel of the patient's oral intake is required to prevent dehydration. In order to remobilize the patient, skilled rehabilitation services to regain function are needed.

If a patient was admitted for skilled observation but did not develop a further acute episode or complication, the skilled observation services still are covered so long as there was a reasonable probability for such a complication or further acute episode. "Reasonable probability" means that a potential complication or further acute episode was a likely possibility.

General Comment to Skilled Physical Therapy

It will be the provider's responsibility to demonstrate in all forms of documentation that skilled physical therapy services were provided to the patient. The documentation should support and justify the services billed. If the documentation is inadequate and does not comply with all requirements applicable to the payer's policy, claims could be denied. All therapy provided consists of skilled and medically necessary services and is appropriate to each patient's plan of care.[16]

Author's Note

The documentation guidelines in Medicare Benefit Policy Manual Chapter 15, Sections 220 and 230 identify the *minimal expectations of documentation by providers or suppliers or beneficiaries submitting claims for payment of therapy services to the Medicare program.* State or local laws and policies, or the policies or professional guidelines of the relevant profession, the practice, or the facility may be more stringent.[14]

Some examples where complete documentation outlining the need for skilled physical therapist services include:

- The existence of a plaster cast on an extremity generally does not indicate a need for skilled care. However, a patient with a preexisting acute skin problem, preexisting peripheral vascular disease, or a need for special traction of the injured extremity might need skilled nursing or skilled rehabilitation personnel to observe for complications or to adjust traction.
- Whirlpool baths do not ordinarily require the skills of a PT. However, the skills, knowledge, and judgment of a PT might be required where the patient's condition is complicated by circulatory deficiency, areas of desensitization, or open wounds.

General. Per the Medicare Benefit Policy Manual Chapter 15, Section 220.2(B),[14] skilled physical therapy services must meet all of the following conditions to be considered reasonable and necessary:

- The services shall be considered under accepted standards of medical practice to be a specific and effective treatment for the patient's condition. Acceptable practices for therapy services are found in:
    - Medicare manuals (such as this manual and Publications 100-03 and 100-04),
    - Contractors' local coverage determinations and national coverage determinations (LCDs and NCDs) are available on the Medicare Coverage Database.[17] The Medicare Coverage Database contains all National Coverage Documents, LCDs, and articles. The National Coverage Documents include NCDs, national coverage analyses (NCAs), coding analyses for labs (CALs), Medicare Evidence Development & Coverage Advisory Committee (MEDCAC) meetings, and Medicare coverage guidance documents.[17]
    - Guidelines and literature of the professions of physical therapy, occupational therapy, and speech-language pathology.
- The services shall be of such a level of complexity and sophistication or the condition of the patient shall be such that the services required can be safely and effectively performed only by a therapist, or in the case of physical therapy and occupational therapy, by or under the supervision of a therapist. Services that do not require the performance or supervision of a therapist are not skilled and are not considered reasonable or necessary therapy services, even if they are performed or supervised by a qualified professional. Medicare coverage is based upon the beneficiary's need for skilled care. Continuation of skilled services is based on the presence or absence of a beneficiary's potential for improvement from the therapy.
- While a patient's particular medical condition is a valid factor in deciding if skilled therapy services are needed, a patient's diagnosis or prognosis cannot be the sole factor in deciding that a service is or is not skilled. The key issue is whether the skills of a therapist are needed to treat the illness or injury, or whether the services can be carried out by nonskilled personnel.
- The amount, frequency, and duration of the services must be reasonable under accepted standards of practice.

EXAMPLE

An 80-year-old, previously ambulatory, postsurgical patient has been bedbound for 1 week and, as a result, has developed muscle atrophy, orthostatic hypotension, joint stiffness, and lower extremity edema. To the extent that the patient requires a brief period of daily skilled physical therapy services to restore lost functions, those services are reasonable and necessary.

Author's Note

Based on progress, this patient would probably qualify for continued services on a home health and possibly outpatient basis to return to independence.

Example

A patient with congestive heart failure also has diabetes and previously had both legs amputated above the knees. Consequently, the patient does not have a reasonable potential to achieve ambulation, but still requires daily skilled physical therapy to learn bed mobility and transferring skills, as well as functional activities at the wheelchair level.

Author's Note

If the patient has a reasonable potential for achieving those functions in a reasonable period of time in view of the patient's total condition, the physical therapy services are reasonable and necessary.

If the expected results are insignificant in relation to the extent and duration of physical therapy services required to achieve those results, the physical therapy would not be reasonable and necessary, and thus would not be covered skilled physical therapy services.

Author's Note

Medicare Benefit Policy Manual, Chapter 1—Inpatient Hospital Services Covered Under Part A. Centers for Medicare & Medicaid Services states:[18]

For detailed guidance on the required qualifications of a therapist, required skills of a therapist, and medically necessary and appropriately documented therapy services, see Pub. 100-02, Medicare Benefit Policy Manual, Chapter 15, Sections 220 and 230. The policies in those sections describe a standard of care that should be consistent throughout the therapy disciplines, regardless of the setting of care.

MACs frequently rely on the language in the Medicare Benefit Policy Manual, Chapter 1 to require therapists and therapist assistants who furnish care in the SNF Part A setting to comply with the documentation requirements in the Medicare Benefit Policy Manual, Chapter 15, Sections 220 and 230, such as the progress report. PTs and PTAs should be aware of Medicare Benefit Policy Manual, Chapter 1, in addition to the setting-specific chapters (Medicare Benefit Policy Manual Chapter 7 is applicable to HHAs, Chapter 8 is applicable to SNFs, etc.)

TELEHEALTH

Telehealth is the use of electronic information and telecommunication technologies to remotely provide healthcare information and services. *The Health Resources and Services Administration (HRSA) of the U.S. Department of Health and Human Services (HHS) defines telehealth as "the use of electronic information and telecommunications technologies to support and promote long-distance clinical health care, patient and professional health-related education, and public health and health administration. Technologies include videoconferencing, the internet, store- and-forward imaging, streaming media, and landline and wireless communications.*[19] Medicare at this time does not recognize physical therapy for telehealth payment, but during the COVID-19 public health emergency, Medicare temporarily recognizes physical therapy providers as eligible to furnish and bill telehealth services. *Two-way, real-time interactive communications, e-visits, virtual check-ins, remote evaluation of visual recordings, and telephone assessment and management services all are telehealth services covered under Medicare when furnished by PTs in response to the COVID-19 public health emergency.*[20] See Chapter 13 for more information. These telehealth services may also be covered by commercial payers. For all payers, you'll need to first determine if your state practice act enables you to legally provide services via telehealth and, second, check with each payer policy to see if PTs and PTAs are included as providers eligible to be paid for telehealth services.[20] Different states have regulations on the ability to practice telehealth. For example, in Florida one must register to be able to provide telehealth services

Applications of telehealth in physical therapy have expanded throughout patient care and consultation, as it allows PTs to better communicate with patients and provide more flexible care.[19] Telehealth gives PTs and PTAs the flexibility to provide quality services in a greater capacity, especially for patients that have transportation issues or who are looking for a modified type of services in their home.

Examples of physical therapy practitioners using telehealth technologies include the following:

- Physical therapy practitioners use telehealth technologies to conduct evaluations or provide quicker screening, assessment, and referrals that improve care coordination.
- Physical therapy practitioners provide interventions using telehealth by observing how patients move and perform exercises and activities. Physical therapy practitioners then provide verbal and visual instructions and cues to modify how patients perform various activities. They also may change the environment to encourage more optimal outcomes.
- Physical therapy practitioners use telehealth technologies to provide prehabilitation and conduct home safety evaluations.
- Physical therapy practitioners use telehealth technologies to observe how patients interact with their environment and/or other caregivers and provide caregiver education. Physical therapy practitioners are able to assess the carryover of the activity modification strategies and activities to determine effectiveness.
- Physical therapists provide consultative services by working with other physical therapists, physical therapist assistants, and other health care providers to share expertise in specific movement-related activities to optimize the patient's participation.

Physical therapy practitioners use telehealth for quick check-ins with established patients.[20]

TWO-WAY, REAL-TIME INTERACTIVE COMMUNICATION

This form of telehealth entails real-time two-way interaction between the provider and patient or caregiver using audio and video communication technology. Eligible services are reported using the same CPT codes that describe in-person services. When billing Medicare during the COVID-19 public health emergency, also required are: (1) place of service code that reflects where the service would have been furnished in person; (2) modifier 95 to attest that the service was furnished via telehealth; and (3) the GP modifier.[20]

E-VISITS

CMS has waived certain Medicare restrictions on digital communication in light of the COVID-19 pandemic, including "e-visits." In CMS' 2021 Physician Fee Schedule proposed rule, the agency has proposed to permanently allow PTs to furnish and bill these services after the public health emergency (PHE) ends. APTA's article "Furnishing and Billing E-Visits: Addressing Your Questions" states:[21]

E-visits are *"non face-to-face patient-initiated digital communications that require a clinical decision that otherwise typically would have been provided in the office." The code descriptors for the HCPCS codes related to e-visits indicate that the codes are intended to cover short-term (up to 7 days) assessments and management activities that are conducted online or via some other digital platform and include any associated clinical decision-making.*

An e-visit can comprise more than one communication between you and your patient, and includes all activities that you perform to meet the assessment and management needs as identified by the patient. The maximum duration of an e-visit is 7 days.

An e-visit is not a treatment session, and it does not meet the Medicare definition of telehealth.

The 7-day period begins when you respond to the patient's request to initiate the e-visit and ends 7 calendar days after that response.

You cannot bill an e-visit if you saw the patient in a face-to-face visit fewer than 7 days before the e-visit or if you see the patient in a face-to-face visit fewer than 7 days after the e-visit.

Documentation of an e-visit should include all communication and actions that you take, as well as the following:

- That the e-visit was initiated by the patient.
- That the patient consented to the e-visit.
- The clinical decision-making that occurred as a result of the e-visit.
- For Medicare, bill the e-visit once for the 7-day period. The code billed is based on the total time spent in that period (see Chapter 13 for more information).

For outpatient claims, the place-of-service code is determined by place where you furnished the service. It does not matter where the corporate address of the billing provider is, nor does it matter what the beneficiaries' addresses are. It matters where the service was rendered; that is, where the biller is located.

For institutional billing, the DR condition code and CR modifier both are required. For noninstitutional billing, only the CR modifier is required. The March 18 CMS MLN Matters article explains further. See also MCPM Chapter 38.

EXAMPLES OF E-VISITS

In each of these scenarios, an established patient initiates contact with the PT:

- *The patient contacts the PT through the online portal and reports having difficulty performing one or more of their home exercises.*

  Using the portal, the PT asks the patient to provide details regarding the difficulty. The PT re-evaluates the program and makes a clinical determination to modify, replace, eliminate, or downgrade one of the exercises. The PT sends the updated program to the patient through the portal.

  The patient contacts the PT through the portal and reports being able to perform their home exercise program with ease and not feeling challenged.

  Using the portal, the PT reviews the patient's home exercise program and makes a clinical determination to progress several of the exercises in intensity and add two new exercises. The PT sends the updated program to the patient through the portal.

- *The patient contacts the PT through the portal and reports an increase in neck and shoulder pain.*

  Using the portal, the PT asks the patient to provide details about factors that may have contributed to the increased pain. The PT determines that the pain is associated with the patient spending more time sitting and working at a home computer. The PT develops an activity plan that calls for increased periods of physical activity and stretching exercises to perform throughout the day. The PT sends the program to the patient through the portal and asks the patient to report any changes.

- *The patient, having missed several in-person appointments, contacts the PT through the portal and reports a concern regarding decreased flexibility in their postoperative knee.*

  Using the portal, the PT asks the patient to describe any movement-related changes, such as more difficulty getting out of a chair and not being able to get their foot back as far when sitting in a chair. The PT also asks the patient to provide, through the portal, a diary of activity and exercise throughout the day. The PT determines that the patient is sitting too long throughout the day and is not performing ROM exercises as frequently as prescribed. Using the portal, the PT provides the patient with a specific schedule of exercise and activity and advises the patient to check back in through the portal in 2 days unless the patient experiences any other changes or difficulty before then.

Author's Note

Attachments such as photos and patient handouts may be uploaded to the portal. This is an example of asynchronous, or store-and-forward, technology. The code descriptors for the HCPCS codes related to e-visits (depending on the payer, it is either HCPCS G2061, G2062, and G2063 or CPT 98970, 98971, and 98972) suggest that the codes are intended to cover short-term (up to seven days) assessments and management activities that are conducted online or via some other digital platform and include any associated clinical decision-making.[20]

VIRTUAL CHECK-IN

Virtual check-ins are brief, real-time remote communication services for an established patient. In the 2021 Physician Fee Schedule proposed rule, CMS has proposed to permanently allow PTs to furnish and bill virtual check-ins and remote evaluation of recorded video or images services when furnished by PTs. CMS is proposing to adopt two new HCPCS codes to describe these services and would classify them as "sometimes therapy" services.

CMS allows audio-only real-time telephone interactions (meaning cell phone video calls are not allowed) in addition to synchronous, two-way audio interactions that are enhanced with recorded video or other kinds of data transmission. The HCPCS code related to a virtual check-in is G2012 and explicitly describes (and requires) direct interaction between the patient and the billing PT.[20]

REMOTE EVALUATION OF RECORDED VIDEO OR IMAGES

When a PT reviews a prerecorded video or image that an established patient has submitted, it's considered a remote evaluation of recorded video or images. This is another example of asynchronous technology, although when the PT follows up with the patient after evaluating the video or image, the discussion could be in real time over the telephone or other audio, as well as not in real time via texting, email, or patient portal. The HCPCS code related to remote evaluation of these visual recordings is G2010. Learn more about remote evaluation of recorded video and/or images.[20]

Telephone Assessment and Management Services

Telephone assessment and management services are initiated by the patient or, for a child, the parent or guardian and involves a real-time discussion with the PT over the telephone. The CPT codes for these services are 98966-98968.[20]

SUMMARY

Proper medical records should be maintained for all patient care episodes, regardless of the payer source, including self-pay or pro bono. In some states, record keeping is mandated by statute. All therapy professionals must be aware of their practice act and accompanying rule requirements, as well as other applicable state and federal regulations. CMS mandates specific documentation requirements for all Medicare beneficiaries across all settings. APTA has some recommendations and tips to assist in meeting these requirements.[22] All third-party payers require documentation that accurately reflects the physical therapy services rendered and justifies medical necessity, although they may not dictate format or content (however, many mandate provider compliance with CCI edits and other coding and billing policies).

The categories are Initial Examination and Evaluation/Consultation, Diagnosis, Prognosis, Plan of Care, Authentication, Daily Visit Note, Progress Report, Re-examination/Re-Evaluation, and Discharge/Discontinuation/Documentation of Summation of Episode of Care. The Medicare requirements fit into these categories. Adherence to the APTA and CMS Medicare guidelines will assist in producing effective documentation that withstands scrutiny by any reader.

Attention must be paid to consistent terminology and the matching of all elements: billing dates, treatment dates and times, diagnostic codes (ICD-10), medical services and procedures (CPT and HCPCS), identified patient problems, established goals, interventions, initial examination results, all visit entries, and discharge information. All entries must indicate the necessity for skilled physical therapy. If progress plateaus or stops at any point in the care, consideration must be made to discharge the patient. All care must be reasonable and necessary. The documentation content is the only supporting evidence of medical necessity and the justification of reasonable and necessary care.

REVIEW QUESTIONS

1. What are the basic requirements for Medicare documentation?
2. Identify 10 content elements required in the initial examination and evaluation.
3. Provide five categories of systems review with two examples of content for each.
4. What is the relationship between the patient's prior level of function and physical therapy?
5. What are the basic content requirements for a plan of care?
6. From a Medicare perspective, what is recertification, and what is the relationship to continuing physical therapy?
7. What does the APTA describe as the continuum of care? Provide examples.
8. What is authentication, and what is its relationship to documentation?
9. What is the APTA-recommended frequency of documentation?
10. What is a problem summary?
11. What are the advantages of using premade forms for documentation and billing purposes?
12. Provide four examples of terms that should be avoided in documentation.
13. Can Medicare be billed by the PT for restorative services? Defend your answer.
14. In order for physical therapy services to be considered reasonable and necessary, what criteria have to be met?
15. What is co-treatment? Can more than one service bill for co-treatments? Explain your answer.
16. Compare and contrast certification and recertification in the Medicare context.
17. Under what circumstances is gait training skilled versus unskilled?
18. What constitutes an evaluation?
19. What is the use of a CMS-1500 form?
20. What are duplicate services? Provide examples of a procedure that might be considered duplicative unless the documentation indicates otherwise.
21. What are the advantages and disadvantages of utilizing telehealth?

REFERENCES

1. *APTA Elements of Documentation Within the Patient/Client Management Model*. Alexandria, VA: American Physical Therapy Association. Available at https://www.apta.org/your-practice/documentation/defensible-documentation/elements-within- the-patientclient-management-model. Accessed July 27, 2020.
2. *National Provider Number*. National Plan and Provider Enumeration System (NPPES). Baltimore, MD: Centers for Medicare & Medicaid Services. Available at https://nppes.cms.hhs.gov/#. Accessed July 20, 2020.
3. *CMS 1500 Form*. Baltimore, MD: Centers for Medicare & Medicaid Services. Available at https://www.cms.gov/Medicare/CMS-Forms/CMS-Forms/CMS-Forms-Items/CMS1188854. Accessed July 20, 2020.
4. *CMS Publication 100-04 Internet Only Manual Medicare Claims Processing Manual Chapter 26 Section 1*. Baltimore, MD: Centers for Medicare & Medicaid Services. Available at https://www.cms.gov/regulations-and-guidance/guidance/manuals/internet-only-manuals-ioms-items/cms018912. Accessed July 20, 2020.
5. *Professional Paper Claim Form Instructions CMS 1500*. Baltimore, MD: Centers for Medicare & Medicaid Services. Available at https://www.cms.gov/Medicare/Billing/ElectronicBillingEDITrans/1500. Accessed July 20, 2020.
6. *Proper Use of 59 Modifier*. Baltimore, MD: Centers for Medicare & Medicaid Services. Available at https://www.cms.gov/Outreach-and-Education/Medicare-Learning-Network-MLN/MLNMattersArticles/Downloads/SE1418.pdf. Accessed July 20, 2020.
7. *National Correct Coding Initiative*. Alexandria, VA: American Physical Therapy Association. Available at https://www.apta.org/your-practice/payment/coding-billing/correct-coding-initiative-cci. Accessed July 20, 2020.
8. Baeten AM, Moran ML, Phillippi LM. *Documenting Physical Therapy: The Reviewer Perspective*. Woburn: Butterworth-Heinemann; 1999:215. ISBN: 0 7506 9950 7.
9. *Guide to Physical Therapist Practice*, 3.0. Alexandria, VA: American Physical Therapy Association. Available at https://www.apta.org/Guide/. Accessed July 20, 2020.
10. *Summary of the HIPPA Social Security Rule*. Health Insurance Portability and Accountability Act, HIPPA. U.S. Department of Health and Human Services. Available at https://www.hhs.gov/hipaa/for-professionals/security/laws-regulations/index.html. Accessed July 20, 2020.
11. *International Classification of Diseases, Tenth Revision, ICD-10*. Centers for Disease Control and Prevention. Available at https://www.cdc.gov/nchs/icd/icd10.htm. Accessed February 20, 2020.
12. *ICF: International Classification of Functioning, Disability and Health*. Geneva: World Health Organization. Available at https://www.who.int/classifications/icf/en/. Accessed July 20, 2020.
13. Guccione AA, Mielenz TJ, DeVellis RF, Goldstein MS, Freburger JK, et al. Development and testing of a self-report instrument to measure actions: Outpatient Physical Therapy Improvement in Movement Assessment Log (OPTIMAL). *Phys Ther*. 2005;85(6):515-30. Available at https://academic.oup.com/ptj/article/85/6/515/2805026?searchresult=1.
14. *Medicare Benefit Policy Manual Chapter 15 Section 220.1.3*. Baltimore, MD: Centers for Medicare & Medicaid Services. Available at https://www.cms.gov/Medicare/Prevention/PrevntionGenInfo/Downloads/bp102c15.pdf. Accessed July 20, 2020.
15. *Physical Therapy Outcomes Registry*. Alexandria, VA: American Physical Therapy Association. Available at https://www.apta.org/your-practice/outcomes-measurement. Accessed July 20, 2020.
16. *11 Part B Billing Scenarios for PTs and OTs*. Baltimore, MD: Centers for Medicare & Medicaid Services. Available at https://www.cms.gov/Medicare/Billing/TherapyServices/Downloads/11_Part_B_Billing_Scenarios_for_PTs_and_OTs.pdf. Accessed July 20, 2020.
17. *Medical Coverage Database*. Baltimore, MD: Centers for Medicare & Medicaid Services. Available at http://www.cms.hhs.gov/mcd. Accessed July 20, 2020.
18. *Medicare Benefit Policy Manual, Chapter 1—Inpatient Hospital Services Covered Under Part A*. Baltimore, MD: Centers for Medicare & Medicaid Services. Available at https://www.cms.gov/Regulations-and-Guidance/Guidance/Manuals/Downloads/bp102c01.pdf. Accessed July 20, 2020.
19. *Telehealth Programs*. Health Resources & Services Admnistration (HRSA). Available at https://www.hrsa.gov/rural-health/telehealth. Accessed July 20, 2020.
20. *Telehealth Modalities PTs and PTAs Can Use During the Public Health Emergency*. Alexandria, VA: American Physical Therapy Association. Available at https://www.apta.org/your-practice/practice-models-and-settings/telehealth-practice/telehealth-modalities-that-pts-and-ptas-can-use-during-the-public-health-emergency. Accessed July 27, 2020.
21. *Medicare and E-Visits: What You Need to Know*. Alexandria, VA: American Physical Therapy Association. Available at https://www.apta.org/patient-care/public-health-population-care/coronavirus/covid-19-events/medicare-and-e-visits-what-you-need-to-know. Accessed July 27, 2020.
22. *Documentation Tips*. Alexandria, VA: American Physical Therapy Association. Available at https://www.apta.org/your-practice/documentation/tips. Accessed July 27, 2020.

6 Documentation for Pediatrics

OBJECTIVES

Following completion of this chapter, the reader will be able to:

- Compare and contrast pediatric and adult documentation.
- Explain what information should be included in a treatment plan for a child.
- List examples of behaviors/activities that should be assessed and documented in pediatrics.
- Describe the concept of rehabilitation potential.
- Discuss the role of the problem list in the initial examination.
- Explain the difference between rehabilitation potential and prognosis.

PEDIATRIC DOCUMENTATION

Documentation and payment for physical therapy services when working with the pediatric population present some unique challenges. This section will address the nuances of documentation, billing, and payment issues in the context of documentation specific to pediatric physical therapy. However, the basic contextual guidelines are applicable to the adult population as well.

INITIAL EXAMINATION

Many of the major categories for examination of the pediatric patient are the same as for the adult patient. In general, physical therapists (PTs) must examine range of motion (ROM), muscle tone, muscle performance/strength, sensation, posture, and function regardless of whether the child has a musculoskeletal or neurologic/neuromuscular pathology. However, the focus and content of each of these categories are unique for the child who has a neurologic impairment. In particular, young children require increased emphasis on assessment of their developmental motor skills. This section will focus primarily on conducting and documenting the content for a developmental evaluation of an infant or young child. Pediatric clients with specific diagnoses such as spina bifida warrant a more directed examination. However, the major categories described in this chapter will serve the PT well for the general pediatric population.

During the initial examination and evaluation, recording by video recording or other electronic recording can be beneficial to both the PT and the child's parent or guardian. For the PT, reviewing the recording may allow examination of the child's movement at a pace more conducive to reflective observation. For the parent or guardian, the video recording or other recording may be a helpful reminder of the progress a child has made, which may be difficult to appreciate otherwise. Before recording a session, the therapist should obtain express written permission from the parent or legal guardian by means of a consent form. From a risk management perspective, the video recording becomes a part of the medical record and must be afforded the same confidentiality as dictated by the Health Insurance Portability and Accountability Act (HIPAA). Consult with a risk manager or attorney to ensure HIPAA compliance.

HISTORY

As with any patient, the history should be the first assessment (see Figure 6-1). The most efficient way to obtain a history is with a form developed specifically for the parent/caregiver or legal guardian to complete prior to the first session. The PT can then use the information to obtain clarification during the initial session. If a medical record is available, the information included could be useful and may indicate information that might otherwise be difficult to obtain, such as whether there is any history of maternal drug or alcohol abuse. However, when a medical record is not available, one should be conscientious yet sensitive in questioning a parent about this history because of the emotional stress that may be associated with these questions. Although the question is included in the history prototype form included for reference, the information in the history is the discretion of the facility. In practices that use secure portals for communication and to obtain information needed prior to, during, or after treatment, histories can be completed through the portals. Tablets can be used onsite with preloaded forms or formats that communicate with the electronic medical record (EMR) system.

OBSERVATION

Before conducting the objective tests, the therapist should allow the child to play independently without assistance, if the child has the ability to engage in play. This provides the therapist with the opportunity to observe how the child moves and what the child is able and unable to accomplish motor-wise. In addition, it allows the child time to warm up to the therapist. General comments about motor control and movement patterns can be recorded as observed in a designated section on an evaluation form. As with adults, general observations regarding movement as well as the history drive the decision-making for the performance of specific tests and measures. If the child is too young to engage in play or too involved to engage in play, the therapist should engage in a communicative, interactive process consistent with the child's abilities. A parent or caretaker may on may not be present depending on the situation, environment or other indicators.

OBJECTIVE DATA

Information gathered while observing the infant or child move independently and while taking the history from the parent or guardian will help narrow the focus of the objective assessment. For example, if the therapist notices that the child tends to scissor (cross) the legs when crawling on the floor, the therapist will want to assess hip adductor tone for possible spasticity. Recommendations for categories of objective assessment are provided in the following sections. However, specific categories may be more indicated in a child with a neuromuscular disorder than a musculoskeletal disorder. Examination and evaluation of the child with an acute musculoskeletal pathology, such as post fracture or surgery, may resemble that of an adult.

State of Alertness: document in the appropriate section on the record if the infant or child is awake, happy, angry, agitated, drowsy, or exhibits stranger anxiety or separation anxiety, with specific descriptions of the behaviors (e.g., smiling, crying, hiding face). Because the

Pediatric History

Child's:
Last name: First name: Middle initial: DOB: Age:

Gestational age: ______________________________ Gender: ____ female ____male

ID#: Tel#: Address:

City: State: Zip:

If client is minor: name of parent or responsible party:

Telephone and address if different than minor's: Primary language: ______________

Second language: ______________

Social : Parents are: ____married ____separated ____divorced ___single

Child lives with: ______________________________

Does the child have siblings? ______no ______yes If yes, number and ages ______________________________
Was this child one of a multiple birth? _______no ________yes If yes, please indicate: ____twins ____triplets ____quads ____quints

Is primary caregiver responsible for the care of others in the home? ____no ____yes Explain:

Dwelling: Do you have to negotiate stairs into or inside your home? ____no ____yes

Do you have transportation available? ________yes ________no

Reason for PT: Please indicate if you know the child's medical diagnosis:

Did the physician indicate there were problems? ____yes ____no

Did the caregiver perceive there were any problems? ____yes ____no

Please indicate if birth mother had any of the following problems during the pregnancy:

_____pre-eclampsia _____excessive weight gain : ______pounds gained

_____diabetes _____dehydration

_____thyroid problems _____premature labor

_____edema

How many pregnancies did the birth mother have? ___________ How many live births? _______________

Did the birth mother:
Smoke during the pregnancy?

Drink alcohol during the pregnancy?

Take drugs during the pregnancy that were over the counter?

Take drugs that were prescribed?

Take dietary supplements? Please indicate: ______________________________

Please indicate the type of diet the birth mother was on during the pregnancy:

Figure 6-1. Pediatric history form.

Does the child have: vision impairment _____no _____yes If yes, describe: ________________________

hearing impairment _______no ____yes If yes, describe: ______________

Family history: Are there any other family members with similar problem? ________yes ________no

If yes, please describe:

Please check as appropriate for each category:

Birth history	Where did the birth take place? ________hospital _______home ________birthing center _______other: Please explain:

Type of delivery: ________vaginal __________C-section Did the baby present breech? _______yes ________no

Were forceps used? ______yes ______no Was vacuum extraction used? __________yes _________no

What was the baby's birth weight? ____________	What was the baby's APGAR score?	How long was the baby in the hospital? Was the baby in the NICU?
What was the baby's birth length? ____________	Did the baby need ventilator support? ______yes _________no	How long was the mother in the hospital?

Please indicate any diagnostic tests the baby/child has had:

Please check as applicable	No	Yes	Describe
Respiratory Problems			
Seizures			
Muscle spasms			
Head injury			
Falls			
High fevers			
Hear problems			
Shunt placement			
Failure to thrive			
Loss of consciousness			
Dehydration			
Abnormal bleeding &/or bruising			
Abnormal growth			
Loss of weight			
Diabetes			
Thyroid dysfunction			
Urinary or bowel problems			
Gastrointestinal			
HIV			

Figure 6-1. (Continued)

Wheezing, coughing during or after activity			
Agitation			
Excessive sleeping			
Allergies			
Other			
Development of child: ___normal ___delayed			
Recent weight changes: ____weight gain ____weight loss Describe:			
Recent memory or cognitive changes: ____yes ____no If yes, please describe:			
Medications: Prescription: Over the counter:			
General nutrition: Is the child breastfed: now _____yes _____no Was the child breastfed? _____yes _____no How long?_____ Is the child bottle fed? _____yes _____no Combination breast?bottle: _____yes _____no If on formula, what type? ________________________ Diet/dietary supplements: Please indicate if child is on solid food: _____yes _____no Other:			
Please indicate any other information that may be important or you wish to discuss:			
The above information is accurate and true to the best of my knowledge, and I give my consent for the evaluation to be performed. Signature of responsible party if client is a minor: ______________________________Date: ________________ Printed Name: Relationship to the child:			

Figure 6-1. (Continued)

behavioral or emotional states of the infant or child will affect muscle tone and motor performance, it is important to note these levels of alertness.

Asymmetries Related to Movement: To record any asymmetry, document in the appropriate section if the infant or child prefers to weight-bear on one side or prefers to reach with one arm more than the other, if the child shifts weight better to one side than the other, and if the child primarily transitions (changes position) only in one direction.

Postural Alignment: Recording postural alignment in a child includes documenting the presence of orthopedic deformities, rib flaring, scapular winging, cortical thumb posture, frog leg posturing, opisthotonus, ankle pronation or supination in standing, genu valgus, genu varus, genu recurvatum, hip subluxation or dislocation, scoliosis, or leg length discrepancy.

Muscle Tone: Assess and document muscle tone during functional and passive movement. Describe the muscle tone according to location. For example, is there a difference between trunk and lower extremity tone? If so, indicate which may be low tone compared to high tone. Document if the muscle tone is different distally compared to proximally. Muscle tone should also be quantified either using a standardized scale, such as the Ashworth or modified Ashworth scale, or with more generic terms, such as mild, moderate, or severe increased or decreased muscle tone. Position of assessment is also critical, as tone may fluctuate with position changes (e.g., sitting versus standing).

MODIFIED ASHWORTH SCALE

5/5: Normal tone: no increase or decrease
4/5: Slight tone increase, catch and release, or minimal resistance at end of range
3/5: Slight increase in tone manifested by catch, followed by minimal resistance
2/5: More marked tone through most of the range of motion, but affected part(s) easily moved
1/5: Considerable increase in muscle tone; passive movement is difficult
0/5: Affected part(s) rigid in flexion or extension

Author's Note

Although the Modified Ashworth Scale includes fractions from 0/5 to 5/5, the numbers alone should be avoided, since they may be confused for strength. The numbers should be accompanied by the appropriate verbiage.

Range of Motion (ROM): Both passive and active ROM should be assessed and documented objectively. The ranges should be expressed as fractions (i.e., passive hip flexion 100/140), in which the finding is documented above the "normal" range of a joint. In addition, goniometric measurements of contractures should be documented. Flexibility should be assessed for the following muscles in particular: hip flexors, hip internal and external rotators, hip abductors and adductors, hamstrings, sartorius, plantarflexors, shoulder girdle musculature, and forearm pronators and supinators.

Muscle Performance/Strength: Although standard muscle testing should not be performed in infants and young children under the age of 7 years old, inferences regarding strength may be made based on the child's ability to move against gravity. For example, a child who has difficulty walking down stairs may have eccentric quadriceps femoris weakness. In addition, inferences regarding adequacy of muscle strength can be made based on postural alignment. For example, a child who displays lower rib flaring often has weakness of the oblique abdominal muscles. Pediatric patients may present difficulty "grading" muscle movements as well. For example, assessment must be made whether the child exhibits an ability to accomplish a motor task smoothly through the range or has difficulty controlling mid or end ranges. Therefore, functional strength assessment may be the most appropriate.

Sensation and Perception: Assess and document how the infant or child responds to touch and if any self-calming techniques are used. Also observe whether the child exhibits any primitive reflex activity that interferes with functional skills, such as sitting independently, and if the child displays any evidence of tactile defensiveness. For example, determine from the child's parents/caretakers if the child dislikes walking on the grass, complains about tags in clothing, or dislikes certain textures of food. Visual tracking and hearing should also be screened.

Skin Integrity: Assess and document if the child has any scars, pressure sores, unusual temperature of the skin and extremities, circulation problems with the fingers and toes, or discoloration on the skin or mottling. Also check the child for the presence of birth marks or any bite marks, burn marks, or bruising that may be evidence of child abuse or neglect. Consideration should also be given to self-stimulation behaviors that may be resulting in harm.

Author's Note

Physical abuse signs and symptoms include unexplained injuries, such as bruises, fractures, or burns. These are usually injuries that do not match the given explanation. In many cases, child abuse is done by someone the child knows and trusts, who is often a parent or other relative. Any intentional harm or mistreatment to a child under 18 years old is considered child abuse. If abuse, neglect, or human trafficking is suspected, the therapist is obligated to report it to authorities in a manner consistent with state law.

Cardiopulmonary Status: Determine and document if the infant or child has any unrepaired heart defects or cardiopulmonary pathology, precautions, or contraindications. Indicate if the child requires oxygen or ventilator support, and note the child's aerobic capacity/endurance, including any shortness of breath observed. If the child has a history of cardiopulmonary issues, the therapist should be prepared to take the child's vital signs, including heart rate (HR), blood pressure (BP), and oxygen saturation levels.

Reflexes and Reactions: Assessment and documentation of the following reflexes or reactions are of particular importance with regard to functional ability: primitive reflexes such as asymmetric tonic neck reflex (ATNR) and postural reactions like righting, equilibrium, or protective reactions in sitting and standing. The presence of any tremors or clonus should also be noted. Clonus is considered significant if it lasts for more than four beats. The muscle group exhibiting clonus should be documented. In addition to developmental reflexes, deep tendon reflex assessment may in some cases be indicated and require documentation.

Gross Motor Development: Infants and toddlers should be assessed for the presence of motor milestones in supine, prone, sitting, and standing positions. In addition, an infant's ability to roll, commando crawl, creep on hands and knees, and transition in and out of positions should be assessed and documented. The therapist should note whether the infant or young child can perform gross motor milestones (which are standard and found easily in the literature), as well as the quality of the movement used when performing the milestones. In addition, each of the following should be assessed and documented as age and developmentally appropriate: head control, quadruped, gait, stair climbing, primary method of mobility, balance in all positions, length of time able to maintain standing on one leg, running, jumping, hopping, skipping, kicking a ball, catching a ball, and use of assistive devices or orthotics if present.

In addition to assessing these gross motor skills, evaluating the child for patterns or trends in movement can be helpful. For example, indicate if the child exhibits difficulty initiating, sustaining, or terminating movement as an adult with Parkinson might, or if the infant tends to only initiate movement with the extensor muscles rather than demonstrating a balance between the flexors and the extensors. Determine and document if there are any stereotypical movement patterns, such as scissoring gait or posturing of the arms into shoulder flexion with internal rotation, forearm pronation, and wrist and finger flexion.

The PT that works with occupational therapists (OTs) and speech therapists/speech language pathologists (SLPs) or any interprofessional team member also needs to screen the infant or child for difficulty with fine motor or oral motor skills in order to refer the patient for services that may be indicated but have not yet been consulted. The following sections provide suggestions for screening and documenting fine motor and oral motor development.

Fine Motor Development: Assess and document if the infant or child is able to reach grasp, play at midline, cross midline, or transfer an object hand to hand.

Oral Motor Development: Indicate and document if the infant makes any vocalizations or if the parent or guardian is having any difficulty feeding the child (i.e., if the child gags or chokes when feeding). Determine if the young child is eating age-appropriate food, such as baby food or table food, and if there are any foods the child refuses to eat. Also determine if the child drools often or regurgitates. In infants, note if the sucking reflex is absent or weak.

ASSESSMENT

Summary Statement

After gathering the subjective and objective components of the evaluation, the PT should develop a summary statement of the patient's status in order to establish functionally oriented goals. One strategy for beginning the assessment portion of an evaluation is to begin with a one-sentence summary of the therapist's findings. For example, "9-month old male born at 28 weeks gestational age (with an adjusted chronological age of 6 months) with history of grade IV intraventricular hemorrhage recently diagnosed with cerebral palsy." This provides the reader a brief overview of the significance of the patient's possible impairments and functional limitations.

Author's Note

The beginning summary statement example may also be the way the patient history is presented in the report, as in adult documentation.

PROBLEM LIST

Many healthcare settings also require a "problem list," which may, in actuality, be the summary statement in some organizations. In the functional outcome record, identification of the problems assists all that need access to the record by providing a clear indication of what the challenges are. In the American Physical Therapy Association's (APTA) *Guide to Physical Therapist Practice,*[1] the Nagi disablement model was used to categorize the summary into pathology, impairment, functional limitations, and disabilities. The International Classification of Disease, Disability, and Function (ICF) Model is used to categorize the summary into body structure and function, activities, and participation. Each category in the body of the evaluation documentation will contain the objective assessment. The problem need not repeat the details, but should contain the problems in a summative manner. The following is an example of a general problem list:

- Moderate increased tone in plantar flexors, hamstrings, hip adductors
- Decreased strength in abdominals
- Decreased dorsiflexion ROM bilaterally
- Requires moderate assistance with posterior walker, nonfunctional distance
- Dependent for transfers (rolling, bed)

REHABILITATION POTENTIAL/PROGNOSIS

As with adults, a statement regarding the infant's or child's rehabilitation potential should be included. Rehabilitation potential refers to the prospect of the child to make progress with intervention. This is further elaborated on in the plan of care (POC) summary with descriptive examples of the child's response to handling by the therapist. Prognosis, as described in the *Guide to Physical Therapist Practice,*[1] refers to a more long-term determination of progress, and is not usually required in documentation unless specifically requested by a payer source.

When rating a pediatric patient's rehabilitation potential, it is helpful to include a rationale for the rating. For example, "good rehab potential as evidenced by ability to achieve quadruped with facilitation today." The statement may also include a reference to the child's level of motivation, including an example. For example, "good rehab potential as evidenced by child's strong desire to interact with environment while observed reaching for objects and babbling to therapist" or "good rehab potential based on established goals."

Patients who are rated as having either "excellent" or "poor" rehabilitation potential may experience difficulty with payment for physical therapy services. This results from the belief that patients with "excellent" rehabilitation potential can get better without physical therapy. In contrast, patients with "poor" rehabilitation potential are viewed as receiving very little benefit from therapy services, and therefore, declared ineligible. If the PT is setting the goals with the parents or responsible party and has considered all relevant information, the rehabilitation potential should be successful.

GOALS/FUNCTIONAL OUTCOMES

From a payment perspective, perhaps the most important component of the evaluation process is the goals section. In pediatrics, many outpatient physical therapy settings will develop specific, measurable, short-term goals and less specific or objective long-term goals. For example, with Medicaid payment, the POC is usually set at a 6-month interval for re-evaluation and goal setting. Short-term goals are designed to be achieved in 1 to 3 months, whereas long-term goals are designed to be achieved in 3 to 6 months, although the time frame should be designated. As Medicaid differs from state to state, the PT should comply with the specific state practice act and payer requirements for goal-setting time intervals.

Regardless of the time frame preferred in the pediatric practice setting, goals should be documented in the same fashion as physical therapy goals for adults. Goals should include what is to be achieved, the time frame for achieving it, and under what conditions or criteria. Similar to goals for adult patients with neurologic disorders, goals for pediatric patients should be listed in functional terms and should include what goals the parent/caretaker or guardian has for the child. This may mean listing the parent's goal as a long-term goal and using the short-term goal as components necessary to achieve the parent's goal. For example parents of infants often state they want their child to be able to walk. This can be listed as the long-term goal, and the therapist can use this as a "teachable moment" for helping the parents understand what component skills the child needs before being able to walk. At times, this may mean discussing that ambulating with an assistive device qualifies as "walking."

Author's Note

As walking is not considered a skilled term and does not correspond to a Current Procedural Terminology (CPT) code, the terms "walk or walking" should only be used when quoting the parents/caretakers or guardian. The PT should, for interventions in the POC and other documentation, use the term gait training, as it corresponds to the CPT billing code, or ambulation training.

The following are some examples of goals for the child described in the earlier problem list:

Example

Short-term goals (to be achieved in 3 months): The child will be able to:

1. Stand with support of walker and minimal assistance with feet flat (address dorsiflexion range of motion and standing balance for pre-ambulation).
2. Ambulate or achieve gait 25′ with posterior walker, minimal assist of 25% (also describe pattern and what physical therapy skill constitutes the 25%).

Long-term goals (to be achieved in 6 months): The child will be able to:

1. Assume a deep squat position with moderate assistance for 60 seconds (addresses dorsiflexion range of motion, balance, functional strength, and inclusion of skilled physical therapy input [i.e., stabilization of trunk]) to engage in play.
2. Ambulate or achieve gait, 100′ with posterior walker and contact guard assistance to prevent loss of balance with directional changes on even surface.

Regardless of whether a therapist is writing goals for a child or an adult, the word "maintain" should not be used for restorative care. Third-party payers are much more critical in the payment for therapy services designed to assist a patient in maintenance of a certain skill or ability. It is believed that maintenance activities do not require the skills of a PT or physical therapist assistant. Instead, the therapist should write goals to indicate what the child will be able to do as a result of physical therapy and why they need to have that specific skill.

Here are some questions and answers on maintenance versus restorative care:

What's the difference between "maintenance" and "medically necessary"?
"Medical necessity" is required for all services covered under Medicare, as is the requirement that the services be skilled. The services can be rehabilitative, maintenance, or slowing of decline based on the physical therapist's ability to justify they are reasonable and necessary and require the skills of the physical therapist. It is considered skilled to instruct caregivers and to periodically determine if they are carrying out an unskilled service.[2]

Do you have to "label" a patient as restorative versus maintenance?
Yes, for patients in need of skilled maintenance therapy, you should establish a maintenance program and in your documentation clearly show that the services are being provided for maintenance goals as opposed to restorative.

If a patient's skilled restorative care is completed and the therapist opts to keep the patient on a skilled maintenance level, must they document that the patient is being transitioned to a skilled maintenance program?
Yes, the transition from restorative therapy to maintenance therapy should be documented, as the goals for treatment will be different. The POC should be updated to reflect the new treatment goals for the patient.

In maintenance therapy, you are not trying to improve function but just maintain or decrease the decline in status, so what type of long-term goals would one use?
You should be using functional measures to track the patient's status and use your clinical judgment and knowledge of the patient's various conditions to determine what reasonable expectations are. The patient may be able to maintain a certain level of function based on a functional measure, or with a disease that is progressive, you may have goals to decrease the decline of status with a slow decline of the results of the functional measures.

When considering a patient for a maintenance program, is it essential that they have a chronic, progressive diagnosis in order to see them under maintenance therapy?
No, it is not a requirement for maintenance therapy coverage that the patient have a certain diagnosis. Coverage is based on individualized assessment of the patient's condition and the need for skilled care to carry out a safe and effective maintenance program. Skilled maintenance therapy is covered in cases in which needed therapeutic interventions require a high level of complexity.[2]

Can a patient with a chronic diagnosis be put straight onto maintenance program from findings from the initial evaluation?
Yes, the therapist can develop a maintenance program from the findings in an initial evaluation as long as the documentation justifies the need for skilled therapy to maintain function or prevent/slow deterioration. It is not necessary to establish rehabilitation/restorative therapy prior to the maintenance program.[2]

In outpatient therapy, is it necessary for the physician to sign off on the maintenance POC?

Yes, a POC must be certified by the physician within 30 days of the initial treatment date and must be recertified every 90 days or when the POC duration has expired (whichever is sooner).

PLAN OF CARE

When compiling the findings, the therapist should consider the techniques that can be used to help the child achieve the established goals. The "plan" portion of the evaluation should include the frequency and duration the child will be treated, any recommendations for additional consultations, such as referral to an OT, SLP, or orthotist; what treatment methods will be used; and how the findings and plan will be communicated to the referring physician.

Regarding treatment methods, general references indicating the focus of therapy are usually sufficient. For example, "Therapeutic exercise: instruction to parents of home exercise program and strengthening, functional activities: developmental activities, gait training" indicates what the focus of the therapy session will be. The setting for physical therapy may need to be stated as well. Indicate where the child will receive physical therapy (i.e., in the home setting, in an outpatient clinic, at day care, or at school). As with adults, the interventions should be identified using the CPT code verbiage (i.e., therapeutic exercise, neuromuscular re-education, therapeutic activities, gait training, etc.) before listing specifics in each category. This will help ensure that when billing for services, the codes and verbiage match the information for each treatment session.

Author's Note

The therapist should know, based on payer source, what codes may not be covered for physical therapy or need to be bundled. Medicaid services often have their own designated codes for evaluation and physical therapy treatment. It is the responsibility of the therapist to know the idiosyncrasies of coding for billing purposes depending on the payer and state. Additionally, depending on the payer source, the therapist may need a specific provider number or approved provider status.

DOCUMENTATION OF THE CONTINUATION OF CARE

Requirements for documentation of treatment sessions, treatment notes, progress notes, and progress reports vary between facilities and payers. While some facilities require a complete note regarding the treatment session, other facilities may utilize a flow sheet method of recording attendance, treatment goals for the day, and significant findings for each therapy session. Inpatient rehabilitation facilities for children may only require weekly documentation. However, from a health information perspective and medical records "rules," entries should be made for each visit. Failure to do so may result in denial of payment. As a result, it is prudent for each physical therapy practitioner to be aware of the facility's requirements, as well as the requirements of the paying agency. The format of the entry (e.g., SOAP, narrative, or other, manual or electronic) should be consistent throughout the organization. Payer sources do not usually dictate format unless specific forms are required. It is the therapist's responsibility to know if a payer does have specific requirements.

In general, treatment notes and reports may contain the following:

- Date of the treatment
- Number of units or time

- Specifics regarding the treatment that was provided, including any parent education or home exercise instruction that was provided in skilled terms, stressing training and CPT codeable verbiage (i.e., "therapeutic exercise" or "gait training")
- Child's response to treatment (was the child able to complete the task with assistance, or was the child still unable to complete the task even with the skill of the therapist or assistant?)
- Length of the session
- Goals of the session
- Plan for the next visit
- Presence of family members, caretakers, or others
- Progress note that includes all of the components listed in addition to the progress made relative to a prior report; the initial examination/evaluation or previous progress note or report objectively stated

Regardless of the frequency of documentation, PTs should provide regular written updates to the referring physician indicating the child's progress and the treatment plan. Similar to the initial examination, the treatment plan should include the frequency and duration of physical therapy services, the type of treatment, the treatment setting, and any recommendations for additional services or consultations. As indicated in the payment section, written physician authorization may be necessary to continue therapy services.

DISCHARGE SUMMARY/DOCUMENTATION OF SUMMATION OF CARE

When a child has achieved maximal outcome for a specified time, completed a preauthorized number of visits, or is no longer receiving services for any reason and is being discharged from physical therapy, a discharge summary or documentation of the summation of the episode of care must be completed. Ideally, a discharge summary contains a statement of all the changes and significant findings addressed in the initial evaluation. The current functional status, method of mobility, and adaptive equipment should be addressed. A statement regarding progress toward the short- and long-term goals and whether or not the goals were achieved should be included. If some goals were not achieved, reasons for modifying or not achieving the goals should be stated. A plan should also be included such as "Parent will continue with home exercises as instructed and will call if they have any questions." The discharge summary is particularly valuable if the child requires additional services in the future, as the summary serves as a record of progress gained and function that may have been lost or not achieved during that episode of care. Medicaid continuation-of-care requests will require that the summation of goals and their modification for the next episode of care be included. In addition, Medicaid will want a restatement of the child's rehabilitation potential or prognosis. This request for continued physical therapy will require the referring physician's signature prior to submission. A copy of the discharge summary should be sent to the referring physician regardless of discharge or continuation of care. (See Appendix E for documentation guidelines.)

PAYMENT

Pediatric physical therapy providers have several primary methods for obtaining payment: through federal regulations under the Individuals with Disabilities Education Act (IDEA), including Early Intervention under Part C; school-based services under Part B; state Medicaid; private insurance; cash payments; and philanthropic and professional organizations. A description of each of these methods of funding is provided in the following sections. Qualifications for providers, requirements for the provision of services, and procedures for payment are also discussed. Table 6-1 contains a summary of the requirements for provider eligibility for each of the funding agencies.

Table 6-1 Provider Eligibility Requirements

REQUIREMENTS	IDEA PART C	IDEA PART B	MEDICAID	INSURANCE
Current state license	Yes	Yes	Yes	Yes
Provider application	Yes	Local education agency specific	Yes	Only for network providers
Specific provider number	Depends on state	No	Yes	Depends on insurance company
Resume	Yes	Depends on local education agency	Yes	Depends on insurance company
Background check	Depends on state	Depends on state and local education agency	Yes	No
Occupational license	Depends on state	No	Depends on state	Depends on insurance company
Liability insurance	Yes	Yes	Yes	Yes
Specific pediatric training	State-specific training modules	Local education agency specific	No	No
Contract	Yes	Local education agency specific	Yes	Yes, for network providers
National Provider Identification number	Yes	No	Yes	Yes or Social Security number
Federal identification number	Yes	Depends on local education agency	Yes	Yes or Social Security number for individual provider

Individuals with Disabilities Education Act (IDEA) Early Intervention—Part C[3]

- *The Individuals with Disabilities Education Act (IDEA) of 2004 (Public Law 108-446) is a federal law that supports the provision of public education for all children regardless of the nature or severity of their disability.*
- *Part C of IDEA is an optional federal program that supports early intervention for infants and toddlers (birth up to 3 years). All states currently are participating in Part C. IDEA interacts with other legislative mandates, such as the Americans With Disabilities Act, Section 504 of the Rehabilitation Act, and the Technology-Related Assistance for Individuals With Disabilities Act.*
- *Implementation of IDEA Part C is the responsibility of each state through a lead agency appointed from education, health, human services, public health, or another related state agency.*
- *Part C requires that multiple agencies work together and collaborate on meeting the needs of infants and toddlers and their families in their states and communities.*

- *Eligible children have a developmental delay or a medical diagnosis that has a high probability of a developmental delay.*
- *States define the eligibility criteria for developmental delay by addressing the child's development in cognition, physical, communication, social/emotional, and adaptive (self-help) domains or areas.*
- *Eligible infants and toddlers are entitled to early intervention services in natural environments where children live, learn, and play.*
- *Early intervention services are provided, as necessary, to meet the developmental needs of the child and needs of the child's family related to the family's ability to enhance the child's development.*

Qualification for this program does not depend on the family's income. Early intervention services are available for any child who meets the eligibility requirements up until the child's third birthday. To determine eligibility of children, the lead agency for each state establishes a team of professionals to screen birth to 3-year-old children who have been identified as possibly needing early intervention services. The team consists of the family in conjunction with some combination of the following professionals: psychologist, nurse, physician, PT, OT, or SLP/speech therapist. A service coordinator from the team is designated and assigned to the family and child to assist with the provision of services as determined by the team. Ultimately, the family makes the final decision regarding recommendations that will affect their child.

The team of professionals that evaluates the child often uses a standardized assessment tool to determine the presence and severity of developmental delay and to determine eligibility for services under Part C. There are a variety of evaluation tools that compare the child's performance with other typically developing children. Two commonly used standardized assessment tools are the Bayley Scales of Infant Development II and the Battelle Developmental Inventory for Young Children. However, specific tests or standardized assessments are not required to determine eligibility. An objective narrative therapy assessment addressing delays is acceptable for documenting a child's developmental needs.

Following the developmental evaluation, an Individual Family Support Plan (IFSP) is written to document the treatment plan based on the results of the team assessment and family input. This plan is driven by the family and identifies specific concerns, priorities, and resources available to the families. The plan must be reviewed every 6 months in addition to an annual IFSP meeting to determine what services are still needed.

IDEA mandates that therapy services must be provided in the natural environment for the child. A "natural" environment for a child may be the child's home, day care, or other community settings. In some states, professionals trained to provide these services in the home may be limited. Under these circumstances each state handles this dilemma differently.

Qualifications for Providers. Table 6-1 outlines the requirements for providers of early intervention physical therapy services. In order to provide therapy services for children and families covered by Part C, professionals must have the following:

1. Current state license
2. Occupational license
3. State Medicaid provider number
4. Resume
5. Liability insurance
6. National Provider Identification (NPI) number

Additional requirements may include:

1. One year of postdegree professional experience
2. Level II background is now referred to as Fingerprint background checks.
3. Early intervention–specific Continuing Education Units (CEUs)
4. Current certifications in area of practice

5. Completion of orientation and training modules covering such topics as:
    a. The family-centered philosophy
    b. An introduction to service coordination
    c. Transitioning the child from early intervention to public school
    d. IFSP

Professionals must agree to sign an annual contract to provide services to Part C clients. This contract may include a procedural safeguards statement and a memorandum describing services and methods for payment. However, having appropriate credentials does not guarantee approval as a provider. Some states may require a renewal procedure for the provider to continue to offer services to Part C clients.

Requirements for Providing Services: Once the professional has met all of the qualifications to provide therapy services, the therapist must obtain a referral from the developmental evaluation intervention team, a current IFSP, and a physician's referral for physical therapy services. Therapy services may then be provided in the natural environment consistent with that particular state's provisions, understanding that the natural environment could be the home setting, day care, or other.

When the IFSP is updated, a recommendation for continuation of therapy services must be provided. Any changes in the services must be cleared through the service coordinator. Services should not be initiated without the IFSP, which provides authorization for coverage through Part C. In addition, there may be an initial time frame to contact the family for the start of services.

Procedures for Payment: In order to receive payment for therapy services through Part C, the therapist must first bill the family's primary funding source if the family has agreed to have their private insurance or other source billed. The family may have to assume responsibility for applicable co-payments and deductibles depending on the state. For example, if there is private insurance, the private insurance agency must be billed first. If services are not covered by the family's insurance company, the services may be covered by Part C. The services would have to be documented as medically necessary and approved by the local agency that manages Part C prior to initiation of services.

Similarly, if the family has Medicaid, the therapist must first bill Medicaid for therapy services. If the services are not covered by Medicaid, then they may be provided with approval from the local Part C agency. Services must also be deemed medically necessary with submission of required documentation. Co-payments and deductibles may not apply to these recipients.

Part C is considered the payer of last resort in relationship to all other third-party payers. Payment rates and claim submission time frames are determined by each state agency. After receiving payment from the family's insurer, the therapist can then bill Part C for the remaining balance up to the allowable state Medicaid rates or the agreed-upon allowable rate as determined by each state. When Part C funding for a service is accepted, this reimbursement must be considered the full payment for the services, and the provider may not bill the balance of services to the family or third-party payers. Progress notes and recommendations must be submitted when billing Part C. Providers are required to maintain records and information related to the provision of covered services, the cost of the services, and the payments received by the provider on behalf of the client. Table 6-2 contains a summary of requirements for payment for each of the three major types of funding sources.

IDEA—PART B

The provision of therapy services to children ages 3 to 21 is covered by Part B of IDEA. The federal legislation stipulates that all children deserve a quality education alongside their peers. The legislation allows for all children and youth in this country the right free appropriate public education (FAPE) in the least restrictive environment (LRE).

IDEA is a federal law, with state education agency oversight, that supports the provision of public education for all children—regardless of the nature or severity of their disability. Part B of IDEA mandates the education of children 3 to 21 years old who have a disability

Table 6-2 Payment Requirements

REQUIREMENTS	PART C	MEDICAID	INSURANCE
Physician referral	Required or from IEP team	Required	Depends on state practice act and/or insurance company
Medically necessary	Yes	Yes	Yes, for continued service
Assessment	Provided by team	Yes	Often required
Plan of care	Yes	Yes	Often required
Progress notes	Yes	To be on file	Often required
Renewal of prescription	Annually	Every 6 months	Dictated by insurance company and/or state practice act
Reassessment	Annually	Every 6 months	Depends on insurance company and/or as condition changes (i.e., surgery)
Billing forms	CMS-1500	CMS-1500	CMS-1500

that interferes with their educational performance and their ability to benefit from their educational program.[4]

Implementation of IDEA, Part B, is the responsibility of each local education agency or school district.

- *Children with disabilities are entitled to a free, appropriate public education.*
- *Special education and related services are provided, as necessary, to meet the unique needs of each child.*
- *"Special education" means specialized instruction linked to a measurable annual goal. Students taking an alternate assessment should have benchmarks or short-term objectives.*
- *Special education and related services are to be provided in the least restrictive environment.*
- *IDEA—in conjunction with such other legislative mandates as the Americans With Disabilities Act, Section 504 of the Rehabilitation Act, and the Technology-Related Assistance for Individuals With Disabilities Act—provides appropriate school-based services for children.*
- *Physical therapy is one of the related services under Part B of IDEA.*
- *Physical therapy is provided to support the student's individualized education program (IEP).*
- *Physical therapists work collaboratively with a student's IEP team and participate in screening, evaluation, program planning, and intervention.*
- *As a member of the IEP team, physical therapists design and implement physical therapy interventions—including teaching and training of family and education personnel and measurement and documentation of progress—to help the student achieve his/her IEP goal.*
- *Physical therapists assist students in accessing school environments and benefiting from their educational program.*
- *Physical therapists may be hired through the school district, an intermediate unit, or a contract with an outside agency or private practice.*[4]

Under IDEA, planning and service delivery must be provided by a multidisciplinary team of professionals that must include a standard classroom teacher, a special education teacher, a representative of the local education agency (LEA), and the parents or guardian of the child. At the discretion of the parents or guardian and LEA representative, other individuals who have knowledge or special expertise regarding the child may also be included, such as physical, occupational, or speech therapists. Every child receiving special education must receive an IEP that is developed by this multidisciplinary/interprofessional team.

A parent or guardian, state agency, or LEA can refer a child for evaluation to determine if a child has a disability as defined under IDEA. The referral for a related service, such as physical therapy, can be initiated by anyone on the team for a child who has an IEP in place. The IEP team decides if the goals they developed need the support of a related service. PTs may screen a child before a referral is made by the IEP team. In states where the practice act for physical therapy requires physician referral, it must be obtained to perform the evaluation. In states where there is direct access, the physical referral may not be necessary unless required by third-party payers. In all cases, a physical referral is recommended in order to maintain communication with others outside the educational environment who are involved in the child's care.

Once a referral is made to determine if the child has a disability, a full and individualized initial evaluation must be performed. This evaluation requires parental consent and must be completed within 60 student attendance. The physical therapy evaluation can be part of the initial evaluation to determine eligibility for special education or can be performed after eligibility has been established.

Payment for Providing Services:

IDEA statutes and regulations mandate FAPE to eligible individuals with disabilities. There are specific formulas for the grants awarded to each state that depend on the number of children who receive special education and related services. School districts in each state may have specific funding criteria for the allocation of those funds. PTs do not directly bill for the provision of services rendered under Part B of IDEA. However, school districts may enroll as providers of Medicaid services and receive the federal share of Medicaid payments for providing Medicaid-covered services, such as physical therapy, to Medicaid recipients. Medicaid will be discussed further in the next section.

MEDICAID

Medicaid is a dual-funded system, based on federal and state monies, with the states reserving the right to determine service payment. This program is considered a state-funded health insurance plan designed for children from 0 to 21 years of age who meet certain income and disability criteria. Medicaid is administered by each individual state with state-determined eligibility and guidelines. Each state appoints a lead agency to manage Medicaid funding and contracts a fiscal agent to handle provider payment. Medicaid will pay for physical therapy services at the maximal Medicaid fee or the provider's customary fee, whichever is less. In some states, Medicaid has been privatized, and the rate of payment may differ based on capitation or a negotiated percentage of Medicaid fees with these private entities.

Author's Note

34 CFR 300.301:

"(c) Procedures for initial evaluation.

(1) The initial evaluation—(i) must be conducted within 60 days of receiving parental consent for the evaluation; or (ii) if the State establishes a timeframe within which the evaluation must be conducted, within that timeframe.

(2) Must consist of procedures—(i) to determine if the child is a child with a disability under §300.8; and (ii) to determine the educational needs of the child."

https://www.ecfr.gov/cgi-bin/text-idx?SID=eb5dffa33159a4a019c72acadc328c16&mc=true&node=se34.2.300_1301&rgn=div8

Qualifications for Providers for Medicaid: The qualifications for providers of Medicaid are specific to each state. In general, in order to provide therapy services for children and families covered by Medicaid, professionals must:

1. Apply for provider status.
2. Be fingerprinted for a criminal background check.
3. Provide a federal identification number (FIN) for businesses.
4. Provide the Social Security number (SSN) for individual providers.
5. Maintain a current state professional license.
6. Obtain an occupational license (where applicable).
7. Purchase liability insurance.
8. Obtain a business license (where applicable).
9. Have the billing agent sign the provider agreement.
10. Obtain a group Medicaid number if two or more providers are practicing together. Each member of the group must also enroll as an individual provider within the group.

Author's Note

In order to provide services to adults under Medicare, a PT or facility must also obtain a Medicare provider number by enrolling in Medicare.

Requirements for Providing Services: After meeting all of the qualifications to provide therapy services, the therapist must obtain a physician's referral before evaluating a child. The physician's referral should include the recipient's diagnosis, type of evaluation and service requested, the duration and frequency of treatment, and the physician's authorization number (if applicable). After completing the initial examination, the therapist must submit a copy of the evaluation and POC to the referring physician for signature and authorization for treatment. Treatment may not begin until the physician's signature is received on the POC and it has been submitted to Medicaid for authorization.

Each state establishes guidelines regarding the frequency and duration of therapy services. In some states, visits are approved for 6 months, and then the patient must be reassessed with the POC and frequency of therapy again submitted to the physician for authorization prior to the continuation of therapy services.

Each POC must include, but is not limited to, the following:

Author's Note

The information required is the same as that included in any physical therapy treatment plan.

- Child's full name (no nicknames)
- Child's date of birth
- Child's diagnosis
- Child's Medicaid ID number
- Diagnosis code (ICD-10)
- Name of referring physician
- Date of evaluation
- Requested period for treatment (dates)
- Examination/assessment
- Recommendations, including frequency and duration

- Achievable, measurable short- and long-term goals
- Physician's signature and authorization number, Medicaid number, and/or NPI number
- Provider's signature and provider number (license number)

Procedures for Payment

Many states provide software programs for electronic billing and electronic transfer of funds. Health insurance claim forms developed by the Center for Medicare & Medicaid Services (CMS), referred to as CMS-1500 form (see Appendix C) and 1450 (UB-04) form are required (as for most adult physical therapy payment). These claim forms speed optical scanning for quicker turnaround in processing and payment. As outlined by each state, the CPT codes must be used for billing. The physician's and/or Medicaid authorization number may be needed for billing purposes. Accuracy in completion of the form improves efficiency in payment. If the form is not completed accurately, it could result in a technical denial requiring resubmission.

As with all physical therapy services, only services deemed medically necessary, according to each individual state, will be paid. Depending on the state, covered services often include physical therapy, occupational therapy, speech and language therapy, and early intervention. In certain states, Medicaid may also pay for wheelchair evaluations and fittings to recipients age 21 and older. Justification for wheelchairs often requires lengthy documentation specific to the child's need for the chair and the adaptations or type of chair needed. Wheelchair vendors can often be helpful in providing templates for justification on durable medical equipment for the letter of medical necessity. Making sure that the referring physician has also documented the need for a wheelchair in the child's medical record is often required as well. The letter of medical necessity should include a brief summary of the child's medical condition, current status gathered through a wheelchair assessment, and the need for the wheelchair in general (i.e., the patient is nonambulatory). In addition, each individual part of the chair will require justification.

For children covered by private insurance, the private insurance agency must be billed before submitting for payment through Medicaid. Medicaid can then be billed for deductibles, the remaining balance (up to the Medicaid rate), or claims that were denied.

In many states, public schools are allowed to bill Medicaid for therapy services provided at the school. All requirements for providing services and payment apply. Medical necessity in an educational environment must be determined by the school district.

INSURANCE

Insurance is regulated in the state. State legislatures set broad policy for the regulation of insurance. They establish and oversee state insurance departments, regularly review and revise state insurance laws, and approve regulatory budgets. Each health insurance company outlines which therapy services are covered as stated in the individual subscriber's policies. Specific regulations contained in a subscriber's policy may include:

- Preexisting conditions, with legislation passed in March 2010 precluding a payer from denying a child coverage based on preexisting conditions. These rules went into effect for health insurance beginning on or after January 1, 2014.[5]
- Waiting periods.
- Deductibles.
- Allowable charges.
- Percentage of allowable charge covered.
- Co-payment.
- Documentation required from the service provider.

Some insurance companies require therapy providers to have company-specific provider numbers. Other companies require that therapy providers apply to become part of their "network" of providers. This is especially true in managed care organizations such as health maintenance organizations (HMOs), point-of-service (POS) plans, and preferred provider organizations (PPOs).

Author's Note

Some HMOs now have an "any willing provider" clause. This means that a provider need not be a HMO-designated provider, but must accept the HMO rate of payment.

Private insurance companies may also use national credentialing agencies where the therapy provider completes one application for multiple insurance companies. Therapy services that are part of a network must agree to accept a set fee or capitation as the maximum allowable charge for services rendered. This type of insurance appeals to subscribers, since there is either low or no deductibles and reduced co-pay. However, if the subscriber wishes to utilize an out-of-network provider, there is often an increased deductible, increased co-payment, co-insurance, or special permission required.

Requirements for Providing Services: To provide services for private insurance companies, therapists must have a current professional license for that state. To apply to be a network provider, the therapist must have current liability insurance, must have an occupational license, and must submit a resume. Insurance companies may have additional paperwork and requirements.

Procedures for Payment: Most private insurance companies require a referral from a physician in order to pay for therapy services, even in direct-access states. Some companies require an updated physician referral on a monthly basis; others require the referral be updated annually. A copy of the therapy examination may be required in addition to results of a standardized developmental assessment; written narrative addressing prognosis, short-term goals, and long-term goals; and the frequency and duration of therapy sessions. Interim progress notes and recommendations may also be required. Following major surgeries or changes in the child's condition, an updated physician referral and evaluation may be required.

For many insurance companies, CMS-1500 and CMS-1450 (also referred to as UB-04) "claim forms" are the standard requirement. Increasingly, billing is done electronically through the facility/institution billing software or through a clearing house. These forms must include the following information:

- Signature of the subscriber on file.
- Signed assignment of benefits form on file.
- Name and date of birth of the child.
- Child's diagnosis.
- Place of service.
- Subscriber's policy and/or group number.
- Therapy provider's identification number (if applicable).
- Business tax identification number or provider number and/or National Provider Identifier (NPI) number.
- Address of provider.
- Signature of provider or assigned designee and date of services.
- ICD-10 code indicating the child's diagnosis.
- Appropriate CPT codes for services rendered. There are several websites online to assist with making the appropriate decision. Often the referring provider will supply this in the referral.
- Inclusion of appropriate modifiers to identify each discipline and for coding edit requirements (e.g., GP for services delivered under an outpatient physical therapy POC, GN for services delivered under an outpatient speech therapy POC, and GO for services delivered under an outpatient occupational therapy POC, -59 if two services are rendered that require clarification in order to be paid as separate services/interventions).
- Units of service provided.

Schools/school-based therapy providers may also bill private insurance and in some cases Medicaid for payment of therapy services, but must have the permission of the child's family to do so. If the family refuses, the school must still provide therapy services deemed medically necessary in an educational environment.

CASH PAYMENTS

In today's practice, more PTs are accepting cash payments. Fees for the services should be reasonable and consider the setting where they are performed. Providers must adhere to state practice acts and should carry liability insurance. Upon accepting the patient for services, the examination, evaluation, and diagnosis must be made. Completion of documentation of services provided should be maintained. Content and documentation requirements are required by practice acts in many states. The APTA has developed guidelines for physical therapy documentation policies that are considered standard of practice.

PRO BONO/PHILANTHROPIC

Principle 10 of the APTA's *Guide for Professional Conduct*[6] states "A physical therapist shall endeavor to address the health needs of society." As a therapist, provision of services at a reduced or at no cost should be rendered to those lacking the ability to pay for services. Philanthropic organizations exist that will provide pro bono durable medical equipment or therapy services when not covered by other means. There are organizations at the national, state, and local levels. Examples of such organizations are United Cerebral Palsy, Juvenile Arthritis Association, or local charities and churches. Therapists should be knowledgeable and able to provide families with information about such organizations.

HEALTH INSURANCE PORTABILITY AND ACCOUNTABILITY ACT[7]

The HIPAA Privacy Rule created national standards to protect individuals' medical records and other personal health information by:[7]

- Establishing appropriate safeguards that healthcare providers and others must achieve to protect the privacy of health information
- Holding violators accountable, with civil and criminal penalties that can be imposed if they violate patients' privacy rights
- Setting boundaries on the use and release of health records
- Giving patients more control over their health information
- Striking a balance when public responsibility supports disclosure of some forms of data—for example, to protect public health.[7]

Does the HIPAA Privacy Rule allow parents the right to see their children's medical records?[7]

Answer: Yes, the Privacy Rule generally allows a parent to have access to the medical records about his or her child, as his or her minor child's personal representative when such access is not inconsistent with state or other law.

There are three situations when the parent would not be the minor's personal representative under the Privacy Rule. These exceptions are:

1. When the minor is the one who consents to care and the consent of the parent is not required under state or other applicable law
2. When the minor obtains care at the direction of a court or a person appointed by the court
3. When and to the extent that the parent agrees that the minor and the healthcare provider may have a confidential relationship.

However, even in these exceptional situations, the parent may have access to the medical records of the minor related to this treatment when state or other applicable law requires or permits such parental access. Parental access would be denied when state or other law prohibits such access. If state or other applicable law is silent on a parent's right of access in these cases, the licensed healthcare provider may exercise his or her professional judgment to the extent allowed by law to grant or deny parental access to the minor's medical information.

Finally, as is the case with respect to all personal representatives under the Privacy Rule, a provider may choose not to treat a parent as a personal representative when the provider reasonably believes, in his or her professional judgment, that the child has been or may be subjected to domestic violence, abuse, or neglect or that treating the parent as the child's personal representative could endanger the child.[7]

Child abuse takes many forms, which often occur at the same time. This information is from the Mayo Clinic:[9]

- ***Physical abuse.*** *Physical child abuse occurs when a child is purposely physically injured or put at risk of harm by another person.*
- ***Sexual abuse.*** *Sexual child abuse is any sexual activity with a child, such as fondling, oral-genital contact, intercourse, exploitation or exposure to child pornography.*
- ***Emotional abuse.*** *Emotional child abuse means injuring a child's self-esteem or emotional well-being. It includes verbal and emotional assault—such as continually belittling or berating a child—as well as isolating, ignoring or rejecting a child.*
- ***Medical abuse.*** *Medical child abuse occurs when someone gives false information about illness in a child that requires medical attention, putting the child at risk of injury and unnecessary medical care.*
- ***Neglect.*** *Child neglect is failure to provide adequate food, shelter, affection, supervision, education, or dental or medical care.*[5–9]

SUMMARY

The length of time the medical record for a child should be kept differs from that of an adult. As litigation may be involved with a child who has a disability, the PT must know the regulations regarding the time period required for retaining records (see Chapter 11). In some instances, it may be as long as 21 years.

Although there are some differences between pediatric and adult documentation, the same basic components are required. There must be medical necessity with the need for skilled physical therapy evident in the documentation. Emphasis must be on functionally oriented goals, with justification as to why the child needs the skill, if the child never developed it, or why the child needs to relearn the skill, if it was lost secondary to a new injury. Involvement and instruction to the caregivers must also be included. If equipment or adaptive devices are required for the child, it is the responsibility of the PT to determine if payment is available. If it is, the PT must then justify why the device is necessary through appropriate documentation and accompanying letter of medical necessity.

REVIEW QUESTIONS

1. Compare and contrast pediatric and adult documentation.
2. What information should a treatment plan for a child include?
3. What is Part C? How does a child qualify for Part C funding? Explain the role of documentation.
4. In pediatrics, what is the relationship between observation, assessment, and documentation?
5. Give five examples of behaviors/activities that should be assessed and documented in pediatrics, as age and developmentally appropriate.
6. Explain the concept of rehabilitation potential. Why is it better to use "good" rather than "excellent"? Why is it recommended not to use "poor" to rate rehab potential?

7. What are the basic elements of a progress report?
8. Describe the most efficient way to obtain a history for a child. What is the purpose of the history, and how does it relate to the decision-making process for the initial examination session?
9. What aged children are eligible for Medicaid funding? What is the funding source for Medicaid?
10. What is the role of the problem list in the initial examination? How much detail needs to be documented in it?
11. Are specific documentation formats required for most payers? What is required in pediatric documentation for all payer sources?
12. Explain the difference between rehabilitation potential and prognosis.

REFERENCES

1. *Guide to Physical Therapist Practice*, 3.0. Alexandria, VA: American Physical Therapy Association. Available at http://guidetoptpractice.apta.org/. Accessed July 20, 2020.
2. *Skilled Maintenance Therapy Under Medicare*. Alexandria, VA: American Physical Therapy Association. Available at https://www.apta.org/your-practice/payment/medicare-payment/coverage-issues/skilled-maintenance-therapy-under-medicare. Accessed August 10, 2020.
3. *Early Intervention Physical Therapy: IDEA Part C*. Alexandria, VA: American Physical Therapy Association. Available at https://pediatricapta.org/includes/fact-sheets/pdfs/IDEA%20EI.pdf. Accessed July 20, 2020.
4. *Providing Physical Therapy in Schools Under IDEA 2004*. Alexandria, VA: American Physical Therapy Association. Available at https://pediatricapta.org/includes/fact-sheets/pdfs/09%20IDEA%20Schools.pdf. Accessed July 20, 2020.
5. *Pre-existing Conditions*. U.S. Department of Health & Human Services. Available at https://www.hhs.gov/healthcare/about-the-aca/pre-existing-conditions/index.html. Accessed July 20, 2020.
6. *APTA's Guide for Professional Conduct*. Alexandria, VA: American Physical Therapy Association. Available at https://www.apta.org/your-practice/ethics-and-professionalism/apta-guide-for-professional-conduct. Accessed July 20, 2020.
7. *Health Information Privacy*. U.S. Department of Health & Human Services. Available at https://www.hhs.gov/hipaa/for-professionals/faq/227/can-i-access-medical-record-if-i-have-power-of-attorney/index.html. Accessed July 20, 2020.
8. *FERPA and HIPPA*. U.S. Department of Health & Human Services. Available at https://www.hhs.gov/hipaa/for-professionals/faq/ferpa-and-hipaa/index.html. Accessed July 20, 2020.
9. *Child Abuse*. Mayo Clinic. Available at https://www.mayoclinic.org/diseases-conditions/child-abuse/symptoms-causes/syc-20370864. Accessed July 20, 2020.

7 Documentation for Home Health

OBJECTIVES

Following completion of this chapter, the reader will be able to:

- Identify the qualifications for home health services under Medicare Part A and B.
- Discuss what the OASIS is in home health.
- Describe the role of standardized tests and instruments in home health.
- Explain what a MAC is and what role do they serve in home health.

HOME HEALTH DOCUMENTATION

> *Providing physical therapy services in the home health setting involves creativity, flexibility, and solid documentation skills. Physical therapists need to employ their full scope of assessment skills in order to manage a medically complex individual without the support of a medical facility or quick access to individual staff.*[1]

The legal and professional responsibility associated with documentation is an essential component of home health physical therapy. Physical therapists (PTs) and physical therapist assistants (PTAs) must stay current with continuously changing regulations and laws regardless of payer source. According to the Home Health Section of the American Physical Therapy Association (APTA), home healthcare is a medically oriented, skilled, and intermittent service provided in the home that may include nursing, physical therapy, occupational therapy, speech therapy/speech-language pathology, social services, dietary/nutrition counseling, pharmacy services, and/or home health aides.[2] Performing physical therapy in an individual's home can occur within private direct pay (outpatient physical therapy in the home), Medicare Part A (Hospital Insurance), and Medicare Part B (Medical Insurance). The physical therapist evaluates and provides interventions in the patient's place of residence, a noninstitutional setting. These environments include the patient's home, caregiver's home, assisted living facility, independent living facility, group home, residential facility, or the like. Home health offers more autonomy than other settings in which PT is rendered and provides needed skilled services for individuals who have difficulty leaving their homes or prefer to be treated in their own home.[3]

Author's Note

Medicare B services may be available in the home under 2 conditions:

1. As OP services because of challenges of access.
2. An individual has not had a hospital stay or inpatient rehab, but is in need of skilled services and is essentially homebound.

Outpatient PT services covered under Medicare Part B provided in patient homes via private practice or corporate outpatient, as a result of patient preference or lack of transportation, typically follow the same guidelines as outpatient facilities and usually require a co-pay.[4] Non-Medicare or non-Medicare Part B payers may limit or exclude physical therapy as a covered home health service, possibly resulting in the patient paying privately for therapy at home or being forced to obtain outpatient services. In all cases, PTs and PTAs should continue to document using principles consistent with APTA Guidelines: Physical Therapy Documentation of Patient/Client Management [BOD G03-05-16-41].[5] Since documentation regarding pediatrics is covered separately in this chapter, this section will focus primarily on documentation for the geriatric patient receiving services covered by Medicare and provided by home health agencies (HHA), as most payers follow Medicare guidelines.

Patients are typically aging adults, disabled persons, or children with a variety of diagnoses, including orthopedic, neurologic, cardiovascular, medical, and others. Individuals of any age, however, may need to receive home health services for a variety of medical reasons.

HHAs use the Home Health Change of Care Notice (HHCCN, Form CMS-10280) to notify original Medicare beneficiaries receiving home healthcare benefits of plan-of-care changes. HHAs are required to provide written notification to beneficiaries before reducing or terminating an item and/or service.

Over the past decade, home care documentation by PTs and PTAs has undergone a massive transition, which includes revisions to the primary tool used to assess patients and the transitions of electronic records.[7,8] Clinicians must be familiar with specific regulatory requirements from national, regional, and state levels and be aware of medication management, depression screening, case management, and diagnosis coding. Documentation for each treatment is highly scrutinized for skill level, medical necessity, and matching of all information and may be subject to review or audit by a growing number of government agencies and third-party payers, especially with the advent of Patient-Driven Payment Model, (PDGM) reimbursement as of January 2020.

OASIS AND REGULATORY GUIDELINES

See Appendix B for a copy of the OASIS-D.

REPORTING HOME HEALTH QUALITY USING OASIS DATA

The instrument/data collection tool used to collect and report performance data by HHAs is called the Outcome and Assessment Information Set (OASIS). Since 1999, Centers for Medicare & Medicaid Services (CMS) has required Medicare-certified HHAs to collect and transmit OASIS data for all adult patients whose care is reimbursed by Medicare and Medicaid, with the exception of patients receiving prenatal or postnatal services only. OASIS data is used for multiple purposes, including calculating several types of quality reports, which are provided to HHAs to help guide quality and performance improvement efforts.[7]

OASIS-D is the current version of the OASIS data set. It was implemented on January 1, 2019. OASIS-D includes multiple new standardized items to support measurement domains mandated by the Improving Medicare Post-Acute Care Transformation (IMPACT) Act of 2014. New items were also added for standardization to align with assessment sets for other post-acute care settings. Several items were also removed to reduce provider and patient burden. OASIS-D was approved by the Office of Management and Budget (OMB) on December 6, 2018, with an expiration date of December 31, 2021.[7] CMS is delaying expiration of OASIS-D and the release of the updated version of the Outcome and Assessment Information Set (referred to as OASIS-E) needed to support the Transfer of Health (TOH) Information Quality Measures and new or revised Standardized Patient Assessment Data Elements (SPADEs) in order to provide maximum flexibilities for providers of Home Health Agencies (HHAs) to respond to the COVID-19 Pubic Health Emergency (PHE).

The release of the updated version of the OASIS-E will be delayed until January 1st of the year that is at least 1 full calendar year after the end of the COVID-19 PHE. For example, if the COVID-19 PHE ends on September 20, 2020, HHAs will be required to begin collecting data using the updated versions of the item sets beginning with patients discharged on January 1, 2022.[7]

OASIS is used to collect information related to a home care recipient's demographic information, clinical status, functional status, and service needs. The purpose of the OASIS is to provide a standardized assessment tool that would support the reimbursement model and better monitor quality of care. The OASIS is completed at various time points: upon admission, discharge, transfer, and change in condition for all Medicare and Medicaid, nonmaternity, and nonpediatric beneficiaries.[9] OASIS data is collected by a home care clinician (e.g., nurse or therapist) via direct observation and interview of the patient and/or caregiver. The home care clinician may elicit input from the patient, caregivers, and other healthcare personnel, including the physician, the pharmacist, and/or other agency staff to assist in completion of any or all OASIS items (OASIS-D Guidance Manual Effective 1/1/2019 Centers for Medicare & Medicaid Services; Chapter 1).

The initial OASIS assessment is referred to as the start-of-care (SOC) assessment. This assessment is used when a patient is admitted for treatment to an HHA. When nursing services are ordered, either on their own or as part of a multidiscipline referral, the registered nurse (RN) must complete the SOC assessment. If a therapy service is ordered without nursing, a PT or speech-language pathologist (SLP) may complete the SOC assessment. During COVID-19 PHE, CMS allows PTs, OTs, and SLPs to perform the SOC assessment when nursing and PT, OT, and/or SLP is ordered. The SOC assessment must be finished within 5 calendar days of the SOC date. The SOC assessment must be based on the information collected during an actual visit with the patient.

The OASIS tool has undergone numerous revisions based on input from multiple task forces, government agencies, and clinicians. According to the OASIS-D Guidance Manual, published by CMS, the main reason for the revision was "to increase standardization across post-acute care (PAC) setting to enable calculation of standardized, cross settings quality measures (QMs), pursuant to the Improving Post-Acute Care Transformation Act (IMPACT, 2014)" (OASIS-D Guidance Manual Effective 1/1/2019 Centers for Medicare & Medicaid Services).

Throughout this chapter, OASIS-D will be referenced with the unique challenges it presents to physical therapy.

Information on the most recent version of OASIS and Medicare documentation requirements for home health is available at the CMS website at https://www.cms.gov/Center/Provider-Type/Home-Health-Agency-HHA-Center. This site includes CMS updates and the latest user manual for OASIS-D. The Medicare National Coverage Determinations (NCDs) Manual, published by CMS, which describes the specific services and treatments that may be reimbursed by Medicare.[10]

The Medicare Coverage Database contains all NCDs, Local Coverage Determinations (LCDs), and articles. The National Coverage Documents include NCDs, National Coverage Analyses (NCAs), Coding Analyses for Labs (CALs), Medicare Evidence Development & Coverage Advisory Committee (MEDCAC) meetings, and Medicare coverage guidance documents.

An LCD, as defined in §1869(f)(2)(B) of the Social Security Act (SSA), is a determination by a Medicare Administrative Contractor (MAC) regarding whether or not a particular item or service is covered on a contractor-wide basis in accordance with section 1862(a)(1)(A) of the act.

CMS relies on a network of MACs to serve as the primary contact between the Medicare program and the healthcare providers enrolled in the program. MACs regionally manage the policies and medical claims for Medicare Parts A and B, home health and hospice, and durable medical equipment across the country. Among other activities, the MACs establish LCDs and manage policy and payment related to reimbursement. Although all MACs receive the same directives from CMS, interpretation may differ by region and is interpreted for providers through the LCD process. More information about these contractors can be found at their respective websites. For a list of the MACs see: https://www.cms.gov/Medicare/Medicare-Contracting/Medicare-Administrative-Contractors/Who-are-the-MACs.

ELECTRONIC DOCUMENTATION IN HOME HEALTH

Electronic documentation in home care provides clinicians with useful tools to increase accuracy, consistency, and efficiency. The improvement in communication among clinicians and disciplines provides opportunities to review patient records in order to gain a more thorough assessment. Electronic systems have built-in mechanisms to ensure that documentation is more accurately completed. Electronic medical records (EMR) or systems are not, however, standardized in format and may vary among providers.

Although electronic documentation includes the same components as any written record, using electronic resources can reduce many challenges of handwritten communication, including but not limited to legibility, patient scheduling, specificity of patient goals, inconsistent care plans for supportive personnel, and interdisciplinary/interprofessional communication and access to past records and forms. Systems should provide adequate means for physical therapy professionals to enter narratives that distinguish their unique services and skills without records appearing rote from patient to patient, emphasizing the elements that support the skill needed. Depending on the sophistication of the system, clinicians may be able to document and print home exercise programs, search the Internet for information and patient education materials, and locate patients' homes using built-in mapping programs.

Many different models of portable, handheld devices are available. Devices and programs should comply with Health Insurance Portability and Accountability Act (HIPAA), and the individual professional must protect the device and content. The devices currently on the market can be programmed to meet the specific needs of the HHA. Electronic advancements are not limited to documentation alone. One such advancement, telehealth and telemonitoring, which provides live visual and auditory feedback, is a reality for home physical therapy to record exercise programs and compliance, document exertion levels, or respond to patient concerns about their care. Cardiac rehabilitation home programs have already instituted telemonitoring of vital signs and other information from their patients with overwhelming success.[11]

Author's Note

Professionals should not be documenting on personal devices unless they have encryption or access to organizational cloud-based systems that are password protected.

MEETING THE REQUIREMENTS FOR HOME CARE

Medicare covers HHA services when the following criteria are met:

1. The person to whom the services are provided is an eligible Medicare beneficiary.
2. The HHA that is providing the services to the beneficiary has in effect a valid agreement to participate in the Medicare program.
3. The beneficiary qualifies for coverage of home health services as described in §30.
4. The services for which payment is claimed are covered as described in §§40 and 50.
5. Medicare is the appropriate payer.
6. The services for which payment is claimed are not otherwise excluded from payment. See Medicare Benefit Policy Manual Chapter 7 Section 20: https://www.cms.gov/Regulations-and-Guidance/Guidance/Manuals/Downloads/bp102c07.pdf.[12]

According to MBPM Chapter 7:

Where the Medicare criteria for coverage of home health services are met, patients are entitled by law to coverage of reasonable and necessary home health services. Therefore, a patient is entitled to have the costs of reasonable and necessary services reimbursed by Medicare without regard to whether there is someone available to furnish the services.[12]

Table 7-1 Who Is Eligible for Home Health Medicare Part A and B

All people with Part A and/or Part B who meet all of these conditions are covered:

- You must be under the care of a doctor, and you must be getting services under a plan of care created and reviewed regularly by a doctor.
- You must need, and a doctor must certify that you need, one or more of these:
  - Intermittent skilled nursing care (other than drawing blood)
  - Physical therapy, speech-language pathology, or continued occupational therapy services. These services are covered only when the services are specific, safe, and an effective treatment for your condition. The amount, frequency ,and time period of the services needs to be reasonable, and they need to be complex or only qualified therapists can do them safely and effectively. To be eligible, either (1) your condition must be expected to improve in a reasonable and generally predictable period of time, or (2) you need a skilled therapist to safely and effectively make a maintenance program for your condition, or (3) you need a skilled therapist to safely and effectively do maintenance therapy for your condition. The home health agency caring for you is approved by Medicare (Medicare certified).
- You must be homebound, and a doctor must certify that you're homebound.

You're not eligible for the home health benefit if you need more than part-time or "intermittent" skilled nursing care. You may leave home for medical treatment or short, infrequent absences for nonmedical reasons, like attending religious services. You can still get home healthcare if you attend adult daycare.

SOURCE: Home Health Services. Medicare.gov: The Official U.S. Government Site for Medicare. https://www.medicare.gov/coverage/home-health-services. Accessed July 21, 2020.

To qualify for the Medicare home health benefit, under §§1814(a)(2)(C) and 1835(a)(2)(A) of the act, a Medicare beneficiary must meet the following requirements:

- Be confined to the home
- Be under the care of a physician
- Be receiving services under a POC established and periodically reviewed by a physician
- Be in need of skilled nursing care on an intermittent basis or physical therapy or speech-language pathology
- Have a continuing need for occupational therapy

For purposes of benefit eligibility, under §§1814(a)(2)(C) and 1835(a)(2)(A) of the act, "intermittent" means skilled nursing care that is either provided or needed on fewer than 7 days each week or less than 8 hours of each day for periods of 21 days or less (with extensions in exceptional circumstances when the need for additional care is finite and predictable). A patient must meet each of the criteria specified in this section. Patients who meet each of these criteria are eligible to have payment made on their behalf for services discussed in §§40 and 50. See Table 7.1 for who is eligible for Home Health Medicare Part A and B.

According to Medicare Claims Processing Manual (MCPM) Chapter 10, Section 90, HHAs may submit claims for certain medical and other health services, which are paid from the Part B trust fund. The HHA may receive payment for these services outside of the prospective payment system (https://www.cms.gov/Regulations-and-Guidance/Guidance/Manuals/downloads/clm104c10.pdf).

DOCUMENTATION OF HOMEBOUND STATUS

Section 30.1.1 of MBPM Chapter 7 further states:

> *For a patient to be eligible to receive covered home health services under both Part A and Part B, the law requires that a physician certify in all cases that the patient is*

confined to his/her home. For purposes of the statute, an individual shall be considered "confined to the home" (homebound) if the following two criteria are met:

1. *Criterion One: The patient must either: Because of illness or injury, need the aid of supportive devices such as crutches, canes, wheelchairs, and walkers; the use of special transportation; or the assistance of another person in order to leave their place of residence.*

   OR

   Have a condition such that leaving his or her home is medically contraindicated.

   If the patient meets one of the criterion conditions, then the patient must ALSO meet two additional requirements defined in criterion two below.
2. *Criterion Two: There must exist a normal inability to leave home;*

   AND

   Leaving home must require a considerable and taxing effort. If the patient does in fact leave the home, the patient may nevertheless be considered homebound if the absences from the home are infrequent or for periods of relatively short duration, or are attributable to the need to receive health care treatment.

   Absences attributable to the need to receive health care treatment include, but are not limited to:

   - *attendance at adult day centers to receive medical care;*
   - *ongoing receipt of outpatient kidney dialysis; or*
   - *the receipt of outpatient chemotherapy or radiation therapy.*

   Any absence of an individual from the home attributable to the need to receive health care treatment, including regular absences for the purpose of participating in therapeutic, psychosocial, or medical treatment in an adult day-care program that is licensed or certified by a State, or accredited to furnish adult day-care services in a state, shall not disqualify an individual from being considered to be confined to his home. Any other absence of an individual from the home shall not so disqualify an individual if the absence is of an infrequent or of relatively short duration. For purposes of the preceding sentence, any absence for the purpose of attending a religious service shall be deemed to be an absence of infrequent or short duration. It is expected that in most instances, absences from the home that occur will be for the purpose of receiving health care treatment. However, occasional absences from the home for nonmedical purposes, e.g., an occasional trip to the barber, a walk around the block or a drive, attendance at a family reunion, funeral, graduation, or other infrequent or unique event would not necessitate a finding that the patient is not homebound if the absences are undertaken on an infrequent basis or are of relatively short duration and do not indicate that the patient has the capacity to obtain the health care provided outside rather than in the home.

Some examples of homebound patients that illustrate the factors used to determine whether a homebound condition exists are listed here:[13]

- A patient paralyzed from a stroke who is confined to a wheelchair or requires the aid of crutches in order to walk.
- A patient who is blind or senile and requires the assistance of another person in leaving their place of residence.
- A patient who has lost the use of their upper extremities and therefore is unable to open doors, use handrails on stairways, etc., and requires the assistance of another individual to leave their place of residence.
- A patient in the late stages of amyotrophic lateral sclerosis (ALS) or neurodegenerative disabilities. In determining whether the patient has the general inability to leave the home and leaves the home only infrequently or for periods of short duration, it is necessary (as is the case in determining whether skilled nursing services are intermittent) to look at the

patient's condition over a period of time rather than for short periods within the home health stay. For example, a patient may leave the home (meeting both criteria listed earlier) more frequently during a short period when the patient has multiple appointments with healthcare professionals and medical tests in 1 week. So long as the patient's overall condition and experience is such that he or she meets these qualifications, he or she should be considered confined to the home.

- A patient who has just returned from a hospital stay involving surgery, who may be suffering from resultant weakness and pain because of the surgery and therefore their actions may be restricted by their physician to certain specified and limited activities (such as getting out of bed only for a specified period of time, walking stairs only once a day, etc.).
- A patient with arteriosclerotic heart disease of such severity that they must avoid all stress and physical activity.
- A patient with a psychiatric illness that is manifested in part by a refusal to leave home or is of such a nature that it would not be considered safe for the patient to leave home unattended, even if they have no physical limitations.

The aged person who does not often travel from home because of frailty and insecurity brought on by advanced age would not be considered confined to the home for purposes of receiving home health services unless they meet one of the earlier conditions. Although a patient must be confined to the home to be eligible for covered home health services, some services cannot be provided at the patient's residence because equipment is required that cannot be made available there.

If the services required by an individual involve the use of such equipment, the HHA may make arrangements with a hospital, skilled nursing facility (SNF), or a rehabilitation center to provide these services on an outpatient basis. (See §50.6.) However, even in these situations, for the services to be covered as home health services, the patient must be considered confined to the home and meet both criteria listed earlier.

If a question is raised as to whether a patient is confined to the home, the HHA will be requested to furnish the Medicare contractor with the information necessary to establish that the patient is homebound as defined earlier.

At the onset of care, a PT must determine or verify a patient's homebound status and document it thoroughly and specifically. Clear written justification to support homebound status is required at each therapy session.

Examples of documented home absences include:

- Physician appointment
- Dialysis, chemotherapy, and radiation therapy
- Adult daycare
- Religious event
- Hairdresser
- Reunion, funeral, graduation, or unique event

If patients meet the criteria for homebound status, therapists can proceed with an evaluation once an OASIS has been completed by either a nurse or the PT or SLP. In most cases, the functional status of the patient should serve as validation and is critical in the documentation.

Examples of documentation content for homebound status include:

- Confinement to a wheelchair or bed following any injury, or with pathology such as a stroke or spinal cord injury
- Ambulation with a walker or crutches or other assistive devices with assistance or constant supervision
- Vision deficits requiring assistance and training
- Any medical condition limiting stress or activity, such as cardiac surgery
- Physical deficits, such as loss of lower extremity strength or muscle performance, that may limit function and create safety concerns in public settings

In addition to these criteria, the PT should use standard tests and measures to objectively document functional deficits that limit the patient and quantify progress over time. An example is the Borg Rating of Perceived Exertion (RPE), a 15-point scale ranging from no exertion to maximal exertion.[14] A patient could be assessed and then instructed in the use of the RPE scale. If the patient leaves their home for specific events, the events should be documented with the patient's self-reported RPE. Progress can be measured over time by comparing the patient report.

Other standardized instruments or tests and measures that can assess function over time and response to intervention are also critical to use for establishing objective and measurable goals and monitoring patient progress.

Author's Note

Occasional absences from the home for nonmedical purposes, e.g., an occasional trip to the barber, a walk around the block or a drive, attendance at a family reunion, funeral, graduation, or other infrequent or unique event would not necessitate a finding that the patient is not homebound if the absences are undertaken on an infrequent basis or are of relatively short duration and do not indicate that the patient has the capacity to obtain the health care provided outside rather than in the home.[15]

EVALUATION IN HOME HEALTH CARE: OASIS-D START OF CARE

As of January 1, 2019, the revised OASIS tool, OASIS-D, is required at the initial home health assessment, SOC, for all Medicare and Medicaid patients.[16] Answering OASIS questions requires an in-depth understanding of OASIS conventions, inclusion and exclusion criteria, and CMS clarifications via the quarterly Q&A (question and answer) documents. The CMS OASIS-D Guidance Manual and OASIS updates can be found at the cms.gov website.[7]

According to CMS, a registered nurse, PT, or speech therapist/SLP may complete the SOC OASIS.[16] The assessing therapist may need to consult with other clinicians treating an individual patient or individuals more knowledgeable in certain components of the OASIS to ascertain the best responses to each question. CMS also conducts regular webinars to address concerns with the OASIS and responds to questions posted to their website. Most HHAs also provide training and testing on accurate OASIS completion by all professionals who may be required to use it. Individuals with advanced training and certification in OASIS (e.g., Home Care Clinical Specialist—OASIS [HCS-O] Certification, OASIS Specialist—Clinical [COS-C]) are often employed in Medicare-certified HHAs and are available for additional guidance.

For this section, specific components of the SOC that pose unique challenges to the PT are addressed.

DOCUMENTING HISTORY AND DEMOGRAPHICS

The first series of questions involve the background of the patient and include the following:

- HHA provider number and state
- Physician NPI (National Provider Identification) number
- Start of care (SOC) date
- Patient name, state, ZIP code, insurance number (health insurance claim number [HICN]), Social Security number (SSN; as of April 2019, SSNs will no longer be required on the

OASIS claim—the randomly generated Medicare Beneficiary Identifier [MBI] will replace the SSN-based HICN)

- Patient race/ethnicity
- Discipline of person completing the assessment
- Date assessment was completed and the date the assessment was ordered
- Location of patient prior to the assessment (hospital, home, SNF) and discharge date
- Medical and social history
- Inpatient procedure and diagnoses for the past 14 days, if applicable
- Current diagnoses using ICD-10 coding

DOCUMENTING INTERNATIONAL CLASSIFICATION OF DISEASES CODES

International Classification of Disease (ICD-10) codes represent the diagnosis, surgical, history, and procedure codes that are related to the patient being evaluated.[17] Physical therapists should be knowledgeable about the ICD-10 codes in order to accurately plan the care of the patient and reflect the diagnoses being treated (see Chapter 13 for more information about ICD-10cm codes). The medical diagnoses may be the same as or different from the physical therapy treatment diagnoses, as presented in an earlier chapter. PTs should be familiar with the most commonly used functionally oriented and impairment-oriented code verbiage. Although the PT may not be the one assigning the numeric ICD code, if the verbiage is consistent a "coder" employed by the agency can accurately assign it. Many of the electronic documentation systems contain some form of assistance with ICD coding. The order of the documented codes should list the most severe condition being treated first then the lesser severe to the least severe. The home health PT must document all present diagnoses; medical and treatment; prior medical and surgical history, past and recent; all current dietary habits; social history; and medications and supplements, both prescription and over-the-counter. All this information facilitates the assignment and selection of the most appropriate ICD codes.[17]

DOCUMENTING RISK FOR HOSPITALIZATION

CMS included a question in the OASIS to gain a better understanding of the patient's potential for being admitted to a hospital while in home care. Therapists can select none, one, or multiple choices for hospitalization risk. These options include the following:

- Recent decline in mental, emotional, and behavioral status
- Multiple hospitalizations
- History of falls
- Taking five or more medications (which increases the risk for falls)
- Frailty indicators such as weight loss or exhaustion

CMS has placed an intentional focus on reducing the number of avoidable hospital readmissions and subsequent cost to Medicare. HHAs play a significant role in keeping patients safe at home, especially during high-risk care transitions. The readmission reduction programs in place support the national goal of improving healthcare for Americans by linking payment to the quality of care provided. CMS has placed a focus on quality of care to also reduce the number of avoidable readmissions. CMS has adopted the mission of the National Academy of Medicine (formerly the Institute of Medicine), which has defined quality as having multiple properties or domains (see Table 7.2).

CLINICAL DEPRESSION

In 2010, questions were included in the OASIS that concerned clinical depression. The depression component was added to better understand the psychological needs of home

Table 7-2 CMS Quality

CMS has adopted the mission of the National Academy of Medicine (formerly the Institute of Medicine), which has defined quality as having the following properties or domains:
Effectiveness relates to providing care processes and achieving outcomes as supported by scientific evidence.
Efficiency relates to maximizing the quality of a comparable unit of healthcare delivered or unit of health benefit achieved for a given unit of healthcare resources used.
Equity relates to providing healthcare of equal quality to those who may differ in personal characteristics other than their clinical condition or preferences for care.
Patient-centeredness relates to meeting patients' needs and preferences and providing education and support.
Safety relates to actual or potential bodily harm.
Timeliness relates to obtaining needed care while minimizing delays.

health patients, as it was believed that depression was not properly identified and assessed in elderly clients. This requires the HHA to select a standardized tool to screen for depression but not medically diagnose. CMS includes Pfizer's PHQ-2 scale, which asks about frequency of decreased interest in activities and frequency that the patient feels down, depressed, or hopeless. Other commonly used depression screening tools include the Geriatric Depression Scale and the Cornell Scale for Depression in Dementia.[18,19] As depression may interfere with function and progress, early detection and appropriate medical management will benefit the patient. Therapists should include in their documentation descriptions of behaviors that may be indicative of depression, especially if a patient is not achieving appropriate functionally oriented goals in the expected duration of care. Referral to appropriate mental health professionals may be indicated based on the scale results.

DIABETIC FOOT CARE AND HEART FAILURE

In 2010, CMS added two components to the OASIS requiring further assessment and documentation by physical therapy. If a patient has a diagnosis of diabetes, type 1 or type 2 or other, CMS requires information in the POC that is directed to diabetes-related conditions. This includes two items: monitoring for the presence of skin lesions on the lower extremities and feet and providing education on proper foot care. The PT has three choices of response: "no," inferring the patient has diabetes and these interventions are not on the POC; "yes," the patient is a diabetic and these interventions are included; or "NA" the patient is not diabetic.[16] There are other associated diabetes-related conditions that should also be assessed and monitored by the PT in addition to those specified by CMS, such as sensation on the feet, including pressure/touch and proprioception.

CMS also requests information at discharge concerning symptoms of heart failure. If the patient has a diagnosis of heart failure, CMS wants to know if the patient exhibited any symptoms of heart failure since the last OASIS assessment. As in diabetes, there is the option of three responses: "no," has the diagnosis without symptoms; "yes," has diagnosis and has symptoms; or "NA," the patient has no diagnosis of heart failure.[16] Both of these questions, although simply stated, can be easily misinterpreted and answered incorrectly by the PT. Someone may hastily select "no" to a question if the patient does not have the diagnosis of diabetes or heart failure when the appropriate response is NA. If an appropriate history is obtained or medical record review conducted, the PT should be able to respond correctly. To be able to respond to the CMS queries or adequately monitor cardiac status, the PT/PTA should be regularly monitoring perceived exertion and vital signs and document all results, as well as observed responses to exertion.

PAIN ASSESSMENT AND MANAGEMENT

Medicare regulation requires that clinicians use a standardized assessment tool for the evaluation of pain.[16] The tool should be appropriate for the communication and cognitive level of the patient in order to record an accurate response. The tool should also allow the patient to express the range of answers from *no pain* to *severe pain*. Examples of such tools include:

1. Numeric Pain Intensity Scale: Patients use a 0/10 to 10/10 scale to assess the degree of pain
2. Simple Descriptive Pain Intensity Scale: Patients choose words like "mild," "moderate," and "severe" to describe the pain intensity
3. Visual Analog Scale (VAS): Patients select a point on a 10-cm vertical or horizontal line that indicates pain intensity
4. Wong-Baker Faces Pain Intensity Scale: Patients can select a picture of a facial expression that best matches their pain level. This scale is used more in pediatrics or with adults who are unable or unwilling to use other types of scales.

The initial examination and evaluation should include appropriate questions that best help to describe their experience with pain, including locations, what makes the pain better or worse, a description of the quality of the pain (i.e., sharp, dull ache, throbbing, stabbing), what interventions help manage the pain, if the pain wakes them up at night or disturbs sleep, and how often they experience pain.

In addition to using a standardized tool, clinicians must document pain intensity and the frequency with which the pain interferes with the patient's activity level.[16] A patient may report a decreased pain rating because they are NOT performing an activity, whereas, a patient may not perform an activity, such as gardening, if he or she experiences knee pain. Therefore, the clinician must ask and document what behaviors (including frequencies) would be performed if pain was reduced. However, leisure activities such as gardening are not justification for skilled PT. Clinicians should also observe and document their clients' facial expressions during activities to further evaluate pain. Pharmacologic and/or nonpharmacologic interventions may control the pain so that it does not interfere with activity or movement. These interventions should be documented, since they could be temporary and limit the patient's activity level. Patients' pain over time and the decrease of the pain should be included in continuum-of-care documentation and should reflect positive progress toward goals as function increases using objective measures and patient self-report.

DOCUMENTING WOUNDS AND PRESSURE ULCERS

The documentation requirements for wounds and ulcers may vary based on payment, practice settings, and by how the skin area is classified. CMS has specific guidelines for recording pressure ulcers to gain a better understanding of the risk and status of their clients.[16] In the OASIS document, the clinician must assess the risk of the patient for developing pressure ulcers. As with other sections in the OASIS, the utilization of a standardized tool (e.g., Norton, Braden, etc.) is preferred to determine risk, or the therapist may base the evaluation of risk on clinical factors such as mobility, incontinence, and/or nutrition. CMS reports their intent is to capture the HHA's best practice regarding the integumentary system.[16] If one or more pressure ulcers are present, the clinician must document how many, the stage of each unhealed ulcer, and the measurements (in centimeters) of the largest ulcer. Standard guidelines for documentation of any open wound include size/measurements, drainage, odor, color, and description of tissue both in the wound and in the periwound area.

The clinician must also document in the OASIS any venous stasis ulcers. These areas are caused by poor venous circulation and are often associated with stasis dermatitis.[16] If a surgical procedure was performed, the clinician must also identify if a surgical wound is present.

For each of these concerns, the therapist is requested to describe the status of the most problematic observable pressure ulcer, stasis ulcer, and surgical wound with one of the following:

- Newly epithelialized (epithelial tissue has completely covered the wound surface)
- Fully granulating (granulating but epithelial tissue has completely covered the wound surface)
- Early/partial granulation
- Not healing ($\geq$25% necrotic or avascular tissue)

  And for pressure ulcers only:
- No observable pressure ulcer if covered by dressing, cast, etc.

The documentation of other types of skin lesions or open wounds that require intervention should be listed.[16] Examples of these lesions include skin tears, burns, peripherally inserted central catheter (PICC) line sites, rashes, diabetic ulcers, trauma wounds, and ostomies (bowel ostomies excluded). PTs should address these lesions in a narrative format to describe the location, intervention, and goals if part of the physical therapy plan of care.

DOCUMENTING MEDICATIONS AND MEDICATION MANAGEMENT

In order to participate in the Medicare program, certain medication standards must be met by the HHA.[12] One of these requirements involves evaluating current medications. According to CMS, all current medications must be reviewed to identify any potential adverse effects and drug reactions, ineffective drug therapy, side effects, drug interactions, duplicate drug therapy, and noncompliance with drug therapy.[16] The HHA Interpretive Guideline for Condition of Participation 42 CFR 484.55(c)(5) states: *The patient's clinical record should identify all medications that the patient is taking (both prescription and non-prescription) as well as times of medication administration and route. As part of the comprehensive assessment the HHA nurse should consider, and the clinical record should document, that the HHA nurse considered each medication the patient is currently taking for possible side effects and the list of medications in its entirety for possible drug interactions. The HHA should have policies that guide HHA clinical staff in the event there is a concern identified with a patient's medication that should be reported to the physician. In rehabilitation therapy only cases, the patient's therapist must submit a list of patient medications, which the therapist must collect during the comprehensive assessment, to an HHA nurse for review. The HHA should contact the physician if indicated.* https://www.cms.gov/Medicare/Provider-Enrollment-and-Certification/SurveyCertificationGenInfo/Downloads/QSO18-25-HHA.pdf. From a prevention of medical errors perspective, the PT should be attentive to behaviors exhibited during therapy sessions, which may be side effects of the medications, potential negative interactions, and whether a drug prescribed for a medical condition has potentially stopped working.

DOCUMENTING FUNCTION: M1800 SECTION

A major component of the patient evaluation and OASIS is documentation of function and ability to perform specific tasks.[16] Accurate reflection of the patient's ability to perform certain tasks assists in the determination of justification of skilled care, reimbursement, and outcome reporting to government agencies. Each task may be limited by physical, cognitive, or sensory impairments or environmental barriers. This is critical in physical therapy documentation for Medicare and all other third-party payers.

The PT must document the patient's ability to perform the following functional tasks in the M1800 section of the OASIS (Note: Some of the activities of daily living [ADL] information may be obtained by interview if either the patient or caretaker is competent to answer appropriately):

- Grooming (washing hands, face, hair, teeth, nails, etc.)
- Ability to dress upper body

- Ability to dress lower body
- Bathing (wash entire body; excludes grooming and shampooing hair)
- Toilet transferring (ability to get to and from toilet or bedside commode)
- Toilet hygiene (ability to maintain perineal area or ostomy site and adjust clothing)
- Feeding or eating (ability to eat, chew, and swallow)
- Ability to plan and prepare light meals (also includes safely reheating delivered meals)
- Ability to use the telephone (access, operate keypad or dial and communicate effectively, based on type of phone available)
- Transitional movement/transferring (ability to move safely from bed to chair, sit to and from stand, transition from supine to and from sit, or position in bed)
- Ambulation/locomotion (ability to walk or use wheelchair safely on a variety of surfaces, including directional changes, negotiating doors, curbs, etc.)

For each functional item, responses are ranked from the most independent to the most dependent. For example, the most dependent response for ambulation is *bedfast*, and the most independent response involves walking on even and uneven surfaces and negotiating stairs (with or without railing), both with neither human assistance nor assistive device. CMS explains that these questions identify the patient's ability and not necessarily actual performance.[16] If the ability fluctuates, the clinician should select the response that describes the ability for the client to safely perform the task over 50% of the time. The best method to determine the correct response, especially for mobility, is observation and assessment of the specific activity. The condition in which the task is performed is critical to evaluating safety. A patient may be able to quickly transfer in and out of a bathtub in dry, clothed conditions but may have difficulty with this task in bare feet with soap and water for longer than 5 minutes. Clinicians should refer to the CMS OASIS-D Guidance Manual for further delineation of each functional question

SECTION GG: FUNCTIONAL ABILITIES AND GOALS

The IMPACT (2014) requires the standardization of patient assessment data reported in each post-acute care setting (inpatient rehab facilities, long-term care hospitals, SNFs, and HHAs). With the implementation of OASIS-D, HHAs began collecting mandatory data items related to functional status (self-care and mobility) in section GG of the OASIS. The data collection is standardized and mandated in all post-acute care settings. The intent of the data collection is to promote communication between settings, measure the effectiveness of rehabilitation care delivered in each setting, measure the effectiveness of the providers themselves, and provide the basis for comparing costs associated with care between settings and longitudinally. Prior to these changes, post-acute care settings were collecting their own data with their own definitions and rating scales, which created a challenge in caring for patients when they were transferred from one setting to another.

The GG and M1800 sections are not identical. M1800 revolves around what the patient can safely do for themselves. The GG questions ask about helper assistance. The rating scales are completely different and are to be answered via their respective CMS guidance.

Self-care items include:

- Eating
- Oral hygiene
- Toileting hygiene
- Showering/bathing self
- Upper body dressing
- Lower body dressing
- Putting on/taking off footwear

Mobility items include:

- Rolling left and right
- Sitting to lying

- Lying to sitting on side of the bed
- Sitting to standing
- Chair/bed to chair transferring
- Toilet transferring
- Car transferring
- Walking 10 feet
- Walking 50 feet with two turns
- Walking 150 feet
- Walking 10 feet on uneven surfaces
- Stepping up/down 1 step/4 steps/12 steps
- Picking up an object
- Wheeling 50 feet with two turns
- Wheeling 150 feet

These items will be collected on all SOC OASIS, Recertification OASIS, and Discharge OASIS. Only a few items will be collected on the Follow-up OASIS.

MEDICAL NECESSITY IN HOME CARE

At least one of the MACs has provided guidelines that outline how to support physical therapy services that are reasonable and medically necessary. These guidelines are designed to assure that the treatment provided requires the unique set of skills of the PT or PTA. For a treatment to be deemed medically necessary, the documentation must provide the "complexity of the treatment" and "why the treatment is medically appropriate, based on the beneficiary's condition."[20]

This is consistent with all venues that provide physical therapy to Medicare beneficiaries. Included in the complexity of the treatment are five components.

Tests, Measures, and Assessment

These can include such procedures as orthopedic special tests, goniometric measurements, manual muscle testing, balance tests, standardized testing, postural assessment, cranial nerve testing, developmental tests, or other tests that require the knowledge of a PT or PTA to complete.

Planning, Interventions, and Changes

This stage demonstrates how the knowledge gained through testing and observation is used to create a treatment plan, select specific interventions, and adapt to changes in the patient's condition. For example, if the patient scored a 10 on a Tinetti gait and balance test, the therapist would conclude that the patient is at a higher risk for falls and decide to select interventions that address balance in the patient's treatment plan.

Author's Note

When using a standardized test and measure such as the Tinetti, in addition to attaching the completed test to the initial examination and evaluation, the identified deficits should be summarized in the body of the evaluation. Goals should be established consistent with the specific functional problem and match the treatment. The standardized test can be readministered throughout care to monitor progress and, at a minimum, should be repeated at discharge.

Teaching and Assessment of a Patient's Ability to Follow Through

The documentation following treatment needs to show an improved ability for the patient or patient's caregiver to continue the treatment plan.

Continued Need for Assessment and Teaching

This component is usually the most difficult for PTs and PTAs to write. The goal is to understand the functional problem and determine what skills are required to change the behavior. Example: Instead of assessing a sit-to-stand transfer as "requires moderate assist," one could report "Patient unable to shift upper body forward in order to stand. Instructed in foot placement and provided verbal instruction/cues and tactile input at shoulders for patient to stand. Patient able to perform sit to stand 5 times, with the 5th repetition requiring contact guard." Although this example is noticeably more lengthy, it provides the skills (verbal cues, tactile cues), the assessment (contact guard), and that more treatment is warranted for the patient to be safe and independent. A patient must be able to repeat a skill multiple times in order to be functional.

Avoid Documenting Repetitive Modalities and Interventions

This documentation practice exists in all settings, but since the home usually contains limited exercise equipment, the tendency to repeat exercises and interventions increases. CMS and the MACs are more concerned with the patient's behavior than a PT documenting "ther ex" every treatment session. If the use of a modality improves function, document the new behavior of the patient, or if the gait pattern of a patient improves, select different surfaces and directional changes for the patient to perform gait and gait-related activities.

Documenting Medical Necessity

In order to better document why PT treatment is medically appropriate, three conditions should be met:

- Patient's needs
- Functional changes
- Changes in condition

Documentation should include the rationale for selecting treatment options. For example, if a patient wants to return to safely bending down to don clothing or pick up objects and safely negotiate in the bathroom for personal hygiene, therapy would include gait and balance training on unlevel or uneven surfaces, positional changes, and upper and lower extremity therapeutic exercise including stretching, strengthening, etc. The narrative should also include what functional tasks may be affected by the patient's diagnoses.

Prior level of function (as immediately prior to the current episode of care as possible)
The determination of past performance is helpful to evaluate changes in behavior.

Document any other conditions that may support need for therapy in situations that would not ordinarily need a therapist. Example: A patient with a pelvic fracture may be able to ambulate with family after being instructed by the therapist. However, the patient requires the therapist to support the trunk and guard the patient because of the fracture and risk for falling.

PLAN OF CARE

If the determination is made that physical therapy treatment is appropriate for a patient and medical necessity requirements are met, the PT can establish a POC. The POC should convey the predicted functional outcome over a specified duration of time.[1] In home care, the time duration determined by the PT may span an entire 60-day episode for patients that have significant medical need, but in 30-day periods of care with the Patient-Driven Groupings Model (PDGM) implemented beginning January 1, 2020. Some clients may only be homebound for 1 to 2 weeks and then discharged to outpatient physical therapy or discontinued from care. The POC may be derived separately from the OASIS, but most electronic documentation systems create the documents simultaneously. One should note that although one clinician is responsible for completing the OASIS, the POC should contain the following information from all disciplines:

- Patient-centered goals written in measurable, functional terms with a projected date of completion.
- All interventions to be provided to the patient by the HHA.
- The duration and frequency of all disciplines. Example: Skilled nursing 1wk1, 2wk2; physical therapy 1wk1, 3wk2, 2wk2, 1wk2; occupational therapy 2wk5; home health aide 3wk4.

Author's Note

1wk1 means that the frequency for week 1 was once. 3wk2 means 3 times a week for 2 weeks.

- The anticipated discharge plan for the patient. Example: Outpatient PT; home with caregiver with appropriate instructions
- For Medicare clients, all the current diagnoses and medications are included on the POC.[12]
- Physician orders that may differ from those listed on the referral to home care. These may include frequency and duration of services, modalities, supplies, and interventions.

According to MBPM Chapter 7 Section 30.2.1:[12]

The HHA must be acting upon a physician plan of care that meets the requirements of this section for HHA services to be covered. For HHA services to be covered, the individualized plan of care must specify the services necessary to meet the patients specific needs identified in the comprehensive assessment. In addition, the plan of care must include the identification of the responsible discipline(s) and the frequency and duration of all visits as well as those items listed in 42 CFR 484.60(a) that establish the need for such services. All care provided must be in accordance with the plan of care. If the plan of care includes a course of treatment for therapy services:

- *The course of therapy treatment must be established by the physician after any needed consultation with the qualified therapist;*
- *The plan must include measurable therapy treatment goals which pertain directly to the patient's illness or injury, and the patient's resultant impairments;*
- *The plan must include the expected duration of therapy services; and*
- *The plan must describe a course of treatment which is consistent with the qualified therapist's assessment of the patient's function.*

Section 30.2.2:[12]

The orders on the plan of care must indicate the type of services to be provided to the patient, both with respect to the professional who will provide them and the nature of the individual services, as well as the frequency of the services.

Initial Percentage Payment

If a physician signed plan of care is not available at the beginning of the 30-day period, the HHA may submit a request for anticipated payment (RAP) for the initial percentage payment based on physician verbal orders OR a referral prescribing detailed orders for the services to be rendered that is signed and dated by the physician. If the RAP submission is based on physician verbal orders, the verbal order must be recorded in the plan of care, include a description of the patient's condition and the services to be provided by the home health agency, include an attestation (relating to the physician's orders and the date received per 42 CFR 409.43), and the plan of care is copied and immediately submitted to the physician. A billable visit must be rendered prior to the submission of a RAP.

Final Percentage Payment

The plan of care must be signed and dated by a physician as described who meets the certification and recertification requirements of 42 CFR 424.22 and before the claim for each 30-day period for services is submitted for the final percentage payment. Any changes in the plan of care must be signed and dated by a physician.

Section 30.2.5:[12]

When services are furnished based on a physician's oral order, the orders may be accepted and put in writing by personnel authorized to do so by applicable State and Federal laws and regulations as well as by the HHA's internal policies. The orders must be signed and dated with the date of receipt by the registered nurse or qualified therapist (i.e., physical therapist, speech-language pathologist, occupational therapist, or medical social worker) responsible for furnishing or supervising the ordered services. The orders may be signed by the supervising registered nurse or qualified therapist after the services have been rendered, as long as HHA personnel who receive the oral orders notify that nurse or therapist before the service is rendered. Thus, the rendering of a service that is based on an oral order would not be delayed pending signature of the supervising nurse or therapist. Oral orders must be countersigned and dated by the physician before the HHA bills for the care in the same way as the plan of care. Services which are provided from the beginning of the 60-day certification period based on a request for anticipated payment and before the physician signs the plan of care are considered to be provided under a plan of care established and approved by the physician where there is an oral order for the care prior to rendering the services which is documented in the medical record and where the services are included in a signed plan of care. Services that are provided in the subsequent 60-day certification period are considered provided under the plan of care of the subsequent 60-day episode where there is an oral order before the services provided in the subsequent period are furnished and the order is reflected in the medical record. However, services that are provided after the expiration of the plan of care, but before the acquisition of an oral order or a signed plan of care are not considered provided under a plan of care.

HHAs should check with their MAC for specific guidelines regarding the POC.

Author's Note

The RAP is going to be phased out and replaced with the Notice of Admission (NOA):

In an effort to make improvements to the health care delivery system and to reduce potential program integrity risks, CMS will reduce the split-percentage payment amount, paid in response to a Request for Anticipated Payment (RAP), to 20 percent for existing HHAs beginning in CY 2020 with elimination of split-percentage payments for all HHAs in CY 2021. For CY 2021, there will be no up-front payment made in response to a RAP; however, RAPs will still be submitted by all HHAs every 30 days to alert the claims processing system that a beneficiary is under a home health period of care. HHAs must submit the zero-pay RAP within 5 calendar days of each 30-day period or be subject to a late penalty. For CY 2021, CMS is reducing administrative burden by streamlining the information required in order to submit the RAP. CMS believes that phasing out the RAP payments will mitigate potential fraud and is an important step in paying responsibly and appropriately for home health services. Finally, CMS is finalizing a requirement for a one-time submission of a Notice of Admission (NOA) beginning in CY 2022 to replace RAP submissions every 30-days to further reduce provider paperwork burden while protecting the Medicare trust funds. HHAs must submit the NOA within 5 calendar days of the home health start of care or be subject to a payment penalty.

https://www.cms.gov/newsroom/fact-sheets/cms-finalizes-calendar-year-2020-payment-and-policy-changes-home-health-agencies-and-calendar-year

WRITING GOALS FOR THE PLAN OF CARE

The home environment provides PTs the opportunity to write realistic and functional goals for their clients. Not only can the therapist observe what tasks the patient is able to perform or not perform but is also able to note the many obstacles that prevent the task from being completed safely. Clinicians often have to simulate environments in the hospital or rehab setting that often provide a poor substitute for the patient's specific needs. One example of this difference involves narrow doorways. In the hospital or other inpatient settings, most rooms have wider doors to accommodate beds and wheelchairs. PTs may encounter narrow doorways in the home where the patient cannot maneuver their walker or wheelchair, or clutter limiting negotiable space. Goals that address these practical conditions may not have been addressed elsewhere.

In the home, therapists should discuss with the patient and their caregivers specific behaviors that are required for the patient to function safely. In the home, goals should focus on what the patient needs to do to function in the home and the immediate surroundings safely. Insurance providers expect physical therapy services to provide a significant change in function in a reasonable amount of time.[1] Therefore, a time frame for each goal and outcome should be determined. Goals may be classified as *short term*, which can be accomplished in a few days or a week, or *long term*, which can be weeks or even months. CMS does not require the headings of short or long term, but rather the identification of the time period. In either case, all goals should involve the collaboration of the patient or caregiver and should be updated at regular intervals as the patient improves (or declines).

When writing goals for homebound patients, the PT should consider:

1. What was the patient's previous level of function?
2. What type of equipment, devices, orthotics, wheeled mobility, prostheses, etc., are needed?
3. Is anyone else available to assist the patient to meet the goal?
4. How long is the patient expected to be homebound?
5. How is this goal going to be measured in order to demonstrate improvement?
6. How many visits are needed to reach the goal?
7. Based on the findings from the evaluation, how much progress or improvement can be expected in a reasonable time frame and still meet the legal requirements for reimbursement?

Examples of measurable short-term goals:

Patient will achieve gait 20 feet from the bed to the bathroom in dim lighting and full weight bearing on both lower extremities with supervision in 1 week to reduce fall risk at night, without the use of an assistive device.
Patient will perform sit to stand at the kitchen table with contact guard assist in 3 days to improve safety at mealtimes and initiate gait.

Some examples of measurable long-term goals:

Patient will negotiate 4 to 6, 6" steps with supervision using a railing on one side only in 3 weeks in order to go from the kitchen to the garage.
Patient will be able to stand for 10 minutes at the bathroom sink without upper extremity support and without loss of balance in 4 weeks in order to perform personal hygiene.

DOCUMENTING INTERVENTIONS IN THE PLAN OF CARE

The PT should include the interventions needed to address the patient's limitations for the duration of treatment.[1] If a PTA will treat the patient, interventions should be appropriate and clearly understood. When selecting interventions for a patient, the PT should consider the patient's medical and social history, cognition and learning ability, and discharge plan. Outside agencies may review this POC, so if a particular treatment that is known only by a select group of people is documented, it needs to be described in detail so that it is easily understood.

Some poor examples of intervention documentation include transfer training, modalities prn, and Back in Action Program. Each of these interventions could be improved by providing more information describing the equipment required, progression of the treatment, or components of the program. The PT should remember, as discussed in previous chapters, that all interventions should be preceded by the Current Procedural Terminology (CPT) code verbiage.

- Therapeutic activities: Training and education for car transfers using a mid-size SUV—progressing to SBA with caregiver
- Electrical stimulation: attended: Functional electrical stimulation to right quadriceps for 1 week to facilitate knee extension in gait
- Therapeutic exercise: Therapeutic strengthening exercises for trunk and hips with gradual progression of trunk extension. Increase resistance by 1 lb when patient is able to perform 10 repetitions of each exercise in order …

TREATMENT/VISIT NOTES AND PROGRESS REPORTS

In home care, each visit requires a written record to be completed on the same day as the visit. Whether handwritten or electronic documentation, each visit note should correlate to one or more goals and interventions from the POC. In addition, visit notes provide the opportunity to explain any training or education that was given and the patient's response to that teaching. Typically, PTs and PTAs also discuss any collaboration with each other and other providers working with this patient and plans for the next visit.[1] The record should also include the communication between the PTs and PTAs. Additionally, there may be a "sign in record" at the patient's home to indicate when the PT/PTA completed a visit and a basic indication of what was performed. This serves as information for the patient and caregivers, and other home health professionals providing services.

For each treatment, therapists and assistants should document measurable progress towards goals.[16] This progress can be in percentages, amount of assistance needed, progression to least restrictive device, etc. Communication to other disciplines working with the client is imperative to prevent any duplication of services and assist in the progression of the patient. For example, if the client can now achieve gait to the bathroom safely, then the occupational therapist or certified occupational therapy assistant may be able to progress from bed/chair baths to tub/shower baths. This may also apply to the home health aide and their ability to mobilize the patient safely to the bathroom. Documenting progress at each treatment allows the clinician to evaluate over time if the treatment is effective.

In most therapy practices and third-party payer organizations, PTs are required to complete a progress report. The progress report differs from a daily note in that it provides a summary of the treatment and the degree of improvement (or lack of improvement) since the last evaluation or progress note or prior progress report, as well as describes the current status of the patient. The report should justify the need for physical therapy and be closely related to the current POC. Progress notes may be requested by third-party payers at any time or by physicians prior to an office visit by the patient. Although PTAs may gather data to be included in the progress note, the note must be written by the PT to comply with APTA recommendations, Medicare guidelines, and applicable state law.[5]

Author's Note

Currently, CMS requires a functional reassessment every 30 days. A "qualified" therapist (i.e. physical therapist, occupational therapist, speech-language therapist) must perform the necessary therapy service, assess the patient, measure, and document the effectiveness of the therapy plan at least once every 30 days during a course of therapy treatment. A functional reassessment should substantiate that effective, reasonable, and necessary therapy services are being provided to the patient.

Unfortunately, not all home health patients improve. Pursuant to Section 20.1.2 of MBPM Chapter 7:[12]

The Medicare contractor's decision on whether care is reasonable and necessary is based on information reflected in the home health plan of care, the OASIS as required by 42 CFR 484.55 or a medical record of the individual patient. Medicare does not deny coverage solely on the basis of the reviewer's general inferences about patients with similar diagnoses or on data related to utilization generally, but bases it upon objective clinical evidence regarding the patient's individual need for care. Coverage of skilled nursing care or therapy to perform a maintenance program does not turn on the presence or absence of a patient's potential for improvement from the nursing care or therapy, but rather on the patient's need for skilled care. Skilled care may be necessary to improve a patient's current condition, to maintain the patient's current condition, to prevent or slow further deterioration of the patient's condition.

Section 40.2.1:

The service of a physical therapist, speech-language pathologist, or occupational therapist is a skilled therapy service if the inherent complexity of the service is such that it can be performed safely and/or effectively only by or under the general supervision of a skilled therapist. To be covered, assuming all other eligibility and coverage criteria have been met, the skilled services must also be reasonable and necessary to the treatment of the patient's illness or injury or to the restoration or maintenance of function affected by the patient's illness or injury. It is necessary to determine whether individual therapy services are skilled and whether, in view of the patient's overall condition, skilled management of the services provided is needed.

If a client does not progress either by reaching a plateau where there is no change or by declining in function, the clinician should consider the following:

1. Has there been a change in the medical condition? Has the disease worsened?
2. Is there a medication complication?
3. Is the treatment provided ineffective?
4. Were the initial goals unrealistic?
5. Should someone else treat the patient?
6. Should the patient be referred to a physician or other healthcare provider?

Author's Note

See Section 40.2.1 of MBPM Chapter 7, which includes the following excerpt:

Coverage of therapy services to perform a maintenance program is not determined solely on the presence or absence of a beneficiary's potential for improvement from the therapy, but rather on the beneficiary's need for skilled care. Assuming all other eligibility and coverage requirements are met, skilled therapy services are covered when an individualized assessment of the patient's clinical condition demonstrates that the specialized judgment, knowledge, and skills of a qualified therapist ***or by a qualified therapist assistant under the supervision of a qualified therapist*** *[emphasis added] ("skilled care") are necessary for the performance of a safe and effective maintenance program. Such a maintenance program to maintain the patient's current condition or to prevent or slow further deterioration is covered so long as the beneficiary requires skilled care for the safe and effective performance of the program. When, however, the individualized assessment does not demonstrate such a necessity for skilled care, including when the performance of a maintenance program does not require the skills of a therapist or by a qualified therapist assistant under the supervision of a qualified therapist because it could safely and effectively be accomplished by the patient or with the assistance of non-therapists, including unskilled caregivers, such maintenance services will not be covered.*[12]

The lack of progress does not automatically indicate that a third-party payer will deny payment. Clinicians should document their decision-making abilities when they evaluate progress and provide comments on why they believe the patient's behavior has a change or plateau. This type of documentation helps demonstrate the level of skill required to manage these clients. It is important to delineate between restorative care and maintenance care and the need for a skilled therapist in either or both situation.

Questions and answers previously addressed by the APTA on maintenance.[2]

If Medicare denies a claim for maintenance therapy, can I then bill the patient for the services provided?

Yes, but make sure that you have first provided the patient with Medicare Advanced Beneficiary Notice (ABN). Physical therapists must issue a valid ABN to patients to collect out-of-pocket payment from Medicare beneficiaries when Medicare deems services not reasonable and necessary.

For Medicare Part B, if you establish a maintenance program and will be seeing a patient every two weeks to adjust the program, do you bill a re-evaluation every two weeks?

No, it is not likely that you could bill for a reevaluation (CPT 97164) each visit during the maintenance program. In fact, the Medicare Benefit Policy Manual for outpatient therapy states that "Continuous assessment of the patient's progress is a component of ongoing therapy services and is not payable as a reevaluation. A reevaluation is not a routine, recurring service but is focused on evaluation of progress toward current goals, making a professional judgment about continued care, modifying goals and/or treatment or terminating services. A formal reevaluation is covered only if the documentation supports the need for further tests and measurements after the initial evaluation. Indications for a reevaluation include new clinical findings, a significant change in the patient's condition, or failure to respond to the therapeutic interventions outlined in the plan of care."

Do you have to "label" a patient as restorative versus maintenance?

Yes, for patients/clients in need of skilled maintenance therapy, you should establish a maintenance program and in your documentation clearly show that the services are being provided for maintenance goals as opposed to restorative.

If a patient's skilled restorative care is completed, and the therapist opts to keep the patient on a skilled maintenance level, must they document that the patient is being transitioned to a skilled maintenance program?

Yes, the transition from restorative therapy to maintenance therapy should be documented, as the goals for treatment will be different. The plan of care should be update to reflect the new treatment goals for the patient.

DOCUMENTATION OF SKILL

Home health, not unlike other settings, requires therapists and assistants to document the unique skills they provide the patient during each visit. Since it is highly unlikely that a clinician would report that they lack skill, the most plausible explanation for the lack of documentation is the knowledge of how to record skill in their documentation. According to CMS, skilled rehabilitation services require the technical or professional knowledge of the clinician or the supervision of the clinician to be safe and effective.[12] If the treatment could be provided by a family member or caregiver of the patient, without supervision, the treatment is most likely nonskilled.

In order to prevent a denial for lack of skill, the PT and PTA should clearly and concisely document the skill he or she provided during the treatment. A typical visit note may include many actions that the patient performed, such as gait, transfers, or exercises, but to meet this objective, there should be no question of what skill the PT or PTA performed. The best way to document would be to precede the patient performance with the interventions preceded by the CPT verbiage, as discussed previously.

Poor examples:

1. Patient ambulated 100 ft with rolling walker without loss of balance.
2. Patient performed HEP as per written instructions.

Good examples:

1. Gait training: Patient able to achieve gait to the mailbox 40' with front wheeled rolling walker with PT facilitating weight shifting at the pelvis to lengthen LLE stride length and L hip flexion. PT assistance required with walker and sequencing to execute 180° turn to return to house.
2. Therapeutic Exercise: Patient required verbal instruction for sequencing and body positioning to complete 25% of exercise program correctly today and able to remember and perform 75% of the exercise with supervision.
3. Therapeutic Exercise: Patient required moderate assistance with tapping and vibration facilitation to the hip flexors to perform right hip flexion exercises secondary to 2/5 muscle strength.
4. Therapeutic Exercise or Therapeutic Activities: Patient able to perform sit to stand from the patient's 20-inch high sofa with tactile cues on bilateral shoulder 3/5 times for adequate forward lean and verbal instructions for foot placement; heels posterior to knees.
5. Gait Training: Patient able to demonstrate gait with large based quad cane, R hand, on deep pile rug 15' forward and negotiate R 180 degree turn with verbal instruction without loss of balance, required moderate assistance with trunk stabilization to prevent secondary to loss of balance with 180 degree turn to L.

In addition to skill, the documentation must stand alone and avoid being repetitive from visit to visit.[1] When utilizing electronic documentation, this is more critical. If the same boxes are checked on the EMR at each visit, the notes will look the same visit after visit, even though the treatment may be different. Programs that allow you to read and edit the visit note prior to submitting may resolve some of these concerns, as do the systems that allow free-style entry. As discussed earlier, if the treatment plan needs to be changed, document the justification and reasons for the change to demonstrate skill. These suggestions may only take a few extra minutes to complete but can save hundreds or even thousands of dollars from third-party denials.

RECERTIFICATION, RESUMPTION OF CARE, AND DISCHARGE

Recertification and resumption of care are two concepts that are closely related to the OASIS document addressed previously and are critical to documentation.[12] 10.3 of MBPM Chapter 7: *While HH PPS payment is now made for each 30-day period, the home health PPS permits continuous 60-day recertifications for patients who continue to be eligible for the home health benefit. Medicare does not limit the number of continuous 60-day recertifications for beneficiaries who continue to be eligible for the home health benefit. Each 60-day certification can include two 30-day payment periods. Recertification is required at least every 60 days when there is a need for continuous home health care after an initial 60-day certification. The recertification visit can be done during the prior certification period. With some minor exceptions, the Medicare Conditions of Participation at 42 CFR 484.55(d)(1), require that the recertification assessment be done during the last 5 days of the previous certification period (for example, during the initial 60-day certification period, the recertification visit is required to be done on days 56-60).*[12]

A resumption of care (ROC) occurs when a patient is within their 60-day episode and is admitted to and discharged from a hospital. The provider would conduct another OASIS document that identifies the current status of the patient and any new diagnoses or procedures from the hospital stay.

Although both of these documents are similar to the OASIS SOC document, the responses should clearly reflect the improvement or decline in function, the update of goals and interventions, the change in patient status, and the revision of diagnoses and procedures. For each of these documents, the assessing clinician is responsible for obtaining and documenting orders for all services to be recertified or resumed.

In any setting, discharge planning begins at the time of the initial examination and evaluation. It must be documented in each visit note and planned and discussed with patient and caregiver and physician. For Medicare patients, a Discharge OASIS is required at the time of discharge from the HHA with a few exceptions such as a hospital admission or death.[16] This document contains nearly identical questions to the SOC OASIS and adds a few questions concerning interventions provided. These additions such as diabetic foot care and depression interventions were described earlier. The responses at discharge are reviewed by CMS and other agencies to determine if the patient improved in various outcome measures.

Individuals may review outcomes of any HHA contracted with Medicare by visiting http://www.medicare.gov/HHCompare. The information is provided in aggregate, not by individual patient. In July 2015, "the Quality of Patient Care Star Ratings and Patient Survey Star Ratings were introduced on the Home Health Compare website as a tool to assist people (e.g., family members, caregivers, payers, healthcare systems and care organizations) in evaluating home health agencies. The Star Rating summarizes the performance of a home health agency's patient care by displaying information from several different measures in one simple format."

The star rating is based on a 1 to 5 scale, with 5 being the best ranking.[21] CMS FACT SHEET: Quality of Patient Care Star Rating (https://www.cms.gov/Medicare/Quality-Initiatives-Patient-Assessment-Instruments/HomeHealthQualityInits/HHQIHomeHealthStarRatings).

Because the last clinician (Skilled Nursing, PT, Speech-Language Pathologist, or Occupational Therapist) treating the patient completes the Discharge OASIS, the other disciplines should each be encouraged to write a discharge summary containing progress achieved to be included in the final OASIS. Frequent communication among disciplines is vital to obtaining the most accurate responses at discharge. The discharge summary, or summation of care, should address all problems identified at in the initial SOC examination and evaluation, the interventions provided, the goals established, the status at discharge and whether the patient met their goals. If the patient did not meet the established goals or interim modified goals, the reason they did not must be addressed. The discharge plan must be documented (i.e., Patient will continue physical therapy as an outpatient. Patient will continue with home exercises as instructed until modified by outpatient therapist. Patient instructed to call agency if any questions.).

COMMUNICATION AND SUPERVISION

The importance of communication is critical in home care, and although it occurs on many levels, every day, for every patient, communication often fails to be documented every time it occurs. Communication involves anyone associated with the care of the patient, including doctors, pharmacists, transportation companies, medical equipment companies, etc., all subject to HIPAA regulations. The opening quote to this section described home health as being "without quick access" to others.[1] Therefore, a concerted effort must be made to conduct regular case conferences with every discipline involved with a particular client and document the discussion and outcome in the medical record. If a patient is being treated by a PT and PTA, routine communication is warranted to ensure that the POC is followed and the appropriate level of supervision is conducted. All intraprofessional and interprofessional communication should also be documented in the record. With the easy access to cell phone technology and computers, it is possible in any home care situation to communicate. It is imperative to remember not to be tempted to discuss patients via phone or e-mail in public places where conversations can be overheard or computer screens can be viewed by others, or to pass on patient information via personal e-mail or text if there are patient identifiers.

The service of a PT, Speech-Language Pathologist (SLP), or Occupational Therapist (OT) is a skilled therapy service if the inherent complexity of the service is such that it can be performed safely and effectively only by or under the general supervision of a skilled therapist. *General supervision* has been described in CMS's Medicare Benefit Policy Manual as being furnished under the supervisor's overall direction and control, but the supervisor's presence is not required during the performance of the service.

HOME HEALTH AUDITS

Audits in home health are regularly performed by the state in which the agency is licensed. Public and private payers also conduct pre- and post-payment review. For example, MACs perform medical review as part of CMS's Targeted Probe and Educate program, wherein MACs focus on specific providers and suppliers that bill a particular item or service, rather than all providers and suppliers billing a particular item or service. The physical therapy profession should anticipate ongoing audits for utilization, as well as those discussed earlier in this chapter: legibility, lack of medical necessity, lack of skill, etc. As the audits are conducted using the documentation, this is additional justification for appropriate, objective, skilled documentation.

Author's Note

Home Health Services Review Choice Demonstration

On April 1, 2017, CMS paused the Pre-Claim Review Demonstration for Home Health Services to consider a number of changes in response to stakeholder feedback. On May 29, 2018, CMS first announced the intention to implement the Review Choice Demonstration for Home Health Services in a few states.

This demonstration includes Home Health Agencies (HHAs) that: provide home health services and are enrolled in the Medicare FFS program; and beneficiaries. The term submitter will be used throughout this document to describe the person or entity that submits the claims, documentation and/or pre-claim review request under the different choices.

The Review Choice Demonstration will be conducted in: Illinois, Ohio, North Carolina, Florida, and Texas. It will apply only to those HHAs located in the states who submit claims to the Palmetto GBA Medicare Administrative Contractor (MAC).

For more information about the demonstration: https://www.cms.gov/Research-Statistics-Data-and-Systems/Monitoring-Programs/Medicare-FFS-Compliance-Programs/Review-Choice-Demonstration/Review-Choice-Demonstration-for-Home-Health-Services https://www.cms.gov/Research-Statistics-Data-and-Systems/Monitoring-Programs/Medicare-FFS-Compliance-Programs/Review-Choice-Demonstration/Review-Choice-Demonstration-for-Home-Health-Services

https://www.cms.gov/Research-Statistics-Data-and-Systems/Monitoring-Programs/Medicare-FFS-Compliance-Programs/Review-Choice-Demonstration/Review-Choice-Demonstration-for-Home-Health-Services

DOCUMENTING MEDICARE AND INSURANCE APPEALS IN HOME CARE

The most common first step by an auditor is issuing an additional documentation request (ADR) to the provider.[22] This is common practice regardless of the practice setting. The provider must submit the requested documentation by a specified date. Depending on the type of audit, the requesting agency may accept the documentation, request additional information, deny payment, or request a full or partial refund if a payment was made. If a denial is issued, the provider has two options: accept the denial and make remuneration or appeal the decision.

When appealing a denial, one must follow the directions of the agency issuing the denial policies and procedures of that agency. If the services were justified and supplemental documentation is available, then an appeal is the appropriate action. When preparing the appeal, any or all of the following documents to support the appeal should be provided:

1. Supportive documentation for other treatment dates not in question
2. Progress reports or summaries
3. Communication with physician or other healthcare professionals
4. Nursing notes or notes from other disciplines
5. State practice act
6. APTA's *Guide to Physical Therapist Practice*
7. Communication with the insurance carrier

For more information concerning Medicare appeals, go to Appeals and Grievances at http://www.cms.gov/home/medicare.asp.[23]

HOME HEALTH VALUE-BASED PURCHASING

In January 2016, the Center for Medicare & Medicaid Innovation (CMMI) of the CMS initiated the Home Health Value-Based Purchasing (HHVBP) Model in nine selected states: Arizona, Florida, Iowa, Massachusetts, Maryland, Nebraska, North Carolina, Tennessee, and Washington. CMS designed the HHVBP Model to test the impact of providing financial incentives to HHAs for higher-quality care and greater efficiency.

All eligible agencies in the nine selected HHVBP states will have their Medicare payments adjusted upward or downward based on their Total Performance Score (TPS), a composite score of an agency's quality achievement or improvement. The model's financial incentive is provided by an adjustment to Medicare HHA payments based on their TPS values relative to other agencies within a state (or state HHA size cohort). The adjustment redistributes Medicare payments among agencies within a state to reward agencies with relatively higher achieved quality or improved quality to provide a penalty to relatively lower-quality agencies.

The HHVBP payment adjustment for any given year is applied to Medicare Home Health Prospective Payment System (HHPPS) payments 2 years after the performance year. Thus, the first payment adjustment occurred in calendar year (CY) 2018 and is based on CY 2016 data. Based on their performance in CY 2016, agencies experienced an upward or downward adjustment of up to 3% of their Medicare payments in 2018, based on their relative quality and up to 8% in 2022. The percentage of Medicare payments subject to the adjustment increases over the course of the model and will ultimately result in 8% of an agency's payments being subject to adjustment based on their relative quality performance.

PATIENT-DRIVEN GROUPINGS MODEL

PDGM is the new Medicare case-mix methodology for HHAs that began January 1, 2020. Implementing PDGM is the biggest reimbursement change to take place in home health in roughly two decades.

> In November 2018, CMS finalized a new case-mix classification model, the Patient-Driven Groupings Model (PDGM), effective beginning January 1, 2020. The PDGM relies more heavily on clinical characteristics and other patient information to place home health periods of care into meaningful payment categories and eliminates the use of therapy service thresholds. In conjunction with the implementation of the PDGM, there was a change in the unit of home health payment from a 60-day episode to a 30-day period.

In the Bipartisan Budget Act of 2018 (BBA) Congress laid out many of the changes to the Medicare payment methodology for home health services to be implemented in CY 2020. CMS was required to implement:

- A 30-day payment unit. The 60-day payment episodes are replaced with 30-day payment periods.

- A case-mix methodology that excludes therapy visits as a factor for payment. Therapy visits are no longer included in determining reimbursement.
- Budget neutrality.
- Behavioral adjustments to be made on a prospective basis.

Each 30-day period is categorized into 432 case-mix groups (compared to 153) with varying levels of reimbursement. Calculating the case-mix weight (case-mix weight is a measure of the acuity or health condition of the patient and is an overall scoring system derived from an HHA's OASIS) under PDGM is significantly different using these four components:

- Admission Source
- Episode Timing
- Clinical Group
- OASIS—Functional Impairment Level
- Comorbidity Adjustment

Medicare is continuing to focus on transitioning from a volume-based system to a value-based system. This means that now, more than ever, HHAs will have to take a close look at operations, billing, clinical oversight, care planning, and overall processes. Optimistically, PDGM can be leveraged to help drive change, strengthen care planning, and improve patient quality outcomes.

SUMMARY

Home health documentation is constantly evolving based on federal and state regulations. This section is not intended to be a substitute for learning the specific requirements for Medicare, nor is it comprehensive in addressing all the documentation concerns in home health. PTs and PTAs must be vigilant in keeping up with these changes to be successful in this field of practice. Though the home health documentation responsibilities may seem overwhelming, it is not dissimilar in content to the requirements for other venues. The benefits and rewards of working with people in the comfort of their homes ameliorate the documentation challenges.

REVIEW QUESTIONS

1. Identify the qualifications for home health services under Medicare Part A and Medicare Part B.
2. What does PDGM stand for? What are the episode of care differences between PDGM and the previous PPS reimbursement system for home health?
3. Describe the ages of patients that qualify for home health services.
4. What is the OASIS? Describe the role of the OASIS in home health.
5. Which healthcare professionals can complete the initial and discharge OASIS?
6. If a PT and PTA are sharing the home health treatment of a patient, what is the process for coordinating patient care?
7. If a PT and PTA are sharing the home health treatment of a patient, at what intervals is the PT reassessment required?
8. To better ensure Medicare-compliant documentation, what coding terminology should precede the following:

   Quadriceps strengthening
   Ambulation with front-wheeled rolling walker

9. Describe the role of standardized tests and instruments in home health.
10. What is a MAC, and what role do they serve in home health?

Overview of the Patient-Driven Groupings Model[24]

The Patient-Driven Groupings Model (PDGM) uses 30-day periods as a basis for payment. Figure 1 below provides an overview of how 30-day periods are categorized into 432 case-mix groups for the purposes of adjusting payment in the PDGM. In particular, 30-day periods are placed into different subgroups for each of the following broad categories:

- **Admission source (two subgroups):** community or institutional admission source
- **Timing of the 30-day period (two subgroups):** early or late
- **Clinical grouping (twelve subgroups):** musculoskeletal rehabilitation; neuro/stroke rehabilitation; wounds; medication management, teaching, and assessment (MMTA) - surgical aftercare; MMTA - cardiac and circulatory; MMTA - endocrine; MMTA - gastrointestinal tract and genitourinary system; MMTA - infectious disease, neoplasms, and blood-forming diseases; MMTA - respiratory; MMTA- other; behavioral health; or complex nursing interventions
- **Functional impairment level (three subgroups):** low, medium, or high
- **Comorbidity adjustment (three subgroups):** none, low, or high based on secondary diagnoses.

In total, there are 2*2*12*3*3 = 432 possible case-mix adjusted payment groups. The remainder of this overview provides more detail on each PDGM grouping category and additional adjustments to payment that are made within the PDGM.

FIGURE 1: STRUCTURE OF THE PATIENT-DRIVEN GROUPINGS MODEL

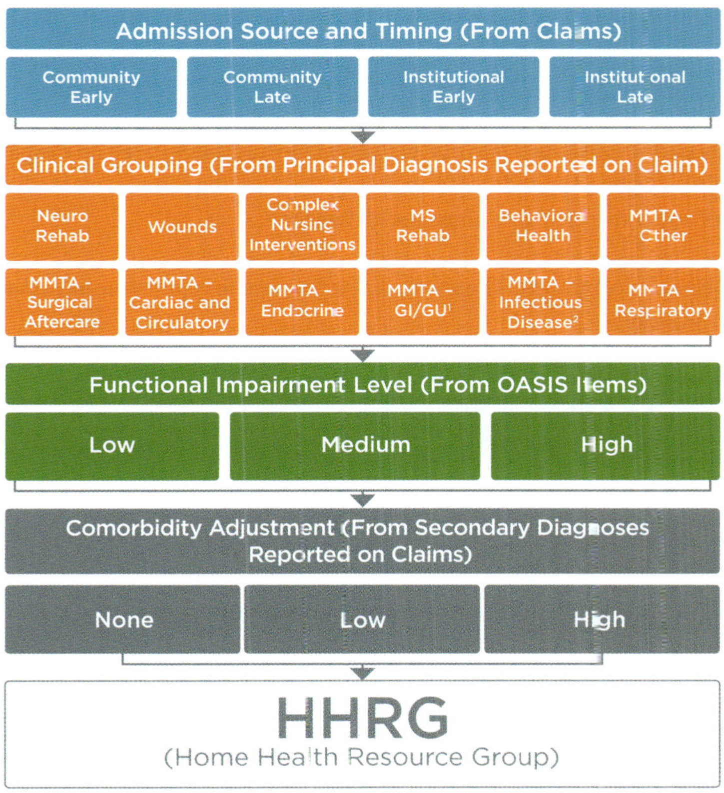

Under the Patient-Driven Groupings Model, a 30-day period is grouped into one (and only one) subcategory under each larger colored category. A 30-day period's combination of subcategories places the 30-day period into one of 432 different payment groups.

1 Gastrointestinal tract/Genitourinary system
2 The infectious disease category also includes diagnoses related to neoplasms and blood-forming

Timing

Under the PDGM, the first 30-day period is classified as early. All subsequent 30-day periods in the sequence (second or later) are classified as late. A sequence of 30-day periods continues until there is a gap of at least 60-days between the end of one 30-day period and the start of the next. When there is a gap of at least 60-days, the subsequent 30-day period is classified as being the first 30-day period of a new sequence (and therefore, is labeled as early). The comprehensive assessment must be completed within five days of the start of care date and updated no less frequently than during the last five days of every 60 days beginning with the start of care date (as currently required by the Medicare Conditions of Participation at 42 CFR 484.55). As a result, information obtained from the Outcome and Assessment Information Set (OASIS) used in the PDGM may not change over the two 30-day periods the OASIS covers. However, if a patient experiences a significant change in condition before the start of a subsequent, contiguous 30-day period, for example due to a fall; a follow-up assessment would be submitted at the start of a second 30-day period to reflect any changes in the patient's condition, including functional abilities, and the second 30-day claim would be grouped into its appropriate case-mix group accordingly.

Admission Source

Under the PDGM, each 30-day period is classified into one of two admission source categories – community or institutional – depending on what healthcare setting was utilized in the 14 days prior to home health admission. Late 30-day periods are always classified as a community admission unless there was an acute hospitalization in the 14 days prior to the late home health 30-day period. A post-acute stay in the 14 days prior to a late home health 30-day period would not be classified as an institutional admission unless the patient had been discharged from home health prior to post-acute stay.

Clinical Grouping

Under the PDGM, each 30-day period is grouped into one of twelve clinical groups based on the patient's principal diagnosis. The reported principal diagnosis provides information to describe the primary reason for which patients are receiving home health services under the Medicare home health benefit.

Table 1 below describes the twelve clinical groups. These groups are designed to capture the most common types of care that home health agencies (HHAs) provide.

TABLE 1: PDGM CLINICAL GROUPS

CLINICAL GROUP	PRIMARY REASON FOR HOME HEALTH ENCOUNTER IS TO PROVIDE:
Musculoskeletal Rehabilitation	Therapy (PT/OT/SLP) for a musculoskeletal condition
Neuro/Stroke Rehabilitation	Therapy (PT/OT/SLP) for a neurological condition or stroke
Wounds - Post-Op Wound Aftercare and Skin/ Non-Surgical Wound Care	Assessment, treatment and evaluation of a surgical wound(s); assessment, treatment and evaluation of non-surgical wounds, ulcers burns and other lesions
Complex Nursing Interventions	Assessment, treatment and evaluation of complex medical and surgical conditions
Behavioral Health Care	Assessment, treatment and evaluation of psychiatric and substance abuse conditions
Medication Management, Teaching and Assessment (MMTA) • **MMTA –Surgical Aftercare** • **MMTA – Cardiac/Circulatory** • **MMTA – Endocrine** • **MMTA – GI/GU** • **MMTA – Infectious Disease/Neoplasms/ Blood-forming Diseases** • **MMTA –Respiratory** • **MMTA – Other**	Assessment, evaluation, teaching, and medication management for a variety of medical and surgical conditions not classified in one of the above listed groups. The subgroups represent common clinical conditions that require home health services for medication management, teaching, and assessment.

Functional Impairment Level

The PDGM designates a functional impairment level for each 30-day period based on the following OASIS items:

VARIABLE #	DESCRIPTION
M1800	Grooming
M1810	Current ability to dress upper body safely
M1820	Current ability to dress lower body safely
M1830	Bathing
M1840	Toilet transferring
M1850	Transferring
M1860	Ambulation and locomotion
M1033	Risk for hospitalization

CMS estimates a regression model that determines the relationship between the responses for the listed OASIS items and average 30-day period resource use. The coefficients from the regression are used to assign points to a 30-day period. Responses that indicate higher functional impairment and a higher risk of hospitalization are associated with having larger coefficients and are therefore assigned higher points. The points are then summed, and thresholds are applied to determine whether a 30-day period is assigned a low, medium, or high functional impairment level. Each clinical group is assigned a separate set of thresholds. On average, 30-day periods in the low level have responses for the listed OASIS items that are associated with the lowest resource use. On average, 30-day periods in the high level have responses on the above OASIS items that are associated with the highest resource use.

Comorbidity Adjustment

The PDGM includes a comorbidity adjustment category based on the presence of secondary diagnoses. Depending on a patient's secondary diagnoses, a 30-day period may receive no comorbidity adjustment, a low comorbidity adjustment, or a high comorbidity adjustment. Home health 30-day periods of care can receive a comorbidity adjustment under the following circumstances:

- **Low comorbidity adjustment:** There is a reported secondary diagnosis that is associated with higher resource use, or;
- **High comorbidity adjustment:** There are two or more secondary diagnoses that are associated with higher resource use when both are reported together compared to if they were reported separately. That is, the two diagnoses may interact with one another, resulting in higher resource use.

A 30-day period can have a low comorbidity adjustment or a high comorbidity adjustment, but not both. If a 30-day home health period of care does not have reported comorbidities that fall into one of the adjustments described above, there would be no comorbidity adjustment applied.

Determining Case-Mix Weights for the Patient-Driven Groupings Model

The case-mix weight for each of the 432 different payment groups under the PDGM are determined by estimating a regression where the dependent variable is the resource use of a 30-day period and the independent variables are categorical indicators representing the five dimensions of the model described above (timing of a 30-day period, admission source, clinical group, functional impairment level, and comorbidities). Case-mix weights are produced by dividing the predicted resource use for each PDGM payment group by the overall average resource use of all 30-day periods. The case-mix weights are then used to adjust the 30-day payment rate. Figure 2 (Page 5) describes how 30-day periods are paid and when payment adjustments are made.

Additional Payment Adjustments for the Patient-Driven Groupings Model

Payments for 30-day periods with a low number of visits are not case-mix adjusted, but instead paid on a per-visit basis using the national per-visit rates. Each of the 432 different PDGM payment groups has a threshold that determines if the 30-day period receives this Low-Utilization Payment Adjustment (LUPA). For each payment group, the 10th percentile value of visits is used to create a payment group specific LUPA threshold with a minimum threshold of at least two for each group. A 30-day period with a total number of visits below the LUPA threshold are paid per-visit rather than being paid the case-mix adjusted 30-day payment rate. A 30-day period with a total number of visits at or above the LUPA threshold is paid the case-mix adjusted 30-day payment rate rather than being paid per-visit.

When a 30-day period of care involves an unusually large number or a costly mix of visits, the HHA may be eligible for an additional outlier payment (See Figure 3). Once the imputed cost of a 30-day period of care exceeds a threshold amount, the HHA receives a payment equal to 80 percent of the difference between the imputed costs and the threshold amount.

Payments would be adjusted if a beneficiary transfers from one home health agency to another or is discharged and readmitted to the same agency within 30 days of the original 30-day period start date. The case-mix adjusted payment for 30-day periods of that type is pro-rated based on the length of the 30-day period ending in transfer or discharge and readmission, resulting in a partial period payment.

FIGURE 2: HOW PAYMENTS AND ADJUSTMENTS ARE CALCULATED FOR THE PATIENT-DRIVEN GROUPINGS MODEL

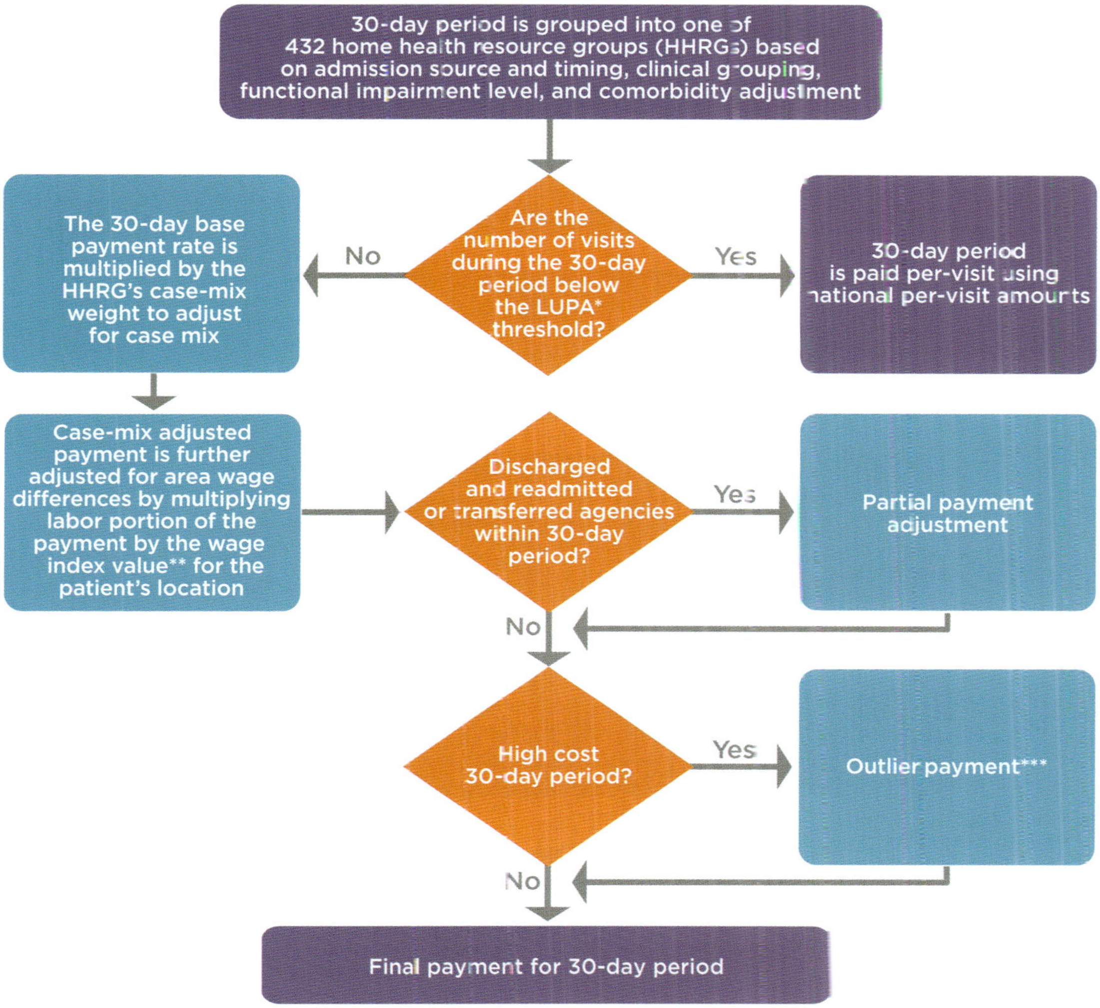

* LUPA = Low Utilization Payment Adjustment

** The wage-adjusted payment for a 30-day period is calculated by taking the case-mix adjusted 30-day payment amount and multiplying 76.1% of that payment by a wage-index value that controls for area wage differences. That value is then added to 23.9% of the case-mix adjusted base-payment to determine the wage-adjusted payment amount.

*** Outlier payment is in addition to the wage-adjusted and case-mix adjusted 30-day period payment

FIGURE 3: CALCULATION OF OUTLIER PAYMENT

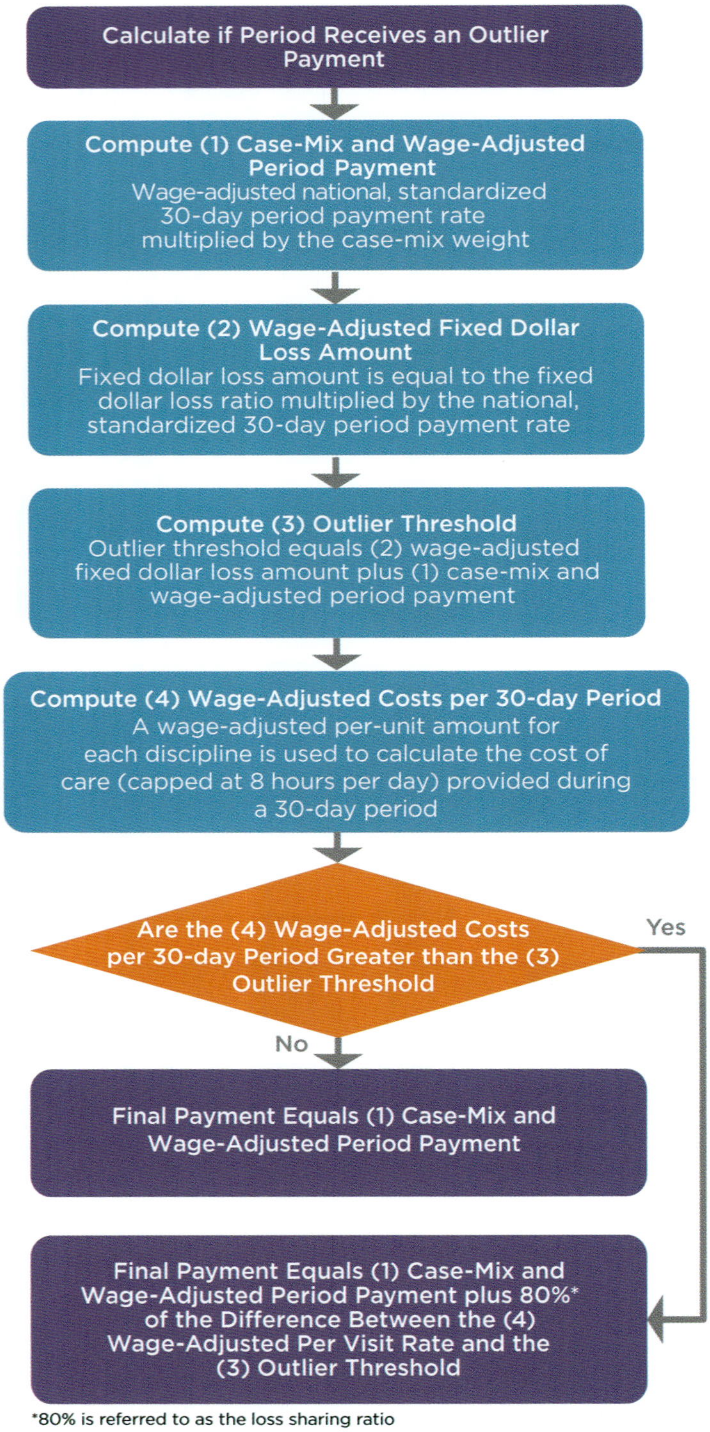

REFERENCES

1. *Physical Therapy Documentation of Patient/Client Management.* Alexandria, VA: American Physical Therapy Association; Available at https://www.apta.org/your-practice/documentation. Accessed July 20, 2020.
2. *Guidelines for the Provision of Physical Therapy in the Home, 3e.* Alexandria, VA: American Physical Therapy Association; Home Health Section; Available at https://iweb.apta.org/Purchase/ProductDetail.aspx?Product_code=P-131. Accessed July 20, 2020.
3. *Information for Consumers and Other Visitors.* Alexandria, VA: American Physical Therapy Association. Home Health Section; Available at https://www.homehealthsection org/. Accessed July 20, 2020.
4. *Medicare Claims Processing Manual Chapter 5—Part B Outpatient Rehabilitation and CORF/OPT Services.* Baltimore, MD: Centers for Medicare and Medicaid Services; Available at http://www.cms.gov/manuals/downloads/clm104c05.pdf. Accessed July 20, 2020.
5. *Guidelines: Physical Therapy Documentation of Patient/Client Management.* (BOD G03-05-16-41). Alexandria, VA: American Physical Therapy Association; Available at https://www.apta.org/uploadedFiles/APTAorg/About_Us/Policies/BOD/Practice/DocumentationPatientClientMgmt.pdf. Accessed July 20, 2020.
6. *Home Health Change of Care Notice (HHCCN, Form CMS-10280).* Baltimore, MD: Centers of Medicare & Medicaid Services; Available at https://www.cms.gov/Medicare/Medicare-General-Information/BNI/HHCCN. Accessed September 18, 2020.
7. *OASIS.* Baltimore, MD: Centers of Medicare & Medicaid Services; Available at https://www.cms.gov/Medicare/Quality-Initiatives-Patient-Assessment-Instruments/HomeHealthQualityInits/OASIS-Data-Sets. Accessed July 20, 2020.
8. *Transform and Modernize the Healthcare System Through Efficient Public Programs.* 2007. Baltimore, MD: Centers of Medicare & Medicaid Services; Available at https://www.aha.org/system/files/content/00-10/0704-uhp-cms.pdf. Accessed July 20, 2020.
9. O'Connor M, Davitt JK. The Outcome and Assessment Information Set (OASIS): A review of validity and reliability. *Home Health Care Serv Q.* 2012;3(4):267-301.
10. *Medicare National Coverage Determinations Manual Chapter 1, Part 1 (Sections 10—80.12) Coverage Determinations.* Baltimore, MD: Centers of Medicare & Medicaid Services; Available at https://www.cms.gov/Regulations-and-Guidance/Guidance/Manuals/Downloads/ncd103c1_Part1.pdf. Accessed July 20, 2020.
11. Cardiovascular monitoring devices. Oximeter. *Federal Register.* 2006;21(8):55733-4. Codified at 21 CFR §870.2700.
12. *Medicare Benefit Policy Manual Chapter 7—Home Health Services.* Baltimore, MD: Centers of Medicare & Medicaid Services; Available at https://www.cms.gov/Regulations-and-Guidance/Guidance/Manuals/Downloads/bp102c07 pdf. Accessed July 20, 2020.
13. *60.4.1—Definition of Homebound Patient Under the Medicare Home Health (HH) Benefit.* Baltimore, MD: Centers of Medicare & Medicaid Services; Available at https://www.cms.gov/Regulations-and-Guidance/Guidance/Manuals/downloads/bp102c15.pdf. Accessed September 18, 2020.
14. Borg G. *Borg's Perceived Exertion and Pain Scales.* Champaign, IL: Human Kinetics; 1998. ISBN: 0-88011-623-4. Available at https://www.researchgate.net/publication/306039034_Borg's_Perceived_Exertion_And_Pain_Scales. Accessed July 20, 2020.
15. Could you clarify CMS' policy about the homebound status of home health patients who can drive? *30.1.1—Patient Confined to the Home.* Available at https://www.cms.gov/Regulations-and-Guidance/Guidance/Manuals/Downloads/bp102c07.pdf. Accessed July 29, 2020.
16. *Home Health Quality Reporting Program.* Baltimore, MD: Centers of Medicare & Medicaid Services; Available at https://www.cms.gov/Medicare/Quality-Initiatives-Patient-Assessment-Instruments/HomeHealthQualityInits/Home-Health-Quality-Reporting-Requirements. Accessed July 20, 2020.
17. *Classification of Diseases, Functioning and Disability.* Centers for Disease Control and Prevention; Available at http://www.cdc.gov/nchs/icd.htm. Accessed July 20, 2020.
18. Yesavage JA, Brink TL, Rose TL, et al. Development and validation of a geriatric depression screening scale: A preliminary report. *J Psychiatric Research.* 1982-1983:17(1);37-49.
19. Alexopoulos GS, Abrams RC, Young RC, Shamoian CA. Cornell Scale for depression in dementia. *Biol Psychiatry.* 1988;23(3):271-284.
20. *Documenting Medical Necessity of Physical Therapy.* CGS, a Celerian Group Company. Available at https://www.cgsmedicare.com/hhh/coverage/hh_coverage_guidelines/9b.html. Accessed July 20, 2020.
21. *Quality of Patient Care Star Rating* (CMS Fact Sheet). Baltimore, MD: Centers of Medicare & Medicaid Services; Available at https://www.cms.gov/Medicare/Quality-Initiatives-Patient-Assessment-Instruments/HomeHealthQualityInits/HHQIHomeHealthStarRatings. Accessed September 18, 2020.
22. *MLNMatters.* Baltimore, MD: Centers of Medicare & Medicaid Services; Available at https://www.cms.gov/MLNMatters Articles/downloads/MM4022.pdf. Accessed July 29, 2020.
23. *CMS Appeals and Grievances.* Baltimore, MD: Centers of Medicare & Medicaid Services; Available at https://www.cms.gov/Medicare/Medicare?redirect=/home/medicare.asp. Accessed September 18, 2020.
24. *Patient-Driven Groupings Model.* Baltimore, MD: Centers of Medicare & Medicaid Services; Available at https://www.cms.gov/Medicare/Medicare-Fee-for-Service-Payment/HomeHealthPPS/Downloads/Overview-of-the-Patient-Driven-Groupings-Model.pdf. Accessed September 18, 2020.

8 Documentation for Certified Nursing Homes

OBJECTIVES

Following completion of this chapter, the reader will be able to:

- Understand who is responsible for completing the Minimum Data Set (MDS).
- Describe the role of the Minimum Data Set (MDS) in patient care in a Skilled Nursing Facility (SNF).
- Explain how each of the 20 Care Area Assessment (CAA) areas is related to physical therapy.
- Describe the Resident Assessment Instrument (RAI) processes and the relationship to the Minimum Data Set (MDS).
- Explain the theory of the Patient-Driven Payment Model (PDPM).

DOCUMENTATION FOR CERTIFIED NURSING HOMES (MINIMUM DATA SET)

The Skilled Nursing Facility (SNF) Patient-Driven Payment Model (PDPM) began October 1 2019 (the start of Medicare's fiscal year 2020), marking a significant difference in the SNF payment system. PDPM replaced the Resource Utilization Group (RUG) reimbursement model.

RESIDENT ASSESSMENT INSTRUMENT

The Resident Assessment Instrument (RAI) consists of three basic components: the Minimum Data Set (MDS) Version 3.0, the Care Area Assessment (CAA) process, and the RAI Utilization Guidelines.

The MDS (see Figure 8-1) is used for an important set of processes beyond the Prospective Payment System (PPS).[1] The MDS is a data collection tool designed to cue facilities to develop care plans that will affect critical components of a resident's health and quality of life. MDS data is also used to assist state agencies in monitoring the quality and safety of skilled nursing facilities.

Resident ____________ Identifier ____________ Date ____________

MINIMUM DATA SET (MDS) - Version 3.0
RESIDENT ASSESSMENT AND CARE SCREENING

Section A	Identification Information
A0050. Type of Record	
Enter Code ☐	1. **Add new record** → Continue to A0100, Facility Provider Numbers 2. **Modify existing record** → Continue to A0100, Facility Provider Numbers 3. **Inactivate existing record** → Skip to X0150, Type of Provider
A0100. Facility Provider Numbers	
	A. National Provider Identifier (NPI): ☐☐☐☐☐☐☐☐☐☐ **B. CMS Certification Number (CCN):** ☐☐☐☐☐☐☐☐☐☐☐☐ **C. State Provider Number:** ☐☐☐☐☐☐☐☐☐☐☐☐☐☐☐
A0200. Type of Provider	
Enter Code ☐	**Type of provider** 1. **Nursing home (SNF/NF)** 2. **Swing Bed**
A0310. Type of Assessment	
Enter Code ☐☐	**A. Federal OBRA Reason for Assessment** 01. **Admission** assessment (required by day 14) 02. **Quarterly** review assessment 03. **Annual** assessment 04. **Significant change in status** assessment 05. **Significant correction** to **prior comprehensive** assessment 06. **Significant correction** to **prior quarterly** assessment 99. **None of the above**
Enter Code ☐☐	**B. PPS Assessment** **PPS Scheduled Assessments for a Medicare Part A Stay** 01. **5-day** scheduled assessment 02. **14-day** scheduled assessment 03. **30-day** scheduled assessment 04. **60-day** scheduled assessment 05. **90-day** scheduled assessment **PPS Unscheduled Assessments for a Medicare Part A Stay** 07. **Unscheduled assessment used for PPS** (OMRA, significant or clinical change, or significant correction assessment) **Not PPS Assessment** 99. **None of the above**
Enter Code ☐	**C. PPS Other Medicare Required Assessment - OMRA** 0. **No** 1. **Start of therapy** assessment 2. **End of therapy** assessment 3. **Both Start and End of therapy** assessment 4. **Change of therapy** assessment
Enter Code ☐	**D. Is this a Swing Bed clinical change assessment?** Complete only if A0200 = 2 0. **No** 1. **Yes**
Enter Code ☐	**E. Is this assessment the first assessment** (OBRA, Scheduled PPS, or Discharge) **since the most recent admission/entry or reentry?** 0. **No** 1. **Yes**

Figure 8-1. MDS 3.0. (Reproduced from MDS 3.0. Centers for Medicare & Medicaid Services; Baltimore, MD. Available at https://www.cms.gov/Medicare/Quality-Initiatives-Patient-Assessment-Instruments/NursingHomeQualityInits/Downloads/MDS-30-SECTIONS-A-AND-GG-DOCUMENT.pdf. Accessed July 20, 2020.)

Resident ______ Identifier ______ Date ______

Section A | Identification Information

A0310. Type of Assessment - Continued

Enter Code [ ][ ]
F. Entry/discharge reporting
01. **Entry** tracking record
10. **Discharge** assessment-**return not anticipated**
11. **Discharge** assessment-**return anticipated**
12. **Death in facility** tracking record
99. **None of the above**

Enter Code [ ]
G. Type of discharge - Complete only if A0310F = 10 or 11
1. **Planned**
2. **Unplanned**

Enter Code [ ]
H. Is this a SNF PPS Part A Discharge (End of Stay) Assessment?
0. **No**
1. **Yes**

A0410. Unit Certification or Licensure Designation

Enter Code [ ]
1. **Unit is neither Medicare nor Medicaid certified and MDS data is not required by the State**
2. **Unit is neither Medicare nor Medicaid certified but MDS data is required by the State**
3. **Unit is Medicare and/or Medicaid certified**

A0500. Legal Name of Resident

A. First name: [ ][ ][ ][ ][ ][ ][ ][ ][ ][ ][ ][ ]
B. Middle initial: [ ]
C. Last name: [ ][ ][ ][ ][ ][ ][ ][ ][ ][ ][ ][ ][ ][ ][ ][ ][ ][ ]
D. Suffix: [ ][ ][ ]

A0600. Social Security and Medicare Numbers

A. Social Security Number:
[ ][ ][ ] – [ ][ ] – [ ][ ][ ][ ]

B. Medicare number (or comparable railroad insurance number):
[ ][ ][ ][ ][ ][ ][ ][ ][ ][ ][ ][ ]

A0700. Medicaid Number - Enter "+" if pending, "N" if not a Medicaid recipient

[ ][ ][ ][ ][ ][ ][ ][ ][ ][ ][ ][ ][ ][ ]

A0800. Gender

Enter Code [ ]
1. **Male**
2. **Female**

A0900. Birth Date

[ ][ ] – [ ][ ] – [ ][ ][ ][ ]
Month Day Year

A1000. Race/Ethnicity

↓ **Check all that apply**

- [ ] **A. American Indian or Alaska Native**
- [ ] **B. Asian**
- [ ] **C. Black or African American**
- [ ] **D. Hispanic or Latino**
- [ ] **E. Native Hawaiian or Other Pacific Islander**
- [ ] **F. White**

Figure 8-1. (Continued)

Resident ______ Identifier ______ Date ______

Section A | Identification Information

A1100. Language

Enter Code [ ]

A. Does the resident need or want an interpreter to communicate with a doctor or health care staff?
- 0. **No** → Skip to A1200, Marital Status
- 1. **Yes** → Specify in A1100B, Preferred language
- 9. **Unable to determine** → Skip to A1200, Marital Status

B. Preferred language:

A1200. Marital Status

Enter Code [ ]

1. **Never married**
2. **Married**
3. **Widowed**
4. **Separated**
5. **Divorced**

A1300. Optional Resident Items

A. Medical record number:

B. Room number:

C. Name by which resident prefers to be addressed:

D. Lifetime occupation(s) - put "/" between two occupations:

A1500. Preadmission Screening and Resident Review (PASRR)
Complete only if A0310A = 01, 03, 04, or 05

Enter Code [ ]

Is the resident currently considered by the state level II PASRR process to have serious mental illness and/or intellectual disability ("mental retardation" in federal regulation) or a related condition?
- 0. **No** → Skip to A1550, Conditions Related to ID/DD Status
- 1. **Yes** → Continue to A1510, Level II Preadmission Screening and Resident Review (PASRR) Conditions
- 9. **Not a Medicaid-certified unit** → Skip to A1550, Conditions Related to ID/DD Status

A1510. Level II Preadmission Screening and Resident Review (PASRR) Conditions
Complete only if A0310A = 01, 03, 04, or 05

↓ **Check all that apply**

- [ ] **A. Serious mental illness**
- [ ] **B. Intellectual Disability ("mental retardation" in federal regulation)**
- [ ] **C. Other related conditions**

Figure 8-1. (Continued)

Resident ____________ Identifier ____________ Date ____________

Section A — Identification Information

A1550. Conditions Related to ID/DD Status
If the resident is 22 years of age or older, complete only if A0310A = 01
If the resident is 21 years of age or younger, complete only if A0310A = 01, 03, 04, or 05

↓ **Check all conditions that are related to ID/DD status** that were manifested before age 22, and are likely to continue indefinitely

	ID/DD With Organic Condition
☐	**A. Down syndrome**
☐	**B. Autism**
☐	**C. Epilepsy**
☐	**D. Other organic condition related to ID/DD**
	ID/DD Without Organic Condition
☐	**E. ID/DD with no organic condition**
	No ID/DD
☐	**Z. None of the above**

Most Recent Admission/Entry or Reentry into this Facility

A1600. Entry Date

☐☐ – ☐☐ – ☐☐☐☐
Month Day Year

A1700. Type of Entry

Enter Code ☐

1. **Admission**
2. **Reentry**

A1800. Entered From

Enter Code ☐☐

01. **Community** (private home/apt., board/care, ass sted living, group home)
02. **Another nursing home or swing bed**
03. **Acute hospital**
04. **Psychiatric hospital**
05. **Inpatient rehabilitation facility**
06. **ID/DD facility**
07. **Hospice**
09. **Long Term Care Hospital** (LTCH)
99. **Other**

A1900. Admission Date (Date this episode of care in this facility began)

☐☐ – ☐☐ – ☐☐☐☐
Month Day Year

A2000. Discharge Date
Complete only if A0310F = 10, 11, or 12

☐☐ – ☐☐ – ☐☐☐☐
Month Day Year

Figure 8-1. (Continued)

Resident Identifier Date

Section A	Identification Information

A2100. Discharge Status
Complete only if A0310F = 10, 11, or 12

Enter Code

01. **Community** (private home/apt., board/care, assisted living, group home)
02. **Another nursing home or swing bed**
03. **Acute hospital**
04. **Psychiatric hospital**
05. **Inpatient rehabilitation facility**
06. **ID/DD facility**
07. **Hospice**
08. **Deceased**
09. **Long Term Care Hospital** (LTCH)
99. **Other**

A2200. Previous Assessment Reference Date for Significant Correction
Complete only if A0310A = 05 or 06

Month – Day – Year

A2300. Assessment Reference Date

Observation end date:

Month – Day – Year

A2400. Medicare Stay

Enter Code

A. Has the resident had a Medicare-covered stay since the most recent entry?
0. **No** → Skip to B0100, Comatose
1. **Yes** → Continue to A2400B, Start date of most recent Medicare stay

B. Start date of most recent Medicare stay:

Month – Day – Year

C. End date of most recent Medicare stay - Enter dashes if stay is ongoing:

Month – Day – Year

Figure 8-1. (Continued)

Resident Identifier Date

Section GG	**Functional Abilities and Goals** - Admission (Start of SNF PPS Stay)

GG0130. Self-Care (Assessment period is days 1 through 3 of the SNF PPS Stay starting with A2400B)
Complete only if A0310B = 01

Code the resident's usual performance at the start of the SNF PPS stay for each activity using the 6-point scale. If activity was not attempted at the start of the SNF PPS stay, code the reason. Code the patient's end of SNF PPS stay goal(s) using the 6-point scale.

Coding:

Safety and **Quality of Performance -** If helper assistance is required because resident's performance is unsafe or of poor quality, score according to amount of assistance provided.

Activities may be completed with or without assistive devices.

06. **Independent** - Resident completes the activity by him/herself with no assistance from a helper.
05. **Setup or clean-up assistance** - Helper SETS UP or CLEANS UP; resident completes activity. Helper assists only prior to or following the activity**.**
04. **Supervision or touching assistance** - Helper provides VERBAL CUES or TOUCHING/STEADYING assistance as resident completes activity. Assistance may be provided throughout the activity or intermittently.
03. **Partial/moderate assistance** - Helper does LESS THAN HALF the effort. Helper lifts, holds, or supports trunk or limbs, but provides less than half the effort.
02. **Substantial/maximal assistance** - Helper does MORE THAN HALF the effort. Helper lifts or holds trunk or limbs and provides more than half the effort.
01. **Dependent** - Helper does ALL of the effort. Resident does none of the effort to complete the activity. Or the assistance of 2 or more helpers is required for the resident to complete the activity.

If activity was not attempted, code reason:

07. **Resident refused.**
09. **Not applicable.**
88. Not attempted due to **medical condition or safety concerns.**

1. Admission Performance	2. Discharge Goal	
↓ Enter Codes in Boxes ↓		
		A. Eating: The ability to use suitable utensils to bring food to the mouth and swallow food once the meal is presented on a table/tray. Includes modified food consistency.
		B. Oral hygiene: The ability to use suitable items to clean teeth. [Dentures (if applicable): The ability to remove and replace dentures from and to the mouth, and manage equipment for soaking and rinsing them.]
		C. Toileting hygiene: The ability to maintain perineal hygiene, adjust clothes before and after using the toilet, commode, bedpan, or urinal. If managing an ostomy, include wiping the opening but not managing equipment.

Figure 8-1. (Continued)

Resident ______ Identifier ______ Date ______

Section GG	Functional Abilities and Goals - Admission (Start of SNF PPS Stay)

GG0170. Mobility (Assessment period is days 1 through 3 of the SNF PPS Stay starting with A2400B)
Complete only if A0310B = 01

Code the resident's usual performance at the start of the SNF PPS stay for each activity using the 6-point scale. If activity was not attempted at the start of the SNF PPS stay, code the reason. Code the patient's end of SNF PPS stay goal(s) using the 6-point scale.

Coding:

Safety and **Quality of Performance -** If helper assistance is required because resident's performance is unsafe or of poor quality, score according to amount of assistance provided.

Activities may be completed with or without assistive devices.

06. **Independent** - Resident completes the activity by him/herself with no assistance from a helper.
05. **Setup or clean-up assistance** - Helper SETS UP or CLEANS UP; resident completes activity. Helper assists only prior to or following the activity.
04. **Supervision or touching assistance** - Helper provides VERBAL CUES or TOUCHING/STEADYING assistance as resident completes activity. Assistance may be provided throughout the activity or intermittently.
03. **Partial/moderate assistance** - Helper does LESS THAN HALF the effort. Helper lifts, holds, or supports trunk or limbs, but provides less than half the effort.
02. **Substantial/maximal assistance** - Helper does MORE THAN HALF the effort. Helper lifts or holds trunk or limbs and provides more than half the effort.
01. **Dependent** - Helper does ALL of the effort. Resident does none of the effort to complete the activity. Or the assistance of 2 or more helpers is required for the resident to complete the activity.

If activity was not attempted, code reason:

07. **Resident refused.**
09. **Not applicable.**
88. Not attempted due to **medical condition or safety concerns.**

1. Admission Performance	2. Discharge Goal	
↓ Enter Codes in Boxes ↓		
☐☐	☐☐	**B. Sit to lying:** The ability to move from sitting on side of bed to lying flat on the bed.
☐☐	☐☐	**C. Lying to sitting on side of bed:** The ability to safely move from lying on the back to sitting on the side of the bed with feet flat on the floor, and with no back support.
☐☐	☐☐	**D. Sit to stand:** The ability to safely come to a standing position from sitting in a chair or on the side of the bed.
☐☐	☐☐	**E. Chair/bed-to-chair transfer:** The ability to safely transfer to and from a bed to a chair (or wheelchair).
☐☐	☐☐	**F. Toilet transfer:** The ability to safely get on and off a toilet or commode.
	☐	**H1. Does the resident walk?** 0. **No**, and walking goal is <u>not</u> clinically indicated → Skip to GG0170Q1, Does the resident use a wheelchair/scooter? 1. **No**, and walking goal <u>is</u> clinically indicated → Code the resident's discharge goal(s) for items GG0170J and GG0170K 2. **Yes** → Continue to GG0170J, Walk 50 feet with two turns
☐☐	☐☐	**J. Walk 50 feet with two turns:** Once standing, the ability to walk at least 50 feet and make two turns.
☐☐	☐☐	**K. Walk 150 feet:** Once standing, the ability to walk at least 150 feet in a corridor or similar space.
	☐	**Q1. Does the resident use a wheelchair/scooter?** 0. **No** → Skip to GG0130, Self Care 1. **Yes** → Continue to GG0170R, Wheel 50 feet with two turns
☐☐	☐☐	**R. Wheel 50 feet with two turns:** Once seated in wheelchair/scooter, can wheel at least 50 feet and make two turns.
	☐	**RR1. Indicate the type of wheelchair/scooter used.** 1. **Manual** 2. **Motorized**
☐☐	☐☐	**S. Wheel 150 feet:** Once seated in wheelchair/scooter, can wheel at least 150 feet in a corridor or similar space.
	☐	**SS1. Indicate the type of wheelchair/scooter used.** 1. **Manual** 2. **Motorized**

Figure 8-1. (Continued)

Resident ______ Identifier ______ Date ______

Section GG | **Functional Abilities and Goals** - Discharge (End of SNF PPS Stay)

GG0130. Self-Care (Assessment period is the last 3 days of the SNF PPS Stay ending on A2400C)
Complete only if A0310G is not = 2 **and** A0310H = 1 **and** A2400C minus A2400B is greater than 2 **and** A2100 is not = 03

Code the resident's usual performance at the end of the SNF PPS stay for each activity using the 6-point scale. If an activity was not attempted at the end of the SNF PPS stay, code the reason.

Coding:

Safety and **Quality of Performance** - If helper assistance is required because resident's performance is unsafe or of poor quality, score according to amount of assistance provided.
Activities may be completed with or without assistive devices.

06. **Independent** - Resident completes the activity by him/herself with no assistance from a helper.
05. **Setup or clean-up assistance** - Helper SETS UP or CLEANS UP; resident completes activity. Helper assists only prior to or following the activity.
04. **Supervision or touching assistance** - Helper provides VERBAL CUES or TOUCHING/STEADYING assistance as resident completes activity. Assistance may be provided throughout the activity or intermittently.
03. **Partial/moderate assistance** - Helper does LESS THAN HALF the effort. Helper lifts, holds, or supports trunk or limbs, but provides less than half the effort.
02. **Substantial/maximal assistance** - Helper does MORE THAN HALF the effort. Helper lifts or holds trunk or limbs and provides more than half the effort.
01. **Dependent** - Helper does ALL of the effort. Resident does none of the effort to complete the activity. Or the assistance of 2 or more helpers is required for the resident to complete the activity.

If activity was not attempted, code reason:

07. **Resident refused.**
09. **Not applicable.**
88. Not attempted due to **medical condition or safety concerns.**

3. Discharge Performance	
Enter Code ☐☐	**A. Eating:** The ability to use suitable utensils to bring food to the mouth and swallow food once the meal is presented on a table/tray. Includes modified food consistency.
Enter Code ☐☐	**B. Oral hygiene:** The ability to use suitable items to clean teeth. [Dentures (if applicable): The ability to remove and replace dentures from and to the mouth, and manage equipment for soaking and rinsing them.]
Enter Code ☐☐	**C. Toileting hygiene:** The ability to maintain perineal hygiene, adjust clothes before and after using the toilet, commode, bedpan, or urinal. If managing an ostomy, include wiping the opening but not managing equipment.

Figure 8-1. (Continued)

Resident ______ Identifier ______ Date ______

Section GG | **Functional Abilities and Goals** - Discharge (End of SNF PPS Stay)

GG0170. Mobility (Assessment period is the last 3 days of the SNF PPS Stay ending on A2400C)
Complete only if A0310G is not = 2 **and** A0310H = 1 **and** A2400C minus A2400B is greater than 2 **and** A2100 is not = 03

Code the resident's usual performance at the end of the SNF PPS stay for each activity using the 6-point scale. If an activity was not attempted at the end of the SNF PPS stay, code the reason.

Coding:

Safety and **Quality of Performance** - If helper assistance is required because resident's performance is unsafe or of poor quality, score according to amount of assistance provided.
Activities may be completed with or without assistive devices.

06. **Independent** - Resident completes the activity by him/herself with no assistance from a helper.
05. **Setup or clean-up assistance** - Helper SETS UP or CLEANS UP; resident completes activity. Helper assists only prior to or following the activity.
04. **Supervision or touching assistance** - Helper provides VERBAL CUES or TOUCHING/STEADYING assistance as resident completes activity. Assistance may be provided throughout the activity or intermittently.
03. **Partial/moderate assistance** - Helper does LESS THAN HALF the effort. Helper lifts, holds, or supports trunk or limbs, but provides less than half the effort.
02. **Substantial/maximal assistance** - Helper does MORE THAN HALF the effort. Helper lifts or holds trunk or limbs and provides more than half the effort.
01. **Dependent** - Helper does ALL of the effort. Resident does none of the effort to complete the activity. Or the assistance of 2 or more helpers is required for the resident to complete the activity.

If activity was not attempted, code reason:

07. **Resident refused.**
09. **Not applicable.**
88. Not attempted due to **medical condition or safety concerns.**

3. Discharge Performance Enter Codes in Boxes	
☐☐	**B. Sit to lying:** The ability to move from sitting on side of bed to lying flat on the bed.
☐☐	**C. Lying to sitting on side of bed:** The ability to safely move from lying on the back to sitting on the side of the bed with feet flat on the floor, and with no back support.
☐☐	**D. Sit to stand:** The ability to safely come to a standing position from sitting in a chair or on the side of the bed.
☐☐	**E. Chair/bed-to-chair transfer:** The ability to safely transfer to and from a bed to a chair (or wheelchair).
☐☐	**F. Toilet transfer:** The ability to safely get on and off a toilet or commode.
	☐ **H3. Does the resident walk?** 0. **No** → Skip to GG0170Q3, Does the resident use a wheelchair/scooter? 2. **Yes** → Continue to GG0170J, Walk 50 feet with two turns
☐☐	**J. Walk 50 feet with two turns:** Once standing, the ability to walk at least 50 feet and make two turns.
☐☐	**K. Walk 150 feet:** Once standing, the ability to walk at least 150 feet in a corridor or similar space.
	☐ **Q3. Does the resident use a wheelchair/scooter?** 0. **No** → Skip to H0100, Appliances 1. **Yes** → Continue to GG0170R, Wheel 50 feet with two turns
☐☐	**R. Wheel 50 feet with two turns:** Once seated in wheelchair/scooter, can wheel at least 50 feet and make two turns.
	☐ **RR3. Indicate the type of wheelchair/scooter used.** 1. **Manual** 2. **Motorized**
☐☐	**S. Wheel 150 feet:** Once seated in wheelchair/scooter, can wheel at least 150 feet in a corridor or similar space.
	☐ **SS3. Indicate the type of wheelchair/scooter used.** 1. **Manual** 2. **Motorized**

Figure 8-1. (Continued)

Under the PDPM (effective October 1, 2019), there are three SNF PPS assessments the 5-day assessment, the Interim Payment Assessment (IPA), and the PPS Discharge Assessment. The 5-day assessment and the PPS Discharge Assessment are required. The IPA is optional and will be completed when providers determine that the patient has undergone a clinical change that would require a new PPS assessment. The goal of this change was to improve payments by focusing on the patient rather than the volume of services provided.[4]

The schedule of PPS assessments under PDPM may be found in Table 8-1.

Two new item sets have been created as a result of PDPM. First, the IPA has its own item set. This contains just payment items and demographic items, as necessary, to attain a billing code under PDPM. Because the IPA is completely optional, there will be no late assessment penalties for that assessment.

Second, for states that rely on the old Resource Utilization Group (RUG)-III or RUG-IV assessment schedule for calculating a case-mix group for NF patients, Centers for Medicare & Medicaid Services (CMS) created the optional state assessment (OSA) so that Medicaid payments were not adversely affected when the PDPM was implemented as of October 1, 2019. States have the ability to determine the policy associated with this assessment to meet their Medicaid payment needs.

MDS PURPOSE AND COMPONENTS

The Minimum Data Set (MDS) is part of the federally mandated process for clinical assessment of all residents in Medicare and Medicaid certified nursing homes. This process provides a comprehensive assessment of each resident's functional capabilities and helps nursing home staff identify health problems. Care Area Assessments (CAAs) are part of this process, and provide the foundation upon which a resident's individual care plan is formulated. MDS assessments are completed for all residents in certified nursing homes, regardless of source of payment for the individual resident. MDS assessments are required for residents on admission to the nursing facility, periodically, and on discharge. All assessments are completed within specific guidelines and time frames.

Table 8-1 Schedule of PPS assessments under PDPM

MEDICARE MIDS ASSESSMENT SCHEDULE TYPE	ASSESSMENT REFERENCE DATE	APPLICABLE STANDARD MEDICARE PAYMENT DAYS
5-day PPS Assessment	Days 1–8	All covered Part A days until Part A discharge (unless an IPA is completed).
Interim Payment Assessment (PA)	The date the facility chooses to complete the IPA relative to the triggering event that causes the facility to chooses to complete the IPA.	ARD of the assessment through Part A discharge (unless another IPA assessment is completed).
PPS Discharge Assessment	PPS Discharge: Equal to the End Date of the Most Recent Medicare Stay (A2400C) or End Date	N/A.

In most cases, participants in the assessment process are licensed health care professionals employed by the nursing home. MDS information is transmitted electronically by nursing homes to the national MDS database at CMS.[1]

The MDS is a core set of screening, clinical, and functional status elements, including common definitions and coding categories, which forms the foundation of a comprehensive assessment for all residents of nursing homes certified to participate in Medicare or Medicaid.[3] The items in the MDS standardize communication about resident problems and conditions within nursing homes, between nursing homes, and between nursing homes and outside agencies. The required subsets of data items for each MDS assessment and tracking document (e.g., Comprehensive, Quarterly, OBRA Discharge, Entry Tracking, PPS item sets) can be found in Appendix H. The MDS is completed for all residents in Medicare- or Medicaid-certified nursing homes and residents in a PPS stay in noncritical access hospitals with Medicare swing bed agreements. States may also establish additional MDS requirements.[1]

The MDS is used as a component of two separate processes. One process is the designation of PDPM categories, for Medicare Part A stays (see Chapter 15 for more information).

PDPM consists of five case-mix adjustment components: physical therapy, occupational therapy, speech-language pathology, nursing, and nontherapy ancillary services. PDPM also includes a variable per diem adjustment that adjusts the per diem rate over the course of the stay.

The other process is designed to provide assessment and reassessment data to be used in the RAI process that was also mandated by the Omnibus Budget Reconciliation Act (OBRA), also known as the Nursing Home Reform Act of 1987, and continues to be used with changes to align with PDPM. MDS data is utilized by state and local agencies to monitor the quality and safety of SNFs.

The MDS has been adjusted to align with the new case-mix methodology. A functional score is calculated as the sum of the scores on 10 Section GG items:[4]

- Two bed mobility items
- Three transfer items
- One eating item
- One toileting item
- One oral hygiene item
- For the two walking items, CMS uses an additional response level to reflect patients who skip the walking assessment due to their inability to walk. This allows CMS to assess the functional abilities of patients who cannot walk and assign them a function score. Without this modification, CMS could not calculate a function score for patients who cannot walk because they would not be assessed on the two walking items included in the function score. MDS item GG0170I1 (Walk 10 feet) responses 07: "resident refused," 09: "not applicable," 10: "not attempted due to environmental limitations," or 88: "not attempted due to medical condition or safety concerns" from MDS item GG0170I1 will be used to identify residents who cannot walk. Patients who are coded as unable to walk receive the same score as dependent patients to match with clinical expectations." **This comes from the CMS Fact Sheet: PDPM Functional and Cognitive Scoring Last Revised: 2-14-19.

Each of the two items for a GG code is valued from 0 to 4.

Nonwalking items are scored for physical therapy (PT), occupational therapy (OT), and nursing with a range in descriptors from dependent; to refused; to not applicable; to not attempted because of environmental limitations, medical conditions, or safety concerns.

Author's Note

Points are assigned to each response level to track functional independence rather than functional dependence, meaning higher points are assigned to higher levels of independence.

Author's Note

When the activity cannot be completed, the equivalent section GG responses ("Resident refused, "Not applicable," "Not attempted due to environmental limitations," "Not attempted due to medical condition or safety concerns") are grouped with "dependent" for the purpose of point assignment." **CMS Fact Sheet: PDPM Functional and Cognitive Scoring Last Revised: 2-14-19.

The primary diagnosis for the MDS under the PDPM uses the ICD-10 code and reflects the primary reason for admission to the SNF. Coding is also required for surgical procedures preceding the SNF admission, if applicable.

PERSONNEL REPORTING ON THE MDS

Nurse assessment coordinators may document all items of the MDS with other interprofessional team members; physicians, speech-language pathologists, occupational therapists, activities professionals, dietitians, and physical therapists may also complete MDS items. Information provided by all of the team members, including the patient, the family, direct care providers such as nursing assistants, and nonancillary and ancillary service personnel, may be used in the assessment process. Signing the MDS denotes legal responsibility for the accuracy of the information documented in the sections that are signed for.

Definitions

Individual services are provided by one therapist or assistant to one resident at a time.

Concurrent therapy is defined as the treatment of two residents at the same time, when the residents are not performing the same or similar activities, regardless of payer source, both of whom must be in line-of-sight of the treating therapist or assistant for Medicare Part A When a Part A resident receives therapy that meets this definition, it is defined as concurrent therapy for the Part A resident, regardless of the payer source for the second resident.

Group therapy is defined for Part A as the treatment of two to six residents, regardless of payer source, who are performing the same or similar activities and are supervised by a therapist or an assistant who is not supervising any other individuals.

Usual performance is defined as a resident's functional status can be impacted by the environment or situations encountered at the facility. Observing the resident's interactions with others in different locations and circumstances is important for a comprehensive understanding of the resident's functional status. If the resident's functional status varies, record the resident's usual ability to perform each activity. Do not record the resident's best performance and do not record the resident's worst performance, but rather record the resident's usual performance.

PPS assessments provide information about the clinical condition of beneficiaries receiving Part A SNF-level care in order to be reimbursed under the SNF PPS for both SNFs and swing bed providers. These assessments are coded on the MDS 3.0 in items A0310B (PPS Assessment) and A0310H (Part A PPS Discharge Assessment). They include:

- Five-day assessment
- IPA
- Part A PPS discharge assessment

Assessment reference dates (ARDs): ARD refers to the last day of the observation (or "look-back") period that the assessment covers for the resident. Since a day begins at 12:00 AM and ends at 11:59 PM, the ARD must also cover this time period. The facility is required to set the ARD on the MDS item set or in the facility software within the required time frame of the assessment type being completed. This concept of setting the ARD is used for all assessment types (OBRA and PPS) and varies by assessment type and facility determination. Most of the MDS 3.0 items have a 7-day look-back period. If a resident has an ARD of July 1, 2011, then all pertinent information starting at 12:00 AM on June 25 and ending on July 1 at 11:59 PM should be included for MDS 3.0 coding.

Assessment timing refers to when and how often assessments must be conducted, based upon the resident's length of stay and the length of time between ARDs.

- For OBRA-required assessments, regulatory requirements for each assessment type dictate assessment timing, the schedule for which is established with the admission (comprehensive) assessment when the ARD is set by the registered nurse (RN) assessment coordinator and the interdisciplinary team (IDT).
- Assuming the resident did not experience a significant change in status, was not discharged, and did not have a Significant Correction to Prior Comprehensive (SCPA) assessment completed, assessment scheduling would then move through a cycle of three quarterly assessments followed by an annual (comprehensive) assessment.

Grace days: Predetermined additional days that may be added to the assessment window for Medicare scheduled assessments without incurring financial penalty. These may be used in situations such as an absence/illness or reassignment of the RN assessment coordinator or an unusually large number of assessments due at approximately the same time. Grace days may also be used to more fully capture therapy minutes or other treatments.

Required OBRA assessments for MDS: If the assessment is being used for OBRA requirements, the OBRA reason for assessment must be coded in items A0310A and A0310F (entry/discharge reporting). PPS reasons for assessment are described in Section 2.9, while the OBRA reasons for assessment are described here. Table 8-2 provides a summary of the assessment types and requirements for the OBRA-required assessments.

Interim payment assessment: There are situations when a SNF provider may complete an assessment after the 5-day assessment. This assessment is an unscheduled assessment called the IPA. When deemed appropriate by the provider, this assessment may be completed to capture changes in the resident's status and condition.

Interrupted stay is a Medicare Part A SNF stay in which a resident is discharged from SNF care (i.e., the resident is discharged from a Medicare Part A–covered stay) and subsequently resumes care in the same SNF for a Medicare Part A–covered stay during the interruption window.

Interruption window is a 3-day period, starting with the calendar day of Part A discharge and including the 2 immediately following calendar days. In other words, if a resident in a Medicare Part A SNF stay is discharged from Part A, the resident must resume Part A services or return to the same SNF (if physically discharged) to resume Part A services by 11:59 PM at the end of the third calendar day after their Part A–covered stay ended. The interruption window begins with the first noncovered day following a Part A–covered stay and ends at 11:59 PM on the third consecutive noncovered day following a Part A–covered SNF stay. If these conditions are met, the subsequent stay is considered a continuation of the previous Medicare Part A–covered stay for the purposes of both the variable per diem schedule and PPS assessment completion.

Discharge assessment: This refers to an assessment required on resident discharge from the facility, or when a resident's Medicare Part A stay ends but the resident remains in the facility (unless it is an instance of an interrupted stay, as defined later). This assessment includes clinical items for quality monitoring as well as discharge tracking information.

Special Treatments, Procedures, and Programs

MDS Section O includes recording the number of days and minutes that the patient receives physical, occupational, speech, respiratory, psychological, and recreational therapy during the 7-day observation period.

The MDS RAI Manual (effective October 1, 2019) Section O-16 states:

Table 8-2 Summary of the assessment types and requirements for the OBRA-required assessments

RAI OBRA-REQUIRED ASSESSMENT SUMMARY										
ASSESSMENT TYPE/ITEM SET	MDS ASSESSMENT CODE (A0310A OR A0310F)	ASSESSMENT REFERENCE DATE (ARD) (ITEM A2300) NO LATER THAN	7-DAY OBSERVATION PERIOD (LOOK BACK) CONSISTS OF	14-DAY OBSERVATION PERIOD (LOOK BACK) CONSISTS OF	MDS COMPLETION DATE (ITEM Z0500B) NO LATER THAN	CAA(S) COMPLETION DATE (ITEM V0200B2) NO LATER THAN	CARE PLAN COMPLETION DATE (ITEM V0200C2) NO LATER THAN	TRANSMISSION DATE NO LATER THAN	REGULATORY REQUIREMENT	ASSESSMENT COMBINATION
Admission (Comprehensive)	A0310A = 01	14th calendar day of the resident's admission (admission date + 13 calendar days)	ARD + 6 previous calendar days	ARD + 13 previous calendar days	14th calendar day of the resident's admission (admission date + 13 calendar days)	14th calendar day of the resident's admission (admission date + 13 calendar days)	CAA(s) Completion Date + 7 calendar days	Care Plan Completion Date + 14 calendar days	42 CFR 483.20 (Initial) 42 CFR 483.20 (b)(2)(i) (by the 14th day)	May be combined with any OBRA assessment; 5-Day or Part A PPS Discharge Assessment
Annual (Comprehensive)	A0310A = 03	ARD of previous OBRA comprehensive assessment + 366 calendar days AND ARD of previous OBRA Quarterly assessment + 92 calendar days	ARD + 6 previous calendar days	ARD +13 previous calendar days	ARD + 14 calendar days	ARD + 14 calendar days	CAA(s) Completion Date + 7 calendar days	Care Plan Completion Date + 14 calendar days	42 CFR 483.20 (b)(2)(iii) (every 12 months)	May be combined with any OBRA or 5-Day or Part A PPS Discharge Assessment
Significant Change in Status (SCSA) (Comprehensive)	A0310A = 04	14th calendar day after determination that significant change in resident's status occurred (determination date + 14 calendar days)	ARD + 6 previous calendar days	ARD + 13 previous calendar days	14th calendar day after determination that significant change in resident's status occurred (determination date + 14 calendar days)	14th calendar day after determination that significant change in resident's status occurred (determination date + 14 calendar days)	CAA(s) Completion Date + 7 calendar days	Care Plan Completion Date + 14 calendar days	42 CFR 483.20 (b)(2)(ii) (within 14 days)	May be combined with any OBRA or 5-Day or Part A PPS Discharge Assessment
Significant Correction to Prior Comprehensive (SCPA) (Comprehensive)	A0310A = 05	14th calendar day after determination that significant error in prior comprehensive assessment occurred (determination date + 14 calendar days)	ARD + 6 previous calendar days	ARD + 13 previous calendar days	14th calendar day after determination that significant error in prior comprehensive assessment occurred (determination date + 14 calendar days)	14th calendar day after determination that significant error in prior comprehensive assessment occurred (determination date + 14 calendar days)	CAA(s) Completion Date + 7 calendar days	Care Plan Completion Date + 14 calendar days	42 CFR 483.20(f) (3) (iv)	May be combined with any OBRA or 5-Day or Part A PPS Discharge Assessment

(Continued)

Table 8-2 Summary of the assessment types and requirements for the OBRA-required assessments (Continued)

RAI OBRA-REQUIRED ASSESSMENT SUMMARY										
ASSESSMENT TYPE/ITEM SET	MDS ASSESSMENT CODE (A0310A OR A0310F)	ASSESSMENT REFERENCE DATE (ARD) (ITEM A2300) NO LATER THAN	7-DAY OBSERVATION PERIOD (LOOK BACK) CONSISTS OF	14-DAY OBSERVATION PERIOD (LOOK BACK) CONSISTS OF	MDS COMPLETION DATE (ITEM Z0500B) NO LATER THAN	CAA(S) COMPLETION DATE (ITEM V0200B2) NO LATER THAN	CARE PLAN COMPLETION DATE (ITEM V0200C2) NO LATER THAN	TRANSMISSION DATE NO LATER THAN	REGULATORY REQUIREMENT	ASSESSMENT COMBINATION
Quarterly (Non-Comprehensive)	A0310A = 02	ARD of previous OBRA assessment of any type + 92 calendar days	ARD + 6 previous calendar days	ARD + 13 previous calendar days	ARD + 14 calendar days	N/A	N/A	MDS Completion Date + 14 calendar days	42 CFR 483.20(c) (every 3 months)	May be combined with any OBRA or 5-Day or Part A PPS Discharge Assessment
Significant Correction to Prior Quarterly (SCQA) (Non-Comprehensive)	A0310A = 06	14th day after determination that significant error in prior quarterly assessment occurred (determination date + 14 calendar days)	ARD + 6 previous calendar days	ARD + 13 previous calendar days	14th day after determination that significant error in prior quarterly assessment occurred (determination date + 14 calendar days)	N/A	N/A	MDS Completion Date + 14 calendar days	42 CFR 483.20(f) (3)(v)	May be combined with any OBRA or 5-Day or Part A PPS Discharge Assessment
Discharge Assessment – return not anticipated (Non-Comprehensive)	A0310F = 10	N/A	N/A	N/A	Discharge Date + 14 calendar days	N/A	N/A	MDS Completion Date + 14 calendar days		May be combined with any OBRA or 5-Day or Part A PPS Discharge Assessment
Discharge Assessment – return anticipated (Non-Comprehensive)	A0310F = 11	N/A	N/A	N/A	Discharge Date + 14 calendar days	N/A	N/A	MDS Completion Date + 14 calendar days		May be combined with any OBRA or 5-Day or Part A PPS Discharge Assessment
Entry tracking record	A0310F = 01	N/A	N/A	N/A	Entry Date + 7 calendar days			Entry Date + 14 calendar days		May not be combined with another assessment
Death in facility tracking record	A0310F = 12	N/A	N/A	N/A	Discharge (death) Date + 7 calendar days	N/A	N/A	Discharge (death) Date +14 calendar days		May not be combined with another assessment

SOURCE: Reproduced from *Long-Term Care Facility Resident Assessment Instrument 3.0 User's Manual Version 1.17.1*. Centers for Medicare and Medicaid Services, Washington, DC; October 2019.

Code only medically necessary therapies that occurred after admission/readmission to the nursing home that were:

(1) *Ordered by a physician (physician's assistant, nurse practitioner, and/or clinical nurse specialist) based on a qualified therapist's assessment (i.e., one who meets Medicare requirements or, in some instances, under such a person's direct supervision) and treatment plan,*

(2) *Documented in the resident's medical record, and*

(3) *Care planned and periodically evaluated to ensure that the resident receives needed therapies and that current treatment plans are effective.*

Therapy treatment may occur either inside or outside of the facility.

Section O-18 further states:

Only skilled therapy time (i.e., requires the skills, knowledge and judgment of a qualified therapist and all the requirements for skilled therapy are met) shall be recorded on the MDS. In some instances, the time during which a resident received a treatment modality includes partly skilled and partly unskilled time; only time that is skilled may be recorded on the MDS.

Therapist time during a portion of a treatment that is non-skilled; during a non-therapeutic rest period; or during a treatment that does not meet the therapy mode definitions may not be included.

In order to capture therapy delivery information over the course of a patient's entire Part A stay as it relates to the concurrent and group therapy limit under PDPM, CMS added Items 0425A1 to 0425C5 to Section O of the MDS. Using a look-back period of the entire FPS stay, providers will report, by each discipline and mode of therapy, the amount of therapy (in minutes) received by the patient. If the total amount of group/concurrent minutes combined comprises more than 25% of the total amount of therapy for that discipline, a warning message will be issued on the final validation report.

Care Area Assessment (CAA) Process

This process is designed to assist the assessor to systematically interpret the information recorded on the MDS. Once a care area has been triggered, nursing home providers use current, evidence-based clinical resources to conduct an assessment of the potential problem and determine whether to plan care for it. The CAA process helps the clinician focus on key issues identified during the assessment process so that decisions whether and how to intervene can be explored with the resident. Specific components of the CAA process include the following:

- Care area triggers (CATs) are specific resident responses for one or a combination of MDS elements. The triggers identify residents who have or are at risk for developing specific functional problems and require further assessment.
- CAA is the further investigation of triggered areas to determine if interventions and care planning are required. The CAA resources are provided as a courtesy to facilities in Appendix C. These resources include a compilation of checklists and web links that may be helpful in performing the assessment of a triggered care area. The use of these resources is not mandatory, and the list of web links is neither all-inclusive nor government endorsed.
- CAA summary (Section V of the MDS 3.0) provides a location for documentation of the care area(s) that have triggered from the MDS and the decisions made during the CAA process regarding whether or not to proceed to care planning.

The MDS does not constitute a comprehensive assessment. Rather, it is a preliminary assessment to identify potential resident problems, strengths, and preferences. Care areas are triggered by MDS item responses that indicate the need for additional assessment based on problem identification, known as "triggered care areas," which form a critical link between the MDS and decisions about care planning.

There are 20 CAAs in Version 3.0 of the RAI, which includes the addition of "Pain" and "Return to the Community Referral." These CAAs cover the majority of care areas known to be problematic for nursing home residents. The CAA (Table 8-3) process provides guidance on how to focus on key issues identified during a comprehensive MDS assessment and directs facility staff and health professionals to evaluate triggered care areas.

Table 8-3 Care Area Assessment

1. Delirium	2. Cognitive Loss/Dementia
3. Visual Function	4. Communication
5. Activity of Daily Living (ADL) Functional / Rehabilitation Potential	6. Urinary Incontinence and Indwelling Catheter
7. Psychosocial Well-Being	8. Mood State
9. Behavioral Symptoms	10. Activities
11. Falls	12. Nutritional Status
13. Feeding Tubes	14. Dehydration/Fluid Maintenance
15. Dental Care	16. Pressure Ulcer/Injury
17. Psychotropic Medication Use	18. Physical Restraints
19. Pain	20. Return to Community Referral

SOURCE: Reproduced from *Long-Term Care Facility Resident Assessment Instrument 3.0 User's Manual Version 1.17.1*. Centers for Medicare and Medicaid Services, Washington, DC; October 2019.

Author's Note

Because the SNF PDPM will not use the minutes of therapy provided to a resident to classify patients for payment purposes, it is possible that SNFs may become incentivized to emphasize group and concurrent therapy over the kind of individualized therapy that is tailored to address each beneficiary's specific care needs, which is generally the most appropriate mode of therapy for SNF patients. In order to mitigate this potential effect of PDPM, CMS imposed a combined limit of 25% on concurrent and group therapy, per discipline.

Under PDPM, providers will be required to complete the PPS Discharge Assessment (Item Set Code = NPE) at the end of an SNF stay for all SNF Part A beneficiaries. As part of this assessment, providers will complete a new section of the MDS, Section O0425, where providers will report the total amount of therapy, broken down by therapy mode (individual, concurrent, and group) and by therapy discipline (PT, OT, speech-language pathology) the patient received during the entire Part A stay.

SUMMARY

Use of the MDS in the SNF setting is challenging. However, it is necessary on an initial and ongoing basis for all SNF patients and residents in order to comply with federal regulations. Although this serves as an introduction to the instrument, clinicians should refer to the MDS 3.0 or the applicable version of the Users' Manual during their first attempts to negotiate the MDS and RAI system. Rehabilitation professionals should appreciate the importance of their contribution to the MDS process and its emphasis on function.

GENERAL SKILLED NURSING HOME BILLING ISSUES

Can a PTA provide skilled maintenance therapy to a Medicare patient under Medicare Part B?

No. Pursuant to the Medicare Benefit Policy Manual, Chapter 15, Section 230.1(C), "The services of PTAs used when providing covered therapy benefits are included as part of the covered service. These services are billed by the supervising physical therapist. PTAs may not provide evaluative or assessment services, make clinical judgments or decisions, develop, manage, or furnish skilled maintenance program services, or take responsibility for the service. They act at the direction and under the supervision of the treating physical therapist and in accordance with state laws."[5]

"Top SNF Therapy Provider Settles DOJ Lawsuit for $125 Million"[6]

The U.S. Department of Justice (DOJ) announced that the nation's largest nursing home therapy provider has agreed to pay $125 million to settle a DOJ lawsuit that alleged the company engaged in a "systematic and broad-ranging scheme" to increase Medicare reimbursements by submitting false claims for rehabilitation therapy.

RehabCare Group Inc, RehabCare Group East Inc, and parent company Kindred Healthcare will pay out the money in response to allegations that they violated the False Claims Act by "providing unreasonable and unnecessary services to Medicare patients," and that they "led … SNF [skilled nursing facility] customers to submit artificially and improperly inflated bills to Medicare that included those services," according to a DOJ press release. RehabCare contracts with more than 1,000 SNFs in 44 states to provide rehabilitation therapy.

The alleged violations include:

- *Placing patients in the highest-possible reimbursement levels, regardless of determinations made through patient evaluation*
- *"Boosting" the amount of reported therapy during "assessment reference periods" and then providing less therapy to those patients outside of those reference periods*
- *Scheduling and reporting the provision of therapy, even after the patients' therapist had recommended discharge*
- *Shifting minutes of planned therapy among disciplines "to ensure targeted therapy reimbursement levels were achieved, regardless of the clinical need for therapy"*
- *Providing higher amounts of therapy near the end of a therapy measurement period to maximize payment*
- *Reporting time spent on initial evaluation as therapy time rather than evaluation time*
- *Reporting that skilled therapy had been provided "when in fact the patients were asleep or otherwise unable to undergo or benefit from skilled therapy"*
- *Reporting estimated or rounded minutes of therapy rather than actual minutes provided*

According to DOJ, the settlement is also linked to 4 other settlements with individual SNFs for their roles in submitting false claims of therapy provided by RehabCare. Those payments range from $3.9 million to $750,000.

SNF billing practices began making headlines late last summer, when the Wall Street Journal *published a report outlining the findings of its study of the use of "ultrahigh" therapy hours, and resurfaced in October when the Office of the Inspector General of the US Department of Health and Human Services (HHS) issued a report highly critical of SNFs. That report was in turn the subject of a* New York Times *article on the issue, an article that prompted a letter to the editor from APTA President Sharon L. Dunn, PT, PhD, OCS, published in the* Times.[6]

REVIEW QUESTIONS

1. Who is responsible for completing the MDS?
2. What is the role of the MDS in patient care in an SNF?
3. An individual is admitted to an SNF as a skilled patient. He remains in the skilled unit 100 days and then becomes a long-term resident for 2 months before being discharged to an assisted living facility. How many MDS reports will be completed in the 160 days? Provide a rationale for your response.
4. How are the minutes of therapy services determined? Is there a difference between the first 5 days and ensuing days? Explain.
5. A patient is admitted to an SNF but following day 1, the patient is unable to participate in any of the therapy services and essentially remains bedbound secondary to low-grade fever and emesis. Explain how this is dealt with in the MDS process.

6. Explain how each of the 20 CAA areas are related to physical therapy.
7. According to MDS and CMS guidelines, who can provide physical therapy services versus assist with physical therapy services?
8. Explain the RAI and RAP processes and the relationship to the MDS.

ADDITIONAL QUESTIONS ON PDPM

See CMS Frequently asked questions for answers and more Q & A.[7]

1. What is PDPM?
2. Why is CMS changing from RUG-IV to PDPM?
3. How are SNF patients classified into payment groups under PDPM?
4. How do providers bill for services under PDPM?
5. What does the HIPPS code represent under PDPM?
6. Is it required that the principal diagnosis on the SNF claim match the primary diagnosis coded in item I0020B?
7. Is it required that the SNF primary diagnosis match the primary diagnosis reported for the qualifying hospital stay?

REFERENCES

1. *Minimum Data Sets 3.0 Tool and Public Reports*. Centers for Medicare & Medicaid Services; Baltimore, MD. Available at https://www.cms.gov/Research-Statistics-Data-and-Systems/Computer-Data-and-Systems/Minimum-Data-Set-3-0-Public-Reports. Accessed July 20, 2020.
2. *MDS 3.0*. Centers for Medicare & Medicaid Services; Baltimore, MD. Available at https://www.cms.gov/Medicare/Quality-Initiatives-Patient-Assessment-Instruments/NursingHomeQualityInits/Downloads/MDS-30-SECTIONS-A-AND-GG-DOCUMENT.pdf. Accessed July 20, 2020.
3. *Social Security*. Compilation of the Social Security Laws. Available at http://www.ssa.gov/OP_Home/comp2/F100-203.html. Accessed February 20, 2020.
4. *SNF Payment Driven Model*. Centers for Medicare & Medicaid Services; Baltimore, MD. Available at https://www.cms.gov/Medicare/Medicare-Fee-for-Service-Payment/SNFPPS/Downloads/MLN_CalL_PDPM_Presentation_508.pdf. Accessed July 20, 2020.
5. *FAQ: Skilled Maintenance: Use of PTA With Skilled Maintenance*. American Physical Therapy Association; Alexandria, VA. Available at https://www.apta.org/your-practice/payment/medicare-payment/coverage-issues/skilled-maintenance-therapy-under-medicare. Accessed July 28, 2020.
6. Nation's largest Nursing Home Therapy Provider, Kindred/Rehabcare, to Pay $125 Million to Resolve False Claims Act Allegations. *Justice News*. The United States Department of Justice. Tuesday, January 12, 2006. Available at https://www.justice.gov/opa/pr/nation-s-largest-nursing-home-therapy-provider-kindredrehabcare-pay-125-million-resolve-false#:~:text=Nation's%20Largest%20Nursing%20Home%20Therapy,Allegations%20%7C%20OPA%20%7C%20Department%20of%20Justice&text=The%20.,government%20websites%20often%20end%20in%20. Accessed July 28, 2020.
7. *Patient Driven Payment Model Q & A*. Centers for Medicare & Medicaid Services. Available at https://www.cms.gov/Medicare/Medicare-Fee-for-Service-Payment/SNFPPS/Downloads/PDPM_FAQ_Final_v5.zip. Accessed July 29, 2020.

SECTION 2

How to Document Clinical Decision-Making

9 Evidence-Based Practice

OBJECTIVES

Following completion of this chapter, the reader will be able to:

- Describe how does evidence-based practice impacts how to treat a patient.
- Understand what does reliability and validity of a test mean.
- Define sensitivity of the test.
- Define specificity of the test.
- Differentiate skilled and non-skilled service.
- Explain the information an outcome measure provides to the clinician.

INTRODUCTION

Ever-increasing healthcare expenditures, both nationally and internationally, have resulted in changes in the healthcare delivery system. In the effort to contain cost while preserving quality, the burden of patient recovery and improvement has been transferred more to clinicians. The United States is currently operating in a functional outcome-based healthcare model. This has resulted in increased research by physical therapists and related rehabilitation professionals to justify and support physical therapy patient management based on evidence. Included in these efforts are patient examination/evaluation and physical therapy interventions to demonstrate that physical therapy has a positive impact on maximizing a patient's functional abilities. The American Physical Therapy Association (APTA)[1] recognizes the need for an evidence-based practice (EBP) (Figure 9-1).

Jette et al[2] demonstrated that within a random sample of 1,000 physical therapists (APTA members) about 72% of clinicians believed that EBP can help in the clinical decision-making process, 79% believed that EBP improves the overall quality of patient care, 90% agreed strongly with the fact that EBP is necessary, and about 82% believed that research literature can help the clinician guide clinical decision-making during patient care.

EBP is based on three equally important pillars: clinical expertise, the patient's belief system, and the research evidence. The challenge for each practitioner is that the effective application of the EBP practice model is based on the ability of the clinician to demonstrate the combination of the best available research evidence and the patient's belief and opinions regarding their medical issues and needs. This combination will be different in each individual case, resulting in variations in treatment interventions for similar medical conditions that should still lead to effective outcomes.

Clinical expertise is the ability of the clinician to be proficient in the clinical assessment, decision making and documentation of proper judgment regarding the case and knowing how to integrate research evidence.

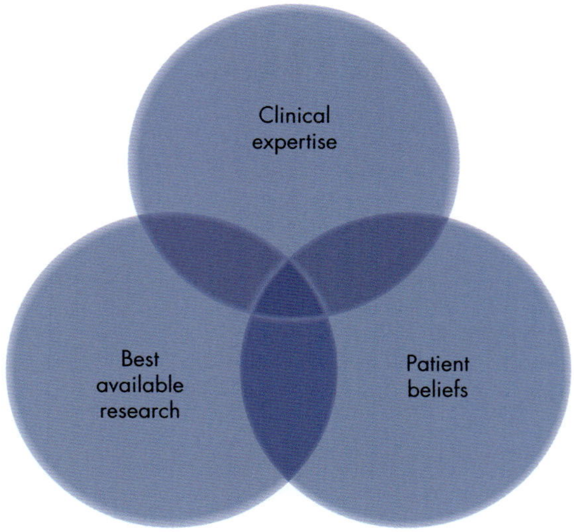

Figure 9-1. Central to the EBP model is the ability to provide and document the need for high-quality care while decreasing unwarranted variation in practice.

Clinical research provides clinicians with the ability to determine the usefulness of traditional clinical tests and results in replacement with more powerful, accurate, and safer tests. Research can inform the clinician about the use of standardized reliable, and valid outcome assessment tools, the interpretation of the score of such tools, and the selection of the optimal therapeutic approaches. Based on research and application of the evidence, clinicians will be able to determine and document if the expected threshold of treatment is achieved and justify selected intervention(s).

In the following sections, EBP will be discussed along with the need to justify physical therapy as a skilled intervention, the use of outcome measures, the dosing of interventions, and progressing patients.

EVIDENCE-BASED PRACTICE

Clinical Testing

In order to document the use and need of physical therapy services, the clinician will have to report the value of clinical testing and how this is used in the clinical reasoning/decision-making process. Consider using the following aspects of clinical testing in documentation, as this will support the need for physical therapy:

- Reliability of a test
- Validity of a test, including:
  - Specificity/sensitivity of a test
  - Likelihood ratios (usefulness) of a test

Realizing the use of clinical diagnostic tests can never provide complete certainty of a clinical diagnosis or provide complete certainty that a specific condition is present is an important consideration for clinicians. However, clinical tests can be used to estimate the probability that the suspected condition or dysfunction might be present in the patient. In order to increase this probability and reach treatment threshold, use only those tests that have been demonstrated to be very accurate in doing so. Reporting both the validity and reliability in your documentation is recommended. *Reliability* of a test identifies the ability of a test to get the same outcome upon repeated testing of the same patient and other patient groups. *Validity* is the ability of a test to measure what it purported to measure. When a clinical diagnostic test is both valid and reliable, it can be used to accurately assess the presence or absence of a specific condition, and this will support the justification for physical therapy intervention.

Sensitivity and Specificity

When further analyzing the clinical importance of a test, it can be expressed with either the sensitivity or specificity of the test. The *sensitivity* of a clinical test is the ability of the test to identify the presence of a condition when it is actually present. Based on this, use tests that have known high sensitivity to rule out the presence of a condition with a negative test.

Example: The upper limb tension test

Subjects: Patients with suspected cervical radiculopathy. Sensitivity of this test is 0.97 (or 97%); therefore, a negative test is a good indicator of a high probability to rule OUT the condition.

The *specificity* of a clinical test is the ability of that test to identify when a condition is actually not present (true negative outcome). Using a test with high specificity, a positive test will identify those patients who actually have the condition.

Example: The use of the Spurling test

Subjects: Patients with suspected cervical radiculopathy. Specificity of this test is between 0.86 and 0.95 (or 86% to 95%) and a fairly low sensitivity; therefore, a positive test could be used to rule IN the condition; however, a negative test CANNOT be used to rule out the condition.

Likelihood Ratio:

Another statistic often used and reported to predict the usefulness of a test is the likelihood ratio.

Likelihood Ratio

The likelihood ratio statistic is used to determine the post-test probability of a condition being present or absent. A positive likelihood ratio indicates an increase in post-test probability for the presence of a particular condition or dysfunction; likewise, a negative likelihood ratio increases the post-test probability that a condition or dysfunction is absent.

POSITIVE LIKELIHOOD RATIO	NEGATIVE LIKELIHOOD RATIO	USEFULNESS OF THE TEST
>10	<0.1	Generate large and often conclusive shifts in probability
5 to 10	0.1 to 0.2	Generate a moderate shift in probability
2 to 5	0.2 to 0.5	Generate a small but sometimes important shift in probability
1 to 2	0.5 to 1.0	Small and rarely important change in probability

Skilled Service

Each clinician assumes the responsibility to demonstrate and document the need for physical therapy interventions and justification for (ongoing) treatment using the evidence-based model. The key aspect of this justification for physical therapy skilled service is that the service should be, and can only be, provided safely and effectively by the physical therapist or physical therapy assistants. This would be based on the unique skills and knowledge physical therapy professionals provide within the patient/client management.physical therapy professionals provide within the patient/client management. The following description of skilled services comes directly from the Centers for Medicare & Medicaid Services (CMS) Publication 100-02 Medicare Benefit Policy Manual Chapter 15[3] and defines clearly what skilled service is:

> *Services must not only be provided by the qualified professional or qualified personnel, but they must require, for example, the expertise, knowledge, clinical judgment, decision making and abilities of a therapist that assistants, qualified personnel, caretakers or the patient cannot provide independently.*[3]

Within the CMS's definition of skilled service, the physical therapist cannot just supervise care, but must actually document that they applied the skills of a therapist. This active participation in the patient's treatment should be documented during each progress report period. The CMS Publication 100-02 Medicare Benefit Policy Manual Chapter 15 provides the following description:

> *In addition, a therapist's skills may be documented, for example, by the clinician's descriptions of their skilled treatment, the changes made to the treatment due to a clinician's assessment of the patient's needs on a particular treatment day or changes due to progress the clinician judged sufficient to modify the treatment toward the next more complex or difficult task.*[3]

As clinicians engage in patient care, they have to keep in mind the fact that when care is delivered by a physical therapist or physical therapist assistant, this does not make it a skilled service. The CMS Publication 100-02 Medicare Benefit Policy Manual Chapter 15 provides the following guidance:

> *If a service can be self-administered or safely and effectively furnished by an unskilled person, without the direct or general supervision, as applicable, of a therapist, the service cannot be regarded as a skilled therapy service even though a therapist actually furnishes the service.*[3]

As part of the EBP model, the clinician has several opportunities to document that services provided are skilled services and are necessary to progress the patient toward better functioning, including but not limited to:

- Appropriate initial evaluation and examination procedures.
- Progress assessments, and patient re-evaluation of functioning.
- Establishment of treatment goals specific to the patient's disability or dysfunction to specifically address each problem identified in the initial or follow-up assessments.
- Design of a plan of care addressing the patient's dysfunction or disorder. This will include what interventional procedures will be used to meet the goals. The plan of care will need to lay out the frequency and intensity of treatment.
- Continued assessment and analysis during implementation of the services at regular intervals.
- Patient-specific instructions that will help them manage the condition or provide compensatory skills.
- The reason and selection of devices to replace or augment a function.
- Training of patient and family to augment physical therapy treatment.
- Training of staff and family should be ongoing throughout treatment and instructions modified intermittently as the patient's status changes.

Necessary Service

In order for physical therapy services to be necessary and reasonable, certain criteria have to be met and documented. Just because services are provided by a physical therapist does not make them necessary. The CMS manual describes this as follows:[3]

> *Services shall be considered under accepted standards of medical practice to be a specific and effective treatment for the patient's condition. Acceptable practices for therapy services are found in: Medicare manuals (such as this manual and Publications 100-03 and 100-04), Contractors Local Coverage Determinations (LCDs), and National Coverage Determinations (NCDs):*
>
> *The services shall be of such a level of complexity and sophistication or the condition of the patient shall be such that the services required can be safely and effectively performed only by a therapist or under the supervision of a therapist. Services that do not require the performance or supervision of a therapist are not skilled and are not considered reasonable or necessary therapy services, even if they are performed or supervised by a qualified professional. Medicare coverage does not turn on the presence or absence of a beneficiary's potential for improvement from the therapy, but rather on the beneficiary's need for skilled care.*[4]

Treatment Dosing

One of the biggest challenges faced clinically is to determine and justify the type of intervention and dosing of this intervention. Treatment parameters being used for patient management must be clearly identified and documented. The CMS Publication 100-02 Medicare Benefit Policy Manual Chapter 15 provides the following insight:

> *Services are of appropriate type, frequency, intensity and duration for the individual needs of the patient. Documentation should establish the variables that influence the patient's condition, especially those factors that influence the clinician's decision to provide more services than are typical for the individual's condition.*[3]

In order to do this, the clinician can use research evidence to support the individual patient treatment plan and dosing. There have been an increasing number of validated clinical prediction rules and clinical practice guidelines published to support the practitioner's decisions. These have facilitated the justification of treatment variables within the patient management model. CMS provides this development as evidenced by the following statement within the Medicare Benefit Policy Manual Chapter 15:

> *Clinicians and contractors shall determine typical services using published professional literature and professional guidelines. The fact that services are typically billed is not necessarily evidence that the services are typically appropriate. Services that exceed those typically billed should be carefully documented to justify their necessity, but are payable if the individual patient benefits from medically necessary service.*[3]

Outcome Measures

As part of the EBP model, the clinician will have to determine if treatment is warranted and assure that continued intervention is indicated. In order to do so, both subjective and objective measures can be used in clinical practice. *Outcome measures* provide the clinician with a baseline to which either progression or regression can be demonstrated. The CMS Medicare Benefit Policy Manual Chapter 15 provides the following description of outcome measures:

> *The use of scientific evidence, obtained from professional literature, and sequential measurements of the patient's condition during treatment is encouraged to support the potential for continued improvement that may justify the patients need for rehabilitative therapy or the patient's need for maintenance therapy.*[3]

Outcomes measures can be particularly useful in situations in which the optimal treatment outcome will not be achieved due to underlying conditions or situations beyond the normal physiology. This is often referred to as the identification of "yellow flags." They typically are psychological, social, and environmental risk factors that may prolong disability or result in pain becoming more chronic in nature.

Yellow flags have often been summarized as psychological in nature and are conditions such anxiety, depression, post-traumatic stress disorder, drug and/or alcohol abuse, and major personality disorders. Although physical therapists are not trained to diagnose these conditions, it is their clinical responsibility to identify and document factors that could lead to the development of chronic disability and chronic pain and therefore prevent normal expected treatment outcomes. The presence of these conditions does not prevent physical therapy intervention, but a concurrent referral should be made to address the possible issues that will prevent normal recovery.

Screening for these yellow flags via history taking has low sensitivity and predictive value for identifying distressed patients; thus, formal screening of some sort, such as with a questionnaire or outcome tool, is recommended. If yellow flags have been identified during the evaluation process, the clinician will have to determine and document the best treatment approach to maximize clinical outcomes.

Examples of the yellow flags one might want to identify and document include the following:

- Clinical depression
- Fear of movement or fear working will increase injury risk or pain
- Poor expectations for treatment outcome
- Worries, anxiety, general fear
- Belief they will never go back to work
- Reliance on passive pain management strategies
- Poor family support
- Litigation for injury

As the CMS description of outcome measures indicates, they can provide guidance in determining and documenting the effectiveness and appropriateness of (ongoing) clinical interventions. Treatment changes that reflect the smallest change in score that are beyond simple chance are reflected in the minimal detectable change (MDC) value of that particular outcome tool. Although the MDC relates to research evidence, it might not directly reflect any change that could be considered clinically meaningful to the patient. In order to capture this change, the minimal clinical important difference (MCID) could be measured and reported. This is a value that should reflect the patient's perception of change that is considered beneficial. In the literature there are various reports on MCID values. Some common MCID values used are shown in Table 9-1.

The MCID and the MDC values might not always be available for the outcome measure used clinically. Another way to document and report change would be to look at the effect size of treatment based on the outcome scores. This should allow the clinician to make a judgment and directly document change as a result of the actual clinical intervention. The effect size is a percentage of change in outcome score over a given time and can be easily calculated with the following calculation: Effect size calculation = Change score / initial score × 100%.

Sample Effect Size Calculation:
Initial visit Visual Analogue Scale (VAS) score is 55 mm, following 6 treatments VAS score is 15 mm; the change in VAS score is 40 mm, which reflects an effect size of about 72% (40 / 55 × 100%).

The CMS manual provides additional support for the use of outcome measures to justify clinical initial and ongoing intervention:

> *Therefore, evaluation, re-evaluation and assessment documented in the Progress Report should describe objective measurements which, when compared, show improvements*

Table 9-1 MCID values

OUTCOME TOOL	MCID VALUE REPORTED IN THE LITERATURE
Oswestry Disability Questionnaire	10 points
NDI (nonradicular)	5 points
VAS for acute pain	3 cm
Lower Extremity Functional Score	9 points
Patient-Specific Functional Scale	2 points
VAS for back pain	1.8 cm

in function, decrease in severity or rationalization for an optimistic outlook to justify continued treatment. Improvement is evidenced by successive objective measurements whenever possible.... If an individual's expected rehabilitation potential is insignificant in relation to the extent and duration of therapy services required to achieve such potential, rehabilitative therapy is not reasonable and necessary.[3]

PROGRESS INTO MAINTENANCE

If the patient has reached a point in which the therapist is no longer able to document a significant change in condition, or does not expect such change, or or establishment of a maintenance program is desired, the therapist will have to document the need for this. The following two examples from the CMS Medicare Benefit Policy Manual Chapter 15 demonstrate demonstrate the development of a justified maintenance program:

EXAMPLE 1: A patient with Parkinson's disease is nearing the end of a rehabilitative physical therapy program and requires the services of a therapist during the last week(s) of treatment to determine what type of exercises will contribute the most to maintain function or to prevent or slow further deterioration of the patient's present functional level following cessation of treatment. In such situations, the establishment of a maintenance program appropriate to the capacity and tolerance of the patient by the qualified therapist, the instruction of the patient or family members in carrying out the program, and such reassessments and/or reevaluations as may be required may constitute covered therapy because of the need for the skills of a qualified therapist.[3]

EXAMPLE 2: A patient with multiple sclerosis needs a maintenance program to slow or prevent deterioration in communication ability caused by the medical condition. Therapy services from a qualified speech-language pathologist may be covered to establish a maintenance program even though the patient's current medical condition does not yet justify the need for individual skilled therapy sessions. Evaluation, establishment of the program, and training the family or support personnel may require the skills of a therapist and would be covered. NOTE: In this example, the skills of a therapist are not required to actually carry out the maintenance program services and, as a result, are not covered.[3]

The key aspect of maintenance therapy is that the therapist can justify the need of skilled physical therapy service and that you can support the justification and reasoning even if services are more extensive than is typical for the condition treated. CMS identifies that no separate statement will be required if your documentation justifies treatment.

CONCLUSION: EVIDENCE-BASED PRACTICE

The current healthcare environment is characterized by escalating costs, emphasis on efficiency and effectiveness, and value based care and documentation. It is the responsibility of physical therapists to justify patient/client management based on the most recent, reliable and valid evidence. Therefore, the choice of validated, appropriate tests and measures based on patient presentation and clinical practice guidelines, is a viable approach for establishing an effective plan of care. This is the initial step in the clinical decision making process. Once the treatment diagnosis is determined, the clinician can employ evidence available to determine specific intervention approaches or justify the medical necessity for skilled physical therapy services. By using tests and measures that can be used at intervals throughout a length of stay, patient progress can be objectively measured. Applying clinical practice guidelines, if available, insures that a treatment approach is evidence-based.

REVIEW QUESTIONS

1. How does evidence-based practice affect how a patient is treated?
2. How does clinical expertise affect how to treat a patient?
3. What does reliability of test tell?
4. What does validity of a test tell?
5. Define sensitivity of the test.
6. Define specificity of the test.
7. What does a positive or negative likelihood ratio indicate?
8. Differentiate between skilled and nonskilled service.
9. What do outcome measures provide to the clinician?

REFERENCES

1. *Evidence-Based Practice and Research*. American Physical Therapy Association; Alexandria, VA. Available at https://www.apta.org/patient-care/evidence-based-practice-resources/components-of-evidence-based-practice. Accessed July 25, 2020.
2. Jette DU, Bacon K, Batty C, et al. Evidence-based practice: beliefs, attitudes, knowledge, and behaviors of physical therapists. *Phys Ther*. 2003;83(9):786-805.
3. *Medicare Benefit Policy Manual Chapter 15—Covered Medical and Other Health Services*. Centers of Medicare & Medicaid Services; Baltimore, MD. Available at https://www.cms.gov/Regulations-and-Guidance/Guidance/Manuals/Downloads/bp102c15.pdf. Accessed July 20, 2020.
4. *Medicare Coverage* Database (MCD). Centers of Medicare & Medicaid Services; Baltimore, MD. Available at http://www.cms.hhs.gov/mcd. Accessed July 20, 2020.

ADDITIONAL RESOURCES

Bury TJ, Mead JM. *Evidence-Based Healthcare: A Practical Guide for Therapists*. Oxford: Butterworth Heinemann; 1998.

Dean E. Physical therapy in the 21st century (Part II): evidence-based practice within the context of evidence-informed practice. *Physiother Theory Pract*. 2009;25(5-6):354-368.

Guyatt G, Evidence Based Medicine Working Group. Evidence-based medicine: A new approach to teaching the practice of medicine. *JAMA*. 1992;268(17):2420-2425.

Guyatt GH, Haynes RB, Jaeschke RZ, et al. Users' guides to the medical literature: XXV. Evidence-based medicine: principles for applying the users' guides to patient care. Evidence-Based Medicine Working Group. *JAMA*. 2000;284(10):1290-1296.

Haynes B, Haines A. Barriers and bridges to evidence based clinical practice. *BMJ*. 1998;317(7153):273-276.

Hammell KW, Carpenter C. *Qualitative Research in Evidence-Based Rehabilitation*. Edinburgh: Churchill Livingstone; 2004.

Herbert R, Jamtvedt G, Mead J, Hagen KB. *Practical Evidence-Based Physiotherapy*. 2nd ed. Edinburgh: Elsevier Butterworth Heinemann; 2012.

Herbert RD, Sherrington C, Maher C, Moseley AM. Evidence-based practice: Imperfect but necessary. *Physiother Theory Pract*. 2001;17(3):201-211.

Koes BW. Now is the time for evidence based physiotherapy. *Physiother Res Int*. 1997;2(2):iv-v.

Maher C, Moseley A, Sherrington C, Herbert R. Core journals of evidence-based physiotherapy practice. *Physiother Theory Pract*. 2001;17(3):143-151.

Maher CG, Sherrington C, Elkins M, Herbert RD, Moseley AM. Challenges for evidence-based physical therapy: Accessing and interpreting high-quality evidence on therapy. *Phys Ther*. 2004;84(7):644-654.

Manske R, Lehecka B. Evidence-based medicine/practice in sports physical therapy. *Int J Sports Phys Ther*. 2012;7(5):461-473.

Richter R, Austin T. Using MeSH to enhance PubMed search strategies for evidence-based practice in physical therapy. *Phys Ther*. 2012;92(1):124-132.

Sackett DL, Rosenberg WM, Gray JA, Haynes RB, Richardson WS. Evidence based medicine: What it is and what it isn't. *BMJ*. 1996;312(7023):71-72.

Sherrington C, Moseley A, Herbert R. Guest editorial. *Physiother Theory Pract*. 2001;17(3):125-126.

Townsend A, Cox SM, Li LC. Qualitative research ethics: Enhancing evidence-based practice in physical therapy. *Phys Ther*. 2010;90(4):615-628.

10 Clinical Decision-Making

OBJECTIVES

Following completion of this chapter, the reader will be able to:

- Define clinical reasoning/clinical decision-making.
- Differentiate the processes used by novice and expert clinicians to make clinical decisions.
- Describe how the elements of evidenced-based practice are used in clinical decision-making.
- Define decision support in electronic medical records and how it is used in clinical decision-making.
- Describe how the patient/client management model is used to guide clinical decision-making.
- Explain the purpose of functional outcome measures, how to choose an appropriate measure, and how they can be used to inform decision-making.
- Describe the elements of clinical decision-making that should be included in documentation.

CLINICAL DECISION-MAKING

Clinical problem solving (CPS), clinical reasoning (CR), and clinical decision making (CDM) and are interconnected terms[1] describing the cognitive process through which physical therapists approach patient care. CDM and CR are important in effective patient and client management to develop an organized process for evaluation and intervention planning. CR is a process whereby knowledge and experience are applied in considering multiple possibilities to achieve the desired goals, while considering the patient's situation.[2] The process involves interacting with patients and others to develop mutually agreed-upon goals, establish prognoses, and develop an appropriate plan of care.[3] CDM is the outcome of the CR process and guides the physical therapist to effectively manage their patients and clients throughout the course of service.[4] Effective CDM is the hallmark of an autonomous professional.[5] A key component of effective documentation is to communicate both the CR and CDM processes.

Reflection will help improve clinical decision-making. Schon describes 3 areas of reflection.[6]

1. Reflection on-action: following an event and thinking back upon the encounter
2. Reflection in-action: during the event making changes in behavior in response to the situation.
3. Reflection for-action: making changes for the future based upon previous.

NOVICE VERSUS EXPERT CLINICAL REASONING AND CLINICAL DECISION-MAKING

Early research into CPS processes originated out of medical education and focused on the processes used by novice clinicians.[1] The hypothetical deductive reasoning process involves collecting a multitude of data from the patient and formulating hypotheses based on this available data. The clinician subsequently tests these hypotheses against prior and new data and formulates the most likely solution to the clinical problem. This process has also been labeled backward reasoning and is especially useful for novice clinicians, as it provides a structured problem-solving approach and requires the clinician to examine the breadth of the data, thereby decreasing errors of omission.

Research into expert reasoning indicates that experts, when solving uncomplicated problems in their field of expertise, do not employ a hypothetical-deductive approach, but instead use rapid pattern recognition approaches, also referred to as forward reasoning.[1] These patterns are based on prior similar clinical experiences that these clinicians have encountered. However, when these experts encounter unfamiliar or complex problems, they will revert back to hypothetical deductive reasoning modes.

Principles of the Dreyfus Model of Skill Development Applied to the Development of a Physician's Competence:[6]

Novice

- Is rule driven
- Uses analytic reasoning and rules to link cause and effect
- Has little ability to filter or prioritize information, so synthesis is difficult at best and the big picture is elusive

Advanced beginner

- Is able to sort through rules and information to decide what is relevant on the basis of past experience
- Uses both analytic reasoning and pattern recognition to solve problems
- Is able to abstract from concrete and specific information to more general aspects of a problem

Competent

- Emotional buy-in allows the learner to feel an appropriate level of responsibility
- More expansive experience tips the balance in clinical reasoning from methodical and analytic to more readily identifiable pattern recognition of common clinical problem presentations
- Sees the big picture
- Complex or uncommon problems still require reliance on analytic reasoning

Proficient

- Breadth of past experience allows one to rely on pattern recognition of illness presentation such that clinical problem solving seems intuitive
- Still needs to fall back to methodical and analytic reasoning for managing problems because exhaustive number of permutations and responses to management have provided less experience in this regard than in illness recognition
- Is comfortable with evolving situations; able to extrapolate from a known situation to an unknown situation (capable)
- Can live with ambiguity

Expert

- Thought, feeling, and action align into intuitive problem recognition and intuitive situational responses and management
- Is open to notice the unexpected
- Is clever
- Is perceptive in discriminating features that do not fit a recognizable pattern

Master

- Exercises practical wisdom
- Goes beyond the big picture and sees a bigger picture of the culture and context of each situation
- Has a deep level of commitment to the work
- Has great concern for right and wrong decisions; this fosters emotional engagement
- Is intensely motivated by emotional engagement to pursue ongoing learning and improvement
- Reflects in, on, and for action

DOCUMENTING CLINICAL DECISION-MAKING AND EVIDENCE-BASED PRACTICE

As described in Chapter 9, evidence-based practice (EBP) is the use of critically appraised and scientifically supported evidence in the delivery of quality care to the patient. Integrating the best available evidence, clinician experience, and patient values and preferences is a critical part of the CR process and is a necessary step toward good clinical decisions. Effective patient care and client service requires integrating the patient and client into the decision-making process. Effective documentation will illustrate how the elements of EBP were included in the decision-making process.

A useful tool to document the CR/CDM process is the Physical Therapy Clinical Reasoning and Reflection Tool (PT-CRT).[7-9] The PT-CRT has 9 Reflection Points: (Questions)

I. Initial Data Gathering/Interview
II. Generation of Initial Hypothesis
III. Examination
IV. Evaluation
V. Plan of Care
VI. Interventions
VII. Reexamination

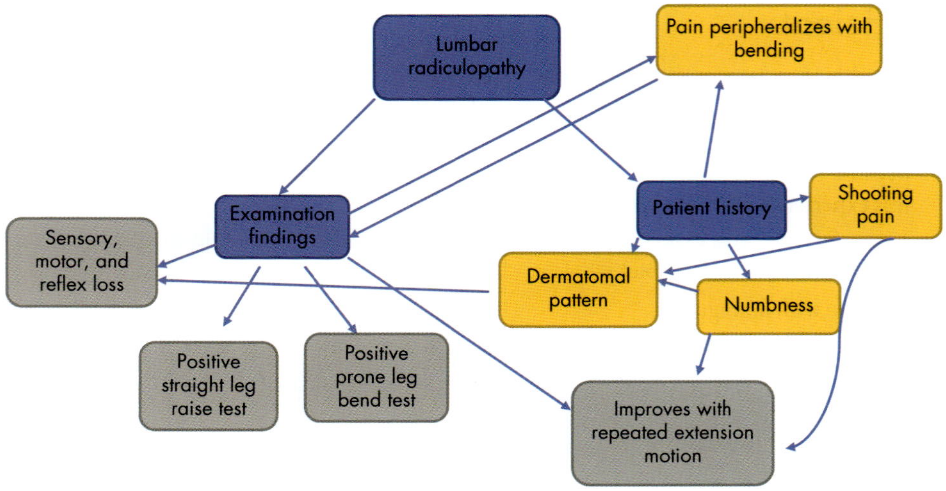

Figure 10-1. Concept map example.

VIII. Outcomes

IX. Mentor Feedback

Clinicians and students can use this tool to document their CDM process within the framework of the International Classification of Functioning, Disability and Health (ICF) model and the Patient and Client Management Model from the American Physical Therapy Association (APTA) *Guide to Physical Therapist Practice*,[10] and this tool provides a mechanism for clinician self-reflection. PT-CRT guides the clinician stepwise through the process of CR, starting with the initial data gathering/interview and progressing to the generation of initial hypotheses, examination, evaluation, plan of care, interventions, re-examination, and outcomes.

The patient management model described in the *Guide to Physical Therapist Practice*[10] can be used as a framework for CDM. In this model, appropriate categories are used as headings in which information can be included, consistent with *Guide* categories such as the systems and subcategories such as aerobic capacity, assistive and adaptive devices, sensory integrity, etc.

Concept mapping can be another useful tool to document the CDM process to differentiate between a good guess and a logical thoughtful problem-solving approach. Concept mapping involves creating a graphic representation of relationships between ideas presented using cells connected by lines or arrows, requiring learners to use active information processes in order to organize reasoning in a graphic format.[11,12] Research has shown that this technique can successfully promote CR and foster meaningful learning.[12] One drawback of this technique is the likely high cognitive load that CPS may impose on the learner, and alternative approaches, such as studying completed concept maps, and especially completing partially completed concept maps, may be useful approaches to learning CDM.[12] Figure 10-1 gives a simplified example of a concept map.

ELECTRONIC MEDICAL RECORDS AND CLINICAL DECISION SUPPORT

The electronic medical record (EMR) has been described in Chapter 4. One aspect of the EMR discussed in Chapter 4 was the term meaningful use. Many EMRs contain clinical decision support (CDS) mechanisms as an example of meaningful use. These CDS mechanisms can be defined as elements designed to assist health professionals with decision-making tasks, linking health observations (signs and symptoms) with health knowledge (best practices and current research) to influence choices made by clinicians to improve care. According to the Agency for Healthcare Research and Quality, the purpose of CDS in the EMR is to help "inform decisions about a patient's care. Clinical decision support tools and systems help clinicians by taking some routine tasks, warning of potential problems, or providing suggestions for the clinical team and patient to consider."[13]

Current iterations of EMRs assist the physical therapist with CDM by prompting the clinician to conduct specific tests, complete and enter an outcome measure score, refer to a clinical practice guideline, or alert the clinician to avoid making an error.

CDS systems may provide provider support based on a patient's diagnosis. In the context of physical therapy practice, someone may have a diagnosis of "History of Falling, Z91.81." One component of a complete exam would be to conduct a test to measure their balance. The EMR with CDS would prompt the user to choose a test to perform (i.e., Berg Balance Scale, Dynamic Gait Index, etc.) and then enter the score in the appropriate place in the EMR. The exact extent and nature of the CDS are dependent on the particular EMR and each clinical facility's policies.

FUNCTIONAL OUTCOME MEASURES

Outcome measures are used to track a patient's improvement and treatment effectiveness, but in some cases, can also be used to guide treatment focus or predict prognosis. Outcome measure differ from many objective measurements taken by physical therapists. For example, a manual muscle test (MMT) will provide an objective measurement of the isolated muscle strength (isometric) but it does not measure the functional ability of the patient to climb stairs. Goniometry will provide information on shoulder range of motion, but it does not provide information on functional reaching that incorporate balance, stability and strength. Relevant outcome measures are selected during the initial examination and evaluation process based on the patient's health condition and region of impairments, as well as the type of impairments and functional difficulties. Outcome measures need to match the goals and interventions. Using validated outcome measures allows the therapist to compare results to normative data and provide a mechanism for determining the extent of impairments, activity limitations, or participation restrictions. Selecting the most appropriate OM enhances clinical practice by (1) identifying and quantifying body function and structure limitations; (2) formulating the evaluation, diagnosis, and prognosis; (3) informing the plan of care; and (4) helping to evaluate the success of physical therapy interventions.[15] The interpretation of measures also allows the therapist to use the results to set goals and informs the choice of other examination techniques. Some outcome measures are also useful predictors of prognosis or for identifying risk of injury, such as falls. Outcome measures are used to evaluate change. It is important to consider the minimal detectable change (MDC) and minimal clinically important difference (MCID). The MDC is considered to be the minimal amount of change that is not likely to be due to error in measurement. See Chapter 9 for more information on MDC and MCID. Other tools provide additional information about psychological status, which can help guide the type of motivational or psychologically informed approaches to prescribing exercises. The number of available functional outcome measures (both self-reported and objective) has dramatically increased, and there are multiple outcome measures for specific diagnoses, patient populations, and regions.[13,16]

Specific functional deficits can be linked with impairments and tracked across treatment sessions, and this helps with the CR associated with treatment choice. Individual rating scores can be used to provide treatment goals and assist with communicating the relevance of treatment to the patient. Using functional outcome measures over the course of rehabilitation is a valid and reliable method of measuring progress over time. Functional measures are being mandated by both public and private payers at increasing rates. Using appropriate outcomes measures consistently, and applying the requisite clinical judgment to interpret them, is essential in order to successfully comply with insurance reporting requirements. Although insurance requirements are an important element of providing care, the primary justification

Author's Note

Factors to Consider When Selecting Outcome Measures for Clinical Practice[14]
What to measure: Body function/structure, activity, participation

Purpose of measure:
- Discriminative
- Predictive
- Evaluative

Type of measure:
- Disease-specific or generic
- Self-report or performance-based

Patient and clinic factors:
- Patient recovery and ability
- Patient goals
- Clinic requirements

Psychometric factors:
- Reliability
- Validity
- Diagnostic accuracy
- Responsiveness

Feasibility:
- Time, space, and equipment
- Training required
- Cost
- Respondent burden
- Culture and language
- Proprietary issue

for functional measures is to inform decision-making and progression of management for optimal care. At the end of the episode of care, the physical therapist measures the global outcomes of the services provided by characterizing or quantifying the impact of the physical therapist intervention on any or all of the following domains, based on suitability for and the circumstances of the patient or client:[17]

1. Pathology or health condition
2. Impairments in body functions and structures
3. Activity limitations
4. Participation restrictions
5. Risk reduction/prevention
6. Health, wellness, and fitness
7. Societal resources
8. Patient or client satisfaction

Figure 10-2 outlines a process for selecting a functional outcome measure and using that measure to evaluate intervention effectiveness and progression toward goals.

ACTIVITY

Given this information regarding Mrs. Alexa, answer the questions after the case.

S: Mrs. Alexa's chief complaint today is that she still tires easily and doesn't have much energy. She is complaining of a bit of a dry mouth. She reports she was walking with a walker

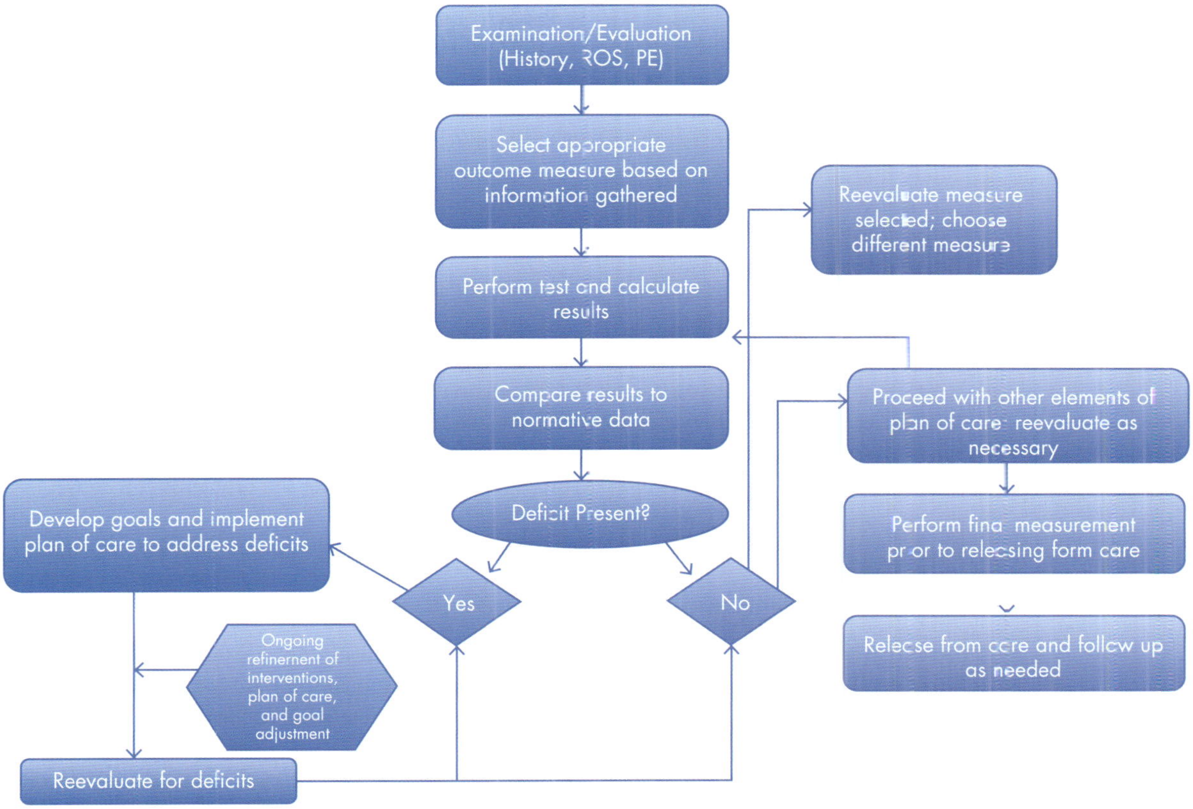

Figure 10-2. Establishing and progressing to goals. (Reproduced, with permission, from Dunleavy K, McGehee W. Evaluation for adjustment of exercise performance and outcomes. In: Dunleavy K, Slowak A, eds. *Therapeutic Exercise Prescription*. St. Louis, MO: Elsevier; 2019.)

with wheels in the hospital the last 2 days she was there but not too much before then. She is very hopeful she can get off of her oxygen soon. She lives with her husband, who is her primary caregiver. They live in a duplex with no stairs inside. It does have a small step to enter the house. Her daughter and son-in-law live nearby and look in on them frequently but don't stay long. She wishes they were able to do more. She is a retired homemaker, been married 50 years, and has three children.

PMH: COPD, CHF, HTN, A-Fib, GERD, obstructive sleep apnea, s/p hysterectomy 1984, s/p cholecystectomy-1990, diverticulitis, depression

Medications: Albuterol nebulizer QID, digoxin, baby aspirin, warfarin, omeprozole, enalapril, furosemide, naproxen, zolpidem, K-tab, levothyroxine, tramadol

O: Mrs. Alexa is alert and oriented to person, place, and time. She is somewhat confused and sometimes doesn't answer your question the first time you ask it. She is sitting in a wheelchair that was used to bring her from her room to the PT department. She is napping in the chair when you get over to her to begin your examination and evaluation. She follows commands intermittently but is very cooperative.

Vital Signs: BP: 130/82; HR: 77, RR: 20 at rest. She is on 2L of O_2 via nasal cannula (note the physician has written that this can be increased to 4L with exercise).

Edema: 2+ pitting edema in bilateral lower extremities distally

ROM: Within functional limits

MMT: 3+/5 throughout except hip extension and hip abduction bilaterally 2+/5, ankle dorsiflexion 3/5.

Transfers: Moderate assist x 2 for sit to stand to sit from her wheelchair. Moderate assist x 1 for supine to sit to supine. She mostly needs help moving her legs up and down off the mat table.

Gait: Moderate assist x 1 with wheeled walker 300 feet before needing to rest. After 5-minute rest she is able to go another 300 feet. Her 6-minute walk test is 600 feet.

Balance: Berg Balance Scale score is 35

Following the examination of a patient, the physical therapist must decide during their evaluation if the patient is appropriate to receive continued physical therapy services and what additional disciplines need to be involved in the care of the patient. Based on the information provided here, would it be appropriate for the physical therapist to continue to be involved in the care of Mrs. Alexa? Besides physicians and nursing, what additional professionals would you recommend be consulted in this case?

Pick two additional outcome measures that would be appropriate to use with Mrs. Alexa and describe why you chose them.

List at least five things that are the most important for you to know about Mrs. Alexa and her current status that you don't know, based on the information you have. Describe the tests or measures you would perform or what you would do to gather that information.

Develop a list of at least five problems (in priority order) that you think you need to address in Mrs. Alexa's plan of care and provide justification for the problems you chose.

SUMMARY

Clinical reasoning and clinical decision-making are critical elements in evidence based physical therapy management. Identification of appropriate tests and measures that include outcome assessment using tools with normative data, lead to appropriate goal development and effective plans of care. Outcome measures can provide motivation to the patient, progress the patient has made, and justify the need for physical therapy services. By re-assessing progress over the course of patient's length of stay (LOS) in any setting using the appropriate outcome measures, determination can be made of the efficacy of treatment, patient response to treatment, functional improvement, and justification of medical necessity.

REVIEW QUESTIONS

1. Define clinical reasoning and clinical decision-making.
2. Differentiate the processes used by novice and expert clinicians to make clinical decisions.
3. Describe how the elements of evidence-based practice are used in clinical decision-making.
4. Define decision support in electronic medical records and how it is used in clinical decision-making.
5. Describe how the patient management model is used to guide clinical decision-making.
6. Discuss the purpose of functional outcome measures, how to choose an appropriate measure, and how they can be used to inform decision-making.
7. Describe the elements of clinical decision-making that should be included in documentation.
8. Generate documentation, using the required elements and tools, that describes clinical decision-making.

Additional Critical Decision-Making Question[9]

1. Who needs treatment and why?
2. What are the expected outcomes of intervention?
3. How should outcomes be measured and documented?
4. What intervention, instructions, services, and number of visits are necessary to meet these outcomes?
5. How should the patient and caregivers be included in the decision-making process?
6. How should the success of the intervention and cost-effectiveness be evaluated?
7. Are referrals needed for other health care services and screenings?

REFERENCES

1. Musolino GM, Jensen GM. *Clinical Reasoning and Decision-Making in Physical Therapy*. Thorofare, NJ: Slack; 2020.
2. Noll E, Key A, Jensen G. Clinical reasoning of an experienced physiotherapist: Insight into clinician decision-making regarding low back pain. *Physiother Res Int*. 2001;6(1):40-51.
3. Edwards I, Jones M, Carr J, Braunack-Mayer A, Jensen GM. Clinical reasoning strategies in physical therapy. *Phys Ther*. 2004;84(4):312-330, discussion 331-335.
4. O'Sullivan SB, Schmitz TJ, Fulk GD. *Physical Rehabilitation*. 7th ed. Philadelphia, PA: FA Davis; 2019.
5. Higgs J, Jones M. *Clinical Reasoning in the Health Professions*. 4th ed. Boston, MA: Butterworth Heinemann; 2018.
6. Schon DA. *The Reflective Practitioner*. Basic Books, 1984. ISBN 0465068782.
7. Carraccio CL, Benson BJ, Nixon J, Derstine PL. From the educational bench to the clinical bedside. translating the Dreyfus Development Model to the learning of clinical skills. *Academic Medicine*. 2008 August;83(8):761-7.
8. Nixon-Cave K, Atkinson H. Chapter 10: The clinical reasoning and reflection tool: Clinical application for clinical decision making. In: Musolino GM, Jensen GM, eds. *Clinical Reasoning and Decision-Making in Physical Therapy*. Thorofare, NJ: Slack; 2020.
9. Atkinson HL, Nixon-Cave K. A tool for clinical reasoning and reflection using the International Classification of Functioning, Disability and Health (ICF) Framework and Patient Management Model. *Phys Ther*. 2011;91:416-30.
10. *Guide to Physical Therapist Practice*, 3.0 edition. American Physical Therapy Association. Alexandria, VA. Available at http://guidetoptpractice.apta.org/content/current. Accessed August 1, 2020. ISBN: 978-1-931369-85-5. doi:10.2522/ptguide3.0_978-1-931369-85-5.
11. Beissner KL. Use of concept mapping to improve problem solving. *J Phys Ther Educ*. 1992;6(1):22-27.
12. Montpetit-Tourangeau K, Dyer JO, Hudon A, et al. Fostering clinical reasoning in physiotherapy: Comparing the effects of concept map study and concept map completion after example study in novice and advanced learners. *BMC Med Educ*. 2017;17:238. doi:10.1186/s12909-017-1076-z.
13. *Evidence Based Decision Making*. Agency for Healthcare Research and Quality. Available at https://www.ahrq.gov/prevention/chronic-care/decision/index.html. Accessed July 20, 2020.
14. Hammel J, Baum CM. Module 2: Using Outcomes in Clinic Assessment and Intervention Planning. National Institute on Disability and Rehabilitation Research. 2013. Available at https://www.sralab.org/sites/default/files/downloads/2018-02/Clinician%20Module%202%20PPT%20Version.pdf. Accessed August 1 2020.
15. Potter K, Fulk GD, Salem Y, Sullivan J. COutcome measures in neurological physical therapy practice: part I. Making sound decisions. *J Neurol Phys Ther*. 2011;35(2):57-64. doi:10.1097/NPT.0b013e318219a51ahttps://pubmed.ncbi.nlm.nih.gov/21934360/
16. Cleland JA, Koppenhaver S, Su J. *Netter's Orthopaedic Clinical Examination: An Evidence-based Approach*. 3rd ed. St Louis, MO: Elsevier; 2015.
17. *Measurement and Outcomes*. Guide to Physical Therapist Practice. American Physical Therapy Association, Alexandria, VA Available at http://guidetoptpractice.apta.org/content/1/SEC3.body#C34. Accessed August 5, 2020.
18. Magee DJ, Manske RC. *Orthopaedic Physical Assessment*. 7th ed. St Louis, MO: Saunders Elsevier; 2020.

11 Legal Issues in the Medical Record

OBJECTIVES

Following completion of this chapter, the reader will be able to:

- Discuss the need for informed consent and explain the relevance to PT documentation.
- Define what HIPAA is and the relevance to medical records keeping and PT documentation.
- Explain what is authentication in documentation.
- Discuss what are the emerging challenges of protection in electronic or computerized documentation.
- Explain the importance of legibility in the medical record.

INTRODUCTION

"Effective patient care documentation is as important as the delivery of care itself."[1] The process of health information management by healthcare professionals presents challenges and legal responsibilities. In all documentation, physical therapists (PTs) and physical therapist assistants (PTAs) must abide by professional standards, ethical codes, accreditation standards, the employer's standards, and legal requirements in creating a permanent record of patient data.

PTs are responsible for all aspects of patient care. PTAs work under the direction and supervision of a PT and can:[2,3]

- Implement selected components of care and interventions in a competent manner
- Instruct and counsel patients effectively in exercises
- Identify a patient's needs and exhibit compassion, caring, and empathy to individual differences
- Recommend options, courses of action, or modifications in selected treatments ensuring a patient's progress, safety, and comfort
- Apply the latest research related to restoring function, reducing symptom frequency, and preventing injury
- Complete documentation to support the delivery of physical therapy services
- Perform selected data collection and obtain accurate information

- Measure performance and report on a patient's medical record
- Participate in patient status judgments
- Adhere to ethical and legal standards
- Ensure continued competence and updated field knowledge

The PT and PTA are responsible for creating, maintaining, and disclosing patient care medical record information as authorized by the patient or as dictated by law. Legally, the records created serve as the best evidence of patient information obtained and shared, the care rendered, the role of the healthcare provider, and whether the professional and legal standards of care were met or breached. For these reasons, PTs and PTAs who document and collect protected health information (PHI) need to understand medical record/health information laws to ensure that they act responsibly and in compliance with applicable laws and identify when expert legal advice is indicated.

The significance of documenting patient care accurately, comprehensively, concisely, objectively, contemporaneously or within a reasonable time, and legibly (although legibility is now best managed by electronic medical records) cannot be overemphasized. The content of the medical record substantiates billing for reimbursement and the need for present and future physical therapy and medical services. The consequences of altered, incomplete, or nonexistent records can be legally and personally catastrophic. Practical application of risk management (prevention of any type of loss—financial or otherwise) and quality care must include proper documentation. The medical record frequently is the most important document available in defending against or preventing legal actions, including but not limited to personal injury suits, criminal cases, workers' compensation actions, disability determinations, and claims of negligent or improper healthcare (medical malpractice), and it is generally admissible at a trial.[4] It also serves to communicate with others as to the patient's status and progress in therapy.

CHANGING ENVIRONMENT

With respect to the constantly changing healthcare environment and the shift from volume-based care to value-based care, the growth of managed care organizations (MCOs), expanded use of technological advances, trend toward national practitioner and patient data banks, and direct access to physical therapy, permitting primary care provision, therapists are assuming new duties and greater responsibilities in their roles as healthcare providers and in healthcare organization delivery systems.

With the dominance of MCOs imposing arbitrary limitations on care delivery, such as requiring visit authorization, working within the stringent allowances for treatment periods has been a continual challenge for clinicians. As a result, PTs need to be effective advocates for their patients to ensure appropriate approval of treatment and payment. The ability to document defensively is essential, as the contents of the medical record affects payment and could negatively affect defensibility against claims.

Documentation may not solve the dilemma of extending treatment for whom continued treatment has been denied by third-party payers, but proper recording of patient care may validate the need for more treatment while protecting against risk of liability.

THE MEDICAL RECORD AS A BUSINESS AND LEGAL DOCUMENT

The medical record is permanent documentation, whether manual or electronic, of substantive and objective evidence of patient information obtained and medical care rendered by providers when legal wrongdoing is alleged. The record forms a basis from which an expert witness can formulate an opinion as to whether acceptable standards of care were met. It also may provide substantive evidence of work or functional capacity in workers' compensation hearings and other administrative proceedings. The recording of informed consent may serve to protect healthcare providers and organizations by demonstrating evidence that a patient understood the risks and benefits of a procedure and made an informed decision to proceed with or terminate care. Inclusion of patient, family, and caregiver goals for therapy and their participation in the decision-making aspects of care will verify patient or caretaker autonomy. In cases where patients have signed advanced directives, appropriate documentation protects providers who must carry out the directives.

Author's Note

Unless physical therapy services are being provided in a hospital, skilled nursing facility, or through a Medicare-certified home health agency, it is not common practice to have a copy of a patient's Do Not Resuscitate (DNR) directives in the medical record. It is recommended that this be included with patient information on the initial patient's visit in all settings, including outpatient.

Generally, laws, regulations, and standards contain requirements for medical recordation relevant to end-of-life decision-making. The medical record should clearly detail pertinent information concerning the patient's decision and plan prior to the physician's order to withdraw or forego life-sustaining treatment.

Healthcare is a multitrillion-dollar industry. The patient care record is a routinely generated business record that serves as the legal record of the nature, extent, and quality of care given the patient, as well as who rendered the care. The medical record has both business and legal significance and serves to protect both the patient and the healthcare professional. Healthcare organizations and healthcare professionals are required by legal, business, and ethical standards to record and safeguard clinically relevant patient history, examination and evaluative findings, and treatment-related information in patient health information records. State and federal laws, organizational policies and procedures, payer policies, and customary practices in the setting should be consulted to determine who could legally record patient health information in the medical record. This information may be entered electronically or manually and the record maintained electronically or in hard copy for the time dictated by state and federal law, as well as payer policy.

THE LAW

The U.S. Legal System

Laws define specific relationships and are classified as public or private. Public laws involve relationships between individuals or businesses and the government and define, regulate, and enforce respective rights of the parties. For example, Medicare is public law and involves the government in its relationship providing health insurance for covered individuals. In comparison, private law involves rules and legal principles defining rights and duties between individuals and/or private businesses. Private laws apply in matters involving contracts or torts such as malpractice. There are four sources of public and private laws: constitutions, statutes, administrative law, and judicial decisions.

The U.S. Constitution defines and establishes the powers of the legislative, executive, and judicial branches of government. It also includes 26 amendments, the first 10 comprising the Bill of Rights. Additionally, every state has a constitution, which is regarded as the highest law of the state but subordinate to the U.S. Constitution. Statutes are laws enacted by state legislatures and U.S. Congress. Accordingly, the Social Security Act and the Health Insurance Portability and Accountability Act (HIPAA) are statutes since the U.S. Congress enacted them.

Administrative rules and regulations are developed by administrative agencies to which Congress has given powers. For example, Congress has directed the Secretary of the U.S. Department of Health and Human Services (HHS) to promulgate rules to carry out the intent of HIPAA. Judicial decisions interpreting the Constitution and statutes form a major source of law and serve as a primary source for private law.

Statutes

Through law, relationships among private individuals, organizations, and government are defined and governed. The four primary sources of law are constitutions, statutes, administrative agencies, and court decisions. The U.S. Constitution is considered the supreme law of the land because it establishes and grants power to the three branches of the federal government (legislative, executive, and judicial) and restricts actions of federal and state governments. As mentioned, the first 10 amendments to the Constitution are called the Bill of Rights. Of significance, the Fourteenth Amendment places due process requirements on state governments, as does the Fifth Amendment on federal government, and as such, they assure equal protection under the law. The power related to the regulation of healthcare traditionally fell upon the states, as protected by "police powers" assured under the Tenth Amendment, which reserves states' rights to regulate behaviors for the general welfare, morals, health, and safety within its boundaries. With respect to regulation of hospitals and healthcare professionals, constitutionally protected rights of privacy and liberty are often at issue.

Laws enacted by legislatures (U.S. Congress, state, and local legislatures) are called statutes and codes. When there is a conflict between federal and state law, federal law supersedes. When state and local laws conflict, valid state law supersedes. Medical records laws are generally governed by state legislation and regulation, and as a result may vary by state. Applicable medical information provisions are found in laws for healthcare information confidentiality, healthcare provider licensure (practice), communicable diseases, child and elder abuse, peer review, fraud, and the dying process.

Courts interpret and determine whether statutes and regulations are constitutional and render decisions in matters not controlled by existing laws.

Administrative Rules and Regulations

The legislature (federal or state) delegates authority to administrative (federal or state) agencies to regulate professionals and professional practices and enforce laws because it lacks the time and expertise to address the complex issues involved. These regulations are enforced as laws, and violation of a regulation is often accompanied by violation of comparable law. Additionally, agencies may provide guidelines related to patient care documentation. The Joint Commission on Accreditation of Healthcare Organizations (JCAHO) and the Centers for Medicare & Medicaid Services (CMS) (the federal agency that administers Medicare and works in partnership with states to administer Medicaid and the Children's Health Insurance Program) expect that documentation in patient medical records be timely, accurate, complete, and legible.

Medical Malpractice

Since the 1970s, there has been a "malpractice crisis" characterized by excessive numbers of lawsuits and verdicts in favor of patients primarily against physicians and large organizations. PTs and PTAs are increasingly vulnerable to lawsuits with the expansion of professional practice into primary care, direct access, clinical specialization, and responsibilities delineated in *The Guide to Physical Therapist Practice.*[5] Effective, systematic communication with patients and other health professionals involved in care, with appropriate documentation, helps reduce risk.

The legal bases for imposing liability on PTs and PTAs include professional negligence, breach of contract, strict product liability, strict liability, and intentional misconduct. Professional negligence or medical malpractice occurs when the delivery of patient care falls below the acceptable standard of care—minimal standards of ordinary, reasonable practitioners acting under similar circumstances. When a therapist performs or fails to perform something during examination, evaluation, treatment, or follow-up that other similarly situated therapists would not find acceptable and harm (adverse outcome) comes to the patient, professional negligence exists. In pursuing a successful action for medical malpractice, the injured party or plaintiff must prove by a preponderance of the evidence or that it is more likely than not that:

1. The therapist (defendant) owed the patient a special duty of care
2. The therapist breached or failed to exercise that duty of care
3. The violation of the standard of care caused physical and/or mental injury to the patient
4. The patient suffered legally recognizable damages for which money can be awarded as compensation to make the patient whole again

The important message is that accurate, complete, timely, and concise documentation not only may save patient lives, but documentation consistent with these criteria may save a professional career. In an action for malpractice, the treatment record may constitute the only objective evidence of whether care to the patient was in compliance with acceptable standards or was a substandard level of care.

TERMINATING CARE/PATIENT ABANDONMENT

In most situations, healthcare providers can decline to initiate care, but the same choice does not apply to discontinuing care that was initiated. When a healthcare provider or organization unilaterally terminates a professional relationship with a patient inappropriately without the patient, his or her representative, or healthcare surrogate's consent when a need for continued service remains, legal abandonment occurs. Legally actionable abandonment based on professional negligence or intentional misconduct may result in a variety of situations ranging from temporarily leaving a patient unattended to terminating service when a patient has not achieved rehabilitative goals or progress toward goals has plateaued.

Patients may unilaterally terminate care without consequence (excluding responsibility for cost of care) because they are not bound by legal or ethical standards. However, the PT must exercise certain steps to avoid potential liability for patient abandonment. Unilateral termination of the professional–patient relationship is legal when the patient voluntarily makes an informed election to end the relationship or there is mutual agreement. Termination of care unilaterally is legal when the patient's medical condition has resolved or therapy goals are met. Discharging a patient at other times places the PT at risk for inappropriate premature discharge. To prevent claims of unjustified, unilateral termination, PTs and PTAs must carefully document all activities in the patient's care record.

Typical situations that result in abandonment include nonpayment of charges, fear of claim denials, failed reimbursement, and personality conflicts between practitioners and patients.[6] Under managed care, practitioners are becoming increasingly liable for patient abandonment due to patient inability to pay for continued intervention. To avoid legal issues of abandonment, good practice would be to advise the patient when a third-party payer has preauthorized a specific number of visits and to record the same in the medical record. If the therapist seeks reconsideration for additional visits, care must be taken not to promise the patient that it will be obtained. If more sessions are not granted but were promised, the therapist may be held responsible for "abandoning" the patient if the patient believed additional care was needed. Alternatively, when permissible by law and payer policy, the therapist can offer the option of private pay. If the patient declines, this can be documented to avoid the appearance or accusation of abandonment.

Author's Note

A recent Supreme Court ruling declared that a health maintenance organization's denial of payment for services rendered does not indicate that care may not be needed. Therefore, an ethical dilemma arises if a professional believed care should be given or continued. CMS regulations governing Medicare indicate that if a professional believes care should be continued even if reimbursement is not, it is incumbent on the professional that care be continued.

When anticipating the need to unilaterally discontinue care, the physical therapist should be honest with the patient in explaining the reasons for terminating care and provide assistance with transferring the patient's care to another provider and providing the patient records if requested in writing by the patient.

PTs and PTAs are held to the same standards of professional performance and abandonment regardless of the form of reimbursement or whether services are provided pro bono (free of charge), and documentation principles should be consistent regardless of payment.[7]

CONFIDENTIALITY, PRIVACY AND SECURITY, AND ACCESS

Confidentiality

State medical record access laws ensure the confidentiality of the patient–provider relationship and impose a duty to guard against unauthorized disclosure of licensed healthcare providers, health plans, and healthcare clearinghouses.[8] Healthcare personnel must access patient medical records for care reasons, administrative purposes, and defense against lawsuits. However, all personnel are legally required to safeguard the confidentiality of the records and prevent unauthorized use of the information. Generally, facilities have established policies and procedures to ensure that confidentiality of health information is maintained. Specific state laws allow reporting of patient health information without patient authorization when reporting vital statistics or matters affecting the public health, safety, or welfare. Some examples include reporting child and elder abuse or neglect, presence of communicable diseases, and victims of violent crimes. Since these requirements vary by state, knowledge and understanding of reporting requirements for the state in which the provider practices is a necessity.

Because insurers and MCOs generally require patient information before making utilization review or reimbursement decisions, some states have instituted patient confidentiality laws or adopted the National Association of Insurance Commissioners Insurance Information and Privacy Protection Model Act (NAIC Model Act), which requires that confidentiality of information be preserved and that disclosure is limited to particular circumstances.[9]

Privacy and Security

The Health Insurance Portability and Accountability Act of 1996 (HIPAA),[8] Public Law 104-191, enacted on August 21, 1996, imposes higher levels of privacy, security, and confidentiality on covered entities than ever before. HIPAA defines covered entities as a healthcare provider (but only if they transmit any information in an electronic form in connection with a transaction for which HHS has adopted a standard), health plan, or healthcare clearinghouse. The HIPAA Privacy Rule establishes national standards to protect individuals' medical records and other personal health information and applies to health plans, healthcare clearinghouses, and those healthcare providers that conduct certain healthcare transactions electronically. The HIPAA Security Rule requires covered entities to protect patients' electronically stored protected health information (known as ePHI) by using appropriate administrative, physical, and technical safeguards to ensure the confidentiality, integrity, and security of this information.[8]

HIPAA privacy standards establish an individual's right to access their health information, limit when access can be denied, and list legal requirements for compilation and storage of patient medical information. HIPAA also requires healthcare organizations to designate a privacy officer to oversee and implement all health information privacy policies and procedures because the standards in their entirety are complex. Prior to the HIPAA privacy rule, there was no generally applicable federal legislation protecting confidentiality of medical or personal information. There also was a lack of conformity with existing regulations governing access, use, and disclosure from state to state.[8]

The HIPAA Privacy Rule requires that healthcare providers and other covered entities must limit use, access, and disclosure to maintain patient privacy. Further, the same standard applies to use of information by individuals working for the facility. Any staff requiring access to the record should be identified in institutional policies.[8]

PHI under the privacy rule is expansive and includes information transmitted or maintained by electronic media or other form or medium. The privacy extends to any health information in any form or medium, including paper, electronic or digital imaging, and oral forms. The privacy standard also refers to designated record sets: health records, billing records, and various claims records used to make decisions about individuals. In addition to HIPAA, accrediting agencies, such as JCAHO, have developed standards to assure security and confidentiality of the patient health data collected.

Computerization of patient information has enabled immediate data exchange among authorized providers, payers, employers, and consumers, both regionally and nationally. The use of electronic format in disclosing patient information is cost-effective and promotes quality (and safety) of patient care. However, protecting patients' privacy and confidentiality of electronic health information can be a challenge. It also is frequently difficult to determine who owns and is responsible for protecting against unauthorized access to the medical content.

To comply with HIPAA rules regarding disclosure, healthcare providers must obtain the patient's consent to access, use, or disclose PHI information for purposes of treatment, payment, and healthcare operations. The HIPAA Privacy Rule, in general, requires that patients have a right to a notice of privacy practice explaining how private health information will be used and disclosed. The notice should explain the individual's rights and covered entity's legal duties with respect to the private information. In most applications, patient consent must be obtained at the time the healthcare services are provided. According to HIPAA, the consent must be in plain language.

Consent for disclosure of PHI should be obtained in writing; ordinarily, the notice does not specify a date of termination or revocation of the consent. With patient consent, only that information minimally necessary to accomplish the intended purpose can be revealed. Patient authorization is required for use or disclosure of information beyond the minimum necessary for treatment, payment, or support of healthcare operations. At a minimum, the disclosure should specify what information is to be disclosed, to whom it is being disclosed, and why it is being disclosed.[8] See table 11.1 For HIPAA Release Form Information.

As with many rules, patients are free to waive their privilege to privacy and nondisclosure of health information. It is recommended that any such waiver be secured in writing. Healthcare providers and facilities may be subject to civil and criminal liability for disclosing patient health information that has not been authorized by the patient or is required by law. HIPAA privacy and security violations may result in a penalty for each violation, ranging from annual limits of $25,000 to $1.5 million, which will be adjusted for inflation (https://www.govinfo.gov/content/pkg/FR-2019-04-30/pdf/2019-08530.pdf).

State and federal laws expressly control access to certain patient records, for example, patients with alcohol and drug abuse problems. Many states also have special laws addressing and limiting staff access to records regarding mental health and patients with human immunodeficiency virus/acquired immunodeficiency syndrome (HIV/AIDS). Only those personnel with a need to know and who are directly involved in a patient's care are permitted access under the law.

Table 11-1

A HIPAA-COMPLIANT HIPAA RELEASE FORM MUST, AT THE VERY LEAST, CONTAIN THE FOLLOWING INFORMATION:
• A description of the information that will be used/disclosed
• The purpose for which the information will be disclosed
• The name of the person or entity to whom the information will be disclosed
• An expiration date or expiration event when consent to use/disclose the information is withdrawn. For example, an expiration event may be when a research study is completed
• A signature and date that the authorization is signed by an individual or an individual's representative. If a representative is signing the form, the relationship with the patient must be detailed along with a description of the representative's authority to act on behalf of the patient
THE HIPAA RELEASE FORM MUST ALSO INCLUDE STATEMENTS THAT ADVISE THE INDIVIDUAL OF:
• Their right to revoke their authorization
• Any exceptions to the individual's right to revoke the authorization
• Details of how the authorization can be revoked
• To the extent that an individual's right to revoke authorization is included in the notice required by § 164.520 (Notice of Privacy Practices)
• That the covered entity may not condition treatment, payment, enrollment or eligibility for benefits on whether the individual signs the authorization
• That there is potential for information disclosed under the terms of the authorization to be redisclosed by the recipient and no longer protected by 45 CFR Part 164, Subpart E

Another federal law, the Privacy Act of 1974, 5 U.S.C. Section 552a (Privacy Act), places restrictions on the type of information a federal agency may collect about citizens and legal aliens, requires that individuals be informed as to the purposes and uses of the information, and limits how the information can be used[10] The Privacy Act also ensures that individuals can access and make copies of their records.

Hospitals operated by the federal government and MCOs that offer health insurance to government employees are subject to the guidelines of the Privacy Act. Healthcare facilities that receive federal funding may be subject to the Privacy Act. Requested changes may be made to the information or explanation provided for denial of the request. Under certain circumstances, the Privacy Act permits the disclosure of information without consent.

Access

The Freedom of Information Act allows public access to information about the operations and decisions of federal administrative agencies.[11] Specific categories of information are available to the public subject to nine specific exceptions. Of the noted exceptions, personnel and medical files that are relevant to healthcare in that disclosure would violate the right to privacy. Requested records must be made available promptly, and there are rules establishing when and where the records can be inspected and the fee for copying. Federal and state laws permit the patient or patient representative to examine and copy the medical record. This requires a written request and payment of reasonable clerical costs for copying the record. State laws provide that records only need to be made available at reasonable times and places.

The American Recovery and Reinvestment Act of 2009 (aka "the Stimulus Bill") amended HIPAA.[12] A portion of this law, called the Health Information Technology for Economic and Clinical Health Act (HITECH Act), was designed to further federal government interests in proliferating the use of electronic health records (EHRs) by healthcare providers and organizations, but maintain confidentiality of PHI. It also imposes a 60-day breach notification for unauthorized disclosures of patient medical information.[13] The HIPAA Breach Notification Rule, requires HIPAA covered entities and their business associates to provide notification following a breach of unsecured protected health information. Similar breach notification provisions implemented and enforced by the Federal Trade Commission (FTC), apply to vendors of personal health records and their third party service providers."[13] The passage of the Patient Protection and Affordable Care Act (ACA), signed into law on March 22, 2010, and more recently, the 21st Century Cures Act of 2016 (21st Century Cures), signed into law on December 13, 2016, have significantly affected how data is accessed, exchanged, and used by healthcare providers and other covered entities.

Author's Note

On March 9, 2020, HHS issued two final rules to address EHR interoperability and information blocking and patient access to EHRs. The rules were issued by the Office of National Coordinator for Health Information Technology and CMS to implement provisions enacted by Congress as part of the 21st Century Cures Act.

RESPONDING TO A PATIENT REQUEST FOR RELEASE OF HEALTH INFORMATION

While a potential malpractice claim may be a reason why a patient requests his or her medical records, there are in fact many reasons for such request. In addition to providing the patient with his or her records, it may be prudent and a good risk management procedure to meet with the patient to answer questions directly and in layperson's terms. This type of meeting may prevent the filing of a claim or avert litigation. It is well-accepted knowledge that the chief complaint among litigants for bringing legal action against providers is the lack of communication between providers and patients. Prior to any patient meeting, it also is wise to consult with appropriate risk management personnel.

Copies of healthcare records and other patient health information should not be disclosed to third parties unless the patient authorizes the release in a signed document. Therapists should request a copy of this signed release from a third-party payer prior to releasing a copy of the patient's record.

Generally, disclosure of the medical record of a minor requires authorization from one parent or legal guardian. Parents typically are permitted access to a child's medical information. Under certain circumstances, the minor may be able to authorize release of medical information.

The Internet is increasingly being used for transmission of clinical information. Every healthcare provider and organization should exercise care to maintain patient confidentiality. Policies and procedures should enforce confidentiality standards and ensure appropriate secure technology. The primary risks in using the Internet are related to unauthorized access and unauthorized disclosure of healthcare information. The American Health Information Management Association (AHIMA) has developed guidelines for Internet use and security concerns.[14] Healthcare providers using the Internet should comply with the AHIMA standards and applicable state and federal laws.

LEGAL REQUIREMENTS FOR MEDICAL RECORDS

Record Security

It is important to safeguard medical records not only to protect patient confidentiality but also to prevent intentional alteration, removal, destruction, or falsification. HIPAA requires that records be stored in a secure, restricted location; not to allow removal of the record from the premises unless court ordered; and to supervise patients and their representatives when examining the record. If a PT or PTA is engaged in home healthcare, they must take care to also safeguard their records and oral communication within the home with individual patients and as they move from patient to patient, home to patient, and home or patient to referring agency. (See Chapter 6 for more information on home health documentation.) With the advent of virtual assistants and smart speakers that automatically record conversations and store them for analysis, a new generation of privacy concerns has developed and will need to be assessed as these systems evolve.

In an EHR or an electronic medical record (EMR), privacy and protections may be accomplished with encrypted cloud-based systems for documentation.

Required Records

Healthcare providers must keep a medical record for each patient, according to proper record-keeping procedures. Failure to abide by this requirement may result in liability. Institutional policies incorporating state laws, when applicable, should designate the types of patient care information to be included in each patient record, the length of time for record retention, and the proper methods for destruction of the record.

Patient medical records consist of personal, financial, social, and medical data. Personal information contains identification information such as full legal name, date of birth (DOB), sex, marital status, next of kin, person to contact in an emergency, occupation, and physician name(s). Information about the patient's employer, health insurance carrier, types of insurance coverage and policy numbers, and Medicare and Medicaid identification numbers (no longer Social Security number based) are considered financial and are used for billing purposes. The patient's race and ethnicity, family relationships, community activities, and information about lifestyle or court orders are considered social data. The continuous recordation of the history of treatment forms the clinical record. This may consist of patient complaint(s), medical and family histories, results of physical or other medically related examinations, course of treatment, diagnosis and therapeutic orders, informed consent, clinical observations, progress notes, consultation reports, nursing notes, reports of diagnostic tests and procedures, and operative reports.

The medical record may be handwritten, typed, dictated, or computer-generated, but should be consistent in format and content data for each discipline within an organization. The record should be a complete, accurate, and current account of the history, condition, and treatment of the patient, including outcomes and all other appropriate information in chronological order.

Content Requirements

Required content in patient healthcare records varies and generally depends on relevant state and federal laws and regulations, accreditation standards, organizational and system requirements, payer policy, patient clinical settings, and professional guidelines, such as those contained in the American Physical Therapy Association's (APTA's) *Guide to Physical Therapy Documentation of Patient/Client Management*.[15]

PTs, PTAs, and other practice personnel responsible for documentation or any information that is incorporated into the medical record should know the rules and regulations for record content as required by the state in which they work and the applicable payer. With the advent of technology, access to state and federal regulations is readily accessible through the Internet.

Healthcare providers who participate in federal reimbursement programs must comply with the federal regulations for record maintenance, which may require a clinical record for each patient be maintained in accordance with professional standards and to be promptly completed, filed, and retained.[16] For providers required to maintain compliance with CMS, specific criteria for record content must be met. While the requirements for CMS records are similar across settings, PTs and PTAs should be familiar with the specific documentation requirements based upon the setting(s) in which they work.

Accrediting organizations also impose maintenance standards for records. JCAHO requires the content of the health record in managed care facilities and hospitals to include member identification; diagnoses; plan of care; medical history; appropriate physical examinations; immunization and screening status; results of treatments, procedures, and tests; referrals or transfers to other practitioners; and evidence of advance directives. For home health accreditation, records must contain the patient's height and weight, dietary restrictions, documentation as to suitability of home for services provided, documentation of patient and family education, and list of individuals and organizations involved in the patient's care, as well as the information required by federal rules and regulations, such as the Home Health Outcome and Assessment Information Set (OASIS), which contains data items developed to measure patient outcomes and to improve home healthcare. Completion of the OASIS is required for all home health agencies certified to accept Medicare and Medicaid reimbursement.

Most facilities have adopted formal written policies concerning the content of medical records. For PTs, it is good practice to adopt and follow the content criteria established in the APTA *Guide to Documentation*[17] (see Appendix E) in conjunction with the most current applicable state, federal, and accreditation requirements associated with medical records, as well as payer policy. As laws and policies frequently change, it is important to continually monitor for updates to pertinent laws, regulations, and guidance.

FORMATS

Healthcare providers should ensure that others involved in the care of the patient understand the content and format used for documentation of patient information. It is up to the facility, department, or therapists to determine which format is selected. In larger organizations, therapists may be using EMR systems that have been customized or are standardized programs that may limit or dictate format and direct content. From an organizational perspective, there should be consistency in content and format within a department and between therapists; however, quality improvement (QI) or quality assurance (QA) initiatives should ensure that content is complete and appropriate to ensure the record will serve all identified purposes. Regardless of the format selected, the content should be objective in nature, with all information matching and relevant. The necessity of the need for skilled intervention should be clear based on identified problems, planned interventions, and relevance of functional goals or outcomes.

Interestingly, written goals represent professional judgment and not necessarily a guarantee or warranty of a specific therapeutic result. Legally, patient intervention goals are generally not actionable. However, actual communication of therapeutic promises, including documentation of said goals, may create contractual obligations to patients and create legal liability if not achieved, so care must be taken to set realistic goals that must be agreed upon by all appropriate parties.

PROBLEMS, ERRORS, AND PRACTICE

Problems with documentation can have serious legal ramifications. Therefore, it is important that therapists familiarize themselves with common errors and the recommendations for averting adverse consequences and employ proper documentation skills.

Illegibility

Illegibility is a common documentation problem and may result in an inability to translate patient care information. The solution is for therapists to write legibly, print, type, or utilize alternative documentation systems not based on handwritten notation. Additionally, the record must be complete. This is reinforced in the Medicare guidelines, which require that all entries be legible and complete.

Patient's Full Name

The patient's full legal name and identifying information should be on every page of the medical record. Failure to correctly identify a patient receiving care is negligence and can lead to liability. When the record is copied, the lack of patient identification on any page can result in inappropriate filing or loss of information.

Date and Time of Patient Care

The date and usually the time of patient care should be included in all records. This will support time billed for that patient and can be used as evidence in any patient dispute regarding date and time of visit. If treatment time is not indicated, total treatment time or units should be included, at a minimum. However, it is important to always check payer policy. For example, as stated in the Medicare Benefit Policy Manual, Chapter 15, Section 220.3(E), documentation requirements for therapy services includes documenting "total timed code treatment minutes and total treatment time in minutes to be documented in the record. … The amount of time for each specific intervention/modality provided to the patient may also be recorded voluntarily, but contractors shall not require it, as it is indicated in the billing."

Standard Forms and Formats

Standard forms and formats that are universally understood by other providers in the same facility or network should be used. Standardization helps ensure appropriate content and consistency. Although many physical therapy practices have adopted their own interpretation of a SOAP note, the SOAP note format is not required by any federal or state regulation, and indeed may be inconsistent between practices or even within a practice (which may be legally challenging). With the advent of commercial EMR programs, the SOAP format is less frequently used than in past decades.

Indelible Black or Blue Ink

If manual entry is being used, indelible black or blue ink should be used for documenting patient care to prevent tampering with entries, especially in the advent of legal action. However, the facility must determine which color will be used by policy and ensure uniformity.

In the event the pen runs out of ink while documenting, a therapist must complete the note. If another ink color is used, an explanation in parentheses should precede the second part of the patient note stating that the original pen ran out of ink. This parenthetical explanation should be initialed. This procedure is necessary to avoid implications of spoilage of records in a potential lawsuit.

Computerized entries should be saved automatically to prevent subsequent loss or alteration of patient content.

Blank Spaces

Blank spaces or lines are unacceptable in the record, as blanks may infer lack of completeness or create the potential to add information. Therapists should use each line to document care, leaving no spaces between lines, or put diagonal lines through large empty spaces. In computerized or electronic records, the format is often preset, and the professional documenting may have to simply comply with what an individual entry field allows.

Signatures

Signatures (or initialing patient care corrections or flow sheets) on entries are required for authentication purposes and to acknowledge legal and ethical responsibility for the information contained in the entry. Entries should bear legible legal signatures followed by professional title to demonstrate a skilled professional rendered care. When signatures are illegible, better practice is to print the name below the signature. In most states, computer signatures constitute legal signatures, but the therapist should seek legal counsel for verification. Licensure number is recommended. If a PT or PTA student is documenting, the designation SPT or SPTA and a co-signature by the supervising therapist must follow their name or "assistant" should follow. Again, it is important to check payer policy for signature requirements. For example, in the Medicare Benefit Policy Manual Chapter 15, Section 230(B), CMS states that because the licensed PT or PTA is responsible for the services and must sign all documentation, a student may also sign, but it is not necessary, since the payment is for the clinician's service, not for the student's services.

Example: Colin Brooks, SPT Eric Shamus, PT, DPT # 12345

Author's Note

APTA supports five categories of abbreviated designations (See Table 11 2 Abbreviated Designation). Note that only the first designation is mandatory—all others are optional, but if you choose to include them, they must be according to the requirements of the APTA position.

Therefore, an individual who wishes to use their professional title and educational level would sign:

Jennifer Shamus, PT, DPT #12234

If a student signature is required and it is not clearly legible, the signature should be followed by the printed name. Although this is good practice for PTs and PTAs as well, the license number would be used as identification if the signature was illegible, providing the numbers were legible.

Stuart Shamus, SPT
Stuart Shamus, SPT

Error Correction

Error correction commonly consists of a single line drawn through the erroneous content, initialed, and dated, preferably with the time. However, in the EMR, there may not be the ability to write over content with a single line or insertion of initials or dates (see "Addendums"). The most important rule is not to hide the mistake by whiting it out, scratching it out, blacking it out, or writing over it or erasing it in the EMR. The addition of the words "error" or "mistake" is controversial and creates an image of sloppy patient care, which may impair a defense in a malpractice claim.

Right DFS, 8/30/20
EXAMPLE: Active ROM of Left shoulder flexion: 100°/180°

Table 11-2 Abbreviated Designations

FIRST designation: PT or PTA
PT, PTA
SECOND designation: Highest earned physical therapy-related degree
DPT, MPT, MSPT, BSPT
THIRD designation: Other regulatory designation(s) issued by government entities
APN, APNR, APRN, ATC, CNS, CPA, CRNP, CS, LAc, LAC, LCMT, LCSW, LDM, LM, LMSW, LMT, LPC, LCPC, LVT, MT, NP, OT, OTR/L, RN, SLP (and others as identified)
FOURTH designation: Other earned academic degree(s)
AuD, BA, BS, CScD, DC, DDS, DEd, DHS, DMD, DMT, DNP, DO, DPM, DSc, DScPT, DVM, EdD, JD, LLM, MA, MBA, MD, MEd, MHS, MLS, MOTR, MPA, MPH, MPP, MS, MSHA, ND, NMD, PharmD, PhD, PsyD, SLPD, SLPM (and others as identified)
Optional FIFTH designation: FAPTA
FAPTA
https://www.apta.org/apta-and-you/leadership-and-governance/policies/appropriate-use-of-designations

Addendums

Addendums can be made or added to the patient record and should always contain the date of the addendum. If the treating professional is entering an addendum to an entry, it should be preceded by the date of entry and state "Addendum to entry of..."

Amendments made at the patient's request should be included as an addendum with a notation explaining that the change was made at the patient's request. Patient amendments that are deemed inappropriate should be discussed with the patient. Generally, if the requested change is not made by the facility, it may be a good idea to permit the individual to insert a statement of disagreement in the record. Some states allow this procedure provided notice of change or statement is given to designated persons within certain time periods.

Intentional alteration of a medical record or writing an incorrect record may subject a provider to statutory sanctions, including license revocation. Altering or falsifying a chart to obtain Medicare or state health reimbursement is a crime under federal law punishable by substantial fine or imprisonment.[18]

Acceptable Abbreviations

Acceptable abbreviations save time and facilitate accurate communication (see Appendix A for a common list of abbreviations). However, problems arise and can result in medical errors when abbreviations have more than one meaning open to multiple interpretations, are illegible and resemble other abbreviations or words, or are not widely known. (Providing a key within the record to a repeating abbreviation may alleviate potential errors.) These are some of the reasons the JCAHO has recommended that in JCAHO-accredited healthcare organizations, abbreviations not be used at all. Physical therapy professionals should only use abbreviations that have been approved or are universally disseminated within their practice or organization. Actionable medical malpractice liability may be attributed to the healthcare provider who authors and/or reads erroneous information conveyed by use of unintelligible abbreviations that result in patient injury.

Improper Spelling and Grammar and Wordiness

Improper spelling and grammar and wordiness create negative impressions of the practitioner and are construed as practitioner carelessness that contributes to findings of liability. All entries should be as accurate and concise as possible to avoid confusion or discrepancy.

Orders or Referrals: Written, Verbal, Telephonic, E-mail, Fax, or Electronic

Illegible or unclear physical therapy referrals must be clarified before seeing the patient or carrying out the referral. Therapists should document all inquiries and physician/nonphysician practitioner responses regarding ambiguities in diagnostic and treatment referrals. State laws, policies of the facility, accreditation standards, payer policy, and customary practices govern whether care is elicited under verbal orders. In direct consumer access states, written referrals from other healthcare professionals may not be required, but reimbursement may be declined without a referral or order or signed plan of care. Medicare and Medicaid require written orders in acute care hospitals, inpatient rehabilitation, home health, and skilled nursing home settings. In the private practice setting, Medicare beneficiaries may be seen without a written order, but a plan of care (POC) must be signed as soon as possible or within 30 days of the first date of treatment, whereas in a Comprehensive Outpatient Rehabilitation Facility (CORF), CORF services must be furnished under a written rehabilitation plan of treatment established and signed by a physician who has recently evaluated the patient, and must be established and signed by a physician prior to the commencement of treatment in the CORF setting and contain the diagnosis; the type, amount, frequency, and duration of skilled rehabilitation services to be performed; and the anticipated skilled rehabilitation goals (42 CFR 410.105).

The person taking a referral verbally, via telephone, e-mail, or fax, should transcribe the orders or referral into the medical record. It is not sufficient to make a copy, for example, of the faxed referral and insert it into the medical record without transcribing the content directly into the record. State law may dictate who can take and transcribe the order, but in most cases, it is the PT and may limit the taking or transcription of orders to physical therapy–related orders or referral only. Payer policy also may dictate who can receive and transcribe a verbal order. The entry should include what the order is for, the time it was taken (i.e., phone, verbal face-to-face, phone message as voice mail, e-mail, fax, other), the prescribing/referring/ordering individual's name, and the name of the person who entered it into the medical record. Verbal, telephone, e-mail, electronic orders, or faxed orders and referrals require authentication, usually within 24 to 48 hours by the prescribing professional, based on organizational and/or accreditation guidelines or requirements. This practice will enhance communication and protect both the referring physician and the therapist. Policies related to verbal orders should require that only personnel qualified to understand physician orders be authorized to receive and transcribe them. Written orders are preferable because they create fewer chances for error. Therapists are responsible for knowing laws regarding the need, if any, to refer patients to a physician or other practitioner. PTs have the professional capability and ability to refer to others in the healthcare system for identified or possible needs that are beyond the scope of PT practice.

Documentation Timeliness

From the legal perspective, timeliness of medical record entries is important. Late entries equate to the records being incomplete for a period of time. Documentation should occur contemporaneously or as closely as possible to when the actual care is rendered. The longer the time lapse between the conclusion of care and the time that the note is written, the less accurate it will be. Untimely documentation that results in prolonged care or extension of patient discomfort is professional negligence and provides opposing attorneys the opportunity to challenge the accuracy of the entire content of the note. In the event a late entry into the medical records must be made, for example, when the record is unavailable, it should be designated as an "addendum" or "follow-up entry." Transcribed or dictated entries (whether transcribed and dictated by external service or directly into a computerized voice-recognition system) should be received within 24 hours and should be reviewed for accuracy. It is unethical to document care before it is given.

Identification of Information Sources

Identification of patient information sources must be recorded. Failing to denote another practitioner's responsibility for clinical information provided might result in legal liability solely to the writer of the note and leads to misinterpretations as to who is responsible for patient care. If a primary care provider receives and documents clinical information regarding an adverse change in patient status, the provider is obligated to re-examine the patient expeditiously and should document accordingly to reduce the risk for legal liability for inappropriate monitoring of the patient.

Blame or Disparaging Comments

Blame or disparaging comments should not appear in the medical record, unless the transcriber is willing to risk potential actions for defamation. However, statements made by patients relevant to the clinical services to be or that were provided must be entered into medical records in quotations. Before documenting a patient statement that appears contradictory to the patient's self-interest, the therapist should have the patient confirm the statement. In such a situation, it is advisable to have a witness, and ethically, the statement must be documented in the patient record when it contains clinically pertinent information.

Objective and Specific Findings

Objective and specific findings should be documented, whereas subjective findings or opinions should not. It is recommended that writing ambiguous statements starting with "it appears" or "apparently" be avoided.

Example

Incorrect: Patient was apparently in pain following therapeutic exercise of the RLE (right lower extremity).

Correct: Patient C/O (complained of) proximal RLE "stabbing pain," 8/10, following therapeutic exercise of the RLE.

Important details should not be presumed. For example, "ROM WNL" (range of motion within normal limits) does not tell the reader what joints were examined or indicate an objective and clear indication of the ROM and is therefore not sufficient. The record is expected to tell a story of the patient's achievement toward his or her goals. The documentation should demonstrate why a skilled service is medically necessary. Treatment notes, progress reports, and other medical record documentation provide important communication among all members of the patient's care team regarding the development, course, and outcomes of skilled observations; treatment; and training.

Informed Consent

Informed consent for examination and treatment must be documented in the patient medical record, preferably as a separate form. However, the therapist may verbally obtain it and then record that it was received. The concept of informed consent originates from the legal and ethical rights that patients have to direct what happens to their own bodies. Medical informed consent generally requires that the patient be given sufficient information concerning the nature and risks of the recommended and alternative treatments to make an educated decision. The general rule is that if patient consent is not given, the patient does not receive services. However, the patient must be competent to make an appropriate decision based on the information received. In some circumstances, such as under emergencies and compulsory treatments when a patient may not be competent to give consent, the law implies consent and temporary consent is proffered.

The Patient Self-Determination Act of 1990 (PSDA),[13] codifies a patient's common law right to control their healthcare decisions and binds all facilities and providers participating in Medicare and Medicaid programs. The PSDA ensures that patients are educated to make "informed decisions" and have rights to make "advanced directives." The PSDA respects the ethical rights of persons to make autonomous decisions about their bodies. In accordance with this law, facilities and organizations should require written informed consent from patients, including written policies and procedures protecting patient rights and documentation of whether a patient executed advanced directives.

A well-written, properly executed consent form is strong evidence that informed consent was given, although it is not legally conclusive. To be a legally effective consent form, the document should be signed voluntarily; indicate that the procedure performed is the same consented to; and demonstrate that the consenting person understood the nature of the procedure, the risks, and probable consequences. This can be done with a short or long form. The short form is generalized and does not contain specific risks and benefits. It is advisable to supplement the short form by writing detailed notes regarding risks and benefits discussed in the patient medical record. The long form includes a detailed description of the medical condition, proposed procedure, consequences, risks, and alternatives. The danger in using this form is that providers rely on and may substitute the form rather than explain the information to the patient to assure understanding. In the absence of a long or short form, at a minimum, a therapist should document that the treatment was explained and consent was given.

Generally, a person's consent constitutes authorization for a particular practitioner to perform a particular procedure, so deviation from that authorization may invalidate the consent. Further, refusal of consent to treatment by a certain practitioner removes that practitioner from engaging in the treatment. For physical therapy specifically, it should be clear to the patient that the treatment includes physical contact or touching.

For situations in which adequacy of information given is disputed, courts will apply standards of the reasonable physician, the reasonably prudent patient, or a subjective standard (i.e., what would this patient need to know and understand). The trend is to apply the reasonable patient standard, wherein the physician's duty to provide information is determined by the information needs of the average patient, not the specific patient or professional practice.

Persons with difficulties understanding English must have the form translated into their native language to avoid any question that the patient understood the content and was able to give an educated consent. Healthcare providers servicing multiple cultural and ethnic populations should have consent forms in primary languages. It is usually sufficient to have a form translated orally. Federal and state laws in all 50 states require covered entities to provide language access services to limited-English-proficient and deaf and hard-of-hearing patients. Pursuant to 45 CFR 92.101(a), any entity operating or administering a health program or activity subject to this part [45 CFR Part 92] shall take reasonable steps to ensure meaningful access to such programs or activities by limited English proficient individuals.

45 CFR 92.101 also incorporates a four-factor test to determine whether the entity has complied with paragraph (a). HHS said in its final rule published on June 19, 2020 that

incorporating such test is meant to strike a balance that ensures meaningful access by LEP individuals to critical services while not imposing undue burdens on small businesses. https://www.federalregister.gov/documents/2020/06/19/2020-11758/nondiscrimination-in-health-and-health-education-programs-or-activities-delegation-of-authority. PTs and PTAs should familiarize themselves not only with relevant federal law but also the of their state.

It is important to have a medically trained translator (not a family or community member) translate the form or certify that the form and discussion of the procedure have been translated for the patient. Pursuant to 45 CFR 92.101(b)(2), when the entity is required to provide language assistance services, such services must be provided free of charge, be accurate and timely, and protect the privacy and independence of the individual with limited English proficiency.

Section 92.101(b)(3) sets forth the specific requirements for interpreter and translation services. https://www.federalregister.gov/documents/2020/06/19/2020-11758/nondiscrimination-in-health-and-health-education-programs-or-activities-delegation-of-authority. Note that under HIPAA, when a covered healthcare provider uses an interpreter to communicate with an individual, the individual's authorization is not required when the provider meets certain conditions:[20]

> *Covered entities may use and disclose protected health information for treatment, payment and health care operations without an individual's authorization, 45 CFR 164.506(c).*
>
> *A covered health care provider might use interpreter services to communicate with patients who speak a language other than English or who are deaf or hard of hearing, and provision of interpreter services usually will be a health care operations function of the covered entity as defined at 45 CFR 164.501.*
>
> *When using interpreter services, a covered entity may use and disclose protected health information regarding an individual without an individual's authorization as a health care operation, in accordance with the Privacy Rule, in the following ways:*
>
> - *When the interpreter is a member of the covered entity's workforce (i.e., a bilingual employee, a contract interpreter on staff, or a volunteer) as defined at 45 CFR 160.103;*
> - *When a covered entity engages the services of a person or entity, who is not a workforce member, to perform interpreter services on its behalf, as a business associate, as defined at 45 CFR 160.103. A covered entity may disclose protected health information as necessary for the business associate to provide interpreter services on the covered entity's behalf, subject to certain written satisfactory assurances set forth in 45 CFR 164.504(e).*
>
> *In addition, a covered health care provider may, without the individual's authorization, use or disclose protected health information to the patient's family member, close friend, or any other person identified by the individual as his or her interpreter for a particular healthcare encounter. In these situations, that interpreter is not a business associate of the health care provider. As with other disclosures to family members, friends or other persons identified by an individual as involved in his or her care, when the individual is present, the covered entity may obtain the individual's agreement or reasonably infer, based on the exercise of professional judgment, that the individual does not object to the disclosure of protected health information to the interpreter. 45 CFR 164.510(b)(2).*

For minors (generally those under the age of 18, although this may vary), parent or guardian consent must be obtained before treatment is given. If the minor needs emergency treatment, a statute gives the minor the right to consent when parents cannot be located or a court order is needed. Legally, either parent can give effective consent for treatment, except when parents are legally separated or divorced, at which time, the consent of the custodial parent is typically required unless there is an agreement or court order permitting the non-custodial parent or requiring both to consent. A provider can rely on the parent(s) to tell them who has authority to consent to the minor's care.

Special consent requirements beyond informing the patient of the risks and benefits are needed when patients undergo experimental treatments or participate in clinical research studies. Federal, state, and local laws, in addition to institutional polices and procedures, impose strict requirements for obtaining patient consent and should be consulted.

When a patient's condition changes significantly, the original consent may no longer be valid, and new consent should be obtained. Patient refusal of consent and withdrawal of consent for treatment should be documented and the physician notified.

Theories of Consent. There are two theories of consent violations. One theory is based on the common law development of battery or violation of an individual's right to be free from harmful or offensive touching. Another theory is based on negligence whereby patients consent to procedures without having sufficient information to make an informed decision.

Refusal of Consent. Refusal of consent is the legal right of competent adults to refuse medical treatment. Legally, courts have upheld these decisions despite the basis of the refusal. It is prudent to seek the advice of legal counsel and institutional legal advisors and ethics committees for situations in which the refusal is a serious threat to health and endangers the patient's life.

When a patient refuses to sign the consent form but is willing to give consent orally, the fact that verbal consent was given and the reason for refusal to sign the form should be documented on the consent form, along with the witnessed signature, and placed in the medical record.

Home Instructions, Independent Exercise Instructions, and Other Instructions

Home instructions, home exercise programs (HEPs), independent exercise programs, other instructions, and the like must be documented, copies maintained, and preferably contain the patient's or responsible party's signature and a statement indicating that they have been received and understand them.

Standardized programs should be kept as part of clinical procedures manuals on site. If the standardized programs are identified by name or number, the name or number should be included in the documentation. As part of the documentation, the therapist should include that the patient, family, or other caregiver understands, safely carries out, and is responsibly complying with home programs of care. All precautions or limitations to activities and follow-up instructions must be documented. Lack of follow-up could be construed as actionable abandonment.

With the advent of smart phones, pictures of the patient performing exercises may be acceptable on the patient's phone. They should not be taken with a healthcare professional's device nor e-mailed or texted through unsecured or encrypted systems.

Noncompliance and Nonadherence

Noncompliance, missed appointments, refusal of care, or nonadherence with given recommendations must be documented. The documentation should be objective, including specific times and dates of violations, and circumstances and descriptions of noncompliance. If a patient fails to comply and goals are not met or they suffer harm and this is documented, contributory negligence may be construed, making the patient partially responsible for an adverse outcome. Depending upon payer policy, if noncompliance, missed appointments, etc., results in any potential for clinical impact upon the patient, the healthcare organization or practitioner may be required to notify the responsible physician of the missed treatment or service. The physician then determines whether the treatment or service may be skipped or whether additional intervention is required by the provider due to the clinical impact on the patient.

Incidence or Occurrence Reports

Incidence or occurrence reports should not be included in the record or identified. It is important to objectively document the incident in the record and obtain quality care for any injuries. Risk management must be notified in order to protect the facility against unwarranted liability and educate to prevent similar future incidents. Incident or occurrence reports preserve memories of incidents. Since the reports are considered more administrative in nature and purpose, they are maintained separately from the patient medical record. In some organizations, formal reports may not be kept. It is up to the organization and risk carrier how an incidence or occurrence should be recorded. The policies and procedures for the organization should identify how incidence/occurrence reports should be recorded. Clinicians should be familiar and comply with their institution's policies and procedures regarding the filing of incidence reports.

Countersignature

A countersignature is expected for student documentation and required by law in some states,[21] as well as payer policy. The reason the note must be co-signed is to authenticate the note and make it legally acceptable. The need for a countersignature is to assure that a professional has reviewed the note and, if appropriate, to indicate approval of action taken by another practitioner. The person who countersigns has the authority to evaluate the entry and typically has more experience or has higher training than the person making the entry. Countersignatures permit delegation of responsibility. Providers who countersign another's notes should carefully proofread the note before co-signing. The countersignature imposes legal responsibility for the information contained in the note. Incomplete or inaccurate notes should not be countersigned until corrected appropriately. PT students' entries must be countersigned by a PT. PTA students' entries must be signed by a PT or PTA. Once countersigned, the PT student's or PTA student's note is legally adopted by the supervising therapist as his or her own note, causing him or her to share the legal responsibility with the student for what is written in the note. Without evidence of that supervision inferred by countersignature, a student might be held as violating and engaging in the unlicensed practice of physical therapy. Also, as discussed previously, always check payer policy regarding co-signature requirements for therapists, assistants, and students.

Authentication

Authentication and signature is made by the provider who delivers the care. Handwritten signatures were traditionally required. More recently, rubber stamps and computer key signatures are accepted and permitted by some states, and state and federal authorities allow computer or electronic signatures.

CMS requires authentication of each entry for Medicare and Medicaid participation. CMS does allow authentication by computer, but not all entities allow this type of "auto-authentication." Failure to obtain a physician's or health care professional's (including PTs and PTAs) signature to the record in its final form constitutes deficiency.

Author's Note

Rubber stamp signatures are not allowed on Medicare documentation. If rubber stamp signatures are allowed in any cases, the therapist or assistant should control the use of the stamp and not leave it behind if they leave the practice.

Record Retention and Destruction

Therapists should check for applicable statutory and regulatory requirements dictating record retention in their particular state. The general period for retention of medical records varies and should minimally cover the statute of limitations or period within which a party may bring a lawsuit. If participating under Medicare, retention of the original record or legally reproduced form must be for a period of at least five years. CMS requires Medicare Advantage providers to retain records for 10 years.[22] Although there are no HIPAA retention requirements for medical records, there is a regulation governing how long HIPAA-related documents should be retained. The regulation requires that documents must be retained for a minimum of six years from when the document was created or the date when it last was in effect, whichever is later.[23] About half of the states require that original medical records be preserved for 10 years. Some facilities require record retention beyond statutes of limitations, including rules for deceased patients and deceased or relocating therapists. For electronic records, backup should be performed regularly and measures taken to preserve and protect the electronic health information.

The statute of limitations on contract and tort actions should also determine how long to maintain records. Statutes of limitation based on various legal causes of actions are not uniform and may vary from state to state. Although most lawsuits brought by minors are filed soon after the incident causing the injury, therapists should retain the records until a minor reaches majority and for an additional time equal to the state statute of limitations for tort actions. Generally, the medical record of a minor should be kept until the patient reaches the age of majority (18 or 21, depending on the state) plus the statute of limitations. For example, for a state in which majority is 21 years and the statute of limitations for medical malpractice is 2 years, records should be preserved for 23 years.

For medical research purposes, it is advisable to establish a long retention period for records. When research involves experimental or innovative patient care procedures, records should be preserved for extended periods of time, typically 75 years. This means that space for storage must be designated and recordation be in a format that will withstand this time. Storage of medical records on computers may be governed by licensure or accreditation laws, federal programs, or rules of evidence associated with admissibility of copies of patient records at trial.

The AHIMA has established record retention guidelines to aid organizations in determining how well they measure up to industry standards.[14] These guidelines include ensuring availability of patient information for continued care; legal requirements; research, education, and other legitimate uses; developing a retention schedule for patients, physicians, researchers, and other user needs; legal, regulatory, and accreditation requirements; specifying what information is saved, for what time period, and how to store the information; establishing compliance programs addressing all types of documentation generated from employee training, hot lines, internal investigations, audits, modifications to compliance programs, and self-disclosures; retaining documentation for a sufficient time to prove compliance with applicable federal and state laws and regulations; and developing policies with legal advice.

AHIMA's recommended minimum time periods for which patient health records be kept are:

- Patient health records (adults): 10 years after the most recent encounter
- Patient health records (minors): Age of majority plus statute of limitations
- Diagnostic images: 5 years
- Disease index: 10 years
- Fetal heart monitor records: 10 years after infant reaches majority
- Master patient index: Permanently
- Operative index: 10 years
- Register of births: Permanently
- Register of deaths: Permanently
- Register of surgical procedures: Permanently

Courts have held facilities liable for an independent act of breaching their duty to make and maintain medical records, and one court permitted an action despite running of the applicable statute of limitations when the plaintiff had insufficient evidence to sustain a medical malpractice action because the patient health record could not be produced.

A patient's health information records may be destroyed in accordance with state law when the retention period expires, the record has been copied onto microfilm or computer, or otherwise converted into readable form. Some states require that an abstract of pertinent information in the medical record be created before destruction. Large facilities generally contract with a commercial enterprise for the destruction of records. It is important that such an agreement contain terms dealing with the method of destruction, safeguards protecting confidentiality of information, indemnification, and certification that the records have been properly destroyed. Failure to apply a uniform policy to all records may result in a jury's interpretation that if the records were available, they would reveal that a patient received substandard care.

Medicare and Medicaid

CMS develops Conditions of Participation (CoPs) and Conditions for Coverage (CfCs) that health care organizations must meet in order to begin and continue participating in the Medicare and Medicaid programs. These health and safety standards are the foundation for improving quality and protecting the health and safety of beneficiaries." https://www.cms.gov/Regulations-and-Guidance/Legislation/CFCsAndCoPs. The conditions relevant to participation in the Medicare and Medicaid programs require that medical records remain confidential. These conditions apply to various types of facilities, including acute care and rehabilitation hospitals, critical access hospitals, long-term care facilities, home health agencies, rehabilitation agencies, substance abuse treatment clinics, and hospices. Although physical therapy private practices are not subject to Medicare and Medicaid conditions of participation, PTs in private practice should have a procedure for ensuring the confidentiality of patient records in accordance with HIPAA and any applicable state or local laws.

Disclosure of Medical Information for Research Purposes

Many states as well as the federal government have laws providing for disclosure of patient information for research projects, especially regarding research using human subjects. Most facilities have established institutional review boards (IRB) that evaluate research protocol, protect the confidentiality of the information obtained, decide whether the research will benefit society, and determine whether adequate safeguards exist to protect the human study subjects placed at risk. With existing HIPAA privacy and security laws, it is required to obtain written patient authorization for any release of the medical record.

SPECIAL DOCUMENTATION CONCERNS

Celebrity Patients

Special care to protect the patient health information records of celebrity patients may be challenging, since the personalities are often subject to the scrutiny of the news media. Some facilities have established policies and procedures to assess the need for anonymity by omitting the patient name from the record or replacing it with an alias or code name and maintaining the record in a special secure file. However, based on the HIPAA guidelines, patient confidentiality is a legal requirement for all.

Hostile Patients

Hostile patients are more likely to take legal action in the event of rendered problematic or perceived problematic healthcare. It is recommended to create a detailed medical record that leaves little ambiguity regarding the medical care given to the patient. Avoid inserting derogatory comments about the patient's behavior in the record, including only objective descriptions and quotes from the patient. Negative remarks may be used in litigation to prove bad faith and/or bias on behalf of the practitioner.

Recording Indicators of Child or Elder Abuse

Documentation in suspected situations of abuse should be detailed and objective, containing a description of all relevant findings. This is important, as the documentation may be used for determination of abuse. The results of any assessments and testing should be included, as well as a detailed history and identities of interviewers or other caregivers or family of the patient. If the danger is not immediate but you suspect that abuse has occurred or is occurring, please tell someone. Relay your concerns to the supervisor, local adult protective services, long-term care ombudsman, or the police. You can reach the Eldercare Locator by telephone at 1-800-677-1116. Specially trained operators will refer you to a local agency that can help. The Eldercare Locator is open Monday through Friday, 9 AM to 8 PM Eastern Time: https://eldercare.acl.gov/Public/Index.aspx.

The laws in most states require helping professions in the front lines—such as doctors and home health providers—to report suspected abuse or neglect. These professionals are called mandated reporters. The HIPAA Privacy Rule permits covered health care providers and other covered entities to disclose reports of child abuse or neglect to public health authorities or other appropriate government authorities. See 45 C.F.R. 164.512(b)(1)(ii). Covered entities may report such information and be in compliance with both state law and the HIPAA Privacy Rule." https://www.hhs.gov/hipaa/for-professionals/faq/406/does-hipaa-preempt-this-state-law/index.html#:~:text=Answer%3A,or%20other%20appropriate%20government%20authorities.&text=Thus%2C%20there%20is%20no%20conflict,Privacy%20Rule%2C%20and%20no%20preemption.

Designation of Healthcare Surrogate or Healthcare Proxy

Most states have adopted a process and form, commonly called the designation of healthcare surrogate or healthcare proxy, that permits an agent of a disabled or incompetent person to make healthcare decisions on behalf of the patient. This document is more flexible than a living will, which is limited to when the patient is terminally ill or comatose and unable to communicate. The healthcare surrogate or proxy can be used whenever a patient is unable to communicate a choice regarding a health decision and is not limited to specific life-sustaining measures.

Do-Not-Resuscitate Orders

It is common practice in inpatient acute care hospital and skilled nursing facility settings to document in writing patient and family desires to "Do Not Resuscitate" (DNR) or "No CPR." The DNR and No CPR (cardiopulmonary resuscitation) are not effective until documented in the orders for patient treatment. Additionally, the patient, patient representative, or family member should sign an appropriate consent form or refusal-of-treatment form. Orders related to DNRs and No CPRs should be prominently displayed in the record so it is common knowledge. Failure to note such orders, resulting in inappropriate action, or inaction, may lead to legal liability. Although not legally mandated, best practices may require documentation of inquiry as to existing DNR or No CPR orders for patients seen in outpatient settings. Failure to respond in accordance with existing advanced directives, although not necessarily known to the treating clinician, could pose liability if determined that the standard of practice would be to obtain this information by patient interview.

Disagreeing Opinions Among Personnel/Staff

All healthcare providers have the duty to take reasonable actions to safeguard the lives of their patients. Using professional judgment, a PT may encounter a situation in which it is necessary to clarify or object to physician orders or inform the physician/nonphysician practitioner of contraindications to treatment. Documentation of professional disagreements should be done in a manner that is objective, factual, nonjudgmental, and could not be used as evidence against the physician or institution in a negligence lawsuit. For example, is it not appropriate to write, "Dr. Joe is negligent again" or "The order is incorrect." Most facilities will have policies and procedures for documenting professional differences of opinion.

Special Disclosures

Records Sought by Managed Care Organizations

MCOs often need access to patient health information to monitor discharge planning, conduct case management and utilization review, and credential healthcare professionals. Requests for access are often established by way of policies and procedures to reduce liability for negligent access. These policies typically adopt applicable laws relating to keeping confidentiality of patient information.

Records Sought by Law Enforcement

The general rule is that healthcare providers and organizations should not release medical records or other patient health information to requesting law enforcement agencies without written authorization of the patient. However, the HIPAA Privacy Rule permits covered entities to disclose protected health information (PHI) to law enforcement officials, without the individual's written authorization, under specific circumstances, such as to comply with a court order or to respond to an administrative request, such as a subpoena. For a full list of disclosures for law enforcement purposes that are permitted, see: https://www.hhs.gov/hipaa/for-professionals/faq/505/what-does-the-privacy-rule-allow-covered-entities-to-disclose-to-law-enforcement-officials/index.html. Be sure to also familiarize yourself with applicable state laws.

LEGAL ISSUES RELATED TO IMPROPER DISCLOSURE

Healthcare providers and facilities may be subject to civil and criminal liability for disclosing patient health information that has not been authorized by the patient, court-ordered, or required by law. State statutes and regulations provide for criminal and professional disciplinary sanctions. State laws and common law usually allow wronged individuals to file civil suits and seek recovery of damages.

Causes of Action for Releasing Information Without Authorization

To sue successfully, a patient must be able to prove the elements of the legal cause of action. The legal theories pertinent to medical information liability are defamation, invasion of privacy, and breach of confidentiality. A suit for defamation is typically based on common law, and the injured plaintiff must prove by greater weight of the evidence that (1) a false and defamatory statement was made about the patient; (2) the statement was published to a third party; (3) the publishing party knew the statement was false or acted with reckless disregard of its truth or falsity; and (4) injury was caused by the statement or the statement by nature was harmful. If accusing invasion of privacy, the patient must show evidence of the improper disclosure of patient information. Another legal theory often governed by state statute and used by patients to sue healthcare providers who disclose medical record information in breach of confidentiality or breach of physician–patient privilege. Generally, a violation of confidentiality results in liability for damages caused by the disclosure that may have resulted in the deterioration of a marriage, loss of a job, and suffering of emotional distress.

Medicare Disclosure

Pursuant to Social Security Act (SSA) Section 1806 (42 U.S.C 1395b-7), if a Medicare beneficiary submits a written request to a health services provider for an itemized statement for any item or service billed Medicare, the provider must furnish this statement within 30 days of the request.[24] Also pursuant to SSA Section 1806 to SSA 1806, a health services provider not furnishing this itemized statement may be subject to a civil monetary penalty of up to $100 for each unfulfilled request unless it can demonstrate that to do so would pose an undue burden.[25] The majority of healthcare organizations and providers have established an itemized billing system for internal accounting procedures and for collecting reimbursement from payers as well as patients. Accordingly, furnishing an itemized statement should not pose any significant additional burden to the provider. Also, other payers/state laws may require providers to disclose itemized statements within certain time frames.

RISK MANAGEMENT

Electronic Health Records

The HHS Office of the National Coordinator for Health Information Technology (ONC) defines an EHR as an electronic version of a patient's medical history. EHRs are real-time, patient-centered records that make information available instantly and securely to authorized users. The EMR is one component of the EHR.

The trend in medicine is to use and rely on technology. The method of maintaining patient medical records in paper files with eventual transfer to microfilm for safekeeping is antiquated. Even facsimile machines are being used much less frequently. An increasing number of providers use computers, computer networks, and optical scanning and storage equipment to create, transmit, store, and retrieve patient healthcare information. Although computerization enhances the quality of patient care, there are risks related to maintaining confidentiality of the information and complex legal issues regarding the duties and rights of providers. For instance, the HIPAA Security Rule requires covered entities to protect patients' ePHI. Covered entities must maintain reasonable and appropriate administrative, physical, and technical safeguards, ensuring the confidentiality, integrity, and availability of all ePHI they create, receive, maintain, or transmit.

Despite the growth in the use of EHRs, due to the lack of interoperability between EHR systems and healthcare providers, information blocking, and other hurdles, patients and practitioners have had little success in accessing, exchanging, and using patient information contained within EHRs. To address these issues, Congress passed the 21st Century Cures Act, signed into law on December 13, 2016, requiring HHS to improve the interoperability of health information. In spring 2019, both CMS and ONC put forward proposed policies to expand patient, clinician, and payer access to electronic health information by breaking down barriers to interoperability. On March 9, 2020, CMS and ONC released final regulations designed to enhance interoperability of electronic health information, increase patient access to health information, and limit information blocking., increase patient access to health information, and limit information block.[26]

Unfortunately, electronic data exchange from the numbers of computer links and electronic fund transfers also has opened the doors to potential healthcare fraud. The legal precedence and laws are not keeping pace with the advances in technology and do not provide much guidance for healthcare providers and organizations. Licensure laws and regulations and Medicare and accreditation standards require providers and facilities to safeguard records and protect against unauthorized access. The legal confidentiality obligations are the same for electronic and paper-based systems. Most legislative protections governing confidentiality of patient health information only apply when the medical record data identifies the patient. Therefore, cleansed—meaning properly de-identified data—may be used with very few restrictions.

There are legal questions regarding which state's law would apply to medical record information transmitted across state lines. Similarly, computerization of patient data increases risk of unauthorized disclosure. A breach of a computer system's security could result in numerous unauthorized disclosures and potentially catastrophic liability, since a system can access, copy, and transmit substantial numbers of records in short times. Therefore, reasonable safeguards employing password access and encryption may set legal standards of what should be built into the systems.

ELECTRONIC CLAIMS

Standards for processing of health claims electronically have been established per HIPAA and mandate compliance. (See the prior discussion in this chapter.)

TELEHEALTH MEDICAL RECORDS

The Health Resources and Services Administration (HRSA) defines telehealth as follows:

The use of electronic information and telecommunications technologies to support and promote long-distance clinical healthcare, patient and professional health-related education, public health and health administration. Technologies include videoconferencing, the Internet, store-and-forward imaging, streaming media, and terrestrial and wireless communications.

Clinicians delivering telehealth services across state lines are subject to applicable state laws and state licensing requirements for healthcare practitioners in both states. Although third-party payer coverage of telehealth services is limited, it is gradually expanding. Generally, state law requires the clinician to comply with the requirements of their home state and the state where the patient is located or fall within an exception as defined by state or federal law.

The practice of using electronic signals to communicate medical information generates potential legal issues regarding accuracy from distortion of data, confidentiality, and security of health information. Airwaves are not secure, and the confidentiality of patient health information cannot be guaranteed. This may include common social media communication platforms, such Skype or WhatsApp, or accidental communication via a virtual electronic assistance, such as Amazon's Alexa or Google Home.

Presently, there are very few legislative or accreditation requirements pertaining to the creation or maintenance of telemedical records. Because there are so few statutory or regulatory guidelines, a covered entity that uses telehealth must take the same precautions to safeguard PHI and establish safeguards to prevent disclosure of patient information to individuals or entities not involved in the patient's care. The documentation standards for telehealth are the same as for in-person services, and that HIPAA's rules and regulations are applicable to telehealth. PHI includes information that relates to the individual's past, present, or future physical or mental health or condition; the provision of healthcare to the individual; or the past, present, or future payment for the provision of healthcare to the individual and that identifies the individual or for which there is a reasonable basis to believe can be used to identify the individual. In addition to name, address, e-mail address, etc., identifiers include biometric identifiers, including finger or voice prints, full-face photographic images and any comparable images, and Internet Protocol (IP) address.

Serious risks of breach are associated with transferring patient information, including photos, through videoconferencing platforms, and the confidentiality of patient health information cannot be guaranteed. There also are concerns associated with the sharing of PHI in the presence of a voice assistant, as discussed later in this chapter. HIPAA requires providers to take reasonable administrative, technical, and physical safeguards to ensure the confidentiality of patient information. Therefore, covered entities should take precautions to prevent any unwanted disclosures of PHI. Covered entities should use remote access technology, such as virtual private networks (VPNs), to ensure the connection is secure and encrypted; password protecting the device being used to communicate with the patient; and, if applicable, password protecting photos or videos on the device.

E-VISIT RECORDS

E-visits do not satisfy the definition of Medicare telehealth services. E-visits are non–face-to-face, patient-initiated digital communications that require a clinical decision that otherwise would be provided in the clinic. An e-visit should have documentation that the e-visit was initiated by the patient, the patient consented to the e-visit, and the clinical decision-making that occurred as a result of the e-visit. Legal issues identified earlier in telehealth pertain to e-visits.[27]

ELECTRONIC MAIL

Electronic mail (e-mail) is increasingly used to transmit sensitive patient health information. Although the modes of e-mail transmission have occurred at a rapid pace, the implementation of related technological safeguards have not developed at a similar pace and are less than adequate, creating more challenges for keeping confidentiality and security of medical records. Providers who send electronic messages must be aware to exercise caution when transmitting patient information to avoid compromising the integrity of the data and to prevent a breach of patient confidentiality. Title III of the Omnibus Crime Control and Safe Streets Act of 1968, commonly known as the federal wiretapping law, provides protection against improper interception of electronic communications, such as e-mail, and imposes civil and criminal liabilities on violators.[28]

If a healthcare provider uses e-mail, it is important to develop policies and procedures addressing recording, retention, and destruction of the communications and implement reasonable safeguards to preserve PHI confidentiality. E-mail communications should be included in patient medical records and follow the guidelines of documentation. Encryption systems can be used to protect electronic communication.

VOICE-ASSISTED TECHNOLOGY

With the proliferation of voice-activated technology and virtual assistants, therapists and assistants are likely to encounter such technology when interacting with patients and may wish to use such technologies to help patients manage their conditions and access services. At the time of this writing, voice-activated assistants, such as Amazon Alexa and Google Home, do not yet fully satisfy HIPAA security and privacy requirements. However, this is likely to evolve in the future. Because HIPAA requires covered entities to take reasonable steps to limit the use or disclosure of, and requests for, PHI to the minimum extent necessary to accomplish the intended purpose, covered entities should take reasonable steps to avoid sharing PHI if there is a voice assistant in the room or near where treatment is being delivered and limit any use of a device to nonidentifiable health information.

MEDICAL RECORDS IN LEGAL PROCEEDINGS

Patient treatment records provide clinical information about the patient to the various healthcare providers involved in that patient's care. As a business record, it justifies to third-party payers the billing for services provided, allows for monitoring of quality patient care, sets forth needs for risk management, and provides a basis for clinical research and educational training. Legally, the records protect the patients, healthcare providers and organizations, and support staff. In litigation proceedings, the records may be the only written record of what transpired. As such, it could be effective for a positive defense against a claim of professional negligence or be the reason for an unfavorable decision against a provider. Failure to create or maintain the records is a breach of the duty owed the patient. If a breached duty results in a patient injury, then actionable malpractice may ensue.

Intentional failure to maintain records, or spoliation, is typically a criminal matter of fraud and obstruction of justice. A charge of spoliation can result in suspension or revocation of licensure and imposition of a fine. Healthcare providers must resist the urge to correct records that appear obviously erroneous. Changes to a record should be implemented in a manner as previously described. It is not difficult to spot an altered patient care entry. Common signs indicating alteration of a hard copy manual record include differences in handwriting, use of different writing instruments, erasures and/or obliteration or correction liquid, and nonuniform crowding of words particularly between lines or in margins. Similarly, signs of rewritten patient care entries may include differences in paper type, binder holes or other markings that do not match the rest of the record, date and/or time discrepancies, subsequent entries that seem out of context or confusing, findings not known at the time, and handwriting style or quality inconsistent with the writer. To avert dangers of spoliation, facility risk managers routinely segregate original patient records involving patients in litigated claims.

In EMRs, audits can be made to determine if changes have been based on electronic record access identification and times and dates on the access. EMR content should not be erased and written over once electronically signed.

DEFENSE: USE OF HEALTH RECORDS IN JUDICIAL PROCEEDINGS

Patient health records containing relevant information are usually admissible into evidence in judicial proceedings when someone is involved in the legal action. Under these circumstances, a court order by way of a *subpoena duces tecum* is issued to require production of the medical information. State regulations governing court procedure indicate whether original or copies of the health records, as routine business records, will suffice. A records custodian will need to testify as to the authenticity of any records produced.

Legal Proceedings

Plaintiffs file complaints against an individual or organization, called the defendant(s), and bring lawsuits against healthcare providers. The next phase of the litigation is discovery, at which time medical records are often produced and utilized to determine the strength or weakness of each party. In depositions, subpoenaed individuals, including the records custodian and authors of the records, may be required to produce records and other patient information, testify that health records were compiled in the normal course of business, and that they have not been altered in any manner. At trial, the medical records often are entered into evidence. Should a verdict or court decision be appealed, an appellate court may review medical records that were admitted into evidence at trial. If a PT or PTA is deposed as part of a legal action, they will be asked a series of questions. It is always best to answer with only the content read from the record, which should be legible and easy to read. The PT or PTA should not "try to remember." As this process, from the filing of a lawsuit to the actual trial could occur years after the injury to the patient, proper documentation may prove helpful in refreshing the memory of what transpired and is very important for defending the claim.

PROFESSIONAL LIABILITY

Medical malpractice refers to the professional liability of healthcare providers involved in the delivery of patient care. Professional liability may arise from breach of contract, intentional tort, and negligence theories.

The provider–patient relationship is established by either an express or an implied contract. Under either type of contract, a legal, contractual obligation arises from the relationship created and a promise to provide services at a certain standard of care, whereby the healthcare provider agrees to diagnose and/or treat the patient in accordance with standards of acceptable practice and to continue treating until the natural termination of the relationship, such as patient gets well or dies, mutual agreement to terminate, patient terminates, or healthcare provider withdraws from providing care. When the provider–patient relationship exists, failure to diagnose or treat using reasonable care and skill may give the patient cause to sue for breach of contract.

Healthcare providers can also be held liable when they intentionally harm a person under the legal theory of tort or strict liability. Intentional torts are wrongful acts that result in injury to another.

Negligence occurs when a healthcare provider commits a wrongful act by failing to do what another prudent reasonable healthcare provider would do under similar circumstances. Other causes of action against healthcare providers may include assault and battery, defamation, invasion of privacy, wrongful disclosure of confidential information, and abandonment.

RISK MANAGEMENT

AHIMA has published guidelines on health information management, health record documentation, and content based on the practice setting.[14] To reduce risk, all facilities providing patient care should have policies ensuring uniformity of content and format of healthcare records based on applicable accreditation standards, federal and state regulations, payer requirements, and professional practice standards. To satisfy legal requirements, many guidelines should be followed, including systematic organization of health records to facilitate retrieval and compilation of information and quantitative and qualitative analysis of health records to confirm that state law, regulation, or healthcare facility licensure standards are upheld as related to documentation.

COMPUTERIZED, PHOTOGRAPHIC, AND VIDEOTAPED PATIENT CARE RECORDS

Increasingly, more facilities are using computers to record patient data. Electronic records, however, pose a challenge to preserving patient confidentiality and create temptations to alter or erase prior patient entries. Therefore, facilities must develop safeguards to protect access to and unauthorized alteration of records generated.

Photographic documentation is also used by PTs and PTAs to memorialize before and after treatments. The photographic evidence—hard copy, video, digital, electronic or other—must be preserved in accordance with statutory retention requirements. Copying of photographs is more expensive and more time-consuming than paper, although computer scanning may reduce the cost.

Video documentation or digital recording memorializing patient status and treatment is also used by PTs. Provided the videotape meets certain legal standards, it may be admitted into evidence if needed. Videotapes must be retained in accordance with statutory requirements. Photography or videotaping typically requires explicit prior written informed consent. Please check state law for specific additional requirements.

SPECIAL CIRCUMSTANCES REQUIRING DOCUMENTATION: SEXUAL ASSAULT AND BATTERY

It is important to obtain and safeguard results of examinations and care given to victims of sexual assault or battery. Most facilities have written policies addressing recordation, storage, and transfer of patient health information to law enforcement authorities. Any statements made by a victim should be included in quotation marks in the documentation and may be admissible in a future court proceeding. Records of patients who are sexually assaulted should be maintained separate from the general patient care records. Facility policies and appropriate laws should be followed regarding reporting.

DOCUMENTATION OF PATIENT RESTRAINT USE

Providers must document certain things before using physical or chemical or pharmacological restraints on patients. This requirement resulted from the danger of misuse and neglect related to the use of such restraints, particularly in skilled nursing facilities. Practitioners must document clinical justification (patient behaviors) for using restraints by including documentation demonstrating that less restrictive alternatives were inadequate, other health providers have been consulted, and that the patient's physical and mental conditions have been considered. The potential for harm must be documented if the patient is not restrained. Documentation and policy for the use of physical and chemical restraints must be consistent with federal and applicable state laws. If not properly documented, there may be cause for legal action based on false imprisonment.

REIMBURSEMENT AND DOCUMENTATION

Documentation requirements for reimbursement are generally administratively controlled and constantly change. For this reason, it is important for therapists and assistants to familiarize themselves on an ongoing basis with applicable requirements. Legal issues involve whether the documentation constitutes larceny (theft) by fraudulent or deceptive practices. Healthcare fraud occurs when there is an untruthful representation of a material fact. Billing for services not rendered, waivers of patient co-payments and deductibles under Medicare Part B, violations of anti-kickback and self-referral laws, overutilization or unbundling of services, upcoding, or miscategorizing coding to enhance payments by third-party payers, if done knowingly, can result in an allegation of fraud. Inadequate patient care documentation may support or create a claim for fraud leading to investigation, sanctions, and liability with HHS. The penalties for reimbursement fraud range from civil fines to criminal convictions, administrative penalties, exclusion from the Medicare and Medicaid programs or other third-party payer systems, suspension or revocation of licensure, and professional association actions for ethical violations. Ignorance is not considered a reasonable explanation if a treating professional is unaware of changed regulations.

PROFESSIONAL GUIDELINES

The APTA's *Guide for Professional Conduct* illustrates ethical principles for therapists relative to documentation practices.[29] Professional conduct standards require that the PT–patient relationship is confidential and cannot be communicated to others without prior written consent from the patient, that peer-reviewed information cannot be released without written permission of the therapist, and that disclosure of medical information without patient consent may be done when necessary to protect the welfare of others in compliance with applicable laws. PTs cannot delegate to less qualified persons activities requiring the skill, knowledge, and judgment of a therapist. Ideally, documentation interpreting health information, examinations, diagnosis, development of the plan of care and goals, identification of precautions and contraindications, reevaluations, discharges, readjustments to plans of care, and follow-up planning are best done when the PT personally records the information. However, if support staff is used purely to transcribe or act as a scribe and the PT signs and/or countersigns such notes, it may be legally sufficient depending on state laws and payer policy. Ethically, the code specifies that the supervising therapist perform "identification and documentation of precautions, special problems, contraindications, goals, anticipated progress, and plans for reevaluation."

SUMMARY

Healthcare professionals will be held accountable for knowing, comprehending, and applying relevant state and federal laws and regulations to their specific practice settings. As pertinent laws and regulations are constantly evolving and changing, a practitioner has a professional responsibility to continually update their knowledge. Documentation that is appropriate, complete, and accurate not only contributes to quality patient care and prevents medical errors but also assists with defense against malpractice actions. Medical records containing inappropriate, incomplete, and inaccurate information may result in verdicts against the healthcare organization and/or practitioner.

REVIEW QUESTIONS

1. What is informed consent? Explain the relevance to physical therapy documentation.
2. What is HIPAA? What is the relevance to medical records keeping and physical therapy documentation?
3. During what stage of litigation are medical records used? What are they used for?
4. While documentation cannot solve the dilemma of extending treatment for those who have been terminated by third-party payers, what role can it play in premature discharge?
5. What is authentication in documentation?
6. What is the "rule" for the use of abbreviations in documentation? What are the risks and benefits?
7. Explain how errors in documentation should be corrected.
8. What is the role of an addendum?
9. What is countersignature or co-signature? In what circumstances is it applicable in PT documentation?
10. What are the benefits of dating and putting the time of treatment on an entry?
11. Are patients entitled to copies of their records? Explain your answer.
12. What are the emerging challenges with protecting electronic or computerized documentation?
13. Explain the importance of legibility in the medical record.
14. A large hospital has physical therapy services in multiple units: cardiac, orthopedic, general medical, trauma, and pediatrics. Although the SOAP note format is used, the PTs and PTAs on each unit put different information in each category. Explain if this is or is not best practice.
15. Outpatient physical therapy facilities have historically not included whether a patient has a DNR. Should this be added to routinely obtain patient information? Provide a rationale for your answer.
16. Jane Smith has just passed her national physical therapy board exam after completing a Doctor of Physical Therapy degree and is licensed in Florida. How should Jane sign her medical record entries?

REFERENCES

1. Scott RW. *Legal Aspects of Documenting Patient Care for Rehabilitation Professionals*. 4th ed. Sudbury, MA: Jones and Bartlett Learning; 2011.
2. *Who Are Physical Therapist Assistants?* American Physical Therapy Association. Alexandria, VA. Available at https://www.apta.org/AboutPTAs/. Accessed August 5, 2020.
3. *Physical Therapist Assistant Job Responsibilities*. Workable. Available at https://resources.workable.com/physical-therapist-assistant-job-description. Accessed August 5, 2020.
4. Pagano MP. *Authoring Patient Records: An Interactive Guide*. Sudbury, MA: Jones and Bartlett Learning; 2011.
5. *Guide to Physical Therapist Practice*. 3.0 edition. American Physical Therapy Association. Alexandria, VA. Available at http://guidetoptpractice.apta.org/content/current. Accessed August 5, 2020. ISBN: 978-1-931369-85-5. doi:10.2522/ptguide3.0_978-1-931369-85-5.
6. Scott RW. *Health Care Malpractice: A Primer on Legal Issues for Professionals*. 2nd ed. New York, NY: McGraw-Hill; 1998.
7. *APTA Code of Ethics*. American Physical Therapy Association. Alexandria, VA. Available at https://www.apta.org/apta-and-you/leadership-and-governance/policies/code-of-ethics-for-the-physical-therapist. Accessed August 5, 2020.
8. *HIPAA Disclosure*. Available at https://www.hhs.gov/hipaa/for-professionals/security/index.html. Accessed August 5, 2020.
9. *National Association of Insurance Commissioners Insurance Information and Privacy Protection Model Act (NAIC Model Act)*. National Association of Insurance Commissioners. Available at http://www.naic.org/. Accessed August 5,2020.
10. *Privacy Act of 1974*. Available at https://www.justice.gov/opcl/privacy-act-1974. Accessed August 5, 2020.
11. *The Freedom of Information Act*. Available at http://www.justice.gov/oip/foia_updates/Vol_XVII_4/page2.htm. Accessed August 5, 2020.
12. *American Recovery and Reinvestment Act of 2009*. Available at https://www.ntia.doc.gov/page/2011/american-recovery-and-reinvestment-act-2009. Accessed August 5, 2020.
13. *Breech Notification Rule*. U.S. Department of Health & Human Services. Available at https://www.hhs.gov/hipaa/for-professionals/breach-notification/index.html. Accessed August 5, 2020.
14. *American Health Information Management Association (AHIMA)*. Available at http://perspectives.ahima.org/PDF/Finished/bok1_038947.pdf. Accessed August 5, 2020.
15. *APTA Defensible Documentation for Patient/Client Management*. American Physical Therapy Association. Alexandria, VA. Available at https://www.apta.org/your-practice/documentation. Accessed August 5, 2020.
16. [42 C.F.R. sect. 482.24 (hospitals); 42 C.F.R. sect. 418.74 (hospices); and 42 C.F.R. sect. 484.48 (home health agencies)]. Available at http://edocket.access.gpo.gov/cfr_2004/octqtr/42cfr482.24.htm. Accessed August 5, 2020.
17. *APTA Guidelines: Elements of Documentation Within the Patient/Client Management Model*. American Physical Therapy Association. Alexandria, VA. Available at https://www.apta.org/your-practice/documentation/defensible-documentation/elements-within-the-patientclient-management-model. Accessed August 5, 2020.
18. *Criminal Penalties For Acts Involving Federal Health Care Programs*. Available at http://www.ssa.gov/OP_Home/ssact/title11/1128B.htm. Accessed August 5, 2020.
19. *H.R.4449—The Patient Self-Determination Act of 1990*. Available at https://www.congress.gov/bill/101st-congress/house-bill/4449. Accessed August 5, 2020.
20. *Health Information Policy*. HHS.gov. Available at https://www.hhs.gov/hipaa/for-professionals/faq/760/must-a-covered-provider-obtain-individual-authorization-to-disclose-to-an-interpreter/index.html. Accessed August 5, 2020.
21. *AHIMA's Long-Term Care Health Information Practice and Documentation Guidelines*. American Health Information Management Association. Available at http://bok.ahima.org/Pages/Long%20Term%20Care%20Guidelines%20TOC/Legal%20Documentation%20Standards/Documentation%20Standards. Accessed August 5, 2020..
22. *Contract Provisions* 42 CFR 422.504. Government Publishing Office. Available at https://www.govinfo.gov/app/details/CFR-2011-title42-vol3/CFR-2011-title42-vol3-sec422-504. Accessed August 5, 2020.
23. *Policies and Procedures and Documentation Requirements*. 45 CFR 164.316(b)(2). Government Publishing Office. Available at https://www.govinfo.gov/app/details/CFR-2011-title45-vol1/CFR-2011-title45-vol1-sec164-316. Accessed August 5, 2020.
24. *Explanation of Medicare benefits: 1806*. Social Security Administration. Available at https://www.ssa.gov/OP_Home/ssact/title18/1806.htm. Accessed October 10, 2020.
25. *Section 4311(b) of the Balanced Budget Act of 1997*. Available at https://www.govinfo.gov/content/pkg/PLAW-105publ33/html/PLAW-105publ33.htm. Accessed August 5, 2020.
26. *HHS Finalizes Historic Rules to Provide Patients More Control of Their Health Data*. U.S. Department of Health & Human Services. Available at https://www.hhs.gov/about/news/2020/03/09/hhs-finalizes-historic-rules-to-provide-patients-more-control-of-their-health-data.html. Accessed October 10, 2020.
27. *Telehealth in PT Practice*. American Physical Therapy Association. Alexandria, VA. Available at https://www.apta.org/your-practice/practice-models-and-settings/telehealth-practice/quick-guide-to-using-e-visits-by-pts. Accessed October 10, 2020.
28. *Title III of the Omnibus Crime Control and Safe Streets Act of 1968*. Available at http://it.ojp.gov/default.aspx?area=privacy&page=1284. Accessed August 5, 2020.
29. *APTA's Guide for Professional Conduct*. Available at http://www.apta.org/uploadedFiles/APTAorg/Practice_and_Patient_Care/Ethics/GuideforProfessionalConduct.pdf. Accessed August 5, 2020.

12 Utilization Review and Utilization Management

OBJECTIVES

Following completion of this chapter, the reader will be able to:

- Explain what utilization review is.
- Describe the difference between utilization review and utilization management.
- Compare and contrast retrospective, concurrent, and prospective review processes.
- Define a technical error and how they can be avoided.
- Compare and contrast first- and second-level denials and their appropriate appeals.
- Compare and contrast internal and external utilization review.
- Explain the benefits of expressing examination findings in numeric terms.

INTRODUCTION

Documentation is the means of communicating information from the professional to all users of the medical record whether electronic or manual. It is the "what" physical therapists and physical therapist assistants do, "how" it is performed, and the outcomes. It is imperative to clearly and concisely communicate only the information that is relevant and necessary about care provided and the resulting condition of the patient or client. Although there are multiple definitions for utilization management (UM), of which utilization review is a component, according to the American Physical Therapy Association (APTA),[1] UM "is based on the information derived from the review process both internal and external to the organization providing services, to ensure quality of service and effective and efficient delivery. Provision of care when looked at through utilization review (UR) should include verification of benefits and applicable co-payments prior to the start of care."[1]

According to Institute of Medicine (now National Academy of Medicine) Committee on Utilization Management, employers or governmental programs that purchase medical care can use UM in one of three ways.[2] The purchaser can:

- *engage in utilization management directly*
- *contract with another organization for utilization management services, as Medicare and many employers do; or*

- *shift some of the financial risk to another party, such as an insurer (HMO, PPO) that is then faced with the same three choices of doing utilization management directly, contracting for the services, or shifting risk to still another party (for example, physicians or hospitals).*

Regardless of who or what entity is performing the UM, it is critical to the process that the treating physical therapist is aware of the third-party payer coverage and benefits a patient or client has to ensure that the length of stay (LOS), interventions, and services provided are included in the benefits available and that the organization or primary treating physical therapist is an approved provider if required by a patient's third-party payer.

APTA[1] defines utilization review as "a system for reviewing the medical necessity, appropriateness and reasonableness of services proposed or provided to a patient or group of patients. This review is conducted on a prospective, concurrent and or retrospective basis to reduce the incidence of unnecessary and or inappropriate provision of services. UR is a process that has two primary purposes: to improve the quality of service (patient outcomes) and to ensure the efficient expenditure of money."[1] To further break this down, the goals are:

- Delivery of value-based, cost effective, high-quality physical therapy services

  Consistent with the patient's benefits (third-party payer), with sensitivity and knowledge about a patient's financial responsibility such as deductibles and amount of co-payment per visit, which has escalated in recent years as third-party payers or employers shift risk to the insured.[3]
- Identification of duplicative, inappropriate, or less effective and less efficient services with corrective action

  Identification of appropriate and effective services, within the context of the patient's benefit plan and financial responsibility. Nonduplication of services that may be billed by other non–physical therapy practitioners using the same physical medicine Current Procedural Terminology (CPT) codes may preclude payment for physical therapy, especially in the absence of skilled supporting documentation clearly describing the physical therapy services and goals
- Assurance of compliance with accreditation and licensing guidelines
- Ensuring the continuum of care in a timely manner
- Assurance that medically necessary and skilled care was delivered
- Avoidance of unnecessary care beyond goals or beyond the point of progress
- Delivery of service not indicated in plan of care (POC)
- Service not rendered for problems identified (or unrelated to diagnosis/es)
- No baseline level of care provision based on information provided
- Referral(s) to other practitioners when out of the physical therapist's scope of "expertise" by training, experience, or otherwise
- Risk management (prevention of all types of loss)
- Appropriate physical therapy personnel provided care for level of skill required or by virtue of third-party payer requirements.

Currently, three areas of UR are identified within the process: retrospective, prospective, and concurrent

HISTORY OF UTILIZATION REVIEW

UR is considered a component of quality assurance and may be referred to as utilization review quality assurance (URQA).[4] In organizations or facilities with ongoing quality improvement or quality assurance programs and monitoring, URQA is often used for monitoring.

Prior to 1965, UR was largely experimental and not performed by many providers. Medicare introduced a new era in accountability with a requirement for all hospitals participating in Medicare and Medicaid programs to also form UR committees and develop written UR plans. Initially, the programs were not successful because the focus was on the fiscal portion of care, the interpretations were inconsistent, and the coordination of benefits was often nonexistent. In 1972, professional standards review organizations (PSROs) primarily for physician services were instituted. PSROs employed nonphysicians and physicians to review the appropriateness and quality of medical services. Although nonphysicians performed the initial review and could affirm care, only a physician could deny services. Little was done with rehabilitation review, however, with the focus instead being on the medical care. Hospitals were required to subscribe to a concurrent review performed during care and a care evaluation program. This process was the precursor to the eventual development of critical pathways in the 1980s and early 1990s associated with the growth of managed care and acknowledgement of the importance of the process.

PSROs evolved into peer review organizations (PROs) in the early 1980s, concurrent with the advent of Medicare inpatient acute care diagnostic related groups (DRGs), with a continued focus on medical services. Based on the Peer Review Improvement Act part of the Tax Equity and Fiscal Responsibility Act (1982), the PSRO program was replaced with the Utilization and Quality Control Peer Review Organization program for utilization and quality monitoring. To increase consistency and effectiveness of quality review organizations, Congress established the PROs to monitor both quality and utilization.[5] The PROs emphasized retrospective reviews with standard pre-established review criteria based on professionally recognized treatment standards versus the concurrent review stressed by the PRSOs. Because of escalating costs to Medicare, there was an increased interest in productivity standards versus quality-of-care standards for physical therapy and other rehabilitation services. The escalating costs to Medicare also started the early growth of managed care organizations such as health maintenance organizations (HMOs) and preferred provider organizations (PPOs), as well as hospital-based Diagnostic Related Group (DRGs). As a result, as organizations focused on physical therapist's productivity versus quality of care, physical therapists practicing in the 1980s experienced some of the first denials for physical therapy services provided to Medicare beneficiaries. Because of cost shifting as a result of the impact of early shorter hospital stays, Medicare UR was expanded to include physical therapy services in skilled nursing facilities: Part A for short-term skilled rehabilitation, Part B for long-term residents, and other outpatient services under Part B. This ultimately extended to Medicare home health as well. This evolved from the Medicare initiative for improvement in efficiency; effectiveness; and skilled, medically necessary care for hospital inpatient care. Initiation of UR by the Centers for Medicare & Medicaid Services (CMS) for the Medicare program created added financial risk for physical therapists (PTs) and organizations providing Part B services.

The practice of UR was and is not exclusive to Medicare. Coincident with the rise in Medicare denials for services, private payer sources looked to the Medicare system for cost containment measures. This is not surprising, as the same companies that contract with CMS to make coverage decisions and pay providers for services they furnish to Medicare beneficiaries (Medicare Administrative Contractors [MACs]) (formerly known as fiscal intermediaries) also provided commercial insurance products. Application of UR practices facilitated examination of medical necessity, effectiveness, and efficiency of care with maximization of outcomes for all services to all patients. In the 21st century, as costs for healthcare continue to grow exponentially, the rise in the interest of evidence-based practice with the alignment to clinical practice guidelines, critical pathways, and algorithms is a result of the need for justification of value-based care.[6] By engaging in UR and UM practices, physical therapists should be able to justify care by clearly identifying medical necessity and the skilled care provided by documenting efficient and effective quality care. These practices can also provide outcome data necessary in a value-based environment to support the efficacy of intervention and the concept of evidence-based practice.

INTERNAL UR/UM PRACTICES

Internal UR and UM practices are based on review of documentation by a UR-designated professional or group of individuals. The physical therapist (PT) and and physical therapist assistant (PTA) must know for whom they are writing, what information must be conveyed and the purpose for which the information will be used. From a UR and medical record perspective, the purposes include reimbursement; effective and efficient utilization of internal resources, such as staff to monitor productivity; determination of staffing needs; consistency of content in the record; consistency and objectivity of goal setting; and effective and efficient selection of interventions and outcome data established by individual physical therapists, as well as effective communication between professionals and others who may view the record. The way the information is recorded should be the same, regardless of the purpose of the review. With the growth of the electronic health record (EHR) and the electronic medical record (EMR), there is evidence of increased standardization of record components. This is a principle of health information management, as described by the American Health Information Management Association (AHIMA).[7] An organization, as part of an ongoing quality management program, can review the content of the medical records for compliance with expectations. Concurrent and retrospective reviews can be utilized to ensure concurrent compliance during an active episode of care, confirm content is error free, confirm content is written in a skilled manner and is legally admissible, revise guidelines for the future, develop clinical pathways or algorithms, ensure effective and efficient care and outcomes, and provide educational input to staff for improvement in documentation process and content. Ultimately, it is the documentation, coding, and billing information that is critical to the UM/UR process. Both CMS and APTA have published guidelines for documentation, and the American Medical Association's CPT coding system should facilitate documentation verbiage for interventions provided.[8] It is also critical that the PT know, prior to the start of care, what a patient's insurance plan and benefits include. If the PT is not responsible for obtaining coverage information, the individual(s) responsible should be communicating information to the treatment team. For example, if a plan limitation is 20 physical therapy visits/year, it is 20 visits, regardless of what the PT, physician, or patient believe is medically necessary or how many episodes of illness or injury an individual may have in 1 year. Some payers allow coverage for physical therapy services for 60 days from the first visit or a predetermined number of days. Therefore, visits and timing should be used appropriately. If preoperative visits are necessary, they should be scheduled with the understanding that fewer visits will be available after the operation.

Ignorance of policy limitations will result in denial of any care rendered beyond the limit. However, once benefits have been exhausted, if additional physical therapy intervention is indicated based on patient goals, additional services may be offered on a cash-pay basis. In this case, although documentation remains a requirement, external UR would not be a factor.

UTILIZATION REVIEW AND PAYMENT

From a payment perspective, documentation must present a clear picture of the episode of care. The elements in the record reviewed are the referral or authorization (if required by the payer), such as the signed POC by a physician or authorized professional; the information included for the initial examination and evaluation, including history; the POC that matches the patient's complaints, problems, and goals, consistent with the International Classification of Functioning, Disability, and Health (ICF) model;[9] all tests, measures, and examinations performed and the objective data; objective and measurable goals with patient agreement; documentation of continued care with daily notes, progress notes, and progress reports; and documentation of summation of episode of care or discharge.[10]

Evidence of continued or continuing care includes documentation of interventions or services provided and current patient status and documentation of re-examination with recording of time of care and total units or minutes. Colloquially, these entries are referred to as treatment notes, progress notes/reports, and periodic summaries (i.e., monthly, weekly, or as designated by policy). They can also be reflected in flow sheet format or variations of checklists with clarifying additional entry, although flow sheets and checklists may be the most likely component of a record to result in denial if they do not include the skill needed by the PT or PTA.

Documentation of summation of the episode of care, or discharge, occurs at the termination or discontinuation of therapy services for a specific episode or LOS. Although

PTAs may enter components of a discharge, the PT is responsible for overall report and discharge recommendations and instructions. Termination or discontinuation may occur for a variety of reasons and must be clearly documented for UR purposes. Based on the APTA definitions,[11] termination of care occurs when a patient or client has met the established physical therapy goals. However, discontinuation may result from reasons, such as lack of progress, illness or change in medical status, hospitalization, patient noncompliance (with specific descriptions of what led to this conclusion), excessive absenteeism (with evidence that the patient was contacted and documented or that an attempt to contact was documented), inappropriate patient behavior, physician decision, decision of third-party payer, decision of a case manager, or patient self-discontinuation of care. Noncompliance in this context is lack of patient compliance with instructions, thus impeding progress in an effective and efficient manner or potentially resulting in harm. Prolonged illness that prevents participation in scheduled therapy must result in discontinuation. However, recovery and renewed ability to participate can result in resumption of care, although if more than 1 or 2 weeks have passed and the physical status has changed, it may be considered a new episode of care or require a new evaluation, revised POC, and communication with the physician (if not a self-referral).

The documentation should emphasize a patient's ability to perform tasks, social roles, and the environment as described in the International Classification of Function by the World Health Organization (WHO),[9] while addressing the disability and function as well as impairments. The APTA has now moved to the ICF model. The impairments are the pathological and physiological consequences of the disease or injury process. The functional limitations are the inability to perform a task in an efficient or competent manner as a result of the impairments. The relationship between the impairments and functional limitations should be clearly identifiable in the documentation as justification for care and appropriateness of intervention in coordination "Body functions and structures" and "activities and participation" replace the previously used terms of "impairment," "disability," and "handicap."[12]

> *Example of application of the ICF Model: "person who has a labeled diagnosis of a cerebral vascular accident (CVA). The labeled diagnosis imparts no information about that person's functioning. In addition, the mere fact that a person requires an assistive device and ambulates less than 500 feet safely does not provide a detailed picture of how this person is able to function in his or her community and chosen role. Does he live alone in a rural community or does she live in an assisted living community with her spouse? The resulting disability in these different scenarios provides rationale for the need to categorize function beyond a diagnostic category."*[12]

The review process takes each documentation element included in the record and examines it for relevancy to the whole picture of the patient's functional needs versus the current functional status. Because this is often based on the level or function of the patient prior to the "recent" functional change, referred to as prior level of function (PLOF), it is imperative to clearly indicate this in the initial examination and evaluation process. If an episode of care has ended or the review is occurring at any point in time during the episode, the information contained in the initial report should be similar in structure and content to allow easy comparison of data. It is important to identify the reason for the referral, whether the examination concurs with the reason for referral (as indicated by the physician) and what the physical therapist's evaluation of the patient's potential for responding to therapeutic interventions will be, or the prognosis when considering the reason for referral, a clear indication should be made of the medical diagnosis versus the treatment or physical therapy diagnosis. Depending on the reason for care, they may be the same or different. Based on the International Statistical Classification of Diseases and Related Health Problems (ICD-10) diagnosis coding, the physical therapy diagnosis is more likely to be functional or impairment based (body function in the ICF model).[13]

There are technical components that can be addressed with an overall review, as described in detail in the APTA *Guidelines for Physical Therapy Documentation* (see Appendix E).[10]

INITIAL EXAMINATION AND EVALUATION/ CONSULTATION

The review of the examination and evaluation/consultation is performed to establish that the documentation provides clear, cohesive data that supports the evaluation conclusions and the need for skilled physical therapy services. It is important to review each document and section as to their relevance to patient management. This documentation should include a clear statement regarding the method of referral (self-referral in states and settings that allow for direct access or a referral from another practitioner) if the services are outpatient. Patients in inpatient facilities receiving inpatient PT services should have this inherent in the documentation and physician orders. If the review is being performed by a third-party payer or by an internal representative, the meaning of all content must be evident.

INITIAL EPISODE OF PHYSICAL THERAPY CARE

Demographic Information

The relating of the demographic information such as full legal name, address, age, gender, date of birth, primary and secondary languages, living environment, family/social support, and potential discharge plans and destinations can affect the rehabilitation potential and overall prognosis. The reviewer should see those items that are relevant to the delivery of service and any additional services (referrals) that may be required to address the patient's desired outcomes. A patient living alone in a home with stairs and the bathroom on the second floor has very different needs than a patient living in a one-bedroom apartment on the ground floor of an apartment building. These should be evident in the documentation of the history. The living situation and type of dwelling may also present barriers to what would otherwise facilitate function (e.g., space limiting use of power mobility, inaccessible bathroom and/or bathing facilities, or inability to function in the kitchen because of space or height limitations).

The history (and interview if possible) is reviewed to determine the patient's medical diagnoses and factors that may affect the length of care/LOS, frequency of intervention, or precautions necessary during the delivery of service, as well as evidence of informed consent. This will also allow the reviewer to determine if the appropriate risks and benefits were reviewed during the informed consent process. The care of the patient will be affected by the comorbidities documented and the demographic information obtained in the history. The information documented in the history, such as living environment, comorbidities and medications, social support/potential caregivers, services (either concurrent or prior), and patient knowledge and expectations (goals), will need to be interpreted in the evaluation to determine the exact effect and relationship to the overall care and specifically to the treatment plan and goals established. Multiple comorbidities and polypharmacy contribute to patient complexity that should be reflected in the initial evaluation. The specific relationship of this information to the POC should be clearly documented and evident to the reviewer, as he or she may make assumptions based on experience or knowledge. The following sections illustrate the elements that should be clearly identified for sound documentation and review purposes.

Diagnosis/Date of Onset

The date of onset and medical and physical therapy diagnoses are important both clinically and for reimbursement purposes. The diagnoses selected from the referral should reflect the medical condition that relates directly to the reason for the functional deficits and should be ICD-10 codable. The diagnosis is the starting point for determining and ensuring appropriate prioritized testing and examination, including standardized outcome measures and, ultimately, appropriate interventions and objective and measurable goals. It is therefore important for the reviewer to see clear documentation of the differentiation between the primary diagnosis and the secondary diagnoses. The selections of the diagnoses are based on the factors surrounding the onset of symptoms/functional problem and, for therapeutic purposes, include functional and body structure and function. The onset could cross provider settings and therefore must reflect the circumstances surrounding the reason for physical therapy, as well as if the patient had previous physical therapy for the same condition. The reviewer may determine that the diagnosis selected reflects a chronic condition or the onset of symptoms that may not reflect an acute condition. This would be a red flag to the payment procedure and would require substantiation within the documentation to support the current provision of skilled services. The physical therapy or treatment diagnosis may be the same as the medical diagnosis in some cases, but it is advisable to also list all functionally based diagnoses, including those directly relating to physical therapy.

Author's Note

There are many questions about the first-listed diagnosis for patients receiving outpatient PT services. The Health Insurance Portability and Accountability Act requires assigning ICD-10-CM diagnosis codes according to the ICD-10-CM Official Guidelines for Coding and Reporting. The ICD-10-CM Official Guidelines for Coding and Reporting for Fiscal Year 2020 state:

"In the outpatient setting, the term first-listed diagnosis is used in lieu of principal diagnosis. In determining the first-listed diagnosis the coding conventions of ICD-10 CM, as well as the general disease specific guidelines take precedence over the outpatient guidelines.

List the first ICD-10 CM code for the diagnosis, condition, problem, or other reason for encounter/visit shown in the medical record to be chiefly responsible for the services provided. List additional codes that describe any coexisting conditions. In some cases, the first-listed diagnosis may be a symptom when a diagnosis has not been established (confirmed) by the provider.

Codes that describe symptoms and signs, as opposed to diagnoses, are acceptable for reporting purposes when a related definitive diagnosis has not been established (confirmed) by the provider."[13]

Example[14]

Musculoskeletal:

Medical diagnosis: M76.61 Achilles tendinitis, right leg

Treatment diagnoses: edema, joint range limitation, gait dysfunction, pain limiting function, impaired strength

Author's Note

If the condition is chronic but there is an exacerbation, exacerbation with remission, a change in function, or need for new instruction or intervention, this must be clearly indicated. In rarer cases, a patient's medical status may actually improve, justifying physical therapy, as in a patient who arouses from a coma or whose cardiac or respiratory status may stabilize enough for functionally oriented intervention.

The UR process is key for ensuring that supportive documentation is in place because this drives the process for payment purposes and internal and external decisions regarding appropriateness of services. The documentation must reflect why specific skilled intervention at this time is critical to the patient's functional status.

Secondary Diagnoses/Comorbidities

The review includes consideration of the secondary diagnoses/comorbidities, as these can affect the selection of and response to therapy. The documentation should reflect the complexity of the medical conditions pertinent to the therapeutic process. The complexity of the medical condition is often omitted and can prevent the reviewer from accurately assessing the true needs of the patient.

Example

Initial referral and WB instructions: PT Eval and Treat: Medical: Fx R hip/ORIF, NWB × 6 weeks

PT/Treatment Diagnosis: difficulty in walking (ICD-10 R26.2), functional decline, weakness right and left lower extremities, R hip joint, range of motion limitations in R hip, pain in R hip, edema R hip with bruising, balance instability, life management difficulty, fatigue and endurance limitations

Medical history: CAD s/p CABG × 3 years, HTN, DM type 2, osteoporosis

Author's Note: Based on the underlying cardiac pathology, DM (diabetes mellitus), and osteoporosis, monitoring of this patient's vital signs, blood glucose levels, and activity tolerance should be included in the plan.

Medications

Documentation of the patient medication regimen is important to the review process because it can affect the interventions performed during patient care. UR should ensure that the medications and their complicating effects to the therapeutic process are clearly documented. Once identified, the reviewer should look for the precautions and modifications to the treatment interventions that are related to the medications identified. In addition, polypharmacy may result in balance issues, with risk increasing with four or more medications. This may support justification for physical therapy.[15]

Example

Medications: atenolol, furosemide, diltiazem, zolpidem

Note: Monitor pulse (observe for physical signs and symptoms (S&S) of distress as atenolol-beta blocker, will keep pulse lower than otherwise expected), monitor blood pressure (diuretics and diltiazem), monitor for need to urinate (furosemide) without signs of incontinence or urgency, schedule mid to late morning or later in day (zolpidem—for sleep), balance and fall precautions with appropriate intervention based on testing secondary to polypharmacy including diuretic, beta blocker, dilitazem, and zolpidem

History of Prior Treatment

Beware of duplication of services, especially with simultaneous patient management.[16] A patient's history of prior treatment may include prior intervention for the same diagnosis by physicians, chiropractors, physical therapists, adjunctive treatments, or alternative practitioners. This history can support the rehabilitation potential for return to prior function. It is important to relate what has benefited the patient in the past and/or current episode of care, especially in the prior therapy interventions for exacerbations of the same diagnosis. However, even if the interventions were primarily palliative without active patient involvement, although they may have helped, they may result in denial of physical therapy. The utilization of previously unsuccessful modalities and interventions would be hard to support. Utilizing interventions that have been successful are easily supported, as the reasonable expectation would be substantiated by the prior response to the treatment. If no treatment has been provided for this diagnosis or if it is a new problem, documentation of this can be beneficial as well. If the condition is recurring or episodic in nature, the reviewer may also look for instruction in techniques that may alter the potential for recurrence or exacerbation.

A red flag, however, may occur when different professionals are treating the same patient simultaneously. CPT billing codes, with the exception of the physical therapy evaluation codes and the re-evaluation code, are physical medicine and rehabilitation codes that can be used by different professionals. Documentation must include clear justification of the skill needed by the PT or PTA with goals specific to physical therapy.

DIAGNOSTIC TESTING AND EXAMINATION

Documentation of the performed diagnostic testing and examination assists in the determination of the value of care, medical necessity, and rehabilitation potential of patients. All appropriate categories should be included with objective findings. Reducing data to numbers, and in numeric format when possible, is universally understood. Reliable and valid tests and measures that can be administered at initial examination, periodically throughout care as indicated, and at the end of care will facilitate justification. Standardized tests and measures establish baselines for patient performance and function. Over time, they can be used to demonstrate successful, value-based outcome measures based on established norms or overall improvement. Standardized self-reports can also be used as valuable outcome tools to justify intervention, such as longer periods of uninterrupted sleep at night, which cannot be observed in the clinical setting.

APTA's Outpatient Physical Therapy Improvement in Movement Assessment Log (OPTIMAL) is an instrument that measures difficulty and self-confidence in performing 22 movements that a patient needs to accomplish in order to do various functional activities.[7] It is an example of a potential standardized assessment tool with patient self-reporting that can be used to assess function over time.[17]

Cognition

Recording data on the cognitive ability of the patient is often a difficult task for the physical therapist. However, it is extremely important to the UR process and can, when well written, justify the necessity of the frequency and duration of the program determined by the PT.

Documentation of confusion or disorientation is often done in a vague manner and lacks sufficient information to determine the appropriate utilization of services. No payment source would pay for services with a patient who is unable to follow the therapeutic program or clearly be able to benefit from the program. Most PTs document orientation with a person, place, time scale, or statement of ability to follow a number of step directions. This can be augmented indicating the type of direction or instruction: verbal, tactile, or visual, with the time needed to respond to the directions given or the need for repetition. Appropriate utilization of services may need to be expanded due to the skill required to determine and present the appropriate stimulus to elicit the desired response.

Local medical review policies or Local Coverage Determinations (LCDs) by Medicare Administrative Contractors[18] and many other payers have established guidelines that may limit coverage for certain diagnoses that affect cognition. These guidelines may require short interventions with more frequent assessments to clearly justify the appropriate utilization of services. In these cases, providing documentation that the patient has appropriate cognition to participate in therapy and to benefit is important to assure that the cognitive status will not interfere with the rehabilitation.

PATIENT GOALS

The patient goals should be written in objective and measurable language in order to determine, as the treatment progresses, that the physical therapist and patient are working toward the same outcomes. In cases in which prevention of functional decline is the goal versus improvement, or when a patient is declining and goals are being revised to maximize function with the therapeutic intervention, it is up to the physical therapist to clearly document the purpose and medical status. All goals must match problems identified in the initial exam or re-examination or reassessment, as indicated, utilizing the appropriate interventions to achieve reasonable goals. The PT should include the patient and family and/or caregivers as appropriate in the discussion of anticipated goals to ensure compliance with interventions and home instructions, as family members or caregivers may need to be involved in the administration of these. If the patient has been provided a home exercise plan (HEP) or other instructions, they should be clearly documented and incorporated into the time for the activity instructed (i.e., HEP should be included with therapeutic exercise).

Example

Instruction to caregivers should be clearly stated in the goals with demonstration of achievement, such as:

Wife will demonstrate safe and independent wheelchair to car transfers of husband in order to provide safe transport upon discharge from __________.

All immediate caretakers participating in care for patient will be able to independently transfer patient to and from wheelchair to bed.

PROFESSIONAL TERMINOLOGY

Although the language in the medical record must be professional and indicate the need for skilled care, it must also be universally understood by anyone who has reason to review the record. Choice of word combinations can influence payment and determination of medical necessity (see Tables 12-1 and 12-2 for a list of nondescriptive and descriptive phrases and common physical therapy terms and their functional phrase alternative). The concept of "training" should be emphasized relative to functional activities such as gait training, balance training, and transfer training. The verbiage that is consistent with CPT codes should precede the entry content.

Example

Therapeutic Exercise: LLE: strengthening with manual resistance, PNF

Therapeutic Activities: transfer training bed to and from chair, sit to and from stand

The results of the tests and measures in any examination should identify the link between the information gathered in the history to specific tests and measures, determining baselines

Table 12-1 Nondescriptive and Descriptive Phrases[19]

NONDESCRIPTIVE PHRASES	DESCRIPTIVE PHRASE ALTERNATIVES
1. Poor quad contraction	Per manual muscle test right quadriceps strength is poor; 2-/5, with minimal palpable contraction limiting ability to stabilize LE in standing and transfers
2. Patient unable to balance unsupported in sitting	Patient exhibits sitting balance loss to the left and posteriorly with postural instability in unsupported sitting when attempting to lean for positional shifts and reaching for objects in all directions, requiring tactile cueing and manual external positional repositioning (contact guard with verbal cueing to correct).
3. Ambulation: Distance is improved from 30 feet to 200 feet × 3 in hallway	1. Neuromuscular electrical stimulation applied to facilitate quadriceps and dorsiflexor contraction bilaterally during gait training; single forearm or R for gait stability due to L knee buckling, facilitating ability to increase gait distance on even and uneven surfaces from 30′ to 200′ in past week with verbal instructions/cues to contract quads and minimal assist for balance with directional changes and to prevent balance loss on even surface 2. Gait training: 4-wheeled walker, supervision and verbal instruction for balance, 200 feet × 3 reps (previously 30 feet with minimal/moderate assistance for balance) on even surface without directional change. Base of support 4 inches with equal stride length, infrequent verbal instruction/cues (previously moderate verbal instruction required). Directional changes with turns R/L, side stepping R/L and backwards stepping requires moderate assist
4. Patient currently complains of a constant ache in the low back radiating into the right lateral leg, right anterior thigh, and right shin	Patient reports LBP of, 8 on a scale of 0 to 10, (or 10/10, at rest and 10/10 with movement, radiating through the posterior and lateral right lower extremity, resulting in interrupted sleep and difficulty falling asleep. CO 10/10 pain in sitting for greater than 15 minutes, necessitating use of BUEs and lateral lean to L for sit to stand.
5. Initially, PROM R extremities WFLs, LLE: hip ext –20°, knee extension –20°; presently, ROM R extremities WFLs, LLE: –20° hip extension(s), –20° knee extension(s)	Therapeutic exercise: static stretch performed with manual pressure, LLE within patient tolerance to increase hip extension to facilitate active rolling and supine positioning in bed. Left hip and knee extension –20° /0 (previously –30°). Note: Avoid use of the term WFL, which is not objective. Neither "within full limits" nor "within functional limits" is an objective measure and requires clarification.

for precautions and limitations or any contraindications, and interventions. The reviewer should be able to discern the relationship between the selection and appropriateness of the tests and measures and the problems identified, including impairments or body functions and structures and the resulting functional limitations or activity and participation and disabilities, which are described in the ICF Model used globally and developed by the WHO.[9,12]

Table 12-2 Common Physical Therapy Terms and Functional Phrase Alternatives[19]

COMMON PHYSICAL THERAPY TERMS	FUNCTIONAL PHRASE ALTERNATIVES
Ambulated/walked	Gait training (consistent with CPT coding)
Confused	Attention span deficit; with redirecting, verbal, tactile and demonstration, able to attend to task and duplicate
Debility/deconditioning	Functional strength/motor performance deficit with inability to ________________
Declined	Functionally regressed as evidenced by inability to...
Did not appear to understand	Following ____ minutes of gestured and tactile facilitated training, demonstrated inconsistent, but effective . . .
Difficulty walking	Gait deviation/abnormality evidenced by...
	Front wheeled rolling walker: Unable to execute functional gait; maximally dependent to maintain required NWB on RLE as needed to preserve integrity of surgical repair of ____________
Endurance	Aerobic capacity, Functional activity tolerance limited, preventing ________________
	RPE (rate of perceived exertion) level of 10/10 with supported standing, preventing functional gait
	Record of vital signs in table format correlated to activity
Helped	Verbally and tactilely facilitated at __________
Improved	List comparative data such as:
	Presently ____ (Previously ____)
Observed/monitored	Evaluated/analyzed
Pacing of activity	Instructed in energy conservation techniques; provide time intervals and RPE reporting
Patient unable to	Patient exhibits . . . . (describe)
Performed lower extremity exercises	Performs individualized therapeutic exercise: lower extremity exercise program with manual cueing and facilitated muscle contraction with tapping to activate the ____________
Poor gait	Gait abnormality or gait disturbance evidenced or characterized by...
Practiced	Instructed patient in ...
Reminders	Verbal instructions (avoid use of "cues" per CMS transmittal, although the term is commonly used)
Some drainage	Indicate specific amount of drainage and characteristics, such as color, as well as any odor, and condition of skin surrounding the wound and description of dressing if there is one

(*Continued*)

Table 12-2 Common Physical Therapy Terms and Functional Phrase Alternatives[19] (Continued)

COMMON PHYSICAL THERAPY TERMS	FUNCTIONAL PHRASE ALTERNATIVES
Stable	Beginning to respond to verbal input and instructions as evidenced by...
Stays in bed	Bed confined, requiring repositioning to prevent skin breakdown
Strengthening	Therapeutic exercise; progressive resistive exercise
Walked	"Gait training" is preferred Note: Because nurses use the term "ambulation," the PT should concentrate on using the term "gait training," which indicates skill and is the term used for CPT coding
Wound cleansing	High pressure irrigation directed to wound in order to...
Weakness	Strength deficit; motor control or muscle performance deficit with inability to ____________
Went to doctor	Transported to physician's office with specialized transportation to accommodate wheelchair

The examination should include documentation of the physiologic and anatomic status of the cardiovascular/pulmonary system or body function and vital signs, including blood pressure, O_2 saturation, pulse rates, respiratory rate, and quality of breathing. Although vascular signs are not consistently seen as important across provider venues, they can be significant in monitoring the response to interventions. Therefore, baselines done at the time of the examination are significant in the UR process. This is especially important when there are comorbidities such as any cardiac, circulatory, or respiratory condition; diabetes; hypertension; sarcoidosis; or autoimmune conditions identified in the history that may necessitate monitoring. Observable skin status on the lower extremities such as edema, lipedema, lymphedema, neuropathy, cramping, claudication, shininess, redness, dryness, flakiness, hemosiderin, integrity, or other skin abnormalities such as bruising, may also be indicative of conditions requiring monitoring. The interpretation of the relevance and significance should be documented and the limitations and precautions identified for the safe performance of functional activities. At a minimum, monitoring of vital signs should be at the start of intervention for baseline, midway through intervention, and following intervention with increased frequency as indicated. This requires the skills of the PT to determine the specific and individualized program that will safely progress the patient to their desired outcomes. The tests and measures expected in this area include aerobic capacity measured objectively during functional activities or standardized exercise protocols, cardiovascular and/or pulmonary signs and symptoms and the response to increased oxygen uptake in exercise or functional activity, oxygen saturation, ventilation/respiration, and physiologic responses to positional changes (i.e., orthostatic hypotension). Borg's Rate of Perceived Exertion scale (RPE) is a good example of a reliable and valid measure of a patient's perception of their exertion or work level. If the patient's primary referring diagnoses are cardiopulmonary, all measurements noted earlier would be expected by the reviewer in determining medical necessity and that skilled care was rendered, tolerated, and associated with objective improvement

Integumentary

The presence of skin integrity issues can often lead to significant compensation of function. The utilization may be affected based on the severity, size, and location of the change in wound or skin integrity. Many skin integrity issues also indicate a loss of sensation locally or regionally. The loss of superficial or deep sensation, proprioception, and pain or temperature sensation can significantly affect the patient's ability to perform functional activities in a safe and effective manner, necessitating teaching compensatory strategies. Therefore, where present or indicated, the reviewer should see assessments and teaching compensation in the POC.

Observable skin status on the distal lower extremities, such as shininess, redness, dryness, plaques, flakiness, hemosiderin, or other skin abnormalities, may also be indicative of conditions requiring monitoring as well as edema, lipedema, or lymphedema. Color changes, rashes, skin temperature, and quality monitoring add to medical necessity validation if being monitored appropriately in response to intervention. This is relevant for cardiovascular and pulmonary conditions as well, as noted earlier.

Musculoskeletal

Range of Motion and Muscle Performance

These categories of examination indicate the patient status in terms of range of motion, flexibility, strength, joint integrity, presence or absence of atrophy, and symmetry of the body (height and weight and other anthropometric measurements may be included as well). Strength can be measured by manual muscle testing (MMT) or instruments developed for the same purpose, which may be more objective. Regardless of the numbering system the PT uses, clear documentation must be made of the strength in numbers expressed as fractions versus verbiage, as in colloquial English, "good" is better than "normal." Percentages should be avoided. It should also be noted that isolated MMT, which is position dependent and isolates muscles, is different from assessment of general muscle performance or strength of a group of muscles or movement across a joint. As the MMT system is colloquially used for a variety of movements against resistance, the PT or PTA should clearly state if MMT has been performed or muscle performance.

Example

Manual Muscle Testing: expressed in terms of the fractions for baselines and goals of strength

Normal	5/5
Good	4/5
Fair	3/5
Poor	2/5
Trace	1/5
None	0/5
	+ and – are also used to denote variations within each numbered strength category.

Author's Note

A variety of systems may be used. That is why it is critical for the PT to clearly and objectively state the finding as a fraction. When gross strength or muscle performance is assessed, it may be a better decision to use verbiage.

It should be noted that unless specifically testing an individual muscle in the prescribed position, most muscle performance tests are actually assessing an individual's ability to move a joint through its range of motion by a group of synergistically acting muscles and tolerate resistance. From a functional perspective, the "tester" should be careful when assigning a specific grade, especially in the 4/5 to 5/5 range, when a patient is clearly impaired in function. The ability to maximally resist one repetition across a joint, which cannot be repeated after activity or at another time during the day, may lead to assignation of a grade that is not realistic and may result in limited therapy or denial of therapy. This is important from a UR perspective, as isolated strength across a joint may not be indicative of functional movement. It may be indicated in some circumstances to describe the ability or inability to repeat a movement across a joint more than once, with a description of the ability to tolerate resistance and the degree of resistance, as well as how it relates to body structure and function.

Example

Clearly indicate what the identified ROM should be

ROM Scale for shoulder flexion:

Shoulder Flexion Active 180°/180°

Exam: R shoulder flexion: 120°/180° actively, which is inadequate to perform overhead work as a house painter

Knee Flexion 135°/135°

Exam: L knee flexion: 80°/135° passively, with inability to effectively........

Cervical Rotation 80°/80°

Exam: L cervical rotation: 40°/80° actively, limiting ability to safely look L while driving

Neuromuscular

The reviewer will be expecting the measurement of tone, synergies, motor control, and the way in which the patient accomplishes gross coordinated movement such as balance, gait, transfers, and transitions and the coordination of these activities, noting compensatory behaviors or movement patterns. Both fine and gross motor control should be included as indicated. The tests and measures expected to be seen in this area include use of assistive and adaptive devices, central nervous system (CNS) integrity, cranial and peripheral nerve integrity, motor function including dexterity, coordination, agility, neuromotor development and sensory integration, pain, and posture as related to position and gravity, and reflex integrity. The relationship to self-care and home management, work, community, and leisure integration or reintegration should appear in the problem summary. In the absence or impairment of peripheral sensation such as proprioception, light touch, or pain, documentation should include compensatory visual compensation strategies with movement, especially gait, as well as visual checking of the feet for skin integrity. This will enhance the likelihood of payment from a UR perspective.

The tests and measures should be carefully chosen to clearly and objectively establish the decline in function seen by the PT and should be apparent to the reviewer to support the practicality, frequency, and duration selected. The measurements should be documented in consistent terminology throughout the examination and should reflect standardized testing methods. Utilization is supported by the comparison of the results to the age-appropriate norms. Where available, disease-specific objective tests and measures, as well as reliable functional tests and measures, should be used at initial exam and discharge. They can also be used as intervention strategies as indicated and to assess progress. This will help the UR reviewer determine appropriateness and effectiveness of care.

DOCUMENTATION OF THE CONTINUUM OF CARE

Whether called progress notes, daily notes, encounters, treatment notes, or progress reports, continuum-of-care documents are reviewed to determine the current and continued need for skilled intervention in prospective review, as well as appropriateness of care that is being rendered in concurrent review. For example, Medicare requires, at a minimum, progress reports/notes for Part B every 10 treatment days. The documentation provides the comparative data to justify the skilled physical therapy services rendered and should reflect measurable, functional progress (progress notes or reports) using standardized measures whenever possible to emphasize the value of the physical therapy. The documents may have different formats, and the EMR systems may have variations; however, all need the same identification information and basic content and should be titled to assist any reader or reviewer in easy identification of a document. The documentation should contain all available information related to the skill required.

Each visit or encounter should be documented and authenticated with the applicable signature and professional designation. This is typically the PT or PTA signature with license held followed by the license number (e.g., *Jennifer Shamus*, PT # 12345 or *Alexa Shamus*, PTA # 12345). Inclusion of the license number ensures that the reviewer can determine a licensed individual rendered skilled care and may avoid a technical denial. In the case of a student PT, the signature should be the student's legal name followed by SPT or SPTA (e.g., *Grant Shamus*, SPT) and then authenticated by the supervising PT or PTA. It is recommended that the student also print their names for easy identification, as signatures are frequently illegible. The licensed professional's license number can be used for determining legitimacy. Electronically generated signatures are the currently acceptable signatures. When a student is documenting, especially for a Medicare beneficiary, there must be clear indication in the documentation that the care was performed with the PT proximally present and not engaged in any other patient care. For Medicare, it needs to be clear that the services were provided by the PT.

Author's Note

As stated in the Medicare Benefit Policy Manual (MBPM) Chapter 15, Section 230:[20]

"Only the services of the therapist can be billed and paid under Medicare Part B. The services performed by a student are not reimbursed even if provided under 'line of sight' supervision of the therapist; however, the presence of the student 'in the room' does not make the service unbillable. Pay for the direct (one-to-one) patient contact services of the physician or therapist provided to Medicare Part B patients. Group therapy services performed by a therapist or physician may be billed when a student is also present 'in the room.'"

Examples[20]

"Physical Therapists may bill and be paid for the provision of services in the following scenarios:

- The qualified practitioner is present and in the room for the entire session. The student participates in the delivery of services when the qualified practitioner is directing the service, making the skilled judgment, and is responsible for the assessment and treatment.

- The qualified practitioner is present in the room guiding the student in service delivery when the therapy student and the therapy assistant student are participating in the provision of services, and the practitioner is not engaged in treating another patient or doing other tasks at the same time.
- The qualified practitioner is responsible for the services and as such, signs all documentation. (A student may, of course, also sign but it is not necessary since the Part B payment is for the clinician's service, not for the student's services)."

Documentation of supervision for treatment provided by PTAs is essential to denote the services were provided under the direction of a PT. This may be done in a variety of ways. The most common may be indication in entries by the PTA that any changes, updates, or progress were discussed (date and time and method; i.e., phone, in person) with the supervising PT. However, there should also be verification that care can be provided by a PTA based on third-party payer guidelines.

Patient self-reporting should be included only as relevant to the therapy rendered. The utilization could be affected by statements documented with either positive or negative reports. If the statements documented are negative, prognosticating statements such as "I don't see anything happening" or "I'm not making progress or don't see any progress," the service will likely not be viewed as appropriate or necessary. Positive, prognosticating statements such as "I am able to bathe myself now" or "I can get my hand over my head now" would support continued services based on a relevant plan established. However, if quotes are included such as "I played a round of golf this weekend" and the patient is being treated for acute bursitis of the shoulder, any treatment rendered after this statement is documented may be denied, especially for Medicare beneficiaries. Leisure activities are not indications for physical therapy under Medicare, and this would be viewed from a UR perspective as not medically necessary unless the patient's occupation was golf specific. The reviewer will look for indications that the patient is an integral part of the review of goals and progress and would expect to see this reflected in the subjective statements documented. Identification of specific interventions in objective, codable terms is also important. The documentation in the continuum of care is one that can create the greatest challenge for the physical therapist. Two areas are affected during the UR of this section. The first is the correlation of the modalities and procedures coded in the billing submitted to the third-party payer. These documents must match. The modalities and interventions also must adhere to the guidelines of the third-party payer in terms of covered services and should be accompanied by the appropriate physician's order for them to be recognized as billable services. Interventions or conditions that are expressly excluded for payment by any third-party payer are non-negotiable. It is the responsibility of the provider to identify these.

Changes in treatment strategies will be reviewed for compliance to the required physician approvals necessary to comply with the procedures for each payer source. Medicare B allows a beneficiary (patient) to be evaluated and treated by a PT without a physician order or referral.

A signed Plan of Care (POC) by the physician or nonphysician provider (NPP) is required. As stated in MBPM Chapter 15, Section 220.1.3,[20] "the physician's/NPP's certification of the plan (with or without an order) satisfies all of the certification requirements for the duration of the plan of care, or 90 calendar days from the date of the initial treatment, whichever is less. The initial treatment includes the evaluation that resulted in the plan. The provider or supplier (e.g., facility, physician/NPP, or physical therapist) should obtain certification as soon as possible after the plan of care is established, unless the requirements of delayed certification are met. 'As soon as possible' means that the physician/NPP shall certify the initial plan as soon as it is obtained, or within 30 days of the initial therapy treatment."[20]

Author's Note

As stated in MBPM Chapter 15, Section 220.1.1:[20] "Payment is dependent on the certification of the plan of care rather than the order, but the use of an order is prudent to determine that a physician is involved in care and available to certify the plan."[20]

The reviewer also looks to see if the treatment strategies are relevant and effective for the problems identified and if the strategies are resulting in the expected progress, as outlined in the goals. A lack of progress, should it be evident, would prompt the reviewer to look for alternative treatment strategies or goal revision to be implemented in a timely manner and not continuation of intervention not resulting in measurable improvement. The expectation of the UR is that the interventions rendered correspond to the services billed, that they are within the coverage guidelines established by the third-party payer, and that they are effective for the problems identified in the POC. All components must match.

Changes in patient status as they relate to the POC (adverse reactions to the interventions and factors that affect the frequency or intensity of the interventions and progression toward goals) are usually documented as part of the patient assessment. Content should reflect the thought process of the PT and should relate the objective information documented with the patient's response and how that affects the progression toward the stated goals. The assessment of the interventions given and the effect they have on the patient's progress relative to function are the only justification allowing the UR to support continued treatment. This provides support for third-party payers to continue to pay for the services rendered. Documentation can support changes in interventions/procedures, frequency/intensity, and continuance/discontinuance.

Communication and consultation with other healthcare providers and family, significant other, or patient is also reviewed for the development of patient-oriented goals and the coordination of interventions to meet those goals. Interprofessional practice is purported to enhance patient outcomes and effectiveness of care. Therefore, it is important that all healthcare professionals are working in concert in an interprofessional manner to achieve the goals established and that there is no duplication of services between the providers, especially if the same CPT code is used on the same day by different therapy disciplines, such as physical therapy and occupational therapy (OT).

DOCUMENTATION OF RE-EVALUATION

Re-evaluation (CPT 97164) is necessary to support continued interventions beyond the original period certified (allowed) by the third-party payer if there is a significant change. This documentation may also require physician approval to be accepted by some third-party payers. State practice acts may require a re-evaluation every so many days, which may or may not be covered by insurance. In addition to the physical therapy initial evaluation codes, this is the only other code exclusive to PT.

As stated in MBPM Chapter 15, Section 220.3,[20]

> *"Continuous assessment of the patient's progress is a component of ongoing therapy services and is not payable as a re-evaluation. A re-evaluation is not a routine, recurring service but is focused on evaluation of progress toward current goals, making a professional judgment about continued care, modifying goals and/or treatment or terminating services. A formal re-evaluation is covered only if the documentation supports the need for further tests and measurements after the initial evaluation. Indications for a re-evaluation include new clinical findings, a significant change in the patient's condition, or failure to respond to the therapeutic interventions outlined in the plan of care. A re-evaluation may be appropriate prior to planned discharge for the purposes of determining whether goals have been met, or for the use of the physician or the treatment setting at which treatment will be continued. A re-evaluation is focused on evaluation of progress toward current goals and making a professional judgment about continued care,*

modifying goals and/or treatment or terminating services. Re-evaluation requires the same professional skills as evaluation. The minutes for re-evaluation are documented in the same manner as the minutes for evaluation."[20]

To effectively advocate for the patient, the re-examination by the PT should assess the effectiveness of the plan given and state the changes to be implemented and the expected outcomes based on the changes made. The documentation should also reflect the positive prognosticating factors supporting the revised POC, including all interventions and outcomes to be carried over from the initial examination or evaluation. Revisions to the plan may be necessary to change interventions or procedures based on patient progress, adverse response to modalities originally planned, or new medical problems occurring during the delivery of service. Patients with multiple comorbid presentations may require modifications to their plan, as their comorbidities may alter the response to treatment, and although every effort should be made to account for this at the time of the evaluation, there may be extenuating circumstances that affect the response.

It is through the re-examination that PTs can advocate for the unique needs of the patient to achieve the desired outcomes that may fall outside the established parameters of the third-party payer standard guidelines. If a specified number of visits were preauthorized and additional visits are indicated from a UR perspective, it is better for the PT to make the request than a nonprofessional, as the PT can communicate professional to professional and respond to questions. It should be noted, however, that if a plan limits the total number of rehabilitation or physical therapy visits per year and it has been met, additional visits will not be approved. It is possible in some cases that care rendered by previous physical therapy providers in the same coverage year, or care rendered by other providers using the same physical medicine codes, may prevent payment of an episode of care even if medically necessary. Denial of payment if a benefit has been exhausted is not denial of services.

DOCUMENTATION OF SUMMATION OF EPISODE OF CARE

Termination of care falls into three general categories: (1) the patient met the goals and expected outcomes; (2) the care was discontinued as a result of a change in the patient desire, medical condition, financial resources, or ability to benefit from intervention as based on the physical therapist's determination; or (3) the patient self-discontinued care without notice. Regardless of the reason for discontinuation of care, the documentation should include a summary of the care from start to finish. Among the items that should be listed are the length of episode; number of visits; the current physical and functional status; the degree of goals achieved or not achieved; complications during the provision of service; and the discharge/discontinuance plan, including any written or verbal directions related to the patient's continued care such as home programs, referrals, follow-up physical therapy, family/caregiver training, and equipment provided.

This report should provide the justification for the skilled intervention from the last progress report. It must also justify the overall progress made from the beginning of care and why this progress could only be made through the interventions provided. The PT should also indicate the expectations for the carryover into the home, work, or play environment and the potential for retaining the achieved functional improvements. The reviewer's ability to determine reasonableness of the POC is dependent on the PT clearly and briefly documenting what happened during the course of treatment.

UTILIZATION MANAGEMENT

UM is the establishment of policies that minimize the occurrence of denial of payment. This starts from the moment a patient walks into the facility. It is important to have policies that will establish important demographic and identifying information with what information is to be verified and who will perform that part of the information gathering. Ensuring that accurate information is received from a patient is critical to the start of care.

Proactive UM should include identifying the need for and presence of a correct referral or authorization (unless self-referral in direct-access states).

Author's Note

Keep in mind that although you may live and work in a state with unrestricted direct access, payers may require an order or referral be secured prior to treatment. Always check each payer's policy for coverage requirements.

The policy should address all applicable guidelines, including state and federal, for your setting, with compliance to the strictest regulation. As previously stated, Medicare does not require an order, but does require that a patient be under the care of a physician and that a physician or NPP sign the POC within 30 days in most instances. The referral process is important, as it is from this point that the patient enters your practice. The referral or POC should have an authorization for physical therapy evaluation, a medical diagnosis that relates to the reason for the problem, and any specific information the practitioner needs to relate to you regarding the patient treatment. In cases of third-party payers with gatekeeper requirements for referral, the referral may be specific and the physical therapy provider may need to be an approved provider for that payer.

Author's Note

MBPM Chapter 15, Section 220 discusses who may certify a therapy POC, stating:[20]

"Nonphysician practitioners (NPP) means physician assistants, clinical nurse specialists, and nurse practitioners, who may, if state and local laws permit it, and when appropriate rules are followed, provide, certify or supervise therapy services. Physician with respect to outpatient rehabilitation therapy services means a doctor of medicine, osteopathy (including an osteopathic practitioner), podiatric medicine, or optometry (for low vision rehabilitation only). Chiropractors and doctors of dental surgery or dental medicine are not considered physicians for therapy services and may neither refer patients for rehabilitation therapy services nor establish therapy plans of care... Certifications and recertifications by doctors of podiatric medicine must be consistent with the scope of the professional services provided by a doctor of podiatric medicine as authorized by applicable state law. Optometrists may order and certify only low vision services. Chiropractors may not certify or recertify plans of care for therapy services."

Author's Note

If the medical diagnosis indicated by the physician is not appropriate, the PT should contact the physician and request a telephone order to change it with a written follow-up For example:

Dx: status post (s/p) total hip replacement (THR) x 6 years. At 6 years post, this is inappropriate.

The referral may specify a body part. If so, the treatment of any other part without physician approval would precipitate a denial. It is therefore necessary for the physical therapist to carefully review the referral and assess the problems to ascertain if further discussion with the physician is necessary. States with direct access allow the provision of therapy services without a physician referral or prescription. However, billing third-party payers may require a physician referral to receive payment for physical therapy services, and Medicare requires a signed POC within 30 days of the first date of treatment.

Ensuring payment also requires the determination of the primary payer and verifying that insurance is active and the extent of the coverage the patient is entitled to. Patients often are lost in the legal language of the insurance policy and may need direction to determine the extent of coverage. This can become a tangled process and result in significant delay, if not outright denial, if done after the treatment has begun. With the changing networks and insurances, it is necessary to know what contracts are current and which types of policies are accepted at a facility. Insurance companies have multiple products, and each may require its own contract to become a provider. A PT could have a valid contract with a company's PPO and not with the HMO program. It is also possible that if you contract with a company's Medicare Advantage product, you may also be agreeing to be an in-network provider for the company's commercial product(s). It is important to read every payer contract carefully so that you understand what is being expected of you when it comes to documentation, coding, and billing. It is important to look at or copy the patient's insurance card, both front and back. Calling to verify insurance or having direct data access can benefit both the patient and the provider, and most insurance cards have customer service and verification phone numbers on the back of the card. The verification process can allow you to determine if there are co-payments or out-of-pocket expenses that need to be met and if there are limits on the number of visits per year. A facility that is not an in-network provider may be able to receive payment, but would need to assist the patient in verifying the insurance allows for out-of-network benefits prior to the start of care or obtain an authorization number for a specific patient. Although the cost may be higher than in-network, the patient may elect to utilize this option. Some insurance companies require preauthorizations. This means the PT must request permission to evaluate and treat the patient. If out-of-network care is rendered, the PT should have a written statement clarifying for the patient that they may be responsible for a portion of their care. A PT should also be able to provide any legally required or provider numbers in order to practice, such as license number, National Provider Identification (NPI) number, Medicare provider transaction numbers, and/or Medicaid provider numbers.

The determination of coverage by the primary insurance is dependent on the reason for referral. One of the common mistakes made by a PT is to verify the health insurance only to complete the history-taking in the examination and determine the major complaint is due to an auto accident. If the patient was in an accident, there may be other insurance that should be billed first (i.e., personal injury protection [PIP], automobile insurance, or homeowner's insurance). Payment from these would take precedence over the individual's health insurance until the policy is exhausted or it is determined no litigation is pending. This would be the same as in workers' compensation. Knowing the correct insurance to bill can avoid delayed payment or no payment at all. With insurance verified, provider number in hand, and examination/evaluation completed, you are ready to submit the billing. However, preauthorization does not guarantee payment. The documentation must support the therapy rendered.

External Review

External review, which includes outsourcing, has expanded since 2010. As physical therapy services have expanded in scope and cost to the healthcare system, as have other healthcare services, the medical loss ratio (MLR) was instituted by the Affordable Care Act of 2010.[1] "MLR is intended to limit insurer profit by requiring that payers spend a minimum percentage of dollars from insurance premiums on medical care, as opposed to administrative costs. ….If an insurer does not achieve the ratio, it must pay a penalty in the form of customer rebates."[2]

"While rebates to consumers may be viewed as beneficial, the MLR also has produced unforeseen consequences, such as the outsourcing of UM/UR. When a payer performs its own UM/UR, the expense is considered administrative under the MLR. If, however, the payer outsources UM/UR to an external vendor that offers quality-improvement services including prospective and concurrent review, UM/UR is considered a medical expense, which can be included in the medical care portion of the MLR. Given this ability to transfer the cost of UM/UR from administrative to medical, the trend toward UM/UR outsourcing can be expected to continue."[1] Therefore, external review may be the primary organization method of review for all phases of the process.

Author's Note

There are many concerns regarding payers' use of utilization management programs, as many of these programs are not grounded in evidence-based medicine; widely accepted best clinical practices; or criteria issued by professional medical associations, accreditation bodies, government agencies, or other nationally recognized healthcare quality organizations. Accordingly, there is a question as to whether these UR programs are, in fact, quality improvement programs intended to ensure appropriate treatment and should be counted as such.

As a result of the MLR initiative, external review may occur retrospectively, concurrently, or prospectively.

Reviews are performed for various purposes: to assist in the improvement of quality and service delivery, to verify the content of the record, and to ensure the efficient expenditure of monies, as well as compliance with the MLR. To make this determination, review organizations employ a variety of nonlicensed and licensed staff. It is important to know who reviews your documentation as the claim is processed and what degrees they hold, as well as their background, training, and experience.

Author's Note

If all efforts are made to ensure appropriate documentation content, justification for skilled services, and elimination of technical errors, regardless of who the reviewer is, the record should withstand any review.

Utilization review organizations (UROs) no longer typically use nurses for the review and screening process. UR is now done more commonly by PTs and occupational therapists for rehabilitation services. If the claim is questionable, a physician may review for approval or denial. There are still UROs employing nurses for denial-level decisions or employing others without medical experience to review services. Knowledge of who reviews the documentation submitted may help determine the expectations. While having a positive relationship with a reviewer is positive, many facilities deal with multiple UROs and can only rely on general expectations. The expectations of any reviewer are to read a clear, legible, coherent, and objective document that relates the physical therapist's efforts to resolve the patient's problems in a timely and efficient manner. The documentation should answer, not create, questions. The focus of the review is on effective use of the dollars spent.

Decisions are made based on the available documentation and how professionally the documentation is presented. Presentation includes legibility if the entry is manual versus electronic and the meaningfulness of the documentation submitted. Documentation sufficient for a favorable decision includes a clear statement identifying the patient's problem in functional terms, a reasonable treatment plan based on medical necessity and significant functionally oriented progress, with measurable changes based on professional and community standards, with clear statement of outcomes and evidence of clinical decision-making. This is also known as reasonable and necessary care. For Medicare, several conditions are identified for "determining whether care is reasonable and necessary:"[21]

1. The treatment is in accordance with accepted standard of practice, with specific and effective modalities for the patient's condition.
2. The documentation denotes the complexity and sophistication of the condition of the patient such that the services of a PT are required to safely perform the program. For instance, therapeutic exercise for a patient with cardiac history may require the skills of a PT to monitor the level and intensity of the exercise program while maintaining cardiac precautions.
3. A reasonable expectation that the condition will improve significantly in a generally predictable and reasonable amount of time is based on the physician's assessment after appropriate consultation with a PT. If this is not the case, it is necessary to establish a safe and effective home exercise program required in a specific disease state. This would be evident if the documentation shows the patient is meeting the goals established on the POC. Note: There is the ability to bill for therapy that is intended to prevent decline or maintain function with appropriate documentation. Therefore, it is critical that the documentation clearly state the results of the intervention.
4. The amount, frequency, and duration are reasonable for the condition and functional deficits documented. The frequency and duration should be established as individualized as the modalities used. A reviewer may see a pattern of frequency and duration that identify the provider for a more intensive review.

Patients who have policies requiring preauthorization may require advocacy through critically documented communication with the payer to receive "reasonable and necessary" treatment from the treating PT. Documentation of specific skilled interventions and measurable gains is necessary in each progress report, and the payer may deny any visit not justified by the specific report. Requests for continuation of care would need to include the skills required to complete the rehabilitation and the specific number of visits required to accomplish the established goals. The expectation of the intermediary or carrier is that the patient take responsibility for their rehabilitation and, once trained in the specific technique, continue the progression on their own.

Management of unfavorable claims requires organization and attention to detail. Most third-party payers use a denial system similar to the Medicare system. Therefore, a basic knowledge of this system is beneficial. Once a claim is submitted, an unfavorable decision may result from the technical or clinical aspect. Technical denials are typically returned to the provider, also referred to as returns to providers (RTPs). RTPs are due to incorrect identification information, illegibility, incomplete information, claim overlap with another provider's claim for the same or similar services, the appropriate qualifier does not accompany the submission, or the intermediary or carrier does not have a record of the provider number or participation identification. Technical errors that result in denial based on review can usually be reversed with the correct information submitted.

Returned claims can be avoided by taking some simple steps. The insurance verification policy of any organization should include copying the beneficiary's insurance card and verifying eligibility before starting treatment. Medicare has eligibility information online through the Direct Data Entry (DDE) system. This system allows a provider to gather information such as exact coverage, other claims currently being billed, and the status of claims. The review of claims to be submitted should also ensure that all handwritten documents are accurate for technical information, including identification numbers and completeness. Names can be a major source of technical denials. The name on the documentation should match the name on the insurance, including the suffix (Jr., Sr., or III), and avoid the use of nicknames. Knowledge of the proper billing codes and value codes can also eliminate RTPs. Claims may also be denied if the services provided were noncovered items. Knowing the coverage of the policy in your particular practice setting will help a provider avoid this type of denial. Additionally, it is always the physical therapist's responsibility to know the laws and guidelines that govern the setting in which they operate in any state or locality and any required coding guidelines. These problems are easily avoided through a process of review and establishment of proper policies.

Claims can also be denied based on the MAC's determination that the service was not medically reasonable and necessary. This is a judgment-based decision made from the documentation submitted with the claim. The appeal of these denials serves the facility and the profession alike, as long as the documentation supports that therapy was necessary for the patient's condition and the patients goals were achieved in a reasonable and predictable time. The appeal is dependent on the documentation and additional supportive statements related to the efficacy of the services provided. The decision to appeal a claim must be made based on an objective review of the services delivered. The procedure should be performed only when the documentation justifies the skilled interventions and the duration of care.

The Medicare program is divided into Part A for inpatient services and Part B for outpatient services. The role of the PT in preparation of the appeal may vary depending on the type of appeal. It could range from collecting and reviewing the documentation to participating in the hearing process, depending on the size, personnel, and policies of the facility. Part A claims management is usually coordinated by administrative personnel, and the PT may have very little to do with the appeal. Part B (outpatient) appeals are highly paperwork intensive and time sensitive. However, if there is a policy outlining the specific responsibilities of each person, the time involved is worth the potential outcome. This process allows you to defend the decisions made during the course of care and can affect future denials. The appeal allows you to advocate for all future patients with a similar condition and care.

Medicare has many types of audit processes; the two most familiar to the physical therapy profession are targeted medical review and targeted probe and educate. The Bipartisan Budget Act of 2018 retains the targeted medical review process that was established in the Medicare Access and CHIP Reauthorization Act of 2015 (MACRA). However, for 2018 through 2028, the targeted medical review threshold is $3,000 for physical therapy and speech-language pathology (SLP) services and $3,000 for OT services—a reduction from $3,700 in previous years. After 2028, the threshold will be indexed annually by the Medicare Economic Index.

The targeted medical review process means that not all claims exceeding the therapy threshold amount are subject to review, as they once were. CMS hired Noridian Healthcare Solutions as the supplemental medical review contractor (SMRC) to conduct these targeted medical record reviews.

Factors used to select claims for review may include the following:

- The provider has had a high claims denial percentage for therapy services or is less compliant with applicable requirements.
- The provider has a pattern of billing for therapy services that is aberrant compared with peers, or otherwise has questionable billing practices for services, such as billing medically unlikely units of services within a single day.
- The provider is newly enrolled or has not previously furnished therapy services.
- The services are furnished to treat targeted types of medical conditions.
- The provider is part of a group that includes another provider identified by the previous factors.

As stated in the Medicare Claims Processing Manual, Chapter 15, Section 10.3.2:

> *"Documentation justifying the services shall be submitted in response to any Additional Documentation Request (ADR) for claims that are selected for medical review. Follow the documentation requirements in Pub. 100-02, chapter 15, section 220.3. If medical records are requested for review, clinicians may include, at their discretion, a summary that specifically addresses the justification for therapy threshold exception."*[20]

CMS's Targeted Probe and Educate (TPE) program is designed to help providers and suppliers reduce claim denials and appeals through one-on-one help. The goal is to help providers quickly improve. MACs work with providers, in person, to identify errors and help you correct them. Many common errors are simple—such as a missing physician's signature—and are easily corrected. Most providers and suppliers will never need the targeted probe and education program. MACs use data analysis to identify:

Providers and suppliers who are targeted are those who have high claim error rates or unusual billing practices, and items and services that have high national error rates and are a financial risk to Medicare. If you are chosen for the program, the goal is to help you quickly improve. The majority of those providers that have participated in the targeted probe and educate program increased the accuracy of their claims. However, any who fail to improve after three rounds will be referred to CMS for next steps.[22]

When claims are denied, the PT or provider should review the documentation and determine if there is sufficient reason to appeal the claim or if it merely requires a request to reopen the claim or appeal.

A reopening is a remedial action taken to change a binding determination or decision that resulted either in an overpayment or an underpayment. Reopenings are separate and distinct from the appeals process. A contractor's decision to reopen a claim determination is not an initial determination and is therefore not appealable. If a claim is suspended for medical review, an additional documentation request (ADR) may be issued to obtain information needed to make a determination. Providers are responsible for supplying the information needed to adjudicate their claims. If no response is received within the specified time frames, the contractor will likely deny the service as not reasonable and necessary due to lack of documentation. Providers should familiarize themselves with the Medicare Claims Processing Manual Chapter 34—Reopening and Revision of Claim Determination and Decisions.

If appealing is the next step, the benefits are not only the recovery of payment but also education of the patient and MAC reviewer, validation of the treatment chosen, and providers' increased understanding of the specific MAC's policy. There are five levels in the Medicare Part A and Part B appeals process. The appellant must begin the appeal at the first level after receiving an initial determination. Each level, after the initial determination, has procedural steps the appellant must take before appealing to the next level.[23]

The levels are:[23]

APPEAL LEVEL	TIME LIMIT FOR FILING REQUEST	MONETARY THRESHOLD TO BE MET(AMOUNT IN CONTROVERSY, OR AIC)
1. Redetermination (MAC)	120 days from date of receipt of the notice initial determination	None
2. Reconsideration (QIC)	180 days from date of receipt of the redetermination*	None
3. Office of Medicare Hearings and Appeals (OMHA);Administrative Law Judge (ALJ)	60 days from date of receipt of the reconsideration	CY 2020: $170
4. Medicare Appeals Council	60 days from date of receipt of the ALJ hearing decision	None
5. Federal District Court	60 days from date of receipt of the Appeals Council decision	CY 2020: $1,670

The decision to appeal is based on several factors, including if the documentation speaks to the reason for the denial; if the provider understands the payer's regulations well enough to clearly explain why the treatment given fits in the guidelines stated; and lack of clear connection of all the factors for the reviewer, such as multiple comorbidities and key symptoms related to the diagnosis. If the facility decides to appeal the claim, a letter of support may accompany the request and can include information supporting the rationale for the interventions and duration. It may not include any new or conflicting information than what was originally submitted. A checklist for the completion of an appeal letter is helpful to target the specific reason for the request. Employing resources such as the state insurance commission, Department of Labor, workers' compensation board, professional organizations, physicians, family members, and the patient can provide support for an appeal. A well-educated physical therapist and patient can be the key ingredients to a successful request. Using the resources and substantiating the rationale for treatment can result in a successful claim review. If the claim is denied at this level, the provider may appeal to the next level. The APTA has information available on its website to assist providers with the appeal process.[20]

If you make it to the third level of appeal, you are entitled to a hearing with an administrative law judge (ALJ). Larger providers who have sufficient claims and wish to set precedence in order to avoid future similar claims being denied usually select this appeal level. If the decision of denial is overturned at any appeal level, payment of the claim is made. If the decision to deny is upheld through the last attempted appeal level, payment is withheld.

In summary, the physical therapist and all involved in the documenting and billing of services should read and understand the regulations and guidelines for all payers before initiating care. The policies and guidelines will assist the PT in determining patient eligibility and the allowable treatment modalities for each payer. The examination/evaluation provides the objective and measurable baseline data, which establishes the need for the skills of a PT to carry out the POC and safely restore the function of the patient. All documentation must use consistent measures and tests that meet standard requirements with established norms for the population being treated. The progress reports must reflect the functional changes occurring as a direct result of the interventions and the critical decision-making performed to alter the program as needed to achieve the goals established. This step is critical when the progress made is not as rapid as predicted by the physical therapist on the evaluation. If events that were not predictable at the time of the evaluation occur, the documentation could show reason to justify continued intervention. It is essential that documentation be complete, accurate, and legible for submission of a good claim. Having this allows for the PT to appeal decisions made by the third-party payers and advocate for the patient and profession.

Denial Templates

Now available to APTA members are customizable template letters that help make the case for payment.[24] The letters target four types of denials:

Denials related to change in practice location. This letter is crafted to address a MAC's denial of payment based on an erroneous conclusion that the provider did not give sufficient notice of a change in practice location.

Denials related to the use of the 59 modifier. The template, applicable to both MAC and private insurer denials, helps make the case for valid use of the 59 modifier, used to represent a service that is separate and distinct from another service it is paired with.

Denials related to medical necessity. Also usable in both Medicare and private insurance–related appeals, this letter helps a member articulate why services were in fact medically necessary.

Denials related to PTA services. Also usable in Medicare and private insurance-related appeals, this letter helps a APTA member articulate why services furnished by the PTA should be covered.[24]

SUMMARY

UR is performed by health insurance companies, hospitals, home health companies, and almost every provider and payer of medical services. CMS requires hospitals to have a UR program.[25] UR can be performed retrospectively if services have already been provided. UR can be performed concurrently or prospectively as part of the prior authorization process. If services have already been rendered, a reviewer must decide retrospectively if the therapeutic intervention was medically necessary, if the skilled services were required, and if so, if they were required for all sessions based on the patient's progress and goals. For a concurrent review, the questions are the aforementioned, as well as if skilled services will be or should be required beyond the point of review based on the information provided. Specific forms can be developed for this purpose (see Table 12-3). In a retrospective review, a reviewer should be

Table 12-3 Therapy Content Review Worksheet

Reviewer:		**Date:**
This is an:	____ **Internal review**	____ **External review**
Record reviewed is for:	___ outpatient	___ inpatient
Review is:	___ retrospective	___ concurrent
Treatment venue		
Acute care hospital:	___ inpatient/acute	____ inpatient/acute rehab
____ outpatient		
SNF:	___ inpatient	____ outpatient
Rehab Hospital:	___ inpatient	____ outpatient
____ CORF	___ PT in private practice	
____ Home health	___ Outpatient	
____ Other: ______________________		

Referral status: ____ self-referral/direct access or ____ physician: If physician referred, status of prescription: ___ in record, written ___ in record, verbal only

General information: Please indicate if the item is present by writing y for yes. If missing or incorrect, please put n for no. If not applicable, please put NA.

____ entries are in ink (single color)

____ informed consent indicated

____ blank spaces are not left in entries

____ co-signature is used for student entries/or for those pending licensure

____ each category of entry is labeled (i.e., PT Evaluation, PT Notes, Discharge Summary)

____ pages are numbered as appropriate (i.e., if multipage evaluation, pages are numbered)

____ indicates release to communicate with family members, caregivers, others

____ treatments rendered are included in the initial plan or interim plans

____ reason(s) for treatment are indicated

____ all required components are included

____ all required components are identified

____ patient response to treatment is indicated

____ consistent attendance is indicated or follow-up is indicated for missed appointments

____ treatment is modified based on changes in function or response to interventions

(Continued)

Table 12-3 Therapy Content Review Worksheet (Continued)

____ outcomes/goals are expected in a reasonable time frame

____ based on the content, care rendered was skilled

____ based on the content, care was reasonable and necessary

____ all entries match: billing dates, visit dates, plan, interventions, goals

____ signatures are original or electronic

____ entry errors are corrected appropriately

Identification:

____ patient's full name (on all pages)

____ other identification as relevant

____ signatures include license #

____ date of birth, age are included

____ all entries are dated/timed

____ signatures include professional designation

Initial Examination/Evaluation with Plan of Care

Please check yes or no to indicate if the item is included or is not included

yes	no	Content item	yes	no	Content item
____	____	Medical history of presenting problem	____	____	Objective measures of systems dysfunction/functional problems
____	____	Primary medical diagnoses	____	____	Problem summary/indication of clinical judgment
____	____	Comorbidities/concurrent problems			
____	____	Physical therapy diagnosis or problem	____	____	Objective, measurable goals that relate to identified problems
____	____	Precautions/contraindications	____	____	Goals are time defined by dates and days or weeks as indicated (circle which)
____	____	Barriers	____	____	Combination of impairment and functionally based goals that are related
____	____	Demographic information: Psychosocial, social, and environmental concerns	____	____	Indication of patient/caregiver participation in goal setting
____	____	Cognition: Ability to communicate/understand	____	____	Treatment plan: Interventions in CPT codable verbiage that matches problems and goals
____	____	Indication of patient's knowledge of problem or responsible party	____	____	Patient/caregiver educational learning goals are included
____	____	Other services patient is receiving related to episode of physical therapy care	____	____	Frequency

Table 12-3 Therapy Content Review Worksheet (Continued)

			___	___	Duration
			___	___	Prognosis: Rehabilitation potential
___	___	Prior level of function relative to presenting problem	___	___	Authentication: PT signature and designation
___	___	Indication of collaboration with other professionals as indicated	___	___	License number

Does the venue require a physician plan of care (POC)?	___ yes	___ no
If yes, is all the information included from the earlier sections (except objective systems data)?	___ yes	___ no
Is the POC signed by the physician?	___ yes	___ no
Is the POC dated?	___ yes	___ no
Is the POC signed on the appropriate date, prior to intervention?	___ yes	___ no

Continuation of care: PT treatment notes, progress notes, progress reports

There is an entry for each encounter/visit	___ yes	___ no	
Each entry is authenticated	___ yes	___ no	
Professional designation is included for all	___ yes	___ no	
License number is indicated for all	___ yes	___ no	
Co-signature as appropriate	___ yes	___ no	___ not applicable

PT Treatment Notes (if applicable; if not, indicate NA)

Please check yes or no to indicate if the item is included or is not included

yes	no	NA	Content item	yes	no	NA	Content item
___	___	___	Each entry is dated	___	___	___	Interventions match POC
___	___	___	Time of visit is indicated	___	___	___	Equipment issued is indicated
___	___	___	Patient self-report in quotes as indicated	___	___	___	Instructions given are indicated
___	___	___	Indication of body areas treated	___	___	___	Response to treatment
___	___	___	Indication of procedures/interventions rendered in CPT codable verbiage	___	___	___	Reflects communication with others as applicable
___	___	___	Parameters of interventions included	___	___	___	Indicates if anyone else was present during sessions

Other

Progress Notes/Reports

Please check yes or no to indicate if the item is included or is not included

yes	no	NA	Content item	yes	no	NA	Content item
___	___	___	Each entry is dated	___	___	___	Interventions match POC

(Continued)

Table 12-3 Therapy Content Review Worksheet (Continued)

___	___	___	Time of visit is indicated if single progress note for single day	___	___	___	Equipment issued is indicated
___	___	___	If entry is for a single or combination of visit days, dates are indicated and frequency of notes is appropriate for acuity	___	___	___	Reflects communication with others as indicated, including caregivers
___	___	___	Indicates where treatment rendered/who accompanied	___	___	___	Instructions given are indicated
___	___	___	Patient self-report in quotes as indicated	___	___	___	Reflects communication with others as indicated (i.e., physicians, other team members), including phone calls, conversations, conferences
___	___	___	Indication of body areas treated	___	___	___	Reflects adjustments in plan
___	___	___	Indication of procedures/ interventions rendered in CPT codable parameters of interventions included	___	___	___	Indicates where treatment rendered
___	___	___	Includes progress toward goals as established in initial examination/evaluation or re-examination	___	___	___	Information matches previous entry information
				___	___	___	Indicates how patient came to PT
___	___	___	Response to treatment is indicated				
___	___	___	Indicates change in status				

Other:

Re-examination

Re-exam is included as applicable to evaluate progress and modify or redirect?____ yes____ no ____NA

Please check yes or no to indicate if the item is included or is not included or NA for not applicable.

yes	no	NA	Content item	yes	no	NA	Content item
___	___	___	Entry is identified as re-exam, recertification, or appropriate designation	___	___	___	Need for continued skilled intervention is included
				___	___	___	Elements from progress notes/ treatment notes included relative to system dysfunction, functional deficits
___	___	___	Timely, every 30 days or as applicable for setting (60 days, then every 30 for CORFs)				

Table 12-3 Therapy Content Review Worksheet (Continued)

___	___	___	Updated functional status, progress toward initial or interim goals	___	___	___	Authentication PT signature, professional designation
___	___	___	Goals modified to reflect changes: up or down				

Other:

Is a recertification signed by the physician required? ____yes____ no

If required, is it in the record? ____yes____ no

If in the record, is it signed and dated? ____yes____ no

Does it contain progress toward goals, interventions provided, and any goal and plan revisions as applicable? ____yes____ no

Summation of Episode of Care

A summation of care/discharge, summary is included?____ yes____ no

Please check yes or no to indicate if the item is included or is not included or NA for not applicable.

yes	no	NA	Content item	yes	no	NA	Content item
___	___	___	Entry is identified	___	___	___	Discharge instructions to patient/caregivers
___	___	___	Summary of interventions				
___	___	___	Time frame of treatment: From : to	___	___	___	Indication of patient/caretaker instruction
___	___	___	Reference to all problems, impairment and functional addressed in initial exam/evaluation	___	___	___	Instructions are signed off on and copy is in record
___	___	___	Goals/outcomes achieved relative to initial plan and revisions	___	___	___	Recommendations/plan regarding condition, communication post-discharge, including:
___	___	___	Indication of current functional status	___	___	___	Referrals for additional services
___	___	___	If goals not achieved, indication of reason	___	___	___	Recommendations for follow-up physical therapy
			Indication that referral source has been informed or communicated with	___	___	___	Equipment provided
				___	___	___	Recommendation for physician follow-up
						___	Indication of where discharged to
				___	___	___	Indication of why being discharged

(Continued)

Table 12-3 Therapy Content Review Worksheet (Continued)

	___	___	___	Authentication: PT signature, professional designation
	___	___	___	Authentication: PT signature, professional designation
Other:				
Additional Comments				
	Signature of Reviewer:		Date:	

able to examine a thorough and complete initial evaluation and compare it to a thorough and complete final discharge note/summary and make a general determination of the quality and value of overall care. The elements should match in the two documentation elements. If they do not, the reviewer may stop the process and deny all care.

There are significant educational opportunities and benefits to having an active internal UR/UM process. This process can range from internal chart audits performed, utilizing a check sheet, to audits by a designated UR department. The results of a strong UR program provide the basis for a strong UM process. Adherence to policies and procedures can result in quality-oriented programs resulting in significant value-based patient outcomes in a cost-effective and efficient manner.

The record or the documentation of services provided will be the primary basis for determination of payment. The term "primary" is used because the reviewer may, depending on the organization, have the opportunity to question the providers or the individuals that actually provided or are providing the care. There may be records to use as a baseline for prospective decision-making. If the documentation reflects the medical necessity of skilled service or intervention, and if the interventions are relevant and appropriate for the physical therapy problems indicated, payment or appropriate continued care can be justified.

The Medicare program consists of a number of payment systems and a network of contractors that process more than 1 billion claims each year submitted by more than 1 million healthcare providers. CMS uses several types of contractors to verify that claims are paid based on Medicare guidelines, including Medicare Administrative Contractors (MACs) and Recovery Audit Contractors (RACs). A RAC's primary task is to review Medicare claims data and determine if a claim was appropriately paid. The national Recovery Audit Program was established in early 2009. Each RAC is responsible for identifying overpayments and underpayments in geographically defined areas, as well as common billing errors, trends, and other Medicare payment issues for CMS.

It behooves physical therapy providers to ensure that if a RAC or other contractor reviews claims that the documentation support the skill and expertise, including value-based objective outcomes, to successfully pass a Medicare audit and avoid recoupment of Medicare payment. All physical therapy providers should appreciate that the best method of success in the UR process is attention to the content needed to justify skilled physical therapy in the documentation. Providers should be able to answer any questions that could be asked before the UR process is initiated.

REVIEW QUESTIONS

1. What is utilization review?
2. How does utilization review differ from utilization management?
3. Compare and contrast retrospective, concurrent, and prospective review processes.
4. What is the continuum of care in physical therapy?
5. How does quality improvement or quality management relate to utilization review programs?
6. What does an external review organization base their decisions for payment on?
7. Define a technical error and give three examples. How can they be avoided?
8. Compare and contrast first- and second-level denials and their appropriate appeals.
9. Compare and contrast internal and external utilization review.
10. Explain the benefits of expressing examination findings in numeric terms.
11. How should a student physical therapist or student physical therapist assistant sign a medical record entry, and how should a PT or PTA authenticate it?
12. Does preauthorization of physical therapy services guarantee payment? Provide a rationale for your answer.

REFERENCES

1. *Utilization Management and Utilization Review*. Alexandria, VA: American Physical Therapy Association. Available at https://www.apta.org/your-practice/payment/coding-billing/commercial-insurance/tpa-umur. Accessed August 10, 2020.
2. Institute of Medicine (US) Committee on Utilization Management by Third Parties, Gray BH, Field MJ. *Controlling Costs and Changing Patient Care? The Role of Utilization Management*. Washington DC; National Academies Press (US); 1989. Available at https://www.ncbi.nlm.nih.gov/pubmed/25144100. Accessed August 10, 2020.
3. Miller S. *For 2019, Employers Adjust Health Benefits as Costs Near $15,000 per Employee*. Society for Human Resource Management (SHRM). Available at https://www.shrm.org/resourcesandtools/hr-topics/benefits/pages/employers-adjust-health-benefits-for-2019.aspx. Accessed August 10, 2020.
4. *Quality Assurance and Utilization Review*. Position paper of the American College of Physicians, American College of Physicians; September 13, 1984. Available at https://www.acponline.org/acp_policy/policies/quality_assurance_utilization_review_1984.pdf. Accessed August 10, 2020.
5. *Peer Review Improvement Act of 1982 (Title I, Subtitle C of the Tax Equity and Fiscal Responsibility Act of 1982) (Public Law 97-248)*. Available at https://www.congress.gov/bill/97th-congress/senate-bill/2142. Accessed August 10, 2020.
6. *Clinical Practice Guidelines*. National Center for Complementary and Integrative Health; 2017. Available at https://nccih.nih.gov/health/providers/clinicalpractice.htm. Accessed August 10, 2020.
7. *American Health Information Management Association (AHIMA)*. Available at http://www.ahima.org/. Accessed February 20, 2020.
8. *CPT® 2020 Professional Edition:* Spiral-bound. American Medical Association; 2020. ISBN#: 978-1-62202-898-6. Available at https://commerce.ama-assn.org/store/ui/catalog/productDetail?product_id=prod2950002&navAction=push. Accessed August 10, 2020.
9. *Towards a Common Language for Functioning, Disability and Health ICF*. World Health Organization; 2002. Available at https://www.who.int/classifications/icf/icfbeginnersguide.pdf. Accessed August 10, 2020.
10. *APTA Guidelines: Physical Therapy Documentation of Patient/Client Management*. Alexandria, VA: American Physical Therapy Association. Available at https://www.apta.org/uploadedFiles/APTAorg/About_Us/Policies/BOD/Practice/DocumentationPatientClientMgmt.pdf. Accessed August 10, 2020.
11. *Guide to Physical Therapist Practice 3.0*. Alexandria, VA: American Physical Therapy Association. Available at http://guidetoptpractice.apta.org/content/current. Accessed August 10, 2020.
12. Bemis-Dougherty A. Practice matters: What is the ICF? *PT in Motion*. 2009. Available at https://www.pacific.edu/Documents/school-pharmacy/Practice%20Matters-What%20is%20the%20ICF.pdf. Accessed August 10, 2020.
13. *ICD-10*. Baltimore, MD: Centers for Medicare & Medicaid Services. Available at https://www.cms.gov/Medicare/Coding/ICD10. Accessed August 10, 2020.
14. *Orthopedics*. Alexandria, VA: American Physical Therapy Association; 2017. Available at https://www.apta.org/contentassets/cc8cc21c17b8431297de80500a2b20c5/commcm-icd-10-cm-orthopaedics.pdf. Accessed August 10, 2020.
15. Zia A, Kamaruzzaman SB, Tan MP. Polypharmacy and falls in older people: Balancing evidence-based medicine against

falls risk. *Postgrad Med.* 2015;127(3):330-337. doi:10.1080/00325481.2014.996112.

16. *The Department of Health and Human Services and the Department of Justice Health Care Fraud and Abuse Control Program Annual Report.* Office of the Inspector General. Available at https://oig.hhs.gov/reports-and-publications/hcfac/index.asp. Accessed August 10, 2020.
17. Guccione AA, Mielenz TJ, Devellis RF, Goldstein MS, Janet K Freburger JK, et al. Development and testing of a self-report instrument to measure actions: outpatient physical therapy improvement in movement assessment log (OPTIMAL). *Phys Ther.* 2005 Jun;85(6):515-530. https://pubmed.ncbi.nlm.nih.gov/15921473/.
18. *Medicare Coverage Database.* Baltimore, MD: Centers for Medicaid & Medicare Services. Available at https://www.cms.gov/medicare-coverage-database/overview-and-quick-search.aspx?list_type=ncd. Accessed August 10, 2020.
19. Baeten AM, Moran ML, Phillippi LM. *Documenting Physical Therapy: The Reviewer Perspective.* Woburn, MA: Butterworth-Heinemann; 1999.
20. *Chapter 15 Covered Medical and Other Health Services.* Medicare Benefit Policy Manual. Baltimore, MD: Centers for Medicare & Medicaid Services. Available at https://www.cms.gov/Regulations-and-Guidance/Guidance/Manuals/downloads/bp102c15.pdf. Accessed August 10, 2020.
21. Medicare Program Integrity Manual. *Chapter 3—Verifying Potential Errors and Taking Corrective Action.* Baltimore, MD: Centers for Medicaid & Medicare Services; 2019. Available at https://www.cms.gov/media/338436. Accessed August 10, 2020.
22. *Targeted Probe and Educate (TPE).* Baltimore, MD: Centers for Medicare & Medicaid Services. Available at https://www.cms.gov/Research-Statistics-Data-and-Systems/Monitoring-Programs/Medicare-FFS-Compliance-Programs/Medical-Review/Targeted-Probe-and-EducateTPE. Accessed August 10, 2020.
23. *Medicare Parts A & B Appeals Process.* MLH Booklet. Baltimore, MD: Centers for Medicare & Medicaid Services. Available at https://www.cms.gov/outreach-and-education/medicare-learning-network-mln/mlnproducts/downloads/medicareappealsprocess.pdf. Accessed August 10, 2020.
24. *Appealing a Denial.* Alexandria, VA: American Physical Therapy Association. Available at https://www.apta.org/your-practice/payment/medicare-payment/denials-and-appeals/appealing-a-denial. Accessed August 10, 2020.
25. *CMS Manual System pub.100-07 State Operations Provider Certification.* Baltimore, MD: Centers for Medicare & Medicaid Services. Available at https://www.cms.gov/Regulations-and-Guidance/Guidance/Transmittals/Downloads/R136SOMA.pdf. Accessed August 10, 2020.

SECTION **3**

Payment and Coding

13 Coding

OBJECTIVES

Following completion of this chapter, the reader will be able to:

- Explain what a Current Procedural Terminology CPT code is and the application of CPT codes in physical therapy.
- Explain what an ICD-10 code is and the application in physical therapy.
- Describe the relationship between the CPT codes and ICD-10 codes.
- Compare the relationship between the medical diagnosis and the physical therapy diagnosis (problem).
- Understand the difference between attended and unattended procedures.

"To be payable, the medical record and the information on the claim form must consistently and accurately report covered therapy services, as documented in the medical record. Documentation must be legible, relevant and sufficient to justify the services billed."[1]

CURRENT PROCEDURAL TERMINOLOGY CODES

The Healthcare Common procedure Coding System (HCPCS) is divided into two principal subsystems, referred to as level I and level II of the HCPCS. Level I of the HCPCS is comprised of Current Procedural Terminology (CPT-4), a numeric coding system maintained by the American Medical Association (AMA). The CPT-4 is a uniform coding system consisting of descriptive terms and identifying codes that are used primarily to identify medical services and procedures furnished by physicians and other health care professionals, including physical therapists. Level II of the HCPCS is a standardized coding system that is used primarily to identify products, supplies, and services not included in the CPT-4 codes, such as ambulance services and durable medical equipment, prosthetics, orthotics, and supplies (DMEPOS) when used outside a physician's office. Because Medicare and other insurers cover a variety of services, supplies, and equipment that are not identified by CPT-4 codes, the level II HCPCS codes were established for submitting claims for these items.[2,3]

The HCPCS has been selected as the approved coding set for entities covered under the Health Insurance Portability and Accountability Act (HIPAA), for reporting outpatient procedures. The HCPCS is based upon the American Medical Association's (AMA) "Physicians' Current Procedural Terminology, Fourth Edition" (CPT-4). It includes three levels of codes and modifiers. Level I contains only the AMA's CPT-4 codes. This level consists of all numeric codes. Level II contains alpha-numeric codes primarily for items and nonphysician services not included in CPT-4, e.g., ambulance, DME, orthotics, and prosthetics.[4]

The CPT contains approximately 10,000 codes.[2] CPT codes are used in the billing process with International Classification of Disease codes (ICD).[2,5]

There are three categories for CPT codes:

- Category 1 is procedures and contemporary medical practices
- Category 2 is clinical laboratory services
- Category 3 is emerging technologies, services, and procedures

ICD codes are numeric codes for diseases and pathologies, medical procedures including surgeries, and functionally oriented deficits or conditions.[5] ICD-10 (10th revision) code versions are in use for physical medicine and physical therapy procedures.[5] The ICD codes were developed by the World Health Organization (WHO) as a way to standardize classification of diseases worldwide (see a sample of ICD-10 codes in Appendix D).[5]

As the CPT codes that describe physical therapy–related procedures have historically been categorized as physical medicine codes, it has been difficult for physical therapists (PTs) to distinguish themselves from others licensed to administer some of the same procedures. The ICD-10 coding needs to be as complete and based on confirmed information identified during the visit. Physical therapists may use codes for signs or symptoms pertinent to the physical therapy services provided and codes that the physician may not have included.

Author's Note

ICD-10-CM was developed and is maintained by the World Health Organization and the National Center for Health Statistics within the Centers for Disease Control and Prevention. It is supplemented by a set of official guidelines that are designated as part of the ICD-10-CM code set by the HIPAA "medical data code set" regulations. The CDC updates these guidelines annually. Use the codes and the guidelines that correspond with the year in which you provide the service.[6]

List first the ICD-10-CM code for the diagnosis, condition, problem, or other reason for encounter/visit shown in the medical record to be chiefly responsible for the services provided. List additional codes that describe any coexisting conditions.

Codes for symptoms, signs, and ill-defined conditions from Chapter 18 are not to be used as principal diagnosis when a related definitive diagnosis has been established.

Codes that describe symptoms and signs, as opposed to diagnoses, are acceptable for reporting purposes when a diagnosis has not been established (confirmed) by the provider.[6]

Although recent changes have resulted in several codes unique to physical therapy, it remains incumbent on the PT to prove medical necessity of the service based on consistent matching of CPT codes, ICD-10 codes, and appropriate documentation of what classifies the intervention as skilled.[2,5]

PTs also must be familiar with the Resource Based Relative Value Scale. (RBRVS), the payment system used by CMS and most other payers. The RBRVS is based on the principle that payments for physician services should vary with the resource costs for providing those services and is intended to improve and stabilize the payment system while providing physicians an avenue to continuously improve it.[7]

Since the introduction of the RBRVS, the AMA has worked with national medical specialty societies to provide recommended updates and changes directly to CMS. The vehicle for this influence is the AMA/Specialty Society RVS Update Committee (RUC), which provides relative value recommendations to CMS annually. In 1992, Medicare significantly changed the way it pays for physician services. Instead of basing payments on charges, the federal government established a standardized physician payment schedule based on RBRVS.[7]

In this system, payments are determined by the resource costs needed to provide them, with each service divided into three components:

Physician work

Practice expense

Professional liability insurance (PLI)

Payments are calculated by multiplying the combined costs of a service times a conversion factor (a monetary amount determined by CMS) and adjusting for geographical differences in resource costs.[7]

Annual updates to the physician work, practice expense and professional liability insurance relative values are based on recommendations from the AMA/Specialty Society Relative Value Scale Update Committee (RUC), which was formed in 1991 to make recommendations to CMS on the relative values to be assigned to new or revised codes in the Current Procedural Terminology (CPT®) code book. The relative values in the RBRVS were originally developed to correspond to the approximately 10,000 CPT procedure codes. The RBRVS is updated annually to reflect new and revised CPT codes.[7]

The MPFS is the primary method of payment for enrolled health care professionals. Specifically, Medicare uses this fee schedule when paying the following services:

- Professional services of physicians and other enrolled health care professionals in private practice;
- Services covered incident to physicians' services (other than certain drugs covered as incident to services);
- Diagnostic tests (other than clinical laboratory tests); and
- Radiology services.

In addition, suppliers such as Mammography Centers are paid according to the MPFS. Institutional providers such as hospitals, Comprehensive Outpatient Rehabilitation Facilities (CORFs), and Skilled Nursing Facilities (SNFs) are paid for some services under the MPFS depending on the institution type and service. For example, hospital outpatient departments are paid for screening mammographies and outpatient rehabilitation services under the MPFS.[8]

Example[8]

Payment = [Work RVU × Work GPCI + PE RVU × PE GPCI + MP RVU × MP GPCI] × Conversion Factor (CF)[8]

The Medicare physician fee schedule pricing amounts are adjusted to reflect the variation in practice costs from area to area. A Geographic Practice Cost Index (GPCI) has been established for every Medicare payment locality for each of the three components of a procedure's Relative Value Unit (i.e., the RVUs for work, practice expense, and malpractice). The GPCIs are applied in the calculation of a fee schedule payment amount by multiplying the RVU for each component times the GPCI for that component.[9]

PRINCIPLES OF CODE USE

One of the challenges of including coding information as a component of documentation is the constant modification of the codes themselves. However, since correct coding is required in order to effect reimbursement, it cannot be ignored. This chapter introduces the concept of coding as it applies to physical therapy. By following the principles and knowing where to obtain the updated information, the PT can ensure that the latest principles and guidelines are consistently applied. Depending on the facility, it may or may not be the PT's responsibility to identify the code numbers. However, in order for a third party such as a billing clerk to correctly code a record, the verbiage must be correct. Based on the size of the CPT and ICD-10 books, learning the verbiage may seem a daunting task. However, many facilities use the same categories of patients on a regular basis. Therefore, it is common for facilities to establish a list of frequently used CPT and ICD-10 codes.[2,5] This list saves time and ensures better consistency throughout facilities. It also eliminates errors if interpretation is left to another party.

Author's Note

For institutional settings, such as acute care, short-term care, long-term care, and psychiatric hospitals; home health agencies; rehab facilities; nursing homes, the ICD-10 code or codes are determined for a single patient's claim; there are not separate codes for each provider within the institution who treats that patient.[6]

INDIVIDUAL CODES

New Codes and Correct Coding Initiatives

It is the PT's responsibility to keep up with the most current coding. Members of the American Physical Therapy Association (APTA) can refer to the APTA website for updates.[6] All healthcare professionals also should have a copy of the *American Medical Association CPT Professional Book,* which is updated on an annual basis.[2]

For CPT and HCPCS, make sure the verbiage in the documentation matches the code that will be used in the billing. Always precede specific types of interventions identified colloquially with abbreviations, with the code terminology.

Example

Incorrect: CPT 97110: General strengthening, PNF

Correct: CPT 97110: Therapeutic exercise: isotonic strengthening, PNF

For ICD-10,[5] the physical therapist must always include the medical diagnosis established by the physician as the referral diagnosis. However, the physical therapy diagnosis for which the therapy is being rendered must be established by the PT, since the physician's diagnosis is not always the same as the PT's diagnosis. Regardless, all diagnoses must have verbiage that specifically matches an ICD-10 code. When appropriate, the physical therapy diagnosis should be functionally oriented and should establish the relevance between the treatment diagnosis, the interventions selected, and the goals established. Do not create "new" diagnoses, and always refer to the ICD-10 list for guidance.[5]

Example

Same:

Medical: 812: closed fracture of humerus, upper end

PT: 812: closed fracture of humerus, upper end

Referred to PT for treatment of humerus to regain functional use

Different:

Medical: 812: closed fracture of humerus, upper end

PT: R26.9 abnormality of gait

Referred to PT for gait training with quad cane, as can no longer use walker secondary to humerus fracture

ICD-10 diagnosis order. List the code for the primary treatment diagnosis first, followed by the others. Comorbidities may help justify the need for skilled services.[5]

MATCHING CODES

ICD-10 and CPT

Once the PT has established the appropriate treatment or physical therapy diagnosis, it should be clear from the verbiage and the code number that they are related. The CMS 1500 form (see Appendix C) allows for services to be specified for each diagnosis.[10]

Example

Incorrect:
Medical: G82.2 paraplegia
PT: G82.2 paraplegia
Treatment: Therapeutic exercise: 97110
Neuromuscular re-education: 97112
Therapeutic activities: 97530

Incorrect:
Medical: I25.2 old myocardial infarction
PT: I25.2 old myocardial infarction
Treatment: Gait training: 97116

Correct:
Medical: I25.2 old myocardial infarction
PT: R26.9 Gait abnormality,
Treatment: Gait training: 97116

PROCEDURE SPECIFICITY

When selecting a code for a procedure, it is important to be as specific as possible. Select the code that best describes the intervention you are using.[2]

Example

Incorrect:
Gait training: CPT 97116
Treatment: Balance and posture training

Correct:
Neuromuscular re-education: CPT 97112
Treatment: Balance and posture training

TIME

Most CPT codes billed by physical therapists are defined in 15-minute increments, with each 15-minute segment described as a unit. Depending on the billing form used, the number of units may be required. The total session time should be recorded in the documentation itself.

For Medicare Part B Outpatient Rehabilitation and Comprehensive Outpatient Rehabilitation Facilities/Outpatient Physical Therapy Providers (also referred to as rehabilitation agencies that are counting minutes for timed codes in 15 minute units, CMS has established what is known as the "8-minute billing rule. CMS describes it as follows:[11]

> *"When only one service is provided in a day, providers should not bill for services performed for less than 8 minutes. For any single timed CPT code in the same day measured in 15 minute units, providers bill a single 15-minute unit for treatment greater than or equal to 8 minutes through and including 22 minutes. If the duration of a single modality or procedure in a day is greater than or equal to 23 minutes, through and including 37 minutes, then 2 units should be billed." Time intervals for 1 through 8 units are discussed in the Medicare Claims Processing Manual Chapter 5 Section 20.2.*[11]

For the purposes of Medicare, the treatment note must include total timed code treatment minutes and total treatment time in minutes. Total treatment time includes the minutes for timed code treatment and untimed code treatment. Total treatment time does not include time for services that are not billable (e.g., rest periods).[12] This is also recommended practice for payers other than Medicare (Non-Medicare) billing purposes as well as liability.

The "8-minute billing rule" is discussed in more detail later on in this chapter.

MODALITIES AND PROCEDURES

Although modalities, such as hot packs or cold packs, are generally not reimbursable alone because application of them is not necessarily considered skilled, they may be when rendered in conjunction with a procedure that is facilitated with their use. It is important to check with the individual payer policy.

MODIFIERS

The use of modifiers allows the therapist to indicate when special consideration is needed to demonstrate the need for specific intervention. Modifiers may be used when treatment and evaluation are being performed on the same day or the patient has seen a physician and the PT. There are two general types of modifiers. Level I, or CPT modifiers, consist of two numeric digits and are updated annually by AMA.[2] "Level II modifiers, also referred to as HCPCS modifiers, consists of two digits and are updated annually by CMS. Some commonly used Level I and Level II modifiers are listed here and can also be found in the AMA CPT Professional Book and CMS HCPCS webpage.[2,12]

- **GP:** Service delivered personally by a physical therapist or under an outpatient physical therapy plan of care.
- **GA:** Patient has been advised in advance beneficiary notice (ABN is issued) that the service is not reasonable and necessary by Medicare standards, and it is anticipated that Medicare will deny it.[13]
- **GZ:** Same as GA, but the Medicare beneficiary has not been advised in advance (no ABN issued).[13]
- **GX:** Notice of liability issued voluntarily.[13]
- **GY:** Item or service is statutorily excluded and does not meet the definition of covered benefit.[13]
- **CQ:** Outpatient physical therapy services furnished in whole or in part by a physical therapist assistant.
- **CO:** Outpatient occupational therapy services furnished in whole or in part by an occupational therapy assistant.
- **25:** Evaluation and management performed on the same day as treatment.
- **59:** Identifies a distinct service. If the physician has evaluated the patient on the same day, this would indicate the physical therapy evaluation was separate and distinct.[14]

Example of Column 1 code/Column 2 code 97140/97530:[14]

- CPT Code 97140—Manual therapy techniques (mobilization/manipulation, manual lymphatic drainage, manual traction), one or more regions, each 15 minutes
- CPT Code 97530—Therapeutic activities, direct (one-on-one) patient contact by the provider (use of dynamic activities to improve functional performance), each 15 minutes

Modifier 59 may be reported if the two procedures are performed in distinctly different 15-minute time blocks. For example, one service may be performed during the initial 15 minutes of therapy and the other service performed during the second 15 minutes of therapy. Alternatively, the therapy time blocks may be split. For example, manual therapy might be performed for 10 minutes, followed by 15 minutes of therapeutic activities, followed by another 5 minutes of manual therapy. CPT code 97530 should not be reported and modifier 59 should not be used if the two procedures are performed during the same time block. *Modifier 59 is used appropriately when two timed procedures are performed in different blocks of time on the same day during separate time intervals.*[14]

Example

59 modifier—the modifier that is used to indicate that a code represents a service that is separate and distinct from another service to which it is paired. The X modifiers (XE, XS, XP, XU) should be used in place of modifier 59 if one of the X modifiers more specifically describes the reason that both codes be paid.[14]

- **76:** Treatment twice a day (BID).
- **96: Habilitative Services:** When a service or procedure that may either be habilitative in nature or rehabilitative in nature is provided for habilitative purposes, the physician or other qualified healthcare professional may add modifier 96 to the service or procedure code to indicate this. Such services help an individual learn skills and functioning for daily living that the individual has not yet developed and then keep or improve those learned skills.
- **97: Rehabilitative Services:** When a service or procedure that may be either habilitative or rehabilitative in nature is provided for rehabilitative purposes, the physician or other qualified healthcare professional may add modifier 97 to the service or procedure code to indicate this. Rehabilitative services help an individual keep, get back, or improve skills and functioning for daily living that have been lost or impaired because the individual was sick, hurt, or disabled.

BUNDLING

Although most procedures and modalities have separate and distinct codes, reimbursement may not be available individually. When a procedure or modality is not paid as distinct and separate, it is considered bundled. Medicare bundles hot packs and cold packs with all other services. CPT code 97602 for nonselective debridement may also be bundled. However, the provider should check with the specific carrier, payer, or fiscal intermediary (FI) regarding bundled procedures and codes.

TELEHEALTH AND REMOTE MONITORING

There are no specific telehealth CPT codes for physical therapists. In 2019, new CPT codes were added in the category of Chronic Remote Physiologic Monitoring. These activities are not face to face. These are not considered telehealth services under the Medicare definition.

Moreover, PTs fit under the Qualified Healthcare Professional (QHCP) designation as applicable by state practice acts to participate in remote monitoring. However, CMS has previously indicated it does not believe PTs are eligible to furnish and bill for these codes. In the 2021 Physician Fee Schedule proposed rule: "The CPT Codebook lists the remote physiologic monitoring codes under the main heading Evaluation and Management (E/M). Currently the Evaluation and Management codes, CPT codes 99453, 99454, 99091, 99457, and 99458, can be ordered and billed only by physicians or non-physician practitioners (NPPs) who are eligible to bill Medicare for E/M services." Thus, CMS is not currently recognizing physical therapists as eligible to furnish and bill these codes.

E-VISITS

For Medicare, when allowed by CMS, the e-visit can be billed once for the 7-day period. The code billed is based on the total time spent in that period. The HCPCS e-visit codes paid under the Medicare Physician Fee Schedule are:

- **G2061:** Qualified nonphysician healthcare professional online assessment and management service for an established patient, for up to 7 days; cumulative time during the 7 days, 5 to 10 minutes.
- **G2062:** Qualified nonphysician healthcare professional online assessment and management service for an established patient, for up to 7 days; cumulative time during the 7 days, 11 to 20 minutes.
- **G2063:** Qualified nonphysician healthcare professional online assessment and management service for an established patient, for up to 7 days; cumulative time during the seven days, 21 or more minutes.

THERAPEUTIC CODES/PROCEDURES

CPT therapeutic codes/procedures are medically necessary only when it requires the professional skills of a physical therapist or physical therapist assistant, is designed to address specific needs of the patient, and must be part of an active treatment plan directed at a specific goal. The patient must have the ability to understand and learn from instructions. Documentation of medical necessity must be included for an unusual frequency or duration of training sessions. Documentation must relate the intervention/training to expected functional goals that are attainable by the patient.

In the case of the timed therapeutic CPT codes, documentation should reflect the thought process and skilled decision making of the licensed therapy provider. As such, documentation of patient/client care needs to be more than a litany of procedures related to a date of service. Documentation must include evidence of knowledge and skill related to the procedures performed. It also should provide verification of professional judgment. This concept of clinical decision making can be incorporated into clinical documentation.[15]

Evaluation and Assessment Codes

PT Evaluation: low-complexity (**97161**), moderate-complexity (**97162**), and high-complexity (**97163**). These codes are used for the physical therapy evaluation, including tests, measures, and analysis and synthesis, to establish a prognosis, plan of care, and appropriate goals based on the findings and anticipated recovery.

PT Re-evaluation: 97164. This code is used for physical therapy re-evaluation, including tests, measures, and analysis and synthesis, to establish a prognosis, plan of care, and appropriate goals based on the findings and anticipated recovery when a complete re-evaluation is needed and not in the course of ongoing treatment and regular reassessment for daily recording.

Physical Performance Test: 97750. Physical performance test covers performance tests, such as functional capacity assessments and other performance measures with written reports (i.e., isokinetic testing).

Limb Muscle Testing, Manual: (95831); Hand Muscle Testing, Manual: (95832); Body Muscle Testing, Manual: (95833–834). Codes 95831 to 95834 are self-explanatory. It is the PT's responsibility to get clarification from the payer regarding the use of these versus the physical therapy evaluation code. In cases such as peripheral nerve injury in a limb, postoperative hand management, or spinal cord injury, these codes may be preferable to the evaluation code.

Range of Motion Measurements: 95851–85852. It is the PT's responsibility to get clarification from the payer regarding the use of these versus the physical therapy evaluation code. In cases such as multiple trauma in which multiple ranges must be obtained, these codes may be preferable to the physical therapy evaluation code.

Motion Analysis, Video 3D: 96000. Justification must be clear in the documentation of the need for motion analysis, video 3D, and the outcomes from the assessment, as well as goals.

Motion Test with Foot Pressure Measurement: 96001. Justification must be clear of the need for motion analysis of dynamic foot pressure measurement during gait. The goals and outcomes from the assessment should also be included.

Dynamic Surface EMG: 96002. Justification must be clear in the documentation of the need for dynamic surface electromyography (EMG) during walking and other functional activities. The goals and outcomes from the assessment should also be included. This is calculated in increments up to 12 minutes.

Dynamic Fine Wire EMG: 96003. Justification must be clear in the documentation of the need for dynamic fine wire EMG during walking and other functional activities for one muscle. The goals and outcomes from the assessment should also be included.

Developmental Test, Limb: 96110; Developmental Test, Extremity: 96111; Neurobehavior Status Exam: 96115. Generally, codes 96110, 96111, and 96115 are covered under the physical therapy evaluation code. With appropriate certification, based on state licensing, PTs with special certification may perform and receive reimbursement for EMG/nerve conduction velocity (NCV) under codes 95860 to 95937 from Medicare.

Intervention Codes

Author's Note

A distinction is made between those modalities that require one-on-one administration by the therapist and those that do not. Additionally, the specific body part(s) must be indicated in the documentation for all procedures and modalities. Deficits must be clearly identified and goals objectively described, with an appropriate treatment plan or plan of care.

Hot Packs/Cold Packs: 97010. For Medicare purposes, this is a bundled code and will not be paid for separately. Justification must be clear in the documentation of the need for the hot pack or cold pack and the expected goal, even if used as an adjunct to another procedure. Specific parameters, including patient position and time, must also be included, as well as the type and shape of the pack. The condition of the skin before and after treatment must be noted.

Mechanical Traction: 97012. Used to describe mechanical traction that is set up for the patient and then requires general supervision and adjustment for a period of time. Justification must be clear in the documentation of the need for traction and the expected goal.

Electrical Stimulation: 97014. This code is used for *unattended* electrical stimulation, once the patient has been set up. Justification must be clear in the documentation of the need for the stimulation and the expected goal. Specific parameters, including patient position and time, must also be included, as well as the type of stimulation, electrode placement, and the machine type. The condition of the skin before and after treatment must be noted. Medicare may reimburse for G0283. G0283 – Electrical stimulation (unattended), to one or more areas for indication(s) other than wound care, as part of a therapy plan of care. When submitting electrical stimulation to Medicare, use G0283. A proper denial maybe given, then a secondary payer can be billed.[16]

Vasopneumatic Device Therapy: 97016. Used for the administration of vasopneumatic compression device therapy instruments that require parameters to be set prior to use (i.e., mmHg based on blood pressure) and then general supervision over a period of time. Justification must be clear in the documentation of the need for vasopneumatic compression and the expected goal. Specific parameters, including patient position and time, must also be included, as well as appropriate measurements of edema using girth or volumetric measurement. It must be clearly stated when using girth where the measurements were taken. Treatment must indicate a linear progression of decreasing edema to enable function. The condition of the skin before and after treatment must be noted.

Paraffin Bath: 97018. Justification must be clear in the documentation of the need for the paraffin bath and the expected goal. Specific parameters, including patient position and time, must also be included. Precautions should be clearly indicated and the patient appropriately supervised. The condition of the skin before and after treatment must be noted.

Microwave Therapy: 97020. Justification must be clear in the documentation of the need for microwave therapy and the expected goal. Specific parameters, including patient position and time, must also be included. Precautions should be clearly indicated and the patient appropriately supervised. The condition of the skin before and after treatment must be noted.

Whirlpool Therapy (non-Hubbard Tanks): 97022. Justification must be clear in the documentation of the need for whirlpool therapy and the expected goal. Specific parameters, including patient position, type of whirlpool used, direction and intensity of jets, water temperature, additives, and time, must also be included. Precautions should be clearly indicated and the patient appropriately supervised at all times. The condition of the skin before and after treatment must be noted. If being used for wound care, specific conditions and measurements of the wound must be included, with clearly stated goals showing linear progression. If being used to facilitate range of motion (ROM) or reduction in limb volume or edema, the justification must be clear.

Author's Note

As there are wound care codes, use of them may be warranted. The use of whirlpool for wound care in the advent of more effective and efficient procedures is questionable.

Diathermy Treatment: 97024. Justification must be clear in the documentation of the need for diathermy treatment and the expected goal. Specific parameters, including patient position, settings, and time, must also be included, as well as appropriate padding to an area and removal of external metals, watches, and the like. Precautions should be clearly indicated and the patient appropriately supervised at all times.

Infrared Therapy: 97026. Justification must be clear in the documentation of the need for infrared therapy and the expected goal. Specific parameters, including patient position, settings, and time, must also be included. Precautions should be clearly indicated and the patient appropriately supervised.

Ultraviolet Therapy: 97028. Justification must be clear in the documentation of the need for ultraviolet therapy and the expected goal. Specific parameters, including patient position, established dosage based on minimal erythemic dosage, and time, must also be included. Precautions should be clearly indicated, such as eye protection, and the patient appropriately supervised.

Electrical Stimulation Manual: 97032. Justification must be clear in the documentation of the need for manual electrical stimulation and the expected goal. Specific parameters, including patient position, settings, type of probe or stimulator, and time, must also be included. Precautions should be clearly indicated and the patient appropriately supervised at all times. The skin should be inspected before and after treatment.

Electrical Current Therapy/Iontophoresis: 97033. Justification must be clear in the documentation of the need for electrical current therapy/iontophoresis and the expected goal. Specific parameters, including patient position and time, must also be included, as well as the medication used. Precautions should be clearly indicated and the patient appropriately supervised at all times. The skin should be inspected before and after treatment.

Contrast Bath Therapy: 97034. Justification must be clear in the documentation of the need for contrast bath therapy and the expected goal. Specific parameters, including patient position, water temperatures, receptacle used, and time in each receptacle and total time, must also be included. Precaution should be clearly indicated and the patient appropriately supervised at all times. The skin should be inspected before and after treatment.

Ultrasound Therapy: 97035. Justification must be clear in the documentation of the need for ultrasound therapy and the expected goal. Specific parameters, including patient position, area treated, type of ultrasound (i.e., pulsed vs. continuous), transmission medium, intensity, and time, must also be included. Precautions should be clearly indicated and the patient appropriately supervised at all times.

Hydrotherapy/Hubbard Tank: 97036. Justification must be clear in the documentation of the need for Hubbard tank hydrotherapy and the expected goal. Specific parameters, including patient position, water temperature, intensity and direction of jets, water additives, and time, must also be included. Precautions should be clearly indicated and the patient appropriately supervised at all times.

Physical Therapy Treatment: 97039. This is a nonspecific code and therefore should be avoided. It should be used only if a procedure is being used that does not fall into any other category.

Manual Therapy: 97140. This code includes manual therapy, mobilization, manipulation, manual lymphatic drainage, and manual traction to one or more regions. Justification must be clear in the documentation of the need for the specific procedure and the expected goal. Specific parameters, including patient position, methodology, and post-therapy procedures such as compression wrapping, must also be included. Precautions should be clearly indicated with the patient constantly attended, as manual therapy is hands-on throughout The coding is by 15-minute increments, regardless of the number of areas treated.

Therapeutic Exercise: 97110. All categories of skilled therapeutic exercise are covered by this code to one or more areas. It covers strengthening (not general in nature) and exercises to develop endurance and flexibility. It is imperative that the documentation and plan of care include the term "therapeutic exercise" before listing the specific types employed with the patient. For justification of the need for skilled exercise, specific exercise parameters, applicable hand placement, technique name, and the patient must be included. The exercises must be appropriate for the level of strength or muscle performance the patient demonstrates and linked ultimately to function. Strength should be expressed in fractions, which are more universally understood by nonprofessionals than verbiage. One of the most common scales expresses strength in a range from 0/5 to 5/5, with 5/5 being the strongest and 0/5 representing no muscle contraction. Avoid using goals for strength that state "increase strength by 1/2 grade." Instead, link the strength to function and state the expectation.

Example

Increase strength from 3/5 to 4/5 in LEs to enable stair climbing into home.

Range of motion (ROM) should also be expressed in numbers. Goniometric measurements, using the appropriate goniometer, are the most reliable compared to visual estimates. ROM is best stated in fractions with the available ROM, active (AROM) or passive (PROM), listed over the total "normal" ROM. If the full AROM should be 180° and the patient demonstrates 90°, it should be recorded as 90°/180°. Avoid using terms such as "increase by 10%." Instead, as in strength, list the numbers and link to function.

Example

Increase ROM from 90°/180° degrees to 160°/180° in order to...

Neuromuscular Re-education: 97112. Justification must be clear in the documentation of the need for neuromuscular re-education. The code is used for re-education of balance, coordination, kinesthetic sense, posture, and proprioception for activities performed sitting and standing.

Aquatic Therapy/Exercises: 97113. This code is intended for individual patient sessions that are in water. For justification of the need for skilled aquatics, specific exercise parameters and why the patient requires a water-based environment must be included.

Author's Note

Medicare's guidance on the use of community pools by different provider types. when therapy services may be furnished appropriately in a community pool by a clinician in a physical therapist or occupational therapist private practice, physician office, outpatient hospital, or outpatient SNF, the practice/office or provider shall rent or lease the pool, or a specific portion of the pool. The use of that part of the pool during specified times shall be restricted to the patients of that practice or provider. The written agreement to rent or lease the pool shall be available for review on request. When part of the pool is rented or leased, the agreement shall describe the part of the pool that is used exclusively by the patients of that practice/office or provider and the times that exclusive use applies. Other providers, including rehabilitation agencies (previously referred to as OPTs and ORFs) and CORFs, are subject to the requirements outlined in the respective State Operations Manual regarding rented or leased community pools.[1]

Gait Training: 97116. Justification must be clear in the documentation for the need for gait training. Although many carriers and fiscal intermediaries allow the term "ambulation" to be used to describe "skilled walking assessment and intervention," the CPT code term is "gait." For consistency, therefore, and indication that the activity is the same, the use of the term "gait" for assessment and training purposes is recommended. The term "walking" is never considered skilled and should be avoided unless the patient is being quoted. "Skilling" gait requires the assessment and training of all gait characteristics with appropriate goals, including base of support (BOS); arm swing; swing phase; initial contact; stance; deviations; level of the pelvis; weight bearing and acceptance of weight on the limb; stride length; cadence; posture; assistive devices; balance; surfaces; safety; ability to change directions and negotiate or avoid obstacles; opening and closing doors; asymmetry; distance; sequencing; leg length discrepancies; extent of total effort patient is exerting if assistance is needed; and speed. Normal gait speed = 82 meters/minute (m/min).

Massage Therapy/Therapeutic Massage: 97124. Massage should be referred to as "therapeutic massage" in the documentation. The body part or area should be clearly stated, as well as the relationship between the therapeutic massage and the expected outcome. It is usually used adjunctively to decrease spasm, increase joint ROM, decrease edema, and restore muscle function. Types of strokes should also be included in the documentation. With appropriate justification, this code may be used for postural drainage techniques if it is necessary for it to be done by a PT.

Group Therapeutic Procedures: 97150. Used when patients are receiving skilled services in a group (two or more) with others requiring similar services (same plan of care). The PT must indicate in the documentation the specific treatment, how it will result in stated goals for the specific patient, and the size of the group.

Author's Note

CMS and Medicare reviewed the group therapy code. They issued a transmittal indicating that even if all patients are not receiving the same treatment, this code should be used if the PT is attending to multiple patients in the same time period. The therapist must be in constant attendance, but not involved in one-on-one physical contact. However, according to the APTA, part of the session may be billed individually for direct one-on-one intervention.[17] (Transmittal: CMS 1753 CR 2126)

Therapeutic Activities, Direct: 97530. This category covers direct functional activities, such as lifting, carrying, reaching, catching, overhead activities, and bending, employed when a patient demonstrates limitations in strength, flexibility, ROM, balance, or coordination. The documentation must show the relationship between the activities and the stated goals.

Transfer training or transitional movements may also be included in this category. Each type of transfer necessary for function should be included (i.e., sit to and from stand, stand and pivot, partial stand and pivot, sliding board use, standing disks, mechanical lifts, sit to and from supine, supine to and from long sit). The degree of patient ability must be stated clearly and reflected in the goals. Colloquially for physical therapy, patient ability has been stated in terms of assistance needed, which translates into patient ability. The terms are independent (I), supervisor(s), minimally dependent or minimal assistance, moderately dependent or moderate assistance, maximally dependent or maximal assistance, and total dependence or total assistance. Medicare recommends the use of the terms limited and extensive, with limited corresponding to minimal, and extensive corresponding to all other more dependent terms. However, percentage (%) of patient effort is required for all descriptions. Percentage should always be expressed in the evaluation to establish a baseline, with goals indicating decreasing percentage in a linear fashion. This covers dynamic activities and assumes one-on-one constant attendance. Essential functional activities—those activities that a patient needs to do rather than wants to do—are applicable in this category.

Sensory Integration: 97533. Justification must be clear in the documentation of the need for sensory integration. The code is used for enhancement of sensory processing, promoting appropriate responses between the patient and the environment. This activity requires constant attendance with one-on-one care, in 15-minute increments.

Selective Debridement: 97601. This code includes removal of devitalized tissue from wound or selective debridement without anesthesia (i.e., high-pressure water jet, sharp debridement). Justification must be clear in the documentation of the need for selective debridement based on the description of the wound and devitalized tissue.

Non-Selective Debridement: 97602. This code includes general, nonspecific removal of tissue. For Medicare purposes, this is a bundled code.

Wheelchair Management Training/Propulsion: 97542. This code is used for skilled instruction and adaptation determination of either temporary or permanent confinement to a manual or power wheelchair or power-operated vehicle (scooter). When documenting for manual chairs, all appropriate aspects must be included, such as ability to transfer in and out of (including falls, bed, toilet, other chairs, other surfaces, ramps, cars/buses/trains), manipulation of any of the parts (brakes or power controls), terrain (even/uneven, indoor/outdoor), door opening and closing, all directions including turns, and folding/unfolding. The training of caretakers in all aspects of wheelchair use may also be applicable to this code. The same parameters are applied for power mobility appropriate for the types of controls and adaptations. Essential functional activities—those activities that a patient needs to do rather than wants to do—are also applicable to this category.[15] What recent event prompted the need for a skilled wheelchair assessment; What previous wheelchair assessments have been completed, such as during a Part A SNF stay; Most recent prior functional level; What intervention was tried by nursing staff, caregivers or the patient themselves; Functional deficit due to poor seating or positioning; Objective assessments of applicable impairments such as range of motion (ROM), strength, sitting balance, skin integrity, sensation and tone.[15]

Cognitive Skills Development: 97532. Justification must be clear in the documentation of the need for cognitive skills development, such as improved memory, reasoning, problem solving, and attention to tasks. This activity requires constant attendance with one-on-one care, billed in 15-minute increments.

Orthosis Training: 97760. Orthotic(s) management and training (including assessment and fitting when not otherwise reported), upper extremity(ies), lower extremity(ies) and/or trunk, initial orthotic(s) encounter, each 15 minutes.

Prosthetic training: 97761. Prosthetic(s) training, upper and/or lower extremity(ies), initial prosthetic(s) encounter, each 15 minutes.

Orthotic and prosthetic management: 97763. *Orthotic(s)/prosthetic(s) management and/or training, upper extremity(ies), lower extremity(ies), and/or trunk, subsequent orthotic(s)/prosthetic(s) encounter, each 15 minutes.*

Author's Note

A durable medical equipment (DME) number may be needed in order to bill for the actual orthosis. Treatment under this code may not be reimbursable for multiple sessions.

Self-Care/Home Management Training: 97535. Justification must be clear in the documentation of the need for self-care/home management training. This includes such things as activities of daily living (ADLs), meal preparation, use of assistive or adaptive devices and technologies, and safety. Precautions should be clearly indicated and the patient appropriately supervised. Billing should be listed in 15-minute increments.

Community/Work Reintegration: 97537. Justification must be clear in the documentation of the need for community/work reintegration. Reintegration includes developing incremental activities of daily living (IADL) skills, such as shopping, negotiating transportation, managing monetary transactions, vocational and avocational activities, work environment and ergonomic considerations, and work task analysis. Precautions should be clearly indicated. This activity requires constant attendance with one-on-one care and should be billed in 15-minute increments. Medicare may not reimburse for all activities covered by this code based on the concept of essential function.

Work Hardening: 97545. Justification must be clear in the documentation of the need for work hardening and the expected goal. Specific parameters, activities, and time must also be included. Precautions should be clearly indicated and the patient appropriately supervised. This code is used for the initial 2 hours of work hardening. Medicare does not reimburse for work hardening.

Work Hardening Add-on: 97546. This code would be used for time beyond the initial 2 hours and is billed in 1-hour increments.

Prosthetic Check-out: 97703. Prosthetic check-out covers check out for an established patient for a prosthesis or orthosis and should be billed in 15-minute increments.

Unlisted Physical Medicine/Rehabilitation Service or Procedure: 97799. This code would be used for an unlisted service.

Apply Neurostimulator: 64550. Application of a neurostimulator may include a bone stimulator or functional electrical stimulation, but not a transcutaneous electrical nerve stimulation (TENS) unit.

Effective CY 2020, the CPT Editorial Panel created two new biofeedback codes to replace CPT code 90911. CMS designated these new codes as "sometimes therapy" to permit physicians and nonphysician practitioners (NPPs), including nurse practitioners, physician assistants, and certified nurse specialists, to furnish these services outside a therapy plan of care when appropriate. The two new "sometimes therapy" codes with their CPT long descriptors are as follows:

Biofeedback Training: 90912. Biofeedback training, perineal muscles, anorectal or urethral sphincter, including EMG and/or manometry, when performed; initial 15 minutes of one-on-one physician or other qualified healthcare professional contact with the patient.

Biofeedback Training, Each Additional 15 Minutes: 90913. Biofeedback training, perineal muscles, anorectal or urethral sphincter, including EMG and/or manometry, when performed; each additional 15 minutes of one-on-one physician or other qualified healthcare professional contact with the patient (list separately in addition to code for the primary procedure).

Needle Insertion(s) without Injection(s) (Dry Needling): 20560 and 20561.[18,19] 20560 — Needle insertion(s) without injection(s); 1 or 2 muscle(s) 20561 — Needle insertion(s) without injection(s); 3 or more muscle(s). CMS has assigned these codes the status of non-covered services under Medicare.

Author's Note

Before using any code to bill for procedures, check each payer's policy to determine if the service is covered. Identification of a procedure by code does not automatically qualify it for payment.

NONCOVERED CONDITIONS AND SERVICES AS LISTED ON THE CMS WEBSITE

It is the responsibility of the therapist to be aware of medical conditions and services not covered by the third-party payer. Regardless of the documentation, noncovered services will not be paid, regardless of therapist efforts or goals. CMS has assigned these codes the status of non-covered services under Medicare. A Medicare beneficiary can be billed directly for the services, but reimbursed will not be provided. Follow these procedures for submitting a claim to Medicare: Provide a voluntary Advanced Beneficiary Notice to the patient, Include the appropriate CPT code (Example: 20560 or 20561) on the claim, Append the GX modifier to indicate that the physical therapist and the patient know the service is non-covered. Examples of noncovered services and conditions in the Medicare program include:

1. Vertebral axial decompression (VAD) therapy is considered "investigational" and is a noncovered service under Florida Medicare
2. General exercises to promote overall fitness and flexibility and activities to provide diversion or general motivation
3. Work hardening/conditioning **(CPT codes 97545-97546)**
4. Electrotherapy performed for the treatment of facial nerve paralysis in the application of electrical stimulation **(97014)**
5. Electrotherapy for the treatment of facial nerve paralysis, commonly known as Bell's palsy **(ICD-10 code G51.0)**
6. Diathermy **(97024)** or ultrasound **(97035)** heat treatments performed for respiratory conditions or diseases **(ICD-10 codes J00-J98.9)** are investigational under the Medicare program
7. General exercise programs to improve a patient's general cardiovascular fitness, pulmonary rehabilitation, cardiac rehabilitation, or a maintenance program of therapeutic activities.
8. Aquatic therapy with therapeutic exercise **(97113)** should not be billed when there is not one-on-one contact between the therapist and patient
9. Diapulse and Rolfing **(97799)** treatment is noncovered

10. Hot packs or cold packs unless bundled and an integral component of other intervention
11. Dry Needling is noncovered. Needle Insertion(s) without Injection(s) (Dry Needling): 20560 and 20561. 20560 — Needle insertion(s) without injection(s); 1 or 2 muscle(s) 20561 — Needle insertion(s) without injection(s); 3 or more muscle(s).[18,19]

CODING GUIDELINES

Providers may report evaluation and management services on the same day as physical medicine treatments, provided the services are separately identifiable.

However, according to the Medicare Claims Processing Manual Chapter 12, Section 30.6.1, Medicare does not pay for CPT evaluation and management codes billed by PTPPs or by occupational therapists in independent practice.[20]

There is a clear relationship between CPT coding,[2] ICD-10,[5] and documentation. In order to receive reimbursement, the ICD code[3] must be related to the treatment rendered. The treatment rendered must be described in verbiage that matches the CPT codes[2] in order to appropriately code the billing. However, regardless of the accuracy of the CPT and ICD coding, the documentation must also support the medical necessity of the skilled physical therapy intervention in an appropriate time frame. Unless there is devastating illness or injury or the patient is in a preapproved program of prescribed time, most care should be planned for episodes of 30 days or less.

Understanding the basic concepts of coding and application of them will not guarantee reimbursement. It is up to the therapist to justify all care by entering into the record that skilled services were required, goals were reasonable and reached (preferably in a linear manner), care was reasonable and necessary, and therapy was both effective and efficient.

CODING MINUTES

Counting Minutes for Timed Codes in 15 Minute Units

When only one service is provided in a day, providers should not bill for services performed for less than 8 minutes. For any single timed CPT code in the same day measured in 15-minute units, providers bill a single 15-minute unit for treatment greater than or equal to 8 minutes, through and including 22 minutes. If the duration of a single modality or procedure in a day is greater than or equal to 23 minutes, through and including 37 minutes, then 2 units should be billed. Time intervals for 1 through 8 units are as follows:[21]

Units Number of Minutes[21]

1 unit: ≥8 minutes through 22 minutes
2 units: ≥23 minutes through 37 minutes
3 units: ≥38 minutes through 52 minutes
4 units: ≥53 minutes through 67 minutes
5 units: ≥68 minutes through 82 minutes
6 units: ≥83 minutes through 97 minutes
7 units: ≥98 minutes through 112 minutes
8 units: ≥113 minutes through 127 minutes

The pattern remains the same for treatment times in excess of 2 hours.

If a service represented by a 15-minute timed code is performed in a single day for at least 15 minutes, which service shall be billed for at least one unit. If the service is performed for at least 30 minutes, that service shall be billed for at least two units, etc. It is not appropriate to count all minutes of treatment in a day toward the units for one code if other services were performed for more than 15 minutes. See Examples 2 and 3 later.

When more than one service represented by 15-minute timed codes is performed in a single day, the total number of minutes of service (as noted on the chart) determines the number of timed units billed. See Example 1 later.

If any 15-minute timed service is performed for 7 minutes or less than 7 minutes on the same day as another 15-minute timed service that was also performed for 7 minutes or less and the total time of the two is 8 minutes or greater than 8 minutes, then bill one unit for the service performed for the most minutes. This is correct because the total time is greater than the minimum time for one unit. The same logic is applied when three or more different services are provided for 7 minutes or less than 7 minutes. See Example 5 later.

The expectation (based on the work values for these codes) is that a provider's direct patient contact time for each unit will average 15 minutes in length. If a provider has a consistent practice of billing less than 15 minutes for a unit, these situations should be highlighted for review.

If more than one 15-minute timed CPT code is billed during a single calendar day, then the total number of timed units that can be billed is constrained by the total treatment minutes for that day. See all examples later.

CMS' Publication 100-02, Medicare Benefit Policy Manual, Chapter 15, Section 220.3(E)[1] Treatment Notes, indicates that the amount of time for each specific intervention or modality provided to the patient is not required to be documented in the treatment note, but can be recorded voluntarily. However, as noted earlier, for Medicare purposes, and as best practice, the total timed code treatment minutes and total treatment time in minutes must be documented. These examples, copied from the Medicare Claims Processing Manual Chapter 5 Section 20, indicate how to count the appropriate number of units for the total therapy minutes provided.

Example 1[21]

24 minutes of neuromuscular re-education, code 97112

23 minutes of therapeutic exercise, code 97110

Total timed code treatment time was 47 minutes

See the chart. The 47 minutes falls within the range for 3 units = 38 to 52 minutes.

Appropriate billing for 47 minutes is only 3 timed units. Each of the codes is performed for more than 15 minutes, so each shall be billed for at least 1 unit. The correct coding is 2 units of code 97112 and 1 unit of code 97110, assigning more timed units to the service that took the most time.

Example 2[21]

20 minutes of neuromuscular reeducation (97112)

20 minutes therapeutic exercise (97110)

40 Total timed code minutes

Appropriate billing for 40 minutes is 3 units. Each service was done at least 15 minutes and should be billed for at least 1 unit, but the total allows 3 units. Since the time for each service is the same, choose either code for 2 units and bill the other for 1 unit. Do not bill 3 units for either one of the codes.

Example 3[21]

33 minutes of therapeutic exercise (97110)

7 minutes of manual therapy (97140)

40 Total timed minutes

Appropriate billing for 40 minutes is for 3 units. Bill 2 units of 97110 and 1 unit of 97140. Count the first 30 minutes of 97110 as 2 full units. Compare the remaining time for 97110 (33 – 30 = 3 minutes) to the time spent on 97140 (7 minutes) and bill the larger, which is 97140.

Example 4[21]

18 minutes of therapeutic exercise (97110)

13 minutes of manual therapy (97140)

10 minutes of gait training (97116)

8 minutes of ultrasound (97035)

49 total timed minutes

Appropriate billing is for 3 units. Bill the procedures you spent the most time providing. Bill 1 unit each of 97110, 97116, and 97140. You are unable to bill for the ultrasound because the total time of timed units that can be billed is constrained by the total timed code treatment minutes (i.e., you may not bill 4 units for less than 53 minutes, regardless of how many services were performed). You would still document the ultrasound in the treatment notes.

Example 5[21]

7 minutes of neuromuscular re-education (97112)

7 minutes therapeutic exercise (97110)

7 minutes manual therapy (97140)

21 Total timed minutes

Appropriate billing is for 1 unit. The qualified professional (see definition in Pub. 100-02/15, section 220) shall select one appropriate CPT code (97112, 97110, 97140).[21]

PATIENT CARE SCENARIOS CODING[17]

(These are only examples of proper coding for billing purposes. They are not intended to establish a standard for clinical practice.) These scenarios involved Medicare patients unless otherwise noted and are applicable only if consistent with the applicable state law.

More Than One patient in the Clinic

PT sees patient A at 9:00 a.m. for 30 minutes of therapeutic exercise. At 9:15 Patient B arrives and begins his visit with 15 minutes on the treadmill focusing on muscular recruitment and posture, assisted by a PTA. At 9:30 the PT sets up patient A to begin electrical stimulation, unattended. Following patient A's set up, the PT begins working with patient B on gait training. At 9:55, the PT briefly returns to patient A for assessment following completion of the electrical stimulation, and patient A leaves the clinic. The PT then completes patient B's gait training and patient B leaves the clinic at 10:10 a.m.

Coding:
Patient A: 97110 (therapeutic exercise) two units; 97014 (electrical stimulation, unattended)
Patient B: 97116 (gait training) two units; 97112 (neuromuscular reeducation) one unit

Rationale:
The PT is one-on-one with patient A from 9 to 9:30 a.m., and therefore two units of 97110 would be billed. Patient A's electrical stimulation is also billable as 97014, as it is a supervised modality.

The time that patient B spends with the PTA from 9:15 to 9:30 is billable as one unit of 97112, as the PTA is providing skilled therapy services under the supervision of the PT. In addition, the time spent with the PT from 9:30 to 10:10 is also billable as two more units of 97116 because the PT is one-on-one with patient B. It is appropriate to bill two units of gait training rather than three units, because there were interruptions during the time frame

Group and One-to-One Procedures

Patients A, B, C, and D are scheduled to see their physical therapist at 9:00 a.m. They have all recently been fitted with lower limb prostheses. Patients A, B, and C have below-knee amputations, and patient D has an above-knee amputation. The PT performs ADL training, including stump management techniques with these four patients for 60 minutes. During the session, each patient demonstrates one-on-one with the PT the techniques they were instructed in individually (for approximately 10 to 12 minutes each), to ensure compliance with the techniques in their home settings.

Coding:
Patient A: 97535 (self-care/home management training); 97150 (group therapy)
Patient B: 97535 (self-care/home management training); 97150 (group therapy)
Patient C: 97535 (self-care/home management training); 97150 (group therapy)
Patient D: 97535 (self-care/home management training); 97150 (group therapy)

Rationale:
Patients A, B, C, and D would be considered as a group with a common, unifying element, making code 97150 appropriate to bill for each patient. In addition, code 97535 would also be billed for each patient, because the PT spends approximately 10 to 12 minutes of one-on-one time with each patient practicing the techniques individually.

SUMMARY

In order to ensure reimbursement, the correct procedural codes must be used for all physical therapy services, many of which are general physical medicine and rehabilitation codes.

The correct combination of CPT codes,[2] ICD-10 diagnostic codes,[5] and CPT matching verbiage describing the procedures rendered in the documentation, with an emphasis on function, ongoing justification of the medical necessity for skilled physical therapy, and matched billing dates will assist the PT in ensuring reimbursement based on the documentation.

In those instances in which the PT is not performing the CPT coding or billing, it is critical that the individual(s) handling the billing understand correct coding. If the PT is familiar enough with the codes and terminology to use them appropriately, an "outsider" can more easily do the coding. Electronic or computerized systems can be designed to facilitate automatic coding, as inclusion of codes with correction description on preprinted forms. The Centers for Medicare and Medicaid Services developed the National Correct Coding Initiative (NCCI) to promote national correct coding methodologies and to control improper coding that leads to inappropriate payment in Part B claims.[22]

REVIEW QUESTIONS

1. What is a CPT code? Explain the application in physical therapy.
2. What is an ICD-10 code? Explain the application in physical therapy.
3. What is the relationship between the CPT codes and ICD-10 codes?
4. What is the medical diagnosis?
5. What is the physical therapy diagnosis or physical therapy problem?
6. What is the relationship between the medical diagnosis and the physical therapy diagnosis (problem)?
7. What is a code modifier? Explain the role of modifiers in the billing process.
8. What are the time increments for CPT code procedures for Medicare billing versus non-Medicare billing?
9. Relative to CPT codes, explain the difference between attended and unattended procedures.
10. What are the risks of billing for noncovered procedures?

REFERENCES

1. *Medicare Benefit Policy Manual Chapter 15—Covered Medical and Other Health Services.* CMS.gov. Available at https://www.cms.gov/Regulations-and-Guidance/Guidance/Manuals/Downloads/bp102c15.pdf. Accessed August 6, 2020.
2. *CPT® Overview and Code Approval.* American Medical Association. Available at https://www.ama-assn.org/practice-management/cpt/cpt-overview-and-code-approval Accessed August 6, 2020.
3. *HCPCS Coding Questions.* Centers for Medicare & Medicaid Services. Available at https://www.cms.gov/Medicare/Coding/MedHCPCSGenInfo/HCPCS_Coding_Questions. Accessed August 7, 2020.
4. *Medicare Claims Processing Manual Chapter 23 - Fee Schedule Administration and Coding Requirements, Section 20.* Centers for Medicare & Medicaid Services. Available at https://www.cms.gov/Regulations-and-Guidance/Guidance/Manuals/downloads/clm104c23.pdf. Accessed August 7, 2020.
5. *International Classification of Diseases, Tenth Revision, ICD-10.* Centers for Disease Control and Prevention. Available at https://www.cdc.gov/nchs/icd/icd10.htm. Accessed February 20, 2020.
6. *Understanding ICD-10 (ICD-10-CM).* American Physical Therapy Association, Alexandria, VA. Available at https://www.apta.org/your-practice/payment/coding-billing/icd-10/faqs. Accessed August 7, 2020.
7. *Resource-Based Relative Value Scale (RBRVS) Overview.* American Medical Association. Available at https://www.ama-assn.org/about/rvs-update-committee-ruc/rbrvs-overview. Accessed August 6, 2020.
8. *How to Use the Searchable Medicare Physician Fee Schedule (MPFS).* Centers for Medicare and Medicaid Services. https://www.cms.gov/apps/physician-fee-schedule/help/How_to_MPFS_Booklet_ICN901344.pdf. Accessed August 7, 2020.
9. *Overview Medicare Physician Fee Schedule (MPFS).* Centers for Medicare and Medicaid Services. Available at https://www.cms.gov/apps/physician-fee-schedule/overview.aspx. Accessed August 7, 2020.
10. *CMS 1500 Form.* Centers for Medicare & Medicaid Services (CMS). Available at https://www.cms.gov/Medicare/CMS-Forms/CMS-Forms/CMS-Forms-Items/CMS1188854. Accessed August 6, 2020.
11. *Medicare Claims Processing Manual, Chapter 5—Part B Outpatient Rehabilitation and CORF/OPT Services.* CMS Claims Processing. Centers for Medicare and Medicaid Services. Available at https://www.cms.gov/media/136366. Accessed August 6, 2020.
12. *Medicare Benefit Policy Manual Chapter 15 – Covered Medical and Other Health Services.* Centers for Medicare & Medicaid Services. Available at https://www.cms.gov/Regulations-and-Guidance/Guidance/Manuals/downloads/bp102c15.pdf. Accessed August 7, 2020.
13. *Medicare Advance Written Notices of Noncoverage. MLN Booklet.* Centers for Medicare & Medicaid Services. Available at https://www.cms.gov/Outreach-and-Education/Medicare-Learning-Network-MLN/MLNProducts/downloads/ABN_Booklet_ICN006266.pdf. Accessed August 7, 2020.
14. *Alpha-Numeric HCPCS.* Centers for Medicare & Medicaid Services. Available at https://www.cms.gov/Medicare/Coding/HCPCSReleaseCodeSets/Alpha-Numeric-HCPCS. Accessed August 6, 2020.
15. *Proper Use of 59 Modifier.* Centers for Medicare & Medicaid Services (CMS). Available at https://www.cms.gov/Outreach-and-Education/Medicare-Learning-Network-MLN/MLNMattersArticles/Downloads/SE1418.pdf. Accessed February 20, 2020.
16. *Medical Billing and Coding - Procedure code, ICD CODE.* Available at http://www.whatismedicalinsurancebilling.org/2010/07/billing-cpt-97530-and-97542.html. Accessed August 7, 2020.
17. *Transmittal AB-03-093. Correction: Coverage and Billing Requirements for Electrical Stimulation for the Treatment of Wounds.* Centers for Medicare & Medicaid Services. Available at https://www.cms.gov/Regulations-and-Guidance/Guidance/Transmittals/downloads/AB03093.pdf. Accessed August 7, 2020.
18. *Coding Interpretations: Group Therapy patient Scenarios.* American Physical Therapy Association, Alexandria, VA. Available at https://www.apta.org/your-practice/payment/coding-billing/coding-interpretations-group-therapy-patient-scenarios. Accessed August 7, 2020.
19. *Busting Payment Myths (and Regulating Your Expectations) Part 4.* American Physical Therapy Association, Alexandria, VA. Available at https://www.apta.org/article/2020/07/29/busting-medicare-part-b-myths-and-regulating-your-expectations-part-4. Accessed August 7, 2020.
20. *Physician Fee Schedule Coding Updates.* American Physical Therapy Association, Alexandria, VA. Available at https://www.apta.org/apta-magazine/2020/02/01/compliance-matters-physician-fee-schedule-coding-updates#:~:text=The%20code%20terminology%20for%20the,3%20or%20more%20muscle(s). Accessed August 7, 2020.
21. *Medicare Claims Processing Manual Chapter 12 Physicians/Nonphysician Practitioners.* Centers for Medicare &

Medicaid Services (CMS). Available at https://www.cms.gov/Regulations-and-Guidance/Guidance/Manuals/downloads/clm104c12.pdf. Accessed August 6, 2020.

22. *Pub 100-04 Medicare Claims Processing Manual.* CMS Claims Processing. Centers for Medicare and Medicaid Services. Available at https://www.cms.gov/Regulations-and-Guidance/Guidance/Transmittals/Downloads/R2121CP.pdf. Accessed August 6, 2020.

23. *Medicare National Correct Coding Initiative.* American Physical Therapy Association, Alexandria, VA. Available at https://www.apta.org/your-practice/payment/coding-billing/correct-coding-initiative-cci. Accessed August 7, 2020.

14 Documentation Content Principles

OBJECTIVES

Following completion of this chapter, the reader will be able to:

- Describe value-based physical therapy.
- Discuss why strength and range of motion are best described in numbers as fractions, but tone, which can also be described in fractions, is preferably described in verbiage.
- Explain rehabilitation potential in the context of physical therapy.
- Identify two components included in muscle performance and provide an example for each.
- Explain the relationship between safety/risk reduction and strength.
- Explain why precautions and contraindications are necessary relative to physical therapy intervention and their relationship to medical necessity.
- Describe the different levels of evaluation.
- Discuss examples of objective descriptions of:

  a. Gait
  b. Range of motion
  c. Balance
  d. Strength
  e. Wheelchair mobility
  f. Motor control

In previous chapters we discussed what should be included when documenting the initial evaluation, daily notes, progress reports, and discharge summary. It is important for the documentation to reflect the need for skilled service. In this chapter we discuss in detail the documentation considerations for the different aspects of the physical therapy evaluation document (including goal writing). This document requires the following components: *History, Examination, Clinical Presentation,* and *Clinical Decision-Making*. These components will be used to demonstrate how the clinician selects the appropriate level of evaluation and the value of physical therapy. It is important to demonstrate the value of physical therapy.

REVIEW OF CENTERS FOR MEDICARE & MEDICAID SERVICES DEFINITIONS

Physical therapists (PTs) have been using a systematic approach to evaluate the patient and to determine the patient dysfunctions that need to be addressed. When documenting on this and subsequent patient encounters, please consider the definitions that the Centers for Medicare & Medicaid Services (CMS)[1] uses and the fact that not all forms of assessment are reimbursable.

Evaluation

The process that the PT uses "that requires professional skills to make clinical judgments about conditions for which services are indicated based on objective measurements and subjective evaluations of patient performance and functional abilities. Evaluation is warranted e.g., for a new diagnosis or when a condition is treated in a new setting. These evaluative judgments are essential to development of the plan of care, including goals and the selection of interventions."[1]

Assessment

Assessment is separate from the evaluation and is included in services or procedures, (it is not separately payable). "Assessments shall be provided only by clinicians, because assessment requires professional skill to gather data by observation and patient inquiry and may include limited objective testing and measurement to make clinical judgments regarding the patient's condition(s). Assessment determines, e.g., changes in the patient's status since the last visit/treatment day and whether the planned procedure or service should be modified. Based on these assessment data, the professional may make judgments about progress toward goals and/or determine that a more complete evaluation or re-evaluation (see definitions later) is indicated. Routine weekly assessments of expected progression in accordance with the plan are not payable as re-evaluations.[1]

PTs participating in the Medicare program are required to identify and document if there are any factors that could potentially affect treatment outcomes. The category used for this is called complexities.

Complexities

These are factors could complicate and may influence treatment, "e.g., they may influence the type, frequency, intensity and/or duration of treatment. Complexities may be represented by diagnoses (ICD codes), by patient factors such as age, severity, acuity, multiple conditions, and motivation, or by the patient's social circumstances such as the support of a significant other or the availability of transportation to therapy."[1]

Currently, PTs need to pick from three different evaluation codes based on the following complexity levels:

CPT 97161 Physical Therapy Evaluation (Complexity Level I: LOW)

The evaluation's complexity is low when there no personal factors or comorbidities in the patient's history that will affect treatment. There are fewer than two exam elements, including body structures, activity limitations, and/or participation restrictions in their exam. Additionally, they are stable and uncomplicated.

CPT 97162 Physical Therapy Evaluation (Complexity Level II: MODERATE)

The evaluation's complexity is moderate when there are either one to two personal factors or comorbidities in their history affecting their current condition. There are three exam elements, including body structures, activity limitations, and/or participation restrictions in their exam and/or they present with an evolving clinical presentation.

CPT 97163 Physical Therapy Evaluation (Complexity Level III: HIGH)

The evaluation's complexity is high when there are three or more personal factors or comorbidities in their history affecting their current condition. There are four or

PHYSICAL THERAPY EVALUATION REFERENCE TABLE

CPT© Code	97161	97162	97163
Required Components (all are required in selecting evaluation level)			
History			
no personal factors and/or comorbidities	X		
1–2 personal factors and/or comorbidities		X	
3 or more personal factors and/or comorbidities			X
Examination of body system(s) (elements include body structures and functions, activity limitations, and/or participation restrictions)			
addressing 1–2 elements	X		
addressing a total of 3 or more elements		X	
addressing a total of 4 or more elements			X
Clinical Presentation			
Stable	X		
Evolving		X	
Unstable			X
Clinical Decision-Making (complexity)			
	low	Moderate	high
Development of Plan of Care			
Additional Guiding Factors			
Coordination, consultation, and collaboration of care with physicians, other qualified healthcare professionals, or agencies is provided consistent with the nature of the problem(s) and the needs of the patient, and/or other caregivers.			
Typical Face-to-Face Time (minutes)	20	30	45

An additional new code, 97164, replaces 97002 for physical therapy revaluation.

NOTE: These codes replace 97001 for Medicare and commercial payers; claims for worker's compensation and auto liability may continue to use 97001.

more exam elements, including body structures, activity limitations, and/or participation restrictions in their exam and/or their current clinical presentation is unstable or unpredictable.

Re-evaluation

Re-evaluation is separately payable and is periodically indicated during an episode of care when the professional assessment of a clinician indicates a significant improvement, or decline, or change in the patient's condition or functional status that was not anticipated in the plan of care. Although some state regulations and state practice acts require re-evaluation at specific times, for Medicare payment, reevaluations must also meet Medicare coverage guidelines. The decision to provide a reevaluation shall be made by a clinician.[1]

INITIAL EXAMINATION AND EVALUATION

PTs treat and manage a great variety of conditions. To assist clinicians, the American Physical Therapy Association (APTA) *Guide to Physical Therapist Practice*[2] has identified 25 categories of tests and measures that need to be used in physical therapy to help determine current patient status, and they can be used to identify a change in patient condition or status.

These 25 categories are aerobic capacity, anthropometric characteristics, arousal/attention and cognition, assistive and adaptive devices, circulation (arterial, venous, lymphatic), cranial and peripheral nerve integrity, environmental/home and work (job, school, play) barriers, ergonomics and body mechanics, gait/locomotion and balance, integument integrity, joint integrity and mobility, motor function (motor control and learning), muscle performance (strength, power, endurance), neuromotor development and sensory integration, orthotic/protective and supportive devices, pain, posture, prosthetic requirements, range of motion (including muscle length), reflex integrity, self-care and home management (activities of daily living [ADL] and instrumental activities of daily living [IADL]), sensory integrity, ventilation and respiration/gas exchange, and work (job/school/play) and community and leisure integration or reintegration.

It is the PT's responsibility to select those tests and measures within each category that are most appropriate to the patient's signs, symptoms, and concerns using the clinical decision-making model.

Essential Function

For Medicare purposes, standardized tests and measures should be focused on activities related to necessary function versus leisure and those problems or impairments directly affecting necessary or essential function. In the outpatient setting, objective standardized tests and measures are required on initial examination. Essential function includes adequate aerobic endurance to perform activities such as transitional movements and transfers, bed mobility, gait on a variety of surfaces or if nonambulatory or limited in gait, other locomotion (i.e., wheelchair, power-operated vehicle, or power wheelchair), negotiating doorways and different surfaces, avoidance of objects, safety, and balance in standing and movements related to effective ADL performance. In some instances, tests and measures include IADL and negotiating public transportation if a beneficiary is still working or receiving treatment on an outpatient basis. Pain in the absence of dysfunction is not a qualifier for skilled physical therapy. However, if the patient is reporting pain and it affects functions not necessarily apparent or measurable in the clinic, close attention must be paid to patient monitoring of improvement external to the clinic as a measure of success. Examples of this are sleeping through the night or if driving is necessary (even if it is to and from medical appointments), the ability to safely turn the head, sit for a prescribed length of time, and operate the vehicle safely. Lack of sleep can result in impairment in judgment and fatigue, endurance limitations, depression, and weakness. Medicare Part B pays for cardiac rehabilitation/intensive cardiac rehabilitation

(CR/ICR) programs and related items and services if specific criteria are met by the Medicare beneficiary, the CR/ICR program itself, the setting in which is it administered, and the physician administering the program. CR/ICR services must be furnished in a physician's office or a hospital outpatient setting (for ICR, the hospital outpatient setting must provide ICR using an approved program). All settings must have a physician immediately available and accessible for medical consultations and emergencies at all times when items and services are being furnished under the program. This provision is satisfied if the physician meets the requirements for direct supervision of physician office services as specified at 42 CFR 410.26, and for hospital outpatient services as specified at 42 CFR 410.27. The CMS Publication 100-02 Medicare Benefit Policy Manual Chapter 15, Section 232[1] discusses the coverage requirements for these services in detail, including the coverage for pulmonary rehabilitation. Individuals with cardiac problems qualify for skilled physical therapy secondary to weakness, functional decline, gait abnormalities, etc.

In the non-Medicare adult context, the concept of function may be more generic in scope, encompassing leisure and lifestyle. However, as in Medicare, pain as a sole diagnosis in the absence of functional limitation may likely not be reimbursable unless the patient has been specifically referred for pain management or a pain program and it has been preapproved by the payer. There may be limited payment to instruct an individual in techniques that may help manage the pain and facilitate function depending on the payer source.

Wellness programs are not paid as skilled physical therapy in Medicare or non-Medicare venues.

Author's Note

According to the Medicare Benefit Policy Manual Chapter 15, Section 220.2:[1]

Services that do not meet the requirements for covered therapy services in Medicare manuals are not payable using codes and descriptions as therapy services. For example, services related to activities for the general good and welfare of patients, e.g., general exercises to promote overall fitness and flexibility and activities to provide diversion or general motivation, do not constitute therapy services for Medicare purposes. Also, services not provided under a therapy plan of care, or provided by staff who are not qualified or appropriately supervised, are not payable therapy services.

Specific respiratory intervention may be covered in non-Medicare venues depending on the payer.

Standardized tests and measures performed at initial examination, depending on the specifics and how long a patient will be treated, should be repeated at intervals and at discharge. In some instances, the test itself can be used as a component of therapeutic intervention. By repeating a test at the time of discharge, significant improvements made as evidenced by improvements in scores facilitate payment and justification of skilled services. This is true for quality-of-life instruments that may be questionnaires, including confidence scales, as well as more movement-related or functional tests and measures.

Example

Questionnaire/survey instrument: Patient-Reported Outcome Measurement Information System (PROMIS),[3] SF36 SF 36 (Quality of Life [QOL]), Oswetry Pain Scale (used frequently for pain assessment related to back pain), disease specific instruments i.e. Parkinson's, Multiple Sclerosis

Standardized Functional Tests: Timed Up and Go (TUG) (for balance), Dynamic Gait Index (DGI) (for gait ability under varied conditions), Romberg and Sharpened Romberg (static balance eyes open and closed; two legs, single leg), Berg Balance Scale (BBS) (14-item objective measure that assesses static balance and fall risk in adults)

Author's Note

Patient-Reported Outcome Measurement Information System (PROMIS)[3] has developed self-report measures for pediatrics and adults for functions, symptoms, behaviors, and feelings. PROMIS asks about the level of confidence in doing the activity, not just whether their health limits the activity.

PROMIS Physical Function (PROMIS PF) measures the outcome of patients or clients with musculoskeletal disorders by assessing physical function through a grading scale of ADLs. PROMIS PF is used as an outcome in research on the effectiveness of interventions. Several variations of PROMIS PF have been developed to better suit target populations.[3]

The overall PROMIS system, of which PROMIS PF is one component, is a comprehensive set of outcome measures that evaluates the physical, mental, and social health of adults and children. PROMIS was designed to improve and standardize measurement of several selected patient-reported outcome measures through both computer adaptive testing and traditional "paper and pencil" instruments.[3]

Example of an Initial Evaluation

Initial examination/evaluation, including plan of care (POC):
Patient demographics, including social history, would precede the information that follows.

Initial Assessment (Fill in Blanks)

Date: Client Name: DOB: Medical DX/Functional DX (ICD-10):
Reason for referral (should be functionally oriented and may match treatment diagnosis if functional):
History of Current Illness/Chief Compliant:
Functional limitations:
Prior level of function (prior to current episode):
Past medical history *(comorbidities/personal factors):*
Current Medications:

Cognition (alert, oriented to person, place, time):
Follows _____ step directions:
Verbal/gesture/combination:
Safety awareness:
Precautions:
Respiratory/cardiac status/aerobic capacity:

Balance:	Sitting: With/ without back supported	Functional activity
If used a device, Type:	Standing: With/ without device	Functional activity

Other categories: Systems

Strength: 0/5 to 5/5 scale:

Other muscle performance:

Range of motion (ROM) (expressed as fraction out of "normal ranges"): Extremities/trunk/cervical:

Tone: low, high, rigidity, spasticity (using Modified Ashworth Scale verbiage) Extremities/trunk/other:

Pain: location/grade 0/10 to 10/10, activity affected:

Level at worst: *(why/when/quality?)*: Least:

What relieves or decreases it?

Willingness to move:

Skin integrity:

Sensation: light touch, pain, proprioception, other:

Coordination:

Motor control/quality of movement:

Bed mobility:

Rolling: L/R:

Supine </> sit: log sit and short sit:

Scooting: side to side, up and down:

Transfers: Sit </> stand:

Stand pivot:

Wheelchair, chair </> bed/mat:

Gait: device, pattern, dependence:

Wheelchair management: manual, electric wheelchair, or power operated vehicle (i.e. scooter)

Posture:

Standardized tests and measures: Summary of results:

Other:

Rehabilitation potential (relative to physical therapy *(e.g., Poor, Guarded, Fair, Good, Excellent)*

Assessment: Related to functional status, level of severity

Goals: Time defined short-term goals (verbiage looking to a long term target date and goals needed to achieve it in increments)

Time defined long-term goals:

(Goals should relate to a client's primary problems and patient's goal, addressing significant objective findings related to a functional activity that is an essential life skill [optional pain]). For example, improve R shoulder flexion to 125 degrees/180 degrees with 50% less pain to 3/10 level to improve ability to reach into cabinets, wash hair, put on shirt/dress, and perform house cleaning.

Sample Plan of Care: Verbiage should match Current Procedural Terminology/Healthcare Common Procedure Coding System (CPT/HCPCS) categories as much as possible. *(CPT codes develop, updated, and copyrighted by the American Medical Association [AMA])*

97110: Therapeutic procedure, on one or more areas, each lasting 15 minutes. Therapeutic exercises are performed in either an active, active-assisted or passive (e.g., treadmill, isokinetic exercise, lumbar stabilization, stretching, strengthening) approach.

97140: Manual therapy techniques, such as mobilization and manipulation, manual lymphatic drainage, and manual traction.

97112: Neuromuscular reeducation, to improve balance, coordination, kinesthetic sense, posture, and proprioception (e.g., proprioceptive neuromuscular facilitation, Feldenkrais, Bobath, BAPs boards, and desensitization techniques). (This category may be challenged by Medicare if Local Coverage Determination [LCD] definition is more specific—check fiscal intermediary's LCD.)

Author's Note

Medicare LCDs and National Coverage Determinations (NCDs) in medical coding and billing medical coders and billers have two types of coverage determinations within Medicare: local and national. When a contractor or fiscal intermediary makes a ruling as to whether a service or item can be paid, it is known as a local coverage determination (LCD).[4]

97530: Therapeutic activities, direct (one on one) patient contact by the provider (use of dynamic activities to improve functional performance), each 15 minutes.
97116: Gait training that's medically necessary for training patients whose walking abilities have been impaired by neurological, muscular, or skeletal abnormalities or trauma (includes stair climbing).
97542: Wheelchair management (e.g., assessment, fitting, training), each 15 minutes and is used to assess a patient's need for a wheelchair as well as teaching the patient wheelchair maneuvering skills.
97535: Self-care/home management training (e.g., ADLs and compensatory training, meal preparation, safety procedures, and instructions in use of assistive technology devices/adaptive equipment) direct one-on-one contact, each 15 minutes
Other CPT codes: (Fill in others as indicated based on AMA CPT codes definitions revised periodically. Interventions selected should refer to the client's primary problems and significant objective findings.)

As all or most of this information using this basic format may be on one or two single pages with standardized tests and measures attached, it is not necessary to write a separate problem summary. However, many clinicians include a problem summary, as this will identify the need for skilled service and will relate to the treatment goals.

Goal formula = Significant objective finding of an essential life skill relating to functional activities.

Example

Improve R shoulder flexion to 125 degrees/180 degrees to improve ability to reach into cabinets, wash hair, put on shirt/dress and perform cleaning.

In some settings the evaluation categories/format may be a facility requirement. Each category with a deficit noted should have a corresponding short-term and long-term goal as indicated. Impairment-based goals should be included but linked to the functional end. Goals should also include what instructions the patient and caretakers need to know.

The categories indicated here may be adjusted depending on the type of clientele a facility sees. Remember that the treatment diagnosis must be consistent with the planned interventions, the deficits identified, and the short- and long-term goals. All categories indicated correspond to the categories in the APTA *Guide to Physical Therapist Practice.*[2]

EXAMPLES FOR CATEGORIES ON INITIAL EXAM AND EVALUATION

Medical diagnosis: Contusions left hip (hematoma), low back pain

Physical therapy diagnosis: Gait abnormality, contusions, low back pain, muscle weakness, abnormal posture

Reason for referral: Dependent for gait, transfers, weakness BLEs, back pain impairing function, dependence for ADL, IADL since she fell

Prior level of function: Lived alone in first floor apartment, I in all ADL & IADL, drove own car, I gait without assistive devices

Strength/quality of movement: BLE: 3+/5 proximal, 3/5 distal, with inability to perform repetitive movement against resistance, movements slow, hesitating

AROM: shoulders 160/180° of flex/abd, fingers maintained in minimal flexion with arthritic changes noted, posture in standing forward flexed ~ 25° and R shifted; unable to extend or flex trunk secondary to CO severe pain 9/10.

PATIENT GOALS

According to the *Guide to Physical Therapist Practice*,[2] goals and expected outcomes are categorized together. Following are the categories of goals (based on increases or improvement) with summaries of the skills that should be considered when writing patient goals. Please note that although categories may be stated in broad, general terms, they must be stated specifically in the actual plan for an individual patient. These are applicable across all settings and are applicable to patients through the lifespan.

Author's Note

The clinician should always remember that goals should address problems (significant objective findings in the evaluation), address essential life skills, and relate to the client's primary problems.

Example

GOALS:

STGs (2 weeks):

Patient will have a reduced Oswestry disability score of 30/100 and a reduced FABQ-W score of 8 in order to return to part time work and leisure activities.

Patient will have reduced pain as indicated by a NPRS score of 2/10 in order to return to part time work and leisure activities.

Patient will increase muscle strength of abdominal and multifidi muscles to 3+/5 and 4+/5 to facilitate active spinal stabilization during sitting and reaching.

LTGs (6 weeks):

Patient will have an Oswestry disability score of 10/100 and a reduced FABQ-W score of less than 5 in order to return to work and leisure activities.

Patient's pain complaints will be resolved as indicated by a NPRS score of 0/10 in order to return to work and leisure activities.

Patient will increase muscle strength of abdominal and multifidi muscles to 4+/5 and 5/5 for active spinal stabilization in order to return to work and leisure activities.

Patient will be independent on HEP to further maintain endurance and strength in spinal posture and stabilization to prevent reoccurrence of injury.

Patient will regain normal spinal mobility through the use of spinal manipulation in order to return to work and leisure activities.

Factors to Consider Regarding Patient Goals

Impact of Pathology/Pathophysiology/Presenting Problems/ Impairments—Body Function and Structures (ICF Model)

The impact of the pathology or pathophysiology on movement is the reason the patient needs physical therapy. This constitutes the physical therapy or treatment diagnosis, physical therapy problems, and the relationship between the medical problem and/or the resulting functional deficits. Patient pathology may lead to the need for reduction of edema or lymphedema, reduction of joint inflammation and swelling, reduction in soft tissue swelling or tone, enhanced wound healing, or tissue restriction reduction, all in order to facilitate movement and function.

Example

Lymphedema: limited AROM, limited use of extremity, pain, limited ADL ability, unable to write, loss of fine motor control in hand

Palpable spasm paraspinals thoracic and lumbar regions limiting trunk movement and ability to stand or sit

Grade IV wound on R heel necessitating NWB gait and inability to drive car

The impact of physical therapy on a patient's impairments, including body function and structures, should be significant. Examples of changes as a result of physical therapy include increased muscle performance endurance and aerobic capacity; decreased energy expenditure or increased energy efficiency; increased ROM/decreased contracture; improved muscle performance (strength, power, endurance); decreased breathing effort or increase in effective breathing effort with ability to sustain longer continuous activity; changes in motor control (synergy, patterns, coordination); stable or improved balance; increased postural control with decreased fall risk; improved integument and joint integrity; increased sensory awareness; improved gait and locomotion; increased weight bearing; optimal joint alignment and use (i.e., prosthesis, orthosis); optimal loading on a body part; increased ability to sit or stand for extended periods; and ability to sleep through the night and enhanced tissue perfusion and oxygenation.

Impact on Functional Limitations and Disabilities/Functioning and Disability (ICF Model)

A PT's impact on a patient's functional limitation includes decreased levels of dependence or need for assistance, improved ability to perform tasks, increased tolerance for positional changes, and increased performance of and independence in ADL and IADL with or without devices, as well as return to work, leisure, school, and other responsibilities (i.e., that of homemaker or caretaker) (in the *Guide to Physical Therapist Practice*[2] gait-related activities are listed under impairments).

As the patient continues physical therapy, his or her disabilities will be affected in several ways, including the patient's ability to resume performance-of-life roles, such as returning to work or school; returning home (if the patient was an inpatient); and resuming those leisure activities once challenging or impossible due to the impairment.

Risk Reduction/Prevention

As a result of physical therapy, the patient should experience a reduction in risk factors associated with nonadherence, as examples, to surgical precautions and weight-bearing limitations. Another area of risk reduction would be enhanced awareness of surroundings for safety, compensation for sensory or vision loss, awareness of potential for skin breakdown, and appropriate awareness of abilities versus inabilities.

Prevention or decreased risk of developing secondary problems may be critical in justifying skilled physical therapy. The necessity of protection of body parts in the absence of sensation or vision impairment, reduction of pressure on tissues to prevent breakdown and infection, and increased understanding of assistive devices to prevent falls or other accidents, as well as prevention of postural syndromes from pain and abnormal protective posturing and loss of function secondary to tissue restrictions, all benefit movement and patient function over time. When prevention of secondary problems/dysfunction are a component of physical therapy, they should be clearly identified in the initial examination/evaluation.

Impact on Health, Wellness, and Fitness

A patient should gradually experience improved movement, health status and increased overall wellness as an outcome of physical therapy. Physical function and capacity are improved, allowing the patient to improve overall fitness and movement-related activity, even in the presence of short-term, long-term, or permanent disability.

Patient Satisfaction

Although there are multiple factors to consider regarding patient satisfaction, the most relevant to goals of physical therapy are improved sense of well-being, decreased stressors, overall improvement in movement and function, and achievement of patient goals. The patient's satisfaction is based on the level and timeliness of goal achievement (see Tables 14-1 and 14-2 for sample patient goals), effectiveness of physical therapy communication, and caring and respect for the patient and significant others.

Patient goals should be established at the initial examination/evaluation, and the PT should incorporate them into the POC.

Plan of Care with Functional Goals

Impairment-based goals should be included but linked to the functional end goal. The following example lists several functionally oriented goals in physical therapy.

Author's Note

Another concept is placing "to-do's" in short-term goals (STGs) and "functional goals" in long-term goals (LTGs). For example, in STGs: Place a 5-mm heel lift in LLE to improve pelvic symmetry, decrease RLE vaulting, improve balance/coordination, and decrease pain. In LTGs: "functional goals" patient to be able to walk prolonged community distances for grocery shopping, community activities as PLF with 1/10 pain.

Table 14-1 Sample Patient Problems and Matching Goals

DEFICIT/FINDING/PROBLEM	SHORT-TERM GOAL 2 WEEKS (INCLUDE DATE)
Aerobic capacity limited to <1-minute continuous activity before becoming short of breath (SOB)	Increase to 3 to 5 minutes continuous activity and eliminate constant respiratory symptoms and fatigue at rest
Impaired static sitting; unable to sustain upright without external support	Increased postural control and muscle performance of trunk stabilizers to reduce fall risk in sitting associated with center of gravity (COG) changes
Dynamic sitting impaired; when perturbed or leans in any direction beyond upright, is unable to resume upright (based on numeric scale)	Increase dynamic sitting balance with ability to return to upright when leans out of COG to prevent falls associated with reaching and bending in sit
Moderate dependence for standing with walker	Decrease dependence to minimal assist with pelvic stabilization to minimize fall risk in standing activities and facilitate activities in standing
Dynamic standing 1+ with rolling walker	Increase to 1 to begin decreasing fall risk on indoor surfaces
Rolling L/R modified with bedrails, limited assist 10% for lower trunk	Progress to limited assist 5% (tactile facilitation at pelvis) without rails to facilitate change of position for skin protection and to facilitate sleep through the night
Supine <> sit limited assist 25% to initiate unweighting of trunk and provide tactile facilitation	Supine <> sit limited assist 10%; tactile facilitation only
Scooting limited assist 25%	Scooting limited assist 10%
Transfers: sit <> stand limited assist 25% to initiate trunk flexion and unweighting	Transfers: sit <> stand limited assist 10% to initiate unweighting
Wheelchair <> bed/mat limited assist 25% to execute pivot	Wheelchair <> bed/mat with supervision/verbal instruction
ROM: bilateral dorsiflexion: 0°	With verbal instruction, will perform exercises to be performed in room and at home to increase ankle ROM in order to facilitate performance of functional activities (i.e., sit to stand)
	Ten degrees of active assistive bilateral dorsiflexion
Strength 3+/5 to 4–/5 throughout extremities with impaired muscle performance; limited ability to perform repetitive activity against gravity or functionally	Strength consistent in 4–/5 range with increased muscle performance and ability to sustain movement and activity against gravity during functional gait, standing

(continued)

Table 14-1 Sample Patient Problems and Matching Goals (Continued)

Gait front-wheeled rolling walker, rear end caps, step to, ↓ knee flexion L with swing, ↓ initial contact L/R, ↓ cadence, forward flexed trunk, limited assist 25% for posture correction, stabilization of walker, tactile facilitation	Gait front-wheeled rolling walker, rear end caps, step through, initial contact with heels L/R, erect posture, limited assist 10%—supervision for stabilization of walker to prevent veering in forward direction
Gait with front-wheeled rolling walker, rear skis, level surfaces moderate (50%) assist to remain upright and propel walker, 10′, forward only	Gait with front-wheeled rolling walker, rear skis, level surfaces 50′ to 80′ with safe/stable directional changes L/R 90° and 180° turns, to enable gait to bathroom and dining
Wheelchair management; moderate dependence, initiates rim movement only; unable to propel effectively	Independent wheelchair management on level and carpeted surfaces to allow safe locomotion and promote I mobility in the short term

Example

Functionally Oriented Goals

- Pain reduction from 8/10 to 1/10 during prolonged sitting for up to 1 hour, to allow resumption of work at computer station, with 10-minute break at end of hour and ability to repeat throughout 6-hour day
- Resolution of disk protrusion with resultant resolution of right-shifted standing posture to allow unguarded, pain-free gait in order to resume ADL and IADL activities, leisure, work, and family responsibilities
- Restore full, stable cervical rotation to allow safe independent driving: checking mirrors, backing up, in order to return to drive to work, etc.
- Increase UE elevation to 160° bilaterally to allow independent dressing including overhead garments, self-care activities, overhead reaching activities in kitchen, adjust auto mirrors

INTERVENTION PLAN

The categories used in the intervention plan or POC should match the categories in the CPT and HCPCS codes. After stating the category, if it includes a variety of activities, such as that for therapeutic exercise, the specific type of exercise would then be listed. This is not necessary in the general POC, but would be in the medical record entries, especially for communication therapist to therapist and therapist to other individuals that require the information, for continuity of care, for continuation of services on subsequent days, and for progression over time. Most facilities use the same categories repeatedly. Remember that the treatment diagnosis must be consistent with the planned interventions, the deficits identified, and the short- and long-term goals. All categories indicated correspond to the categories in the *Guide to Physical Therapist Practice*.[2]

Author's Note

The plan should encompass everything that you may do as a clinician. This avoids you painting yourself in the corner or limiting the ability to perform a variety of interventions based on assessing the client's response to the interventions.

Table 14-2 Sample Patient Goals Based on Time

2 WEEKS (CAN INCLUDE ACTUAL DATE, OR SPECIFY # WEEKS)
1. Contact guard: Gait with standard walker on even (or level) surfaces, WBAT, 50′, with ability to make 180° turn and step backward without toe drag, with single rest of one minute, at half normal speed;~ 40 meters/minute
2. Ability to open and close doors with round handles with limited assistance: 25% for standing balance while using walker
3. Supervision with minimal verbal instructions for safe transfers sit <> stand
4. Supervision with minimal verbal instruction for safe stand pivot transfer bed <> chair
5. Increased R dorsiflexion strength from 3–/5 to 3+/5 with elimination of toe drag to enable safe gait and decrease fall risk
6. Improve standing balance from _____ to _____ without walker to prevent falls when standing for activities that require both upper extremities (UEs) (preclude holding walker) (i.e., dressing, hygiene, kitchen related)
7. Increase aerobic capacity with consistent O_2 saturation of >90, for functional activity from _____ to __________
8. Independent wheelchair mobility on even surface with ability to lock and unlock brakes, flip foot rests and leg rests, and negotiate doorways
9. Patient will demonstrate ability to perform exercises independently
3 WEEKS (CAN INCLUDE ACTUAL DATE, OR SPECIFY # WEEKS)
1. Stable, I gait with standard walker on even and uneven (rugs, concrete, grass) surfaces, with ability to execute turns spontaneously all directions with heel/toe pattern 100′ without rest at normal speed of 82 m/minute
2. Independent ability to negotiate doors (open and close) without loss of balance
3. Improve transfers sit <> stand
4. Improve stand pivot transfers bed <> chair, toilet, shower from moderate (50%) assistance to minimal (25%) assistance with pivot component
5. Increase R dorsiflexion strength from 3–/5 to 4–/5 to eliminate toe drag/drop foot for sustained safe gait up to 100′ on even and uneven surfaces
6. Increase/improve standing balance from _____ to __________ for safe, stable standing for self-care activities, bathroom and kitchen tasks
7. I wheelchair mobility on even and uneven surfaces (rugs, concrete, grass) without need for interrupted propulsion
8. Patient will demonstrate home exercise independently
9. Stabilization of _________spinal segment to facilitate cervical rotation R/L to safely scan environment
10. Eliminate radiating low back pain with centralization to facilitate functional standing

Example

Modalities: E-stim, US, heat/ cold

Therapeutic exercise for UE/LE/Trunk: progressive strengthening/ROM; active, active assistive and passive stretching

Neuromuscular reeducation: balance training, proprioceptive training, coordination training

Soft tissues mobilization: state body area

Gait Training

IMPORTANT CONSIDERATIONS WHEN DOCUMENTING PATIENT-SPECIFIC FINDINGS

The documentation should include baseline or initial examination data, anticipated goals based on the identified patient problems, and the interim status and progress described relative to the baseline and goal. All deficits must ultimately be linked to the function they affect.

Anthropometric

Anthropometric measurement is used in physical therapy to describe overall height, weight, body mass index, and hip-to-waist ratio, as well as overall body type, extremity or extremity segment size, and how size relates to function. The therapist should describe fat distribution as applicable, presence of obesity, and weight control problems. Measurements must be objective. If a scale is not available, record observations and ask the patient his or her height and weight. From a wellness perspective, improvements should be noted over time, and decreases to facilitate movement may be goals, especially in bariatric care or wellness and prevention programs. (Note: wellness and prevention are not usually reimbursable by third-party payers.)

Joint Integrity and Mobility

Joint integrity and mobility in physical therapy are expressed in terms of joint play, end feel, and ROM. The ROM should be listed as a fraction of the measured and full range. These measurements should be taken at baseline, throughout care, and at discharge using the appropriate goniometer. If the measurements are visually estimated, be sure to indicate this in the record. Joint play is usually described with appropriate adjectives such as laxity, and end feel may be described as bone to bone, soft tissue approximation, spasm, empty end feel, capsular end feel, and springy block.

Example

Shoulder flexion: AROM: 80°/180°, PROM 120°/180°

Deviations: from joint and body planes, with excursions in distances

Example

15° L genu valgum

5 inches of spinal excursion in forward flexion

Joint Motion: quality of motion (i.e., end feel, painful arc, bony block, capsular patterns, glide, laxity, or restriction)

Example

Provocation responses/tests:+ anterior drawer test L knee

Patient description/reports of pain (objectively measure) or other during activities and movement

Example

Patient complains of (CO) grinding in shoulders with elevation and functional use

Patient CO clicking in L knee during walking and cycling

Muscle Performance

Strength should be based on a functional performance or expressed as a fraction to indicate the finding is out of the "normal," which is 5 /5 on the most commonly used scale. These measurements should be taken at baseline, progressively throughout care, and at termination of care, based on a predetermined scale of 0/5 to 5/5 or performance activity.

Author's Note

The clinician must think out of the box at times to measure progression. For example, if a client has –3/5 strength of the gluteus medius and cannot rise up against gravity, even if the client improves to rising up 20 cm against gravity, it would still measure as –3/5. Use functional measurements to show improvements as well as ability to stabilize on the limb with single-leg stance in closed chain/balance.

Avoid verbiage only in correspondence regarding muscle performance because it is often misunderstood and considered better than it is.

Example

R quads MMT 3/5 at initial examination

Goal: Increase R quadriceps strength to 4/5 to enable safe standing without device as required for job

Interim statement of progress: Patient's R quad strength has increased from 3/5 to 3+/5 decreasing frequency of buckling with weight transfer on and off limb in standing

Passive tension, length measurement with patient CO pain, pulling, or tenderness during multisegmental movement

However, at times, especially with impaired muscle performance, which may be a primary or secondary problem, strength expressed in numbers, since based frequently on a one-time maximal isometric contraction against resistance, may be misleading. A patient may test at 4/5 on one repetition but be unable to repeat the resistance or use the strength functionally. In this case, clarification is needed in the documentation to ensure that the need for skilled therapy is supported.

Example

R quads/knee extension in sitting: able to tolerate moderate resistance at 4/5 one rep only, unable to functionally extend knee in upright or tolerate repeated resistance

Muscle Tone

When abnormal tone is present, with or without synergy, using the 5/5 scale may also be misleading, and verbiage, including the Modified Ashworth Scale and a description of the patient's ability/inability to tolerate resistance within the range present or with description of the changes in tone, is indicated.

Example

Unable to isolate elbow flexion and extension on table top for support, interfering with eating, writing, self-care; considerable increase in muscle tone of biceps, passive movement difficult and active movement absent

Modified Ashworth Scale:

5/5: Normal tone: no increase or decrease

4/5: Slight tone increase, catch and release, or minimal resistance at end of range

3/5: Slight increase in tone manifested by catch, followed by minimal resistance

2/5: More marked tone through most of the range of motion but affected part(s) easily moved

1/5: Considerable increase in muscle tone, passive movement is difficult

0/5: Affected part(s) rigid in flexion or extension

Sensation impairment: distributions affected and specific sensation

Author's Note

Although the Modified Ashworth Scale includes fractions from 0/5 to 5/5, the numbers alone should be avoided, since they may be confused for strength.

Neuromotor Development and Sensory Integration

Neuromotor development and sensory integration are developed over time in physical therapy and should be documented as such. Neuromotor skills are developed by gradually performing muscle stretch reflexes and deep tendon reflexes (DTRs).

Example

(DTRs):

0 = no response; always abnormal

1+ = a slight but definitely present response; may or may not be normal

2+ = a brisk response; normal

3+ = a very brisk response; may or may not be normal

4+ = a tap elicits a repeating reflex (clonus); always abnormal

Example

R biceps reflex = 2+ (normal)

L patella reflex = 1 (hyporeflexive)

Electrical assessment over time: electromyography (EMG), nerve conduction, etc.

Synergic dominance and tone, abnormal reflexes and ability to initiate and isolate movement in relation to gravity and body position

Example

Sensation absent in RLE L5 dermatome, resulting in potential for injury, skin breakdown

Sensory integration with environment: state of system

Example

Demonstrates tactile defensiveness to all external stimuli, including clothing and touch. Demonstrates increase in observable synergies in response to noise in room, interfering with ability to isolate movement and preventing functional use of extremities.

Developmental reflexes can impact movement patterns and posture.

Example

Right asymmetrical tonic neck reflex (ATNR) dominance preventing neutral supine positioning, unable to roll right or left preventing rolling.

Developmental level: described in terms of milestones usually indicated on standardized forms for standardized assessment.

Motor Function, Motor Control, and Learning

When documenting motor function, motor control, and learning, the PT should describe movement patterns, postural control, and unprovoked movement. Objective tests and measures are encouraged for consistency of assessment and documentation.

Coordination Skills

When evaluating coordination skills, include the quality of the movement, smoothness of movement, and ability to perform a motor task with accuracy and speed in a functional context. Objective tests and measures are encouraged for consistency of assessment and documentation.

Example

Demonstrates severe kyphosis in sitting, limiting UE elevation and diaphragm excursion associated with increased respiratory rate and accessory muscle use. Is able to correct trunk posture approximately 5 degrees with passive positioning.

Example

Time to complete tasks: slowness when it interferes with function is justification of care, especially in tasks that need an immediate response such as toileting.

Example

Patient transferred wheelchair to bed with minimal assist or limited assist of 25% in 5 minutes, stand/pivot to R.

Sequencing and Cuing for Task Accomplishment

Example

Able to perform stand pivot transfer from wheelchair to mat table with supervision; intermittent verbal instructions.

Requires moderate or extensive assist at 50% from wheelchair to bed at same height to unweight buttocks and execute pivot. Response to therapeutic exercise intervention such as rhythmic stabilization and contract-relax.

Example

Able to maintain erect trunk posture in response and maintain for 2 minutes with verbal instructions.

Coma level description using standardized scales such as the Glasgow or Rancho Los Amigos.

Balance

The therapist should describe balance and/or record balance ratings on standardized scales or from computerized equipment. Always use functional terms rather than good, fair, or poor, which are not objective, measurable terms. There are standard instruments such as the Berg Balance and Timed Up and Go and Functional Reach, which assist in qualifying and quantifying balance. One can also use a 0/5 to 5/5 Kansas University Standing Balance Scale for describing balance in sit and stand, static and dynamic, but the scale should be included.

Kansas University Standing Balance Scale (KUSBS)

KUSBS Score Ordinal

Description of Patient Performance for KUSBS Scores

0 Performs 25% or less of standing activity (maximum assist).

1 Supports self with upper extremities but requires therapist assistance. Patient performs 25 to 50% of effort (moderate assist).

1+ Supports self with upper extremities but requires therapist assistance. Patient performs >50% of effort (minimal assist).

2 Independently supports self with both upper extremities.

2+ Independently supports self with one upper extremity.

3 Independently stands without upper extremity support for up to 30 seconds.

3+ Independently stands without upper extremity support for 30 seconds or greater.

4 Independently moves and returns center of gravity 1 to 2 inches in 1 plane.

4+ Independently moves and returns center of gravity 1 to 2 inches in multiple planes.

5 Independently moves and returns center of gravity in all planes greater than 2 inches.

Example

Maintains vertical position in standing for 60 seconds without cues or support. Self-corrects to vertical 50% of time with verbal cues. Requires bilateral UE support to maintain balance during gait. Resting posture is 15° to right of vertical. Falls to left 3 out of 5 times when perturbed from right. Consistently able to reach beyond base of support without falling. Falls to left when changing direction of gait 80% of time and relies on constant cues to sequence. Requires constant physical cues to weight shift during gait or loses balance.

Balance must be specific and described in sitting or standing, with or without support, and type of support, or during a particular movement task or activity, such as gait, rising from a chair, or reaching. Also describe the patient's ability to incorporate spatial relationships during movement.

Example

Patient is able to perform bilateral activities 12 inches to both the right and left of midline in sitting.

Describe behavior or painful reactions during specific movement tasks and the movements that aggravate or relieve pain.

Example

Patient experiences sharp, severe pain in L knee with initial attempt at single leg stand; a necessary gait component (midstance).

Pain

When documenting a patient's pain, use numbers from standardized scales for rating pain, a faces scale (smile versus frown), or any of the other measurement scales such as the Oswetry. The 0/10 to 10/10 scale is most commonly used to indicate no pain to the most severe. It is important to note areas of pain and levels at rest and during activity, as well as what relieves the pain and what increases it and the type of pain described (i.e., dull ache, throbbing, sharp, and stabbing). The Oswetry Scale is a good indicator of how pain affects function. Pain reduction as a goal must be supported in terms of how the reduction in pain is related to a change in functional performance and increased ability to perform specific movement tasks. When documenting pain reduction, it is important to relate interventions to specific goals.

Author's Note

No matter how well you qualify and describe a patient's pain, if pain does not affect function, physical therapy will not, beyond a very brief period, be considered medically necessary unless a patient is specifically in a preapproved pain program.

Describe the patient's expression of sensory and temporal qualities of pain in response to tests of provocation or during rest or movement tasks.

Example

Patient reported stabbing pain with deep friction massage that lingered for 20 minutes after completion of treatment of the R biceps tendon.

Give location of tender or trigger points and determine sensitivity with a pressure point gauge or verbiage such as the following criteria for tenderness to touch or tender or trigger points:

0 = none
1 = mild, expressed, but no withdrawal
2 = moderate, expressed plus withdrawal
3 = severe, immediate exaggerated withdrawal
4 = patient untouchable, withdraws without palpation

Somatosensory

To measure and document a patient's somatosensory functions, describe the patient's expression of sensation during sensory testing. This includes light touch, pain (sharp/dull), deep pressure, hot and cold sensitivity, and proprioception or kinesthetic sensation and any description of reported paresthesias or neuropathic symptoms such as numbness, tingling, burning, or inability to "feel."

Example

Response to light touch is absent on the L side, putting patient at risk for injury.

Document the patient's ability to describe position of body part with eyes closed (proprioception), to identify objects by touch only (stereognosis), to identify use of objects (praxis), neglect of body part, and expression of sensation in absent body part or phantom pain sensation.

Example

Impaired proprioception of L foot; unable to identify positions of the great toe and ankle, impairing balance/postural stability safety in standing and during gait. Unable to identify coin, comb, or pin placed in left hand.

Patient unable to determine hand position for use; experiences severe phantom pain in L residual limb that limiting all mobility.

Cranial Nerve Integrity

To evaluate and record the patient's cranial nerve integrity, describe provoked and unprovoked eye, tongue, and swallowing movements. It is also helpful to list the patient's visual field and hemianopsia and describe the ability to form facial expressions and evaluate the strength of applicable cervical muscles. To complete the cranial nerve integrity evaluation, describe the patient's vestibular problems, such as nystagmus, vertigo, and past-pointing, as well as postural stability/instability.

Posture

The patient's posture should be recorded and evaluated throughout the course of therapy, if impaired, for the following positions: sitting, lying, standing, and during functional activity. In some cases, posture alone, or "postural syndrome," may be the root cause of the patient's functional limitations and correction may be the solution. There are ICD-10 codes related to abnormal posture.

Example

Patient demonstrates flexed trunk posture in unsupported sitting while working on the computer, with inability to correct secondary to trunk weakness, perceptual deficits, etc.

In describing a patient's posture, include limb position, joint limitation, tone, and positions of comfort.

Example

Patient's relaxed standing posture demonstrates forward head, UEs forward of trunk, knee hyperextension, and bilateral pronated feet.

The posture evaluation should also include descriptions of muscle imbalances in relation to the vertebral curves (the cervical lordotic curve, the thoracic kyphotic curve, the lumbar lordotic curve, and scoliosis).

Example

Lordotic curve decreased/flattened, cervical lordosis increased (Include the functional implications)

Mobility

When evaluating a patient's mobility, it is important to consider all applicable aspects and types of mobility, including bed mobility, transfers, gait, and wheelchair mobility (manual, electric, or powered operated vehicles/scooters). For babies or toddlers, the ability to creep, crawl, and cruise should be documented. Bed mobility documentation should include descriptions of rolling left or right with or without bedrails, positioning self cephally or caudally, and shifting body/body segments left and.

Describe assistance required by the patient in terms of the effort the patient is exerting, rather than the exertion by the PT. The terms minimal assist (or limited), moderate assist (extensive), maximal assist (extensive), and total assist are commonly used to describe the amount of assistance needed by the PT/PTA. However, conversely, the terms could be modified to: minimally dependent, moderately dependent, maximally dependent, total dependent. When using the Functional Independence Measures (FIM) terminology, it should be accompanied by the description of what component of the activity requires the assistance.

To better define these subjective terms, a percentage of effort scale serves as the basis of the Functional Independence Measures (FIM), taken from the Uniform Data System, which is available from Data Management Service, Buffalo General Hospital, SUNY at Buffalo, 100 High Street, Buffalo, New York 14203. These percentages are related to the terms as follows:

Total assist (extensive assist) = Patient exerts 0% of total effort.

Maximal assist (extensive assist) = Patient exerts some and up to 25% of total effort.

Moderate assist (extensive assist) = Patient exerts at least 50% of total effort.

Minimal assist (limited assist) = Patient exerts at least 75% of total effort.

Contact guard = Patient requires hands-on guarding in the event assist is needed.

Supervision or standby assist = Patient has safety issues and requires someone close by for safety and occasional verbal instructions.

Independence = Patient is able to perform activity without assistance. If a device is used, it must be identified and may be considered modified independence, as in the FIM grading.

Wheelchair Mobility

Whether temporarily or permanently using a wheelchair, manual or power, instruction in use and determining the ability to maneuver, and type and adaptations are skilled services. The following should be used to describe wheelchair mobility:

- The patient's ability to propel the chair in multiple directions for distances over varied surfaces and elevations, indoors and outdoors. Note: type of controls must be included. Using BUEs to manipulate wheels is significantly different than a joy stick or a sip and puff on a power chair
- Patient's ability to manipulate the parts (i.e., brakes, legrest, and armrests, etc.)
- Chair model selected (including power, power-operated vehicles/scooters) and its fit
- Ability of caretaker to manage the chair, including pushing, folding, braking, and car transfers with patient in the chair and securing versus patient transfer out of chair into vehicle and then placing and securing chair on lift or into vehicle
- Ability of patient to manage the chair, including pushing, folding, braking, and car transfers
- Adaptations made, needed, or recommended, including cushions, backs, head rests, leg rests, seat belts, or other stabilizing adaptations
- Ability to negotiate doors and other entrances and bathrooms/toilets
- Integumentary (skin) condition and ability to change position for protection from breakdown

Transfers

There are many types of transfers with multiple components. Break down the components of these functions to be specific. There are many small goals to be identified and achieved before an end result is evident. Include those components that are applicable to your patient. The following words and phrases should be used to describe transfers:

- Sit to stand, with or without pushing or using UEs
- Stand to sit/sit to stand
- Stand and pivot
- Partial stand to pivot with or without a device
- Full stand to pivot
- Sliding board or standing disk utilization
- Use of mechanical lift, manual ift or assistive device
- Supine to/from sit with roll to side-lying vs. directly to long sit

The direction of the transfer must also be described, such as transfers to the left or the right or both directions, as indicated for the needs of patient.

Although there is normal variation in motor planning for transfer and mobility activities, any posturing or reflexes, weakness, or other impairments that interfere with the patient's activity must be addressed in the documentation and intervention.

Gait

Gait assessment and training are unique to physical therapy and should be documented properly. They are highly skilled services, making it imperative that documentation refer to the normal phases of gait and description of deviations. Any use of a device, including assistive gait devices, prosthetics, or orthotics, must also be included.

TRADITIONAL	RANCHO LOS AMIGOS
• Arm swing	Arm swing
• Heel strike	Initial contact
• Foot flat	Midstance
• Toe off	Terminal stance
• Swing	Preswing/swing

The following terms should be used to describe the gait:

1. Width of base; base of support (BOS) normal = 2 to 4 inches
2. Cadence
3. Stride length
4. Posture
5. Weight bearing/weight acceptance/weight shift
6. Level of pelvis/pelvic movement
7. Stability of hips and knees
8. Trunk movement
9. Leg length discrepancy
10. Varum or valgus in the LEs
11. Assistive devices, prostheses, or orthoses required
12. Distance, directionality
13. Ability to sequence
14. Surfaces and elevations negotiated
15. Quality of movement/motor control

Integument

The initial examination and evaluation documentation should also include a description of any wounds, burns, scars, open areas, rashes, lesions, discoloration, hair patterns, dryness, cracking, or other conditions that affect function and present risk. Open areas must be measured and described. Wound measurements may be obtained with grids, pictures, picture grids, traces of the wounds, readings from a volumeter, water injection, syringe volume, or cotton-tipped applicator inserted to determine depth. Describe drainage, odor, temperature, color, bruising, scabs, skin tears, trophic changes, turgor, pigment, and skin and scar pliability.

Peripheral Vascular

When documenting peripheral vascular conditions, describe color, skin temperature, skin condition, and pain resulting from ischemia or claudication, edema (pitting or nonpitting), capillary refill in fingers and toes, peripheral pulse integrity, and any other pertinent findings.

Lymphatic System

Record edema measurements at selected points throughout the limb. The points for measurement must be recorded, as well as the circumferential measurements at the points. When possible, compare measurements to the uninvolved limb. Avoid terms such as minimal, moderate, severe, and less than or more than. Measurements should be recorded approximately every inch along the involved extremity. If the breast is involved, measurements should be taken around the base of the breast and around the trunk at the nipple line. Lymphatic evaluations should also include descriptions of peripheral pulses (check for their presence and describe their strength), such as lower extremity (LE), femoral, popliteal, posterior tibial, and dorsal pedal. Describe the color, temperature, pain, and skin condition of the patient. Skin temperature and a full integument assessment should also be included.

Record the degree of pitting edema if present, using the following scale:

1+ barely perceptible depression (pit)

2+ easily identified depression (EID) skin rebounds to its original contour within 15 sec

3+ EID skin rebounds to its original contour within 15 to 30 sec

4+ EID rebound >30 sec

Describe the rationale for and use of external elastic supports or intermittent compression, as well as lymphatic drainage and massage techniques and necessity. Describe the overall size of the body, extremity, or extremity segment and how problems with size relate to function. Describe uneven fat distribution and poor weight control, as well as abnormal size. Measurements must be objective by measuring, weighing, or volumetric displacement.

Cardiopulmonary Status, Aerobic Capacity, and Endurance

To record cardiopulmonary status and aerobic capacity and endurance, be as objective as possible, avoiding terms such as poor, fair, and good. Instead, describe the behaviors that led you to the subjective word. Pulse oximeter readings and vital signs; blood pressure sitting, standing, and laying down, if indicated, as well as at intervals during the session; and radial pulse (if a pulse other than radial is used, state which) should be included, as well as respiratory rate, pattern, shortness of breath (SOB), and quality of respiration. Depending on the venue and reason for referral, auscultation of the heart and lungs may be necessary to include as well. The therapist should be able to determine normal heart and lung sounds and deviations from norms or abnormalities and record them. For patients with cardiopulmonary dysfunction, instruction in the Rate of Perceived Exertion Scale (RPE) is an outcome indicator that can be measured over time.

Example

Patient requires 5 minute rest after 3 minutes of therapeutic exercise to return from respiratory rate (RR) of 30 shallow, mouth open, to RR of 22, mouth closed; able to participate for 30 total minutes with appropriate rest.

Note: By describing the time intervals, progression is easier to document as periods of activity tolerance increase and RR stabilizes in the normal range (12 to 20) or SOB decreases. It is helpful to include teaching the Rate of Perceived Exertion as an additional measure of activity tolerance and one the patient can self-monitor.

Establish an objective baseline from which to compare improvement in function. The following should be included in descriptions of aerobic capacity/endurance:

- Autonomic responses to activity
- Breathing patterns/quality
- Need for supplemental O_2 and volume needed
- Patient complaints in quotes
- Ability to increase treatment time or repetitions or tolerance
- Rate of perceived exertion scales (Borg Scale of Perceived Exertion)
- Respiratory rates
- O_2 saturation

Example

Patient is able to accomplish only 10 feet, minimal assist with 4-wheeled rollator before becoming diaphoretic and SOB. Pulse increases from 80 at rest to 120 after stand pivot transfer. After 10 reps of knee extension with a 5-pound weight, patient's breathing became shallow with RR of 32. Patient requires 5 minutes of rest for breathing to return to normal after every 5 minutes of exercise. Patient tolerates only 1 hour sitting in reclined wheelchair. Requires 2 hours bedrest after every hour out of bed.

Describe cardiac status by comparing to baseline measurements at rest to measurements during activity. Examples of words and phrases include heart rate, blood pressure, respiratory rate, and breathing pattern and O_2 saturation. Any abnormalities or complaints such as chest pain, SOB, and pounding in the chest should be recorded. The preexisting need for medications and history of medical problems, such as asthma and myocardial infarction (MI) should also be included in the description. Unusual fatigue and other abnormalities must be described. Patient activity should be modified as necessary by recommending paced activity, energy conservation techniques, and rest periods. Pulse oximetry, electrocardiogram (ECG) readings, and similar tests should be performed during treatment if the patient is specifically referred for cardiac reconditioning. If a patient uses Nitroglycerin, it should be readily available during all activity. Teaching a patient the Angina Scale provides objective and activity related outcomes.

Describe baseline pulmonary function data to compare with data during activity as necessary. Pulmonary function data includes respiratory rate; breath sounds; congestion/cough, sputum color, and consistency (if present); breathing patterns; chest deformity; unusual fatigue; difficulty breathing; abnormal breathing patterns; or chest pain. The pulmonary function data should also include paced activity and energy conservation techniques and pulse oximetry measurements.

EXAMPLE OF AN ENDURANCE SCALE (SOURCE UNKNOWN)

Good: Tolerates normal activity, using moderate to maximal resistance. Activity and position changes with no signs of fatigue, palpitation, dyspnea, or pain. Standing tolerance is 30 minutes.

Good–: Tolerates normal activity, using moderate resistance activity, and positional changes with only occasional or minimal fatigue, no palpitations, dyspnea, or pain increase. Standing tolerance is 15 minutes.

Fair+: Tolerates high to moderate resistive activity and position change with infrequent rest periods (20 to 30 minutes work period) and minimal fatigue noted; longer time or more resistance causes fatigue, palpitations, dyspnea, or pain. Standing tolerance is 15 minutes.

Fair: Tolerates light resistive activity for short to moderate length of times (10 to 15 minutes); needs occasional rest periods; longer time or more resistance causes fatigue, dyspnea, palpitations, or pain. Standing tolerance is 10 minutes.

Fair–: Comfortable at rest; tolerates nonresistive activity for short duration (5 to 10 minutes), needs frequent rest periods; longer time, or more addition of resistance increases fatigue, dyspnea, or pain. Standing tolerance is 5 minutes.

Poor+: Comfortable at rest; tolerates nonresistive activity for short duration (2 to 4 minutes); needs very frequent rest periods of longer time or addition of resistance to exercise causes fatigue, palpitations, dyspnea, or pain. Standing tolerance is 2 to 4 minutes.

Poor: Comfortable at rest; light nonresistive activity of brief duration causes fatigue, palpitation, dyspnea, or pain. Standing tolerance 1 to 3 minutes.

Poor–: Symptoms may be present at rest; if any physical activity undertaken distress is increased. Standing tolerance less than 1 minute.

Body Mechanics

To report on body mechanics, describe posture and movement patterns during all activities performed during the session, which may be ADLs, any transitional movements from position to position, and work-related tasks such as sitting or lifting. Abnormal body mechanics may result in pain and dysfunction. Phrases and words used to describe body mechanics include abnormal body alignment, abnormal movement patterns, and inability to perform specific movement tasks. There are instances in which adaptation of a specific movement task is indicated, but a change in body mechanics is not feasible. This may be the case for specific pathology related to fused spine, limb contracture, or fused or limited joint movements, or movement contraindications such as post-posterolateral total hip arthroplasty.

Orthotics and Prosthetics

Describe orthotics and prosthetics in terms of the need for a device based on impairment in order to facilitate function. At times, a device may be used for cosmetic purposes only, but would not require rehabilitation unless instructions in skin care and application and removal are required. Once prescribed and obtained, describe how the devices are to be monitored for fit and function, and the patient must be appropriately trained to use the device. Documentation should include the type of device if patient already has a device and condition of it, gait, posture, and/or body part description with and without the device; alignment of the device itself relative to the body and its impact on function; ability to perform functional tasks with and without the orthosis/prosthesis and need for assistive or adaptive devices; comfort; ability to apply and remove; skin integrity as a result of wearing the device; proper fit and prescription; and ability for self-care with the device.

Adaptive and Assistive Devices and Equipment

General categories of prostheses and orthoses include ankle foot orthosis (AFO) rigid or dynamic; knee, ankle foot orthosis (KAFO); upper extremity (UE) orthoses; reciprocating gait orthosis (RGO); above the knee (AK) prosthesis; below the knee (BK) prosthesis; above the elbow (AE) prosthesis; below the elbow (BE) prosthesis; myoelectric prosthesis; lumbar supports; trunk orthoses; cervical collars; slings; and bivalve casts. There is a large variety of both custom and off-the-shelf splints and braces/orthoses for the elbow, wrist/hand, fingers, knee, and ankle/foot.

When evaluating the assistive devices, describe the devices and equipment in terms of the need for a device based on impairment and their functionality in facilitating function. Once obtained, documentation must address how devices must be monitored for fit and function, and the patient must be trained to use the device. Phrases and words for this documentation include mobility, posture, ability or inability to use the device functionally, comfort, and self-care.

Types of adaptive and assistive devices and equipment include walking aids such as walkers, canes, and crutches; wheelchairs; cushions; lift chairs; transfer disks; hospital beds; reachers; elastic shoelaces; and lap trays. From a documentation perspective, the devices must be objectively described.

Activities of Daily Living

Due to the multitude of ADLs, it is necessary to describe which ADLs are addressed or identified as impaired in the documentation. ADL specifically relates to self-care and function in the daily environment but excludes work-related activities. Describe ADLs in objective, functional terms that can be addressed and measured for evidence of improvement. ADLs include household chores, personal hygiene, dressing, toileting, and retrieval of articles and items.

Information about ADLs may be dependent on information provided by the patient during the initial interview or through observation. ADL scales, such as the Katz and Barthel's, are helpful and standardized for ADL skills. Depending on the facility and venue, the PT may or may not be actually conducting an ADL examination.

Author's Note

When the patient's main complaint is pain, it may be difficult to justify treatment unless it is related to the inability to perform ADLs. The patient's subjective description of improvement and pain relief may have to be relied on for determination of progress. Whenever possible, try to duplicate the ADL in the clinic to observe actual rather than reported performance.

Functional Capacity

Descriptions of results of functional capacity testing and work hardening and conditioning programs are typically completed on standardized forms or programs for accurate, consistent recording of the performance and behavior of patients. When preparing functional activity data, avoid personal opinion (as in all initial evaluation). In this area—perhaps more than any other—the PT must rely on professional opinion rather than personal conclusions because patients involved in these programs are commonly patients injured on the job who are involved with the workers' compensation system.

DOCUMENTING INTERVENTION AND TREATMENT

An entry into the record should be made for each physical therapy visit on the day the treatment was rendered, as close to treatment time as possible to ensure accuracy, regardless of the payer source. CMS currently refers to daily notes as "treatment notes," which must include the following according to Medicare Benefit Policy Manual Chapter 15, Section 220.3:[1]

Documentation of each treatment shall include the following required elements:

- *Date of treatment;*
- *Identification of each specific intervention/modality provided and billed, for both timed and untimed codes, in language that can be compared with the billing on the claim to verify correct coding. Record each service provided that is represented by a timed code, regardless of whether or not it is billed, because the unbilled timed services may impact the billing;*
- *Total timed code treatment minutes and total treatment time in minutes. Total treatment time includes the minutes for timed code treatment and untimed code treatment. Total treatment time does not include time for services that are not billable (e.g., rest periods). For Medicare purposes, it is not required that unbilled services that are not part of the total treatment minutes be recorded, although they may be included voluntarily to provide an accurate description of the treatment, show consistency with the plan, or comply with state or local policies. The amount of time for each specific intervention/modality provided to the patient may also be recorded voluntarily, but contractors shall not require it, as it is indicated in the billing. The billing and the total timed code treatment minutes must be consistent. See Pub. 100-04, chapter 5, section 20.2 for description of billing timed codes; and*
- *Signature and professional identification of the qualified professional who furnished or supervised the services and a list of each person who contributed to that treatment (i.e., the signature of Kathleen Smith, PTA, with notation of phone consultation with Judy Jones, PT, supervisor, when permitted by state and local law). The signature and identification of the supervisor need not be on each treatment note, unless the supervisor actively participated in the treatment. Since a clinician must be identified on the plan of care and the progress report, the name and professional identification of the supervisor responsible for the treatment is assumed to be the clinician who wrote the plan or report. When the treatment is supervised without active participation by the supervisor, the supervisor is not required to cosign the treatment note written by a qualified professional. When the responsible supervisor is absent, the presence of a similarly qualified supervisor on the clinic roster for that day is sufficient documentation and it is not required that the substitute supervisor sign or be identified in the documentation.*

Pursuant to the Medicare Claims Processing Manual Chapter 5 Section 20.3:

Providers report the code for the time actually spent in the delivery of the modality requiring constant attendance and therapy services. Pre- and post-delivery services are not to be counted in determining the treatment service time. In other words, the time counted as "intra-service care" begins when the therapist or physician (or an assistant under the supervision of a physician or therapist) is directly working with the patient to deliver treatment services. The patient should already be in the treatment area (e.g., on the treatment table or mat or in the gym) and prepared to begin treatment. The time counted is the time the patient is treated. For example, if gait training in a patient with a recent stroke requires both a therapist and an assistant, or even two therapists, to manage in the parallel bars, each 15 minutes the patient is being treated can count as only one unit of code 97116. The time the patient spends not being treated because of the need for toileting or resting should not be billed. In addition, the time spent waiting to use a piece of equipment or for other treatment to begin is not considered treatment time.

The APTA recommends that there should be documentation establishing the "physical therapist of record" who assumes the primary responsibility for the patient's management. The APTA's position[5] is as follows:

Standards of Practice for Physical Therapy HOD S06-20-35-29[5]

Physical Therapist of Record: All patients and clients receiving physical therapist services shall have a physical therapist of record who is responsible for patient and client management.

Whether or not a facility chooses to use a progress note format, usually in the SOAP (Subjective, Objective, Assessment, Plan) format, is an individual one. The significant difference between a daily or treatment note and a progress note is statements about progress relative to previous entries or established goals. Progress reports are episodic summaries that include progress toward goals in addition to a summary of interventions rendered over a prescribed period. For Medicare purposes, progress reports for outpatient therapy providers are required once every 10 treatment days. According to MBPM Chapter 15, Section 220.3:[1]

The day beginning the first reporting period is the first day of the episode of treatment regardless of whether the service provided on that day is an evaluation, reevaluation or treatment. Regardless of the date on which the report is actually written (and dated), the end of the progress report period is either a date chosen by the clinician or the 10th treatment day, whichever is shorter. The next treatment day begins the next reporting period. The progress report period requirements are complete when both the elements of the progress report and the clinician's active participation in treatment have been documented.

CMS further states in the MBPM Chapter 15, Section 220.3:[1]

In many settings, weekly progress reports are voluntarily prepared to review progress, describe the skilled treatment, update goals, and inform physician/NPPs or other staff. The clinical judgment demonstrated in frequent reports may help justify that the skills of a therapist are being applied, and that services are medically necessary.

Author's Note

All PTs and physical therapy assistants (PTAs) should read Medicare Benefit Policy Manual Chapter 15, Sections 220 and 230[1] in their entirety, as well as Medicare Claims Processing Manual Chapter 5. Also, provisions within these manuals are updated every so often, so it is important to continue to review them on a regular basis.

When documenting intervention and treatment, always be specific, using CPT codable terms to precede all interventions, unless the interventions themselves have codes, such as ultrasound or electrical stimulation (qualifying constant attendance versus unattended). This is applicable regardless of the format used: narrative, SOAP, flow charts, manual, or electronic. Include in what location the treatment was rendered (i.e., patient room, physical therapy department, patient home), if anyone accompanied the patient or was present and who that person was and make sure the patient—if not a minor—gave consent, how long, and specific parameters and position for reproducibility. All verbiage used in the content section that preceded this section should be applied in context. In any entry for intervention, it is critical for payment, audits, consistency, and coordination of billing with documentation of patient treatment sessions or visits that the CPT code verbiage be included and precedes the actual descriptions of what was performed.

Improvements should be stated in relation to the functional goals dependent on that improvement. For situations in which physical therapy was administered in the outpatient gym, bedside, or home, clearly identify all intervention(s). Identify the specific equipment as indicated, with specific parameters (settings), time, and patient position. Describe the number of repetitions, dosage, distance, quality of movement/performance, deviations from norms, and degree of assistance needed. These should show progressions or improvements over time. If the same exercises, repetitions, and resistance are administered for several days and the entries lack content that describes the physical therapy skills required, payment is at risk. Also list the specific area of the body treated and target tissues, problems, and purpose, as well as patient position. Include in your entries the start and end time and the duration of the session, noting if rests were needed and, if so, include the length of the rest. The patient's response to treatment should always be included. In some settings, the number of minutes or units for individual interventions is required. The concept of documenting in a skilled manner, always emphasizing the medical necessity, should always be considered.

Example

Minutes for individual interventions:

15 mins (1 unit) Therapeutic Procedures

15 mins (1 unit) Manual Therapy

Include vital signs in the intervention/treatment documentation as required based on history, condition treated, and precautions, taken at intervals during the session. It is also important to include any occurrence out of the "ordinary" or unique to that patient. Patient condition before and after treatment, including response and effect on integument, should also be included.

In the record, the PT should also describe:

- Contraindications and precautions and barriers, if any
- Symptom relief and improved function resulting from interventions
- Specific mode of treatment and parameters for application
- Immediate effects of intervention in terms of change in endurance, pain, sensation, reflexes, strength, and range and quality of joint movement, as well as patient response
- Terminology should be skilled, but not so technical that it cannot be understood by other health professionals and most individuals needing access to the record

The continued use of physical therapy interventions without documentation of meaningful, practical, and sustained benefits related to function is not acceptable and will not, in most cases, especially Medicare, be paid. Use the suggested terminology examples in your continuing care documentation, as well as any progress reports to support your ongoing interventions and progress toward goals. It is not the format of the entry that matters, but the content.

SUMMARY

Regardless of the audience for physical therapy documentation, the content and overall progress toward goals justify the care given and establish medical necessity. The PT must convey what is known to be true relative to the need for care. Historically, although PTs can verbally describe what treatment is being rendered, including the parameters and the medical necessity, the lack of ability to communicate this in writing has proven to be challenging.

The PT must remember to include all areas of patient deficits that would justify the need and value for skilled care to ensure the patient benefits fully from the physical therapy. For example, a patient with a recent amputation required gait and transfer training with and without the prosthesis, wheelchair training (at least early on), training on multiple surfaces in varied environments, adaptive driving, skin care training, prosthetic care training, therapeutic exercise, extensive transfer training including car transfers, ADLs, and IADLs. If patient is working, ergonomic assessment may be indicated as well. If they plan to return to work or continue working while receiving physical therapy services, the ability to do so should be included as a goal at the onset of treatment.

A listing of all of the patient's deficits should be included in inpatient and outpatient documentation, with emphasis on what will be addressed in the context of a specific venue and length of stay (LOS). For example, in a 3- to 4-day acute care LOS, treatment may focus on getting in and out of bed and gait for short distances, with instruction in activity the patient can do at home. In home health, in which a homebound status is a concern, returning the individual to a higher level of function, including aerobic capacity and muscle performance, in addition to safe transfers in the home, progression of gait to a variety of surfaces, and self-care may be emphasized. This continues as the patient progresses to outpatient status. Additionally, emphasis should be placed on all comorbidities because they can potentially affect the need for skilled care and prolong the need for care. Regardless of venue, all components of the record should match. Critical to audits is matching by the PT of patient goals to the goals of therapy, identifying all relevant deficits, and establishing matching goals and interventions. The goals achieved at the end of the therapeutic LOS should match those established either at the initial examination and evaluation or as the patient progressed. If a peer or auditor can compare the initial examination or evaluation with the summation of care or discharge summary and quickly assess the progress, with emphasis on function, the record will more likely be viewed positively as representing skilled care.

The key to successful documentation is not in what the therapist *knows,* but what the therapist or other designated personnel *documents.* Remember, if it is not written, it was not done. Furthermore, if it is not written correctly, it might as well not have been rendered or recorded. Only the therapist can justify the need for care and support the need through appropriate, objective, and functionally oriented documentation.

SUMMARY: PHYSICAL THERAPY EVALUATION COMPLEXITY CODES

https://www.apta.org/your-practice/payment/medicare-payment/coding-billing/tiered-physical-therapy-evaluation-and-reevaluation-cpt-codes and https://www.apta.org/contentassets/ca1bb36814844853812b8a073e79ee3d/guide-to-the-levels-of-physical-therapy-evaluation.pdf

EVAL COMPONENTS	97161 LOW COMPLEXITY	97162 MOD COMPLEXITY	97163 HIGH COMPLEXITY	EXAMPLES
History *Choose one →*	0 personal factors 0 comorbidities affecting POC	1–2 personal factors and/or comorbidities affecting POC	3 or more personal factors and/ or comorbidities affecting POC	*Personal factors represent influences on functioning particular to the individual. (2.6)*
Exam *Choose one →*	1–2 elements Body structures/ function, activity limitations, and/ or participation restrictions	3 elements Body structures/ function, activity limitations, and/ or participation restrictions	4 elements Body structures/ function, activity limitations, and/ or participation restrictions	*Includes all exam elements (e.g., MMT, ROM, VAS, FR instruments, etc.)*
Clinical Presentation *Choose one →*	Stable and/or uncomplicated	Evolving clinical presentation	Unstable or unpredictable	

These components need to be assessed to determine the complexity of your client based on your evaluation.

The "clinical decision" is a summary of these components.

The determination of the patient's evaluation complexity (clinical decision) is an aggregate of the data gathered while taking the patient's history and conducting the examination and based on the clinical presentation of the patient.

In order to code the evaluation at one level or another, each element must be satisfied to select a particular level of complexity. If all elements have not been achieved, then the complexity level will "default" to the level below.

For example:

History 3, Exam 1, Clinical Presentation 2 = Low Complexity 97161 (defaults down with exam)

History 3, Exam 3, Clinical Presentation 2 = Moderate Complexity 97162 (defaults down with Clinical Pres)

History 3, Exam 3, Clinical Presentation 3 = High Complexity 97163

ELEMENTS OF EVALUATION

Relationship of Elements of Evaluation

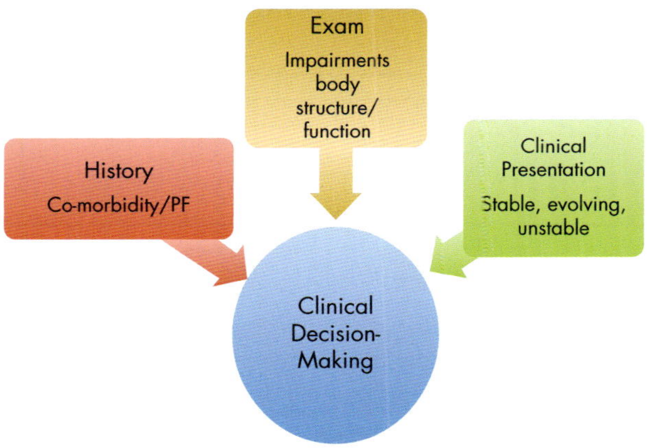

How can I Use the Personal Factors?

What are the Personal Factors?

Personal factors may include gender, age, race, lifestyles, habits, education, and profession. They represent influences on functioning particular to the individual that are not represented elsewhere in the ICF model. An example of this is when an individual cannot get a job due to lack of qualifications, rather than any difficulty in functioning or problem in the environment. One way to include personal factors in the functioning profile is by annotation and description. Population surveys routinely gather such information as part of the survey.

Source: Reproduced, with permission, from World Health Organization. How to use the ICF: A practical manual for using the International Classification of Functioning, Disability and Health (ICF). Exposure draft for comment. Geneva: WHO. October 2013.

BOX 1
THE ICF MODEL: INTERACTION BETWEEN ICF COMPONENTS

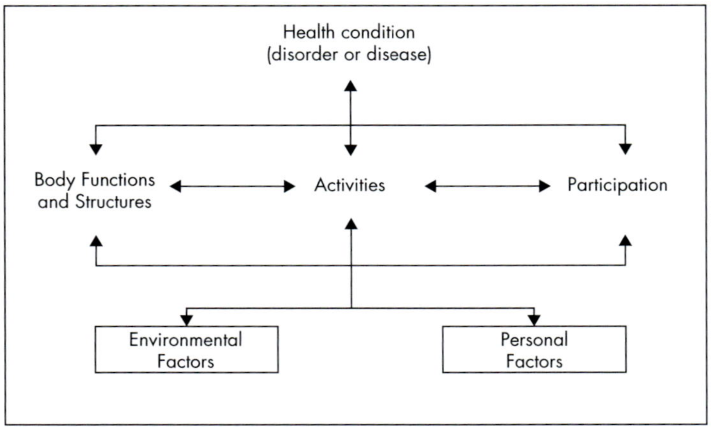

Source: Reproduced, with permission, from World Health Organization. The International Classification of Functioning, Disability and Health (ICF). Geneva: WHO; 2001. (http://www.who.int/classifications/icf/en/).

BOX 2
DEFINITIONS

In the context of health

Functioning is an umbrella term for body function, body structures, activities and participation. It denotes the positive aspects the interaction between an individual (with a health condition) and that individual's contextual factors (environmental and personal factors).

Disability is an umbrella term for impairments, activity limitations and participation restrictions. It denotes the negative aspects of the interaction between an individual (with a health condition) and that individual's contextual factors (environmental and personal factors).

Body functions—The physiological functions of body systems (including psychological functions)

Body structures—Anatomical parts of the body such as organs, limbs and their components.

Impairments—Problems in body function and structures such as significant deviation or loss.

Activity—The execution of a task or action by an individual.

Participation—Involvement in a life situation.

Activity limitations—Difficulties an individual may have in executing activities.

Participation restrictions—Problems an individual may experience in involvement in life situations.

Environmental factors—The physical, social and attitudinal environment in which people live and conduct their lives. These are either barriers to or facilitators of the person's functioning.

Source: Reproduced, with permission, from World Health Organization. The International Classification of Functioning, Disability and Health (ICF). Geneva, WHO; 2001. (http://www.who.int/classifications/icf/en/).

ICF Overview
https://www.cdc.gov/nchs/data/icd/icfoverview_finalforwho10sept.pdf

EXCERPTS FROM APTA GUIDELINES

Relationship of Elements of the Physical Therapy Evaluation

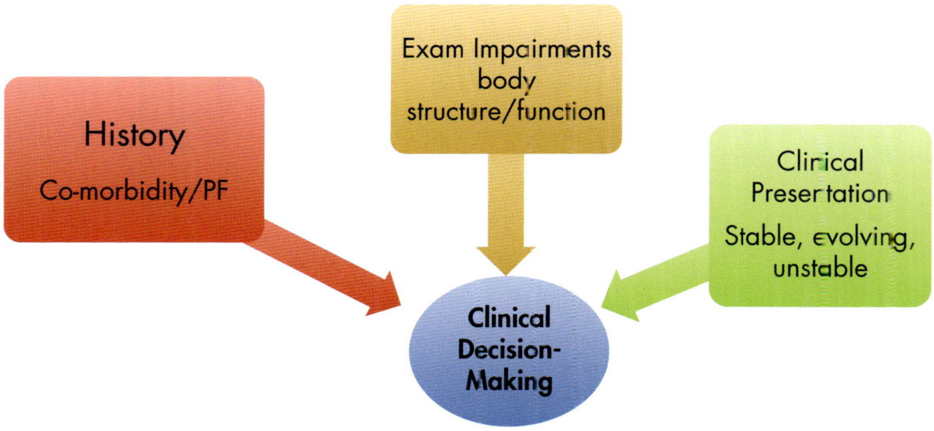

This figure can help visualize how the history, exam, and clinical presentation all inform your clinical decision-making. That's why it is so important to understand all the elements of the evaluation process.

97161—Physical Therapy evaluation: low complexity

History	Examination	Presentation	Decision-Making
A history with no personal factors and/or comorbidities that impact the plan of care;	An examination of body system(s) using standardized tests and measures, patient assessment instrument and/or measurable assessment of functional outcome addressing **1-2 elements** from any of the following: body structures and functions, activity limitations, and/or participation restrictions.	A clinical presentation with **stable and/or uncomplicated characteristics**	**Clinical decision-making of low complexity**

This is language from the AMA CPT manual, but in a visual format. At a minimum, each of the components must be documented in order to report the selected level.

History with no personal factors and/or comorbidities.

The exam is one to two elements of any of the body structures and functions, activity limitations, and/or participation restrictions.

Presentation is stable or uncomplicated.

Low-complexity clinical decision-making using a standardized assessment tool can help in guiding and supporting your decision.

97162—Physical Therapy evaluation: moderate complexity

History	Examination	Presentation	Decision-Making
A history of present problem with **1–2 personal factors and/or comorbidities** that impact the plan of care;	An examination of body system(s) using standardized tests and measures, patient assessment instrument and/or measurable assessment of functional outcome addressing a total of **3 or more elements** from any of the following: body structures and functions, activity limitations, and/or participation restrictions.	An evolving clinical presentation with **changing characteristics;** and	**Clinical decision-making of moderate complexity**

History with one to two personal factors and/or comorbidities.

The exam is three or more elements of any of the body structures and functions, activity limitations, and/or participation restrictions.

Presentation is evolving (changing).

Moderate-complexity clinical decision-making using a standardized assessment tool can help in guiding and supporting your decision.

97163—Physical Therapy evaluation: high complexity

History	Examination	Presentation	Decision-Making
A history of present problem with **3 or more personal factors and/or comorbidities** that impact the plan of care;	An examination of body system(s) using standardized tests and measures, patient assessment instrument and/or measurable assessment of functional outcome addressing a total of **4 or more elements** from any of the following: body structures and functions, activity limitations, and/or participation restrictions.	A clinical presentation with **unstable and unpredictable characteristics;** and	**Clinical decision-making of high complexity**

This is a very involved evaluation.

History with three or more personal factors and/or comorbidities.

The exam is four or more elements of any of the body structures and functions, activity limitations, and/or participation restrictions.

Presentation is unstable and unpredictable.

High clinical decision-making using a standardized assessment tool can help in guiding and supporting your decision.

REVIEW QUESTIONS

1. What activities should tests and measures focus on in the initial examination?
2. Describe tiers for evaluation codes.[6]
3. Explain why strength and range of motion are best described in numbers as fractions, but tone, which can also be described in fractions, is preferably described in verbiage.
4. Explain rehabilitation potential in the context of physical therapy.
5. Identify two components included in muscle performance and provide an example for each.
6. Explain the relationship between safety and risk reduction and strength.
7. Explain why precautions and contraindications are necessary relative to physical therapy intervention and their relationship to medical necessity.
8. Why is pain as the primary diagnosis (in a nonpain program) not an indication for physical therapy?
9. Provide an example of objective descriptions of:
   a. Gait
   b. ROM
   c. Balance
   d. Strength
   e. Wheelchair mobility
   f. Motor control
10. Why is CPT code verbiage necessary when documenting PT?
11. Describe the different levels of evaluation.

REFERENCES

1. *Medicare Benefit Policy Manual Chapter 15—Covered Medical and Other Health Services.* Baltimore, MD: Centers for Medicare & Medicaid Services. Available at https://www.cms.gov/Regulations-and-Guidance/Guidance/Manuals/Downloads/bp102c15.pdf. Accessed August 20, 2020.
2. *Guide to Physical Therapist Practice 3.0.* Alexandria, VA: American Physical Therapy Association. Available at http://guidetoptpractice.apta.org/content/current. Accessed August 20, 2020.
3. *Patient-Reported Outcomes Measurement Information System (PROMIS).* Available at https://www.healthmeasures.net/explore-measurement-systems/promis/intro-to-promis. Accessed August 20, 2020.
4. *Local Coverage Determinations.* Alexandria, VA: American Physical Therapy Association. Available at https://www.apta.org/your-practice/payment/medicare-payment/coverage-issues/local-coverage-determinations-lcds. Accessed August 20, 2020.
5. *Standards of Practice for Physical Therapy, HOD S06-20-35-29.* Alexandria, VA: American Physical Therapy Association. Available at https://www.apta.org/siteassets/pdfs/policies/standards-of-practice-pt.pdf. Accessed August 25, 2020.
6. *Tiered Physical Therapy Evaluation and Reevaluation CPT Codes.* Alexandria, VA: American Physical Therapy Association. Available at https://www.apta.org/your-practice/payment/coding-billing/tiered-evaluation-codes. Accessed August 20, 2020.

ADDITIONAL REFERENCES

Steiner WA, Ryser L, Huber E, Uebelhart D, Aeschlimann A, Stucki G. Use of the ICF model as a clinical problem-solving tool in physical therapy and rehabilitation medicine. *Phys Ther.* 2002;82(11):1098-1107.

Rundell SD, Davenport TE, Wagner T. Physical therapist management of acute and chronic low back pain using the World Health Organization's International Classification of Functioning, Disability and Health. *Phys Ther.* 2009;89(1):82-90.

Escorpizo R, Stucki G, Cieza A, Davis K, Stumbo T, Riddle DL. Creating an interface between the International Classification of Functioning, Disability and Health and physical therapist practice. *Phys Ther.* 2010;90(7):1053-1063.

Helgeson K, Russell-Smith A. Process for applying the International Classification of Functioning, Disability and Health Model to a patient with patellar dislocation. *Phys Ther.* 2008;88(8):956-964.

15 Alternative Payment Models

OBJECTIVES

Following completion of this chapter, the reader will be able to:

- Define and differentiate fee for service, per-diem, per-episode, and capitation payment mechanisms.
- Define value-based payment.
- Analyze alternative payment models and rationale for their development.
- Describe the Improving Medicare Post-Acute Care Transformation (Impact) Act of 2014.
- List the reporting requirements required by the Impact Act of 2014 for physical therapy providers in post-acute care settings.
- Describe the self-care and mobility items that must be rated on patient assessment instruments across post-acute care settings.
- Explain documentation needs for new models of payment.

TRADITIONAL PAYMENT MODELS

Payment for healthcare is rapidly evolving, with healthcare providers and the insured being asked to share more financial risk in the delivery of care. Traditional models of payment that provide incentives for providers to deliver a higher *quantity* of service are being replaced by payment models that provide incentives for providers to deliver higher-*quality* service that is effective and efficient. As these payment models evolve, documentation to demonstrate the delivery of a higher quality of care will be required. This chapter will define the different models of traditional payment schemes, describe alternative payment models and value-based payment, and discuss documentation changes necessary to demonstrate compliance with requirements of new payment models.

Fee-for-Service Payment (Pay for Quantity)

Payment for physical therapy has traditionally been based on the volume of service delivery. The amount of payment a therapist receives for each treatment session is based on the procedures billed indicated by Current Procedural Terminology (CPT) codes, Healthcare Common Procedure Coding System (HCPCS) codes (Medicare), and the number of units billed for each procedure. The monetary value for each procedure is established in a complex process called the Resource-Based Relative Value Scale (RBRVS) that considers multiple factors, including work value, practice expense and malpractice, and a conversion factor in determining the value for each procedure. This system provides financial incentives to providers who perform the most expensive procedures and bill for the highest quantity of units. No consideration is given to the medical value of the service provided or to minimizing the time spent with patients. Furthermore, there is no financial incentive to pushing a patient to achieve his or her goals in fewer sessions. Variations of the fee-for-service (FFS) payment methodology have evolved over time as payers sought to limit their financial risk by placing additional financial risk with the providers.

Per diem Providers receive one lump sum for each episode, regardless of severity.

Per episode of care This is similar to per diem, but accounts for severity and complexity. This payment covers the entire episode of care, regardless of the duration.

Capitation Entire networks of providers pool their resources and receive fixed monthly payments for each enrolled patient.

Cash based The physical therapist accepts payment directly from the client, and no insurance or other party is involved in the transaction.

Value-Based Payment (Pay for Quality)

Value-based payment is defined as a broad set of performance-based payment strategies that link financial incentives to providers' performance on a set of defined measures of quality and/or cost or resource use. The goal is to achieve better value by driving improvements in quality and slowing the growth in healthcare spending by encouraging care delivery patterns that are not only high quality but also cost-efficient.[1]

Payment is evolving to a system that provides financial incentives for providing care based on best practice, producing effective outcomes by measuring them consistently, and doing so as rapidly as possible in the most appropriate setting.

In 2015, the U.S. Department of Health and Human Services (HHS) announced its goal to:

- Base 30% of all Medicare FFS on alternative payment models by the end of 2016
- Increase that proportion to 50% by 2018
- Link 85% of FFS payments to outcome measures by the end of 2016
- Bump that percentage to 90% by the end of 2018[2]

The Department of Health and Human Services (HHS) announced the creation of the Health Care Payment Learning & Action Network (HCP-LAN) aimed at serving as a forum for payers, providers, employers, purchasers, state partners, consumer groups and the individual consumer to discuss how to transition towards alternative payment models emphasizing value. See Figure 15.1 for goals revised in 2020 for HCP-LAN. In March 2016, the U.S. Centers for Medicare & Medicaid Services (CMS) certified they had met the 30% target for all Medicare FFS payments.[3] In 2017, 38.3% of the FFS payments were based on alternative payment models.[3] The transition to value-based payment continues.[4]

With these statements, the federal government made it clear they are serious about getting the healthcare community on track to transition to a value-based payment environment—sooner rather than later by announcing specific measurable goals and timeline to move Medicare and the health care system at large away from payment based on quantity of care towards payment based on quality. Examples of Programs that tie hospital payment to Quality of Value: Hospital Value Based Purchasing (VBP) Program, Hospital Readmission Reduction Program (HRRP) and the Hospital-Acquired Condition (HAC) Program.[4] Payers in the private market are not far behind. As this *Medical Economics* article notes, "the shift from FFS to value-based reimbursement will be even more dramatic."[5] Never before has there

	Medicaid	Commercial	Medicare Advantage	Traditional Medicare
2020	15%	15%	30%	30%
2022	25%	25%	50%	50%
2025	50%	50%	100%	100%

Figure 15-1. Percentage of US health care payments tied to quality and value in each market segment through the adoption of two-sided risk alternative payment models.[4]

been a government-issued call for such a radical healthcare payment overhaul in such a short amount of time—with defined deadlines. This is an example of an established trend that likely will not change: the private health sector's tendency to follow the government's payment policy lead. In fact, some private insurers and provider groups have already jumped on the alternative payment model bandwagon. Eventually, providers in all disciplines—physical therapy included—will receive payment for their services based on their participation in alternative payment models. At this time, the end model is questionable, but expected to be complicated.[5]

The Shared Savings Model (Accountable Care Organizations)

In a shared savings structure, individual providers join together in a group called an accountable care organization (ACO). The group then contracts with a payer to provide care for a particular patient population. As part of that contract, the parties agree on specific cost and quality benchmarks and determine a time frame for measuring performance on those fronts. If the ACO's performance exceeds the predetermined cost and quality goals, the group shares the savings with the payer. If the providers do not meet the benchmark goals, the ACO absorbs the difference.

Essentially, the shared savings model merges traditional FFS with real financial incentives for minimizing healthcare spending by either refraining from providing unnecessary services or prioritizing the delivery of less expensive, similarly effective alternatives—while simultaneously maintaining or improving quality of care. While some ACOs include physical therapy in their organization, others contract the services with external providers.

Quality Payment Program

On November 1, 2018, the final 2019 Medicare Physician Fee Schedule (PFS) was released by CMS. The rule contains changes to the Quality Payment Program (QPP), including the new requirement for certain physical therapists in private practice to participate in the QPP through one of two tracks: either the Merit-based Incentive Payment System (MIPS) or Advanced Alternative Payment Methods (APMs). Advanced APMs are a subset of APMs that let practices earn more rewards in exchange for taking on risk related to patient outcomes.

In the Advanced APM track of QPP, physical therapists may earn a 5% incentive for achieving threshold levels of payments or patients, and participation in the Advanced APM exempts you from the MIPS reporting requirements (the other QPP track).[6]

Merit-Based Incentive Payment System

As mentioned, the other QPP track is the MIPS. MIPS is a large-scale quality program affecting those providers who see Medicare beneficiaries. This is the first such quality improvement program that will include mandatory participation by certain physical therapists. Successful participation in the MIPS program can qualify providers for up to 9% payment adjustment. Conversely, failure to meet the targets for successful participation can result in a downward payment adjustment in Medicare payment of up to 9%.[7]

Advanced Alternative Payment System

Bundled Payment Model

Many episodes of care involve several different types of interprofessional services, delivered by many different providers. Even though they are all working toward the same outcome, theoretically their incentives are not truly aligned because in the traditional payment structure each provider receives payment independently. Essentially, in the traditional payment model every provider is working for himself or herself, which may lead to unorganized, inefficient care and overutilization of services.

The bundled payment model, on the other hand, more effectively gets individual providers better aligned with the same goals, and most importantly, working under the same budget. The payer offers a single lump sum for the entire episode of care related to a particular treatment or condition to the entity they deem responsible. Some bundled payment spin-offs, like the patient-centered medical home model, incorporate some FFS components to supplement the lump sum. All of the providers involved in that episode get a share of the lump sum. For example, for a patient who has knee surgery, such as a total knee replacement, they would incur one single charge to cover the surgery itself, the postoperative rehabilitation, and all follow-up exams and services, with one entity—commonly the hospital—responsible for payment of all related services in all settings.

A few different variations of the lump sum structure fall under the bundled payment umbrella. For example, the per diem structure provides one lump sum for each type of episode, regardless of severity, whereas the episode of care structure accounts for severity and complexity.

Bundled Payment for Care Improvements Advanced

Bundled Payment for Care Improvements (BPCI) Advanced is a voluntary episodic payment model that will test bundled payments for episodes of care related to 35 conditions or procedures, from acute myocardial infarction to urinary tract infection. BPCI Advanced qualifies as an Advanced APM under QPP. An episode of care begins either with an inpatient admission to an acute care hospital—called an anchor stay—or with the start of an outpatient procedure—called an anchor procedure. Anchor stays are identified by Medicare Severity Diagnosis Related Groups (MS-DRGs), and anchor procedures are identified by HCPCS codes. The episode ends 90 days after the end of the anchor stay or anchor procedure. The first group of participants started October 1, 2018; CMS offered a second application period in spring 2019, for a January 2020 start. The program is scheduled to end December 31, 2023. Physical therapists are eligible to participate.[6]

Comprehensive Care For Joint Replacement Model

The Comprehensive Care for Joint Replacement (CJR) model is a payment model being tested for episodes of care related to total knee and total hip replacements (MS-DRG 469 and 470) under Medicare. One track of the CJR model qualifies as an Advanced APM under the QPP. The model began April 1, 2016, and will run through December 31, 2020. In 2020, CMS proposed to extend the model for an additional 3 years.[8] The CJR model holds participant hospitals financially accountable for the quality and cost of an episode of care and incentivizes increased coordination among participating hospitals, physicians, and post–acute care providers such as physical therapists. An episode of care begins with a patient's hospital admission, continues upon hospital discharge, and ends 90 days post-discharge to cover the patient's complete period of recovery.

THE IMPROVING MEDICARE POST-ACUTE CARE TRANSFORMATION ACT OF 2014

CMS is aligning quality measurement across post–acute care assessment instruments to meet the provisions of the Improving Medicare Post-Acute Care Transformation (IMPACT) Act of 2014. The act requires the submission of standardized data in all post–acute care settings: long-term acute care hospitals (LTACHs), inpatient rehabilitation facilities (IRFs), skilled nursing facilities (SNFs), and home health agencies (HHAs). CMS established quality-reporting programs for LTACH, IRF, SNF, and HHA to implement the provisions of the IMPACT Act.[9]

By standardizing quality measures and standardized data collection, CMS intends to enable interoperability and access data across the continuum of care to facilitate coordinated care, improved outcomes, and quality comparisons among institutions.[10] For the first time, these changes will create alignment between the IRHs, SNFs, LTACHs, and home healthcare settings. One tool that is used to standardize data collection across the continuum of care is the intake assessment form for each setting. For example, in SNFs this form is the Minimum Data Set (MDS) 3.0. (See Chapter 8 for additional breakdown of the MDS.) Assessment instruments used in each setting are listed in Table 15-1. Each instrument will contain a common section assessing the same functional tasks (e.g., self-care and mobility items) scored with the same scale. The scale for scoring the self-care and mobility portion of Section GG is listed in Table 15-2.

Each post–acute care setting will collect this information at the start or resumption of care for each patient with a goal for discharge established at the same time. To illustrate in more detail the documentation requirements and nuances for data collection, details of the Patient-Driven Payment Model (PDPM) for SNFs will briefly be discussed below for the new payment models for SNFs and HHAs. See Chapter 7 Documentation for Home Health and Chapter 8 Documentation for Certified Nursing Homes for where they are discussed in more detail. Keep in mind that each post–acute care setting will have similar requirements, but currently are operating under different payment models that rely on different incentives.

Patient-Driven Payment Model for Medicare Beneficiaries

In October 2019, the payment system in SNFs changed from the Resource Utilization Groups-IV (RUGS IV) that has been in place in some form for over 20 years with the PDPM.

Table 15-1 Medicare Assessment Instruments by Setting[11]

SETTING	ASSESSMENT INSTRUMENT
Long-Term Acute Care Hospital	Long-Term Care Hospital Continuity Assessment Record and Evaluation (CARE) Data Set (LCDS)
Inpatient Rehabilitation	Inpatient Rehabilitation Facility-Patient Assessment Instrument (IRF-PAI)
Skilled Nursing Facility	Minimum Data Set (MDS)
Home Healthcare	Outcome and Assessment Information Set (OASIS)

Table 15-2 Section GG Scoring for Self-Care and Mobility[11]

LEVEL OF PERFORMANCE	DESCRIPTION
01-Dependent	Helper does all of the effort. Resident does none of the effort to complete the activity. Or the assistance of two or more helpers is required for the resident to complete the activity.
02-Substantial/Maximal Assistance	Helper does more than half the effort. Helper lifts or holds trunk or limbs and provides more than half the effort.
03-Partial/Moderate Assistance	Helper does less than half the effort. Helper lifts, holds, or supports the trunk or limbs, but provides less than half the effort.
04-Supervision or Touching Assistance	Helper provides verbal cures and/or touching/steadying and/or contact guard assistance as resident completes the activity. Assistance may be provided throughout the activity or intermittently.
05-Setup or Clean-up Assistance	Help set up or clean up; resident completes activity. Helper assists only prior to or following the activity.
06-Independent	Resident completes the activity by himself or herself with no assistance from a helper.
07	Resident refused
09	Not applicable
10	Not attempted due to environmental limitations
88	Not attempted due to medical condition or safety concerns

According to CMS, this new system is an improvement, as it "improves payment accuracy and appropriateness by focusing on the patient, rather than the volume of services provided, significantly reduces administrative burden on providers, and improves SNF payments to currently underserved beneficiaries without increasing total Medicare payments."[12] This system is designed to address concerns that RUG-IV did not produce accurate and appropriate adjustments based on the severity of the patient's condition. It adjusts the payment away from the provision of services (quantity) to verifiable patient characteristics and needs (quality).

Under PDPM, each patient is classified into a group for each of the five case-mix adjusted components: Physical Therapy (PT), Occupational Therapy (OT), Speech Language Pathology (SLP), Nursing, and Non-Therapy Ancillary (NTA). Each component then uses different criteria as the basis for classification. For the PT and OT components, this is based on a clinical category and a functional score derived from elements from the MDS 3.0. Patients are first classified into a clinical category (see Table 15-3) based on their primary ICD-10-CM diagnosis.

Then the PT and OT components use four collapsed clinical categories for patient classification (Table 15-4).

Once these PT and OT component clinical categories are established, a functional score is determined based on the patient's performance on elements of Section GG of the MDS 3.0. Table 15-5 lists those components rated to determine this functional score.

Table 15-3 PDPM Clinical Categories[12]

PDPM CLINICAL CATEGORIES	
Major Joint Replacement or Spinal Surgery	Cancer
Non-Surgical Orthopedic/Musculoskeletal	Pulmonary
Orthopedic Surgery (Except Major Joint Replacement or Spinal Surgery)	Cardiovascular and Coagulations
Acute Infections	Acute Neurological
Medical Management	Non-Orthopedic Surgery

Table 15-4 PDPM Clinical, Physical Therapy and Occupational Therapy Categories[12]

PDPM CLINICAL CATEGORIES	PT AND OT CLINICAL CATEGORIES
Major Joint Replacement or Spinal Surgery	Major Joint Replacement or Spinal Surgery
Acute Neurological	Non-Orthopedic Surgery and Acute Neurological
Non-Orthopedic Surgery	
Non-Surgical Orthopedic/ Musculoskeletal	Other Orthopedic
Orthopedic Surgery (Except Major Joint Replacement or Spinal Surgery)	
Medical Management	Medical Management
Cancer	
Pulmonary	
Cardiovascular and Coagulations	
Acute Infections	

Following the determination of the resident's performance level on each activity, scoring is performed for the purposes of creating a functional score. Each Section GG item will be assigned a score from 0 to 4 based on the scale in Table 15-6.

Six items make up the components of the functional score, thereby producing a total functional score ranging from 0 to 24. Proper rating of the patient's performance and supporting that with documentation is essential for properly classifying the patient to qualify for the necessary level of service to maximize their potential for regaining function prior to their discharge.

The patient's therapy classification (case-mix classification groups) for payment purposes is determined based on the combination of the clinical category and Section GG functional score. The case-mix classification groups are in Table 15-7.

In an effort to better determine the intensity of services delivered to beneficiaries, CMS will add two new therapy reporting requirements to the current discharge assessment.[13] Therapists will have a responsibility to accurately assess the patient's level of performance and support it with their documentation, both on the evaluation and by properly coding Section

Table 15-5 Section GG Items Included in the PT and OT Component Score[12]

SECTION GG ITEM	FUNCTIONAL SCORE RANGE
Self-care: Eating	0–4
Self-care: Oral Hygiene	0–4
Self-care: Toileting Hygiene	0–4
Mobility: Sit to Lying	0–4 (average of 2 items)
Mobility: Lying to Sitting on Side of Bed	
Mobility: Sit to Stand	0–4 (average of 3 items)
Mobility: Chair/Bed-to-Chair Transfer	
Mobility: Toilet Transfer	
Mobility: Walk 50 Feet with Two Turns	0–4 (average of 2 items)
Mobility: Walk 150 Feet	

Table 15-6 Creating the PT and OT Functional Score[12]

RESPONSE ON SELF-CARE AND MOBILITY ITEMS	DESCRIPTION	SCORE
05, 06	Setup assistance, independent	4
04	Supervision or touching assistance	3
03	Partial/moderate assistance	2
02	Substantial/maximal assistance	1
01, 07, 09, 10, 88	Dependent, refused, not applicable, not attempted due to environmental limitations, not attempted due to medical condition or safety concerns, resident cannot walk (for GG item 017011)	0

GG of the MDS 3.0. Additionally, the responsibility to track minutes of therapy delivered will remain in place, although it will no longer be used as the basis for payment.

Linkage to the SNF Quality Reporting Program

The data collected on these assessments will be used to measure performance on meeting the requirements of specific SNF QRP quality measures.[14] Skilled Nursing Facilities can potentially avoid a 2% reduction on their Medicare Fee For Service rates by ensuring they have submitted all necessary MDS data for admissions and discharges as part of the required reporting for the SNF Quality Reporting Program.[15]

Table 15-7 PT and OT Case-Mix Classification Groups[12]

CLINICAL CATEGORY	SECTION GG FUNCTION SCORE	PT-OT CASE-MIX GROUP
Major Joint Replacement or Spinal Surgery	0–5	TA
Major Joint Replacement or Spinal Surgery	6–9	TB
Major Joint Replacement or Spinal Surgery	10–23	TC
Major Joint Replacement or Spinal Surgery	24	TD
Other Orthopedic	0–5	TE
Other Orthopedic	6–9	TF
Other Orthopedic	10–23	TG
Other Orthopedic	24	TH
Medical Management	0–5	TI
Medical Management	6–9	TJ
Medical Management	10–23	TK
Medical Management	24	TL
Non-Orthopedic Surgery and Acute Neurological	0–5	TM
Non-Orthopedic Surgery and Acute Neurological	6–9	TN
Non-Orthopedic Surgery and Acute Neurological	10–23	TO
Non-Orthopedic Surgery and Acute Neurological	24	TP

Patient-Driven Groupings Model

Similar to the changes that occurred in 2019, the payment methodology in the home healthcare setting changed on January 1, 2020, from the Home Health Resource Utilization Group (HH-RUG) system to the Patient-Driven Groupings Model (PDGM). According to CMS, "the PDGM relies more heavily on clinical characteristics and other patient information to place home health periods of care into meaningful payment categories and eliminates the use of therapy service thresholds."[16] The payment periods in PDGM will shift from the HH-RUG 60-day episode of care to a 30-day episode of care to better capture the greater intensity of services typically seen early in the episode of care. The elimination of the therapy thresholds is meant to align payment to the *value* of the services delivered to the patient, rather than to the volume of services delivered to the patient.

After the initial assessment, patients are categorized into one of 432 case-mix groups based on their classification into each of five broad categories, as outlined in Table 15-8.[17]

The clinic grouping categories are described in Table 15-9.

The functional impairment level is determined using items from the OASIS-D assessment (see Appendix B).[18] These items are listed in Table 15-10.

Table 15-8 PDGM Patient Grouping Categories[17]

CATEGORY	CLASSIFICATION LABELS
Admission Source (2 subgroups)	Community or institutional admission source
Timing of 30-day Period (2 subgroups)	Early or late
Clinical Grouping (12 subgroups)	Musculoskeletal rehabilitation; Neuro/stroke rehabilitation; Wounds; Medication Management, Teaching, and Assessment (MMTA): surgical aftercare; MMTA: cardiac and circulatory; MMTA: endocrine; MMTA: gastrointestinal tract and genitourinary system; MMTA: infectious disease, neoplasms, and blood-forming diseases; MMTA: respiratory; MMTA- other; behavioral health; or complex nursing interventions
Functional Impairment Level (3 subgroups)	Low, medium, high
Comorbidity Adjustment	None, low, or high based on secondary diagnoses

Table 15-9 PDGM Clinical Group Categories[17]

CLINICAL GROUP	PRIMARY REASON FOR HOME HEALTH ENCOUNTER IS TO PROVIDE
Musculoskeletal Rehabilitation	Therapy (PT/OT/SLP) for a musculoskeletal condition
Neuro/Stroke Rehabilitation	Therapy (PT/OT/SLP) for a neurological condition or stroke
MMTA: surgical aftercare; MMTA: cardiac and circulatory; MMTA: endocrine; MMTA: gastrointestinal tract and genitourinary system; MMTA: infectious disease, neoplasms, and blood-forming diseases; MMTA: respiratory; MMTA: other	Assessment, evaluation, teaching, and medication management for a variety of medical and surgical conditions not classified in one of the above listed groups. The subgroups represent common clinical conditions that require home health services for medication management, teaching, and assessment.
Wounds-Post-Op Wound Aftercare and Skin/Non-Surgical Wound Care	Assessment, treatment, and evaluation of a surgical wound(s); assessment, treatment and evaluation of non-surgical wounds, ulcers burns, and other lesions
Behavioral Health	Assessment, treatment and evaluation of psychiatric and substance abuse conditions
Complex Nursing Interventions	Assessment, treatment, and evaluation of complex medical and surgical conditions

Unlike in the SNF setting, Section GG items are not used in the calculation of the home health episodic payment. However, providers are required to collect and report the Section GG items for each patient at admission, follow-up, and discharge. They are used in meeting the quality reporting process measures for the Home Health Quality Reporting Program (HH

Table 15-10 OASIS-D Items Used to Calculate Functional Impairment Level[17]

OASIS ITEM NUMBER	DESCRIPTION
M1800	Grooming
M1810	Current ability to dress upper body
M1820	Current ability to dress lower body
M1830	Bathing
M1840	Toilet transferring
M1850	Transferring
M1860	Ambulation and locomotion
M1033	Risk for hospitalization

QRP). The data submitted from the OASIS-D, including the Section GG items, is one element used to measure performance on meeting the requirements of the HH QRP quality measures. 42 CFR 484.225(i) provides that HHAs that meet the quality data reporting requirements are eligible to receive the full home health (HH) market basket percentage increase. HHAs that do not meet the reporting requirements are subject to a two (2%) percentage point reduction to the HH market basket increase.[19]

Documentation Requirements for Alternative Payment Models

Regardless of the payment model for the service (i.e., cash-based, government payer, private insurer) or how the patient entered into the practice (i.e., self-referral, provider referral, direct access), the basic principles of documentation outlined in this textbook must be applied. Physical therapy providers must create documentation that accurately reflects what occurred with the patient during the entire episode and supports the fees that were charged for the services provided. Effective documentation also demonstrates the progress of the patient, leading to better decision-making with future patients and the value of your care to other patients, payers, and referral sources.

Although a patient or client may be paying cash directly for the services provided to them, they may submit the invoice provided to them to their insurance company for reimbursement. The documentation provided to them needs to adhere to specific requirements for that payer and accurately reflect the proper billing practices. Using documentation and facility policies to clearly set expectations about payment terms and clearly listing the charges for each service will help solidify a solid relationship with your patients and ensure their ultimate reimbursement from their payer.

In the case of alternative payment models, physical therapy practices may be involved with public and private insurers, and there may be specific documents that must be completed that are payer required. For example, in the PDPM model described earlier, the MDS, which includes Section GG, must be submitted according to procedures and timing outlined by CMS in order for payment to be rendered. Failure to comply with these requirements will result in a payment delay or denial. These requirements are in addition to the normal notes and outcome measures that are completed with every patient. For the CJR, patient-reported outcomes (PROs) must be reported in order to qualify for the maximum incentive payment for participation. Again, this documentation is in addition to the documentation requirements of the clinic. The Hip Disability Osteoarthritis and Outcome Score (HOOS)[20] is an example of a PRO that patients who undergo a total hip arthroplasty in an institution participating in the CJR must complete.

SUMMARY

The ability to demonstrate value is a necessary prerequisite to participation in the U.S. healthcare system. Physical therapists have successfully positioned themselves to make a meaningful contribution to the health of individuals and society. However, consumers, referral sources, payers, and policy makers no longer accept a profession's anecdotal reports as a demonstration of value. Physical therapists must engage in a coordinated approach to demonstrate that value[21] and must embrace and engage in programs that measure the quality of the care they deliver. Ideally, they will be actively involved in developing those metrics and become active participants in the quality improvement process, including influencing the development of APMs and quality reporting programs. The alternative payment models and quality reporting programs discussed in this chapter are a sampling of the evolving payment methods in our healthcare system and illustrate the continuing move toward more value-based purchasing in both the public and private sector.

ALTERNATIVE PAYMENT MODELS ACTIVITIES

Place the following payment mechanisms in order from *least risk* to the provider to *most risk* to the provider and then explain what each term means in your own words.

(1) Cash Based
(2) Per Episode
(3) Capitation
(4) Fee for Service
(5) Per Diem

According to the requirements of the IMPACT Act, providers in most post–acute care settings are going to be required to set a discharge goal for patients at the time of the initial assessment. What information that you gather during your examination and evaluation will you use to help you determine an appropriate goal for discharge? Other than on the specific form used for the patient's assessment, where would be the appropriate place to document this in a traditional SOAP note?

ACTIVITIES FOR PROPER CODING OF SECTION GG ON THE MDS AND OASIS-D

Mr. B sits on a tub bench as he washes, rinses, and dries himself in the bathtub. A staff member stays with him the entire time to ensure his safety. He also needs minimal lifting assistance from one person as he gets on and off of the tub bench.

How would you code GG0130E. Shower/Bathe Self?

Why did you choose that code?

Mrs. M has diabetes and peripheral neuropathy in her upper and lower extremities. She has a history of a transtibial amputation. Mrs. M needs assistance of one person to don and doff her lower limb prosthesis. She needs no assistance to put on and remove her underwear or pants.

How would you code GG0130G. Lower Body Dressing?

Why did you choose that code?

Mrs. K has degenerative joint disease and recently had a right total knee arthroplasty. During her stay in the SNF, her walking was assessed. She will need to walk on unstable and uneven surfaces when she returns home, so the physical therapist wanted to assess her ability to do this activity. She required the assistance of the physical therapist less than half the time to keep her from falling during her 10-foot walk over an uneven surface.

How would you code GG0170L-Walking 10 Feet on Uneven Surfaces?

Why did you choose that code?

Mr. L has Parkinson's disease and is recovering from a short hospital stay due to pneumonia. He has 12 steps at home that he must use to enter and exit his home. He has a railing on both sides. The physical therapist uses a gait belt around his waist during the examination of his ability to go up and down 12 stairs but does not provide any assistance to Mr. L during the activity.

How would you code GG0170O-12 Steps?

Why did you choose that code?

REVIEW QUESTIONS

1. Define and differentiate fee for service, per diem, per episode, and capitation payment mechanisms.
2. Define value-based payment.
3. Explain alternative payment models and the rationale for their development.
4. Describe the Improving Medicare Post-Acute Care Transformation (IMPACT) Act of 2014.
5. List the reporting requirements required by the IMPACT Act of 2014 for physical therapy providers in post–acute care settings.
6. Describe the self-care and mobility items that must be rated on patient assessment instruments across post–acute care settings.
7. Describe documentation needs for new models of payment.

REFERENCES

1. *Roadmap for Implementing Value-Driven Healthcare in the Traditional Medicare Fee for Service Program*. Baltimore, MD: Centers for Medicare & Medicaid Services. Available at https://www.cms.gov/Medicare/Quality-Initiatives-Patient-Assessment-Instruments/QualityInitiativesGenInfo/downloads/VBPRoadmap_OEA_1-16_508.pdf. Accessed August 10, 2020.
2. Burwell SM. Setting value-based payment goals-HHS efforts to improve US health care. *N Engl J Med*. 2015;372(10):897–899.
3. *Health Care Payment and Learning Action Network. Center for Medicare and Medicaid Innovation*. Baltimore, MD: Centers for Medicare & Medicaid Services. Available at https://innovation.cms.gov/initiatives/health-care-payment-learning-and-action-network/. Accessed August 10, 2020.
4. *APM Measurement Effort*. Health Care Payment and Learning Action Network. Available at https://hcp-lan.org/apm-measurement-effort/. Accessed August 10, 2020.
5. Shifting reimbursement models: The risks and rewards for primary care. *Medical Economics*. Cranbury, NJ: Multimedia Healthcare. April 8, 2014. Available at https://www.medicaleconomics.com/view/shifting-reimbursement-models-risks-and-rewards-primary-care. Accessed August 10, 2020.
6. *An Introduction to Alternative Payment Models*. Alexandria, VA: American Physical Therapy Association. Available at https://www.apta.org/your-practice/payment/medicare-payment/alternative-payment-models/apms-an-introduction. Accessed August 10, 2020.
7. *Merit-Based Incentive Program*. Alexandria, VA: American Physical Therapy Association. Available at https://www.apta.org/your-practice/payment/value-based-payment-models/quality-payment-program/merit-based-incentive-program. Accessed August 10, 2020.
8. *Comprehensive Care for Joint Replacement Model*. Baltimore, MD: Centers for Medicare & Medicaid Services. Available at https://innovation.cms.gov/initiatives/cjr. Accessed August 10, 2020.
9. *Skilled Nursing Facility (SNF) Quality Reporting Program Measures and Technical Information*. Baltimore, MD: Centers for Medicare & Medicaid Services. Available at https://www.cms.gov/Medicare/Quality-Initiatives-Patient-Assessment-Instruments/NursingHomeQualityInits/Skilled-Nursing-Facility-Quality-Reporting-Program/SNF-Quality-Reporting-Program-Measures-and-Technical-Information.html. Accessed August 10, 2020.
10. *Medicare Post-Acute Care Reform*. Alexandria, VA: American Physical Therapy Association. Available at http://www.apta.org/PostacuteCareReform/. Accessed August 10, 2020.
11. *SNF Quality Reporting Training Program*. Baltimore, MD: Centers for Medicare & Medicaid Services. Available at https://www.cms.gov/Medicare/Quality-Initiatives-Patient-Assessment-Instruments/NursingHomeQualityInits/Skilled-Nursing-Facility-Quality-Reporting-Program/SNF-Quality-Reporting-Program-Training.html. Accessed August 10, 2020
12. *Patient Driven Payment Model*. Baltimore, MD: Centers for Medicare & Medicaid Services. Available at https://www.cms.gov/Medicare/Medicare-Fee-for-Service-Payment/SNFPPS/PDPM.html. Accessed August 10, 2020.
13. *What You Should Know About the Patient-Driven Payment Model for Skilled Nursing Facilities*. Alexandria, VA: American

Physical Therapy Association. Available at https://www.apta.org/your-practice/payment/medicare-payment/coding-billing/skilled-nursing-facilities/patient-driven-payment-model/what-you-should-know. Accessed August 10, 2020.

14. *Skilled Nursing Facility (SNF) Quality Reporting Program Measures and Technical Information*. Baltimore, MD: Centers for Medicare & Medicaid Services. Available at https://www.cms.gov/Medicare/Quality-Initiatives-Patient-Assessment-Instruments/NursingHomeQualityInits/Skilled-Nursing-Facility-Quality-Reporting-Program/SNF-Quality-Reporting-Program-Measures-and-Technical-Information.html. Accessed August 10, 2020.
15. *The Skilled Nursing Facility Value-Based Purchasing (SNF VBP) Program*. Baltimore, MD: Centers for Medicare & Medicaid Services. Available at https://www.cms.gov/Medicare/Quality-Initiatives-Patient-Assessment-Instruments/Value-Based-Programs/SNF-VBP/SNF-VBP-Page.html. Accessed August 10, 2020.
16. *Home Health Patient Driven Groupings Model*. Baltimore, MD: Centers for Medicare & Medicaid Services. Available at https://www.cms.gov/Medicare/Medicare-Fee-for-Service-Payment/HomeHealthPPS/HH-PDGM.html. Accessed August 10, 2020, 2020.
17. *CMS Home Health Patient Driven Groups Model*. Baltimore, MD: Centers for Medicare & Medicaid Services. Available at https://www.cms.gov/Medicare/Medicare-Fee-for-Service-Payment/HomeHealthPPS/Downloads/Overview-of-the-Patient-Driven-Groupings-Model.pdf. Accessed August 10, 2020.
18. *OASIS-D All Items*. Baltimore, MD: Centers for Medicare & Medicaid Services. Available at https://www.cms.gov/Medicare/Quality-Initiatives-Patient-Assessment-Instruments/HomeHealthQualityInits/Downloads/OASIS-D_All-Items_final.pdf. Accessed August 10, 2020.
19. *Home Health Quality Reporting Requirements*. PPS Fact Sheet. Baltimore, MD: Centers for Medicare & Medicaid Services. Available at https://www.cms.gov/Medicare/Quality-Initiatives-Patient-Assessment-Instruments/HomeHealthQualityInits/Home-Health-Quality-Reporting-Requirements. Accessed August 10, 2020.
20. Klässbo M, Larsson E, Mannevik E. Hip disability and osteoarthritis outcome score: An extension of the Western Ontario and McMaster Universities Osteoarthritis Index. *Scand J Rheumatol*. 2003;32(1):46–51.
21. Jewell DV, Moore JD, Goldstein MS. Delivering the physical therapy value proposition: A call to action. *Phys Ther*. 2013;93(1):104–114. doi:10.2522/ptj.2012017.

SECTION **4**

Steps and Framework for Coding and Documentation

16 Documentation Writing Examples and Worksheets

OBJECTIVES

Following completion of this chapter, the reader will be able to:

- Explain documentation activities that reinforce appropriate content.
- Identify prior level of function (PLOF) in cases provided.
- Describe components of the initial examination in cases provided.
- Define the plan of care (POC) in cases provided.
- Discuss improvements to daily notes, progress notes, and summaries in cases provided.
- Discuss how the physical therapy intervention affect the patient and discharge instructions.

Documentation is key to communication between professionals involved in the care of a patient and communication with any individuals needing access to a patient's record, including the patient. Other than a patient's or therapist's word, it is the only permanent record of the therapy or intervention a patient received and patient response to treatment. Although billing is also a written record, billing without the required documentation does not stand alone.

According to the American Physical Therapy Association (APTA),[1] documentation is:

- A planning tool for physical therapy
- Communication among providers

- Record of care provided
- Evidence of compliance with federal, state, payer, and local regulations
- An historical account of physical therapist (PT)/patient encounters that serves a legal purpose
- Vehicle for third-party payers to determine appropriateness of services
- Information that can be used for policy or research purposes, including outcome analysis

When Medicare was instituted in 1966, records were required to indicate physical therapy was rendered. The details required of services provided by PTs and physical therapist assistants (PTAs) today must, in alignment with the International Classification of Functioning, Disability, and Health model (ICF), include the following:[2-4]

- Clear identification of the patient
- Referral source and mechanism (self-referral, physician, other)
- Psychosocial information, including the patient's history with identified pathology, medical diagnosis(es) and comorbidities, and physical therapy or treatment diagnoses in ICD-10[5] codable terminology and code
- Current complaints
- Precautions and barriers
- Justification that physical therapy is medically necessary
- Be timely, objective, and descriptive
- Articulation of the skill needed
- General systems screening
- Inclusion of objective tests and measures that can be performed at the initial visit and repeated over the length of stay (LOS) with appropriate explanation of functional relevance
- Prognosis for the patient relevant to the physical therapy
- A plan of care (POC) that indicates interventions in Current Procedure Terminology (CPT)[6] codable verbiage and clear intent
- Inclusion of time-defined objective and measurable goals, focusing on function, that reflect the problems and POC in CPT[6] descriptive and codable verbiage identified in the initial examination and evaluation
- Treatment on a session-by-session basis, with specific skilled intervention (International Statistical Classification of Diseases [ICD][5] codable verbiage, skill required by the treating PT/PTA (including patient response to treatment/tolerance), rationale for change or reflection of decision-making, ensuring there is ongoing change
- Plan from visit to visit or session to session
- Description of progress over time
- On every entry: signature of the evaluating or treating PT/PTA is required, preferably legible (electronic in the electronic medical record [EMR]), and it is recommended that the treating professional include their license number for the state in which they practice
  - For billing purposes, the PT's National Provider Number (NPI)[7] must be available

Although entry-level curricula include content and training in documentation to PT and PTA students, and the APTA has published guidelines, complete and accurate documentation across settings and the lifespan continues to be a challenge for practitioners at all levels of practice. In recent years, EMRs have provided templates and drop-down options for improved content inclusion, but challenges continue if skill is not clearly identified.

This chapter includes a series of documentation exercises with a sample guideline to facilitate more effective and accurate documentation

SAMPLE PRINCIPLES

The PT/PTA documents the treatment preceding all descriptions with CPT[6] verbiage. As therapeutic exercise is a timed code, the actual time should be included. Terminology used in the

documentation must be universally understood by all possible record "readers," yet sophisticated enough to justify the skilled care rendered. Colloquial spoken language, unless quoting a patient, should be avoided.

1 unit: 15 minutes: Therapeutic exercise: passive stretching; × reps × 15 secs of the L hamstrings, manual reciprocal inhibition quadriceps/hamstrings to facilitate hamstring lengthening, manual resistive exercise with progressive resistance knee extension/flexion for facilitation of strengthening.

Objective measurements must be provided indicating available active or passive range of motion (ROM) measured over normal ranges for the joint. They should be stated in fractions, and ultimately relate to lack of function as the reason for care because of the limited ROM. This is also relevant to muscle performance. In some cases, manual muscle test grading may be misleading, and muscle performance, describing performance—including inability to repeat a movement against resistance or sustain a position—may be more indicative of the relevancy to function.

NOTE WRITING EXERCISES: DAILY TREATMENT OR DAILY ENCOUNTER

Author's Note

According to Medicare Benefit Policy Manual Chapter 15, Section 220.3(e):[8]

Documentation of each treatment shall include the following required elements:

- Date of treatment;
- Identification of each specific intervention/modality provided and billed, for both timed and untimed codes, in language that can be compared with the billing on the claim to verify correct coding. Record each service provided that is represented by a timed code, regardless of whether or not it is billed, because the unbilled timed services may impact the billing;
- Total timed code treatment minutes and total treatment time in minutes. Total treatment time includes the minutes for timed code treatment and untimed code treatment. Total treatment time does not include time for services that are not billable (e.g., rest periods). For Medicare purposes, it is not required that unbilled services that are not part of the total treatment minutes be recorded, although they may be included voluntarily to provide an accurate description of the treatment, show consistency with the plan, or comply with state or local policies. The amount of time for each specific intervention/modality provided to the patient may also be recorded voluntarily, but contractors shall not require it, as it is indicated in the billing. The billing and the total timed code treatment minutes must be consistent. See Pub. 100-04, chapter 5, section 20.2 for description of billing timed codes; and
- Signature, professional identification, and license number of the qualified professional who furnished or supervised the services and a list of each person who contributed to that treatment (i.e., the signature of Kathleen Smith, PTA, #1234, with notation of phone consultation with Judy Jones, PT, supervisor, when permitted by state and local law). The signature and identification of the supervisor need not be on each treatment note, unless the supervisor actively participated in the treatment. Since a clinician must be identified on the plan of care and the progress report, the name and professional identification of the supervisor responsible for the treatment is assumed to be the clinician who wrote the plan or report. When the treatment is supervised without active participation by the supervisor, the supervisor is not required to cosign the treatment note written by a qualified professional.

When the responsible supervisor is absent, the presence of a similarly qualified supervisor on the clinic roster for that day is sufficient documentation and it is not required that the substitute supervisor sign or be identified in the documentation.

If a treatment is added or changed under the direction of a clinician during the treatment days between the progress reports, the change must be recorded and justified on the medical record, either in the treatment note or the progress report, as determined by the policies of the provider/supplier. New exercises added or changes made to the exercise program help justify that the services are skilled. For example: The original plan was for therapeutic activities, gait training and neuromuscular re-education. "On Feb. 1 clinician added electrical stim. to address shoulder pain."

Documentation of each treatment may also include the following optional elements to be mentioned only if the qualified professional recording the note determines they are appropriate and relevant. If these are not recorded daily, any relevant information should be included in the progress report.

- Patient self-report;
- Adverse reaction to intervention;
- Communication/consultation with other providers (e.g., supervising clinician, attending physician, nurse, another therapist, etc.);
- Significant, unusual or unexpected changes in clinical status;
- Equipment provided; and/or
- Any additional relevant information the qualified professional finds appropriate.

See Pub. 100-04, Medicare Claims Processing Manual, Chapter 5, Section 20.2[9] for instructions on how to count minutes. It is important that the total number of timed treatment minutes support the billing of units on the claim, and that the total treatment time reflects services billed as untimed codes.

For the following entries, rewrite the content to correct the elements that demonstrate skilled physical therapy:

1. In SOAP format with skilled, codable verbiage
2. In narrative format with skilled, codable verbiage

Note # 1: OP
S: "Fixed lawnmower over weekend, able to mow front and back lawns:
O: Seen in dept. for cont with Isokinetic protocol to BLEs 2 cycles R, 1 cycle L. Followed by balance beam, kicking ball, unilateral stance 15 sec. L unable to maintain L. Side <> side stepping. Side <> side gallop. Fast walking length of hall leasing to office and back, 15′, 45 sec 1st trial, 43 in 2nd, 36 in 3rd with encouragement. Kneeling–1/2 kneeling on mat 2 sets 10 reps. Amb 60′ with 8 hyperextensions at knee: 1st time; 4, 2nd time; 8, 3rd time.
A: Tolerated treatment well, although fatigued. Improving.
P: Continue with plan.

Note #2: OP
S: Good spirits
O: Gait + advanced gait + balance techniques; required instruction, repetitive practice.
A: Demonstrating good gait and balance with some proprioceptive L/E deficit. Therefore, contact guard to stand-by assistance for safety at present at all times.
P: Continue as above

Note #3: OP
S: Patient stated that he "played golf over the weekend"
O: LUE: massage L shoulder, stim, stretching and strengthening; progressive

A: Improving
P: Modalities as indicated, massage, exercise

Write an appropriate entry for the following situations:

1. A patient did not show up for their scheduled physical therapy appointment and there is no record of cancellation.
2. A patient is transported to physical therapy by a transporter, but the patient refuses to do anything and is disrupting other patients in the gym.
3. A pediatric patient is accompanied to therapy by his grandmother, who is the legal guardian. She repeatedly corrects the therapist, interrupts the session, and is distracting the child.

Rewrite the following entries with appropriate elements and terminology:

a. Patient now able to don long pants with dressing stick with min to mod asst LLE; but unable to don L sock or shoe. With min asst able to don button shirt using RUE, 20° L neglect. Poor follow through.
b. Patient able to lean forward in unsupported sitting but unable to reach to floor without losing balance.
c. Can now rotate neck 25° and 10° to the left from midline with pain at end range.
d. Lunges with RLE forward; limited rear leg shaky, forward leg limited in flexion, can't maintain.
e. Able to extend and flex L knee with 5# weight 3 sets of 10 reps with assistance counting, resting as needed.
f. Gait in hallway, leans forward, bent at waist, short steps, CO SOB constantly, hemiwalker R, min asst with hemiwalker for 25′.
g. Spasm in low back decreasing; patient pain now 5/10 when sitting.
h. Active ROM increasing R hip in standing.
i. Taught husband how to transfer wife into bed.
j. Patient able to walk on even surface without directional changes × 1 rep, 50′, front wheeled rolling walker. Occasional verbal cues for attempts of step through pattern, flat footed.
k. Patient transfers have improved from max assist to mod assist; weakness persists in all extremities. Patient has difficulty sequencing components, preventing further progress at this time.
l. Now able to go up four 6-inch steps holding on to rails, with minimal assist, needs a lot of help to descend.
m. Patient goes from supine to side-lying using bedrail and mod asst. Mod asst to assume short sitting; minimal improvement.
n. IV L forearm, indwelling catheter, NG tube; ambulation training bedside chair to door of room and back, FWRW, shuffled, mod asst walker forward, constant instructions.
o. Child is able to roll R, using LUE and R head turning, no LE use; LE extensor tone.
p. Ambulation with posterior walker, bilateral AFOs, flexed in standing, drags legs forward laboriously, moderate asst for balance.
q. Exercise in prone to decrease extension and facilitate reaching.

DOCUMENTATION CONTENT EXERCISE

For the following intervention entries, based on documentation principles and codable CPT verbiage, determine the following and rewrite accordingly:

1. Is it written objectively with all appropriate objective information included?
2. Is the terminology correct for payment and billing?
3. Is the intervention billable or reproducible based on the information provided?
4. If there is enough information to reproduce the treatment, defend your decision.

5. If there is not enough information to reproduce the treatment, what other information is needed?
   a. Strengthening exercises to the LEs.
   b. Massage to neck
   c. Electrical stimulation to low back
   d. Joint mobilization lumbar region
   e. Gait
   f. Intermittent cervical traction in supine, head in neutral × 20 minutes, 25 pounds, 30-second hold, 15-second release
   g. Stretching to R heelcords
   h. Biofeedback for R UE
   i. US to L calf
   j. Back exercises
   k. Transfers
   l. Bed mobility
   m. PNF for bilateral upper extremities
   n. CORE training
   o. Teach to use wheelchair
   p. Show patient how to put on and take off prosthesis
   q. Teach patient how to look at feet when walking
   r. Control incontinence
   s. Bowel train to prevent incontinence
   t. Decrease post mastectomy swelling

GOAL WRITING EXERCISE

According to CMS Medicare Benefit Policy Manual (MBPM) Chapter 15, Section 20.2.1,[8] the Center for Medicare & Medicaid Services (CMS) requires the Medicare outpatient therapy POC include "long-term goals for the entire episode of care in the current setting. Goals should be measurable and pertain to identified functional impairments. Therapists typically also establish short term goals, such as goals for a week or month of therapy, to help track progress toward the goal for the episode of care. If the expected episode of care is short, for example therapy is expected to be completed in 4 to 6 treatment days, the long term and short term goals may be the same." Initial examination and evaluation should also include a prognosis for the therapy response and progress. When physical therapy is being delivered over a period of time or specified LOS, patient skills and function are being mastered over that time, and the interventions should be progressive and skilled.

As a patient makes progress toward the long-term goals, they are indeed achieving short-term goals in the process that can be specified by date or week. It is the PT's responsibility to determine, in coordination with the patient, caretakers, family, and others proximally involved, what goals are practical to achieve during the specified LOS. While impairment-based goals are important, it is ultimately how they contribute to function that makes them reimbursable and practical to the patient and demonstrates the value basis of the care provided.

Assuming a patient's goal is realistic relative to their diagnosis(es) and medical status and is not leisure focused if the patient is a Medicare beneficiary, including the patient's goals is motivating. However, it is the PT's responsibility to translate the goals into appropriate therapeutic verbiage and skills. LOS also has to be considered and included for determination of treatment over a designated time for each treatment venue over the continuum of care by the evaluating and treating PT. The LOS, however, may be dictated by external utilization review, preauthorization by a third-party payer, or predetermined policy visit limits. In the case of total limited physical therapy visits over the course of a year, sensitivity to the number of visits in an episode of care or LOS should be considered and discussed with the patient.

A common error in goal writing is confusing interventions with goals. This can result in denial of services. It is the PT's responsibility to ensure that goals are goals and not procedures or interventions.

- **Identify:**
  - Which of the following are goals (G) and which are interventions (I)
  - For items that are interventions, provide the CPT code identifier

1. Wheelchair (WC) management
2. Functional gait training
3. Propulsion of manual WC with verbal instructions
4. Soft tissue mobilization
5. Transfer training
6. Therapeutic exercise
7. Neuromuscular re-education
8. Manipulation of buttons for donning of shirt
9. Mobility training with power mobility device
10. Independent gait with standard walker, weight bearing as tolerated (WBAT)
11. Prosthetic instruction
12. Able to perform spontaneous unweighting

The ABCD Method of Goal Writing

All patient care goals should start with:

- Patient will be able to: or Patient will demonstrate: (The phrase can be stated once, followed by a colon, with all goals appearing after that.)
- Caretaker/family will be able to: or Caretaker/family will demonstrate:
- Child will be able to:
- Appropriately named or identified individual will be able to or will demonstrate:
- Patient will be able to provide verbal instruction to ____________to assist him or her in assisting patient transfers from ____ to ______

Using the ABCD method, please note the following:

A = Audience: patient, caretaker, husband, wife, daughter, son, sister, brother, etc.
B = Behavior: will be able to perform, do, achieve, negotiate, navigate, etc.
C = Condition: under what conditions the activity is to be performed
D = Degree: should include clarification of patient contribution to the activity and the skilled input from the PT/PTA described for each category. *The description of the skilled assistance or facilitation from the PT/PTA is key to justification of the intervention to be skilled. For each of the statements of assistance and dependence, write an example of what skilled level of assistance the % translates to.*

- **Total or 100% assistance/dependence**
  - Ex: Patient is unable to offer any assistance and requires total assistance to stabilize head, trunk, and extremities to transfer from the bed to reclining WC
- **Maximal or 75% assist/dependence** with clarification of patient contribution described and how the therapist facilitated the activity
- **Moderate or 50% assist/dependence** with clarification of patient contribution described
- **Minimal assist or 25% assist/dependence**
- **Contact guard or less than 25% assist** with occasional physical assistance to assist with occasional loss of balance or other
- **Supervision or standby** for safety without manual guarding, but may need verbal instruction or cues, independence: requires no assistance with any component of an activity

In the Functional Independence Measure (FIM)[10] developed in 1993, there is also a modified independent category which indicates an individual is independent but uses a device such as assistive gait device, dressing device, or other. In the FIM, this could also indicate that an activity takes more time than is average or expected. As of fiscal year 2020, in the inpatient rehabilitation facility (IRF) setting, the FIM is being discontinued and replaced by alternate functional measurement. The modified independence description, however, continues to be used.

For the D category, it is critical that the therapist indicate what component of an activity led him or her to the description provided and indicate the time frame (i.e., 2 weeks or specified date).

Example:
Daily treatment/encounter note that incorporates degree of assist verbiage:

CPT Code Verbiage: Therapeutic Activities: Transfer training: Patient required moderate assistance; 50% during stand pivot transfer training from wheelchair (WC) to mat table/bed in order to facilitate unweighting the patient's buttocks to partial standing, execute trunk/hips pivot and facilitation of controlled descent to sit. Patient was able to demonstrate head control and assist with brief stabilization in static stand prior to pivot.

For each of the following, using the ABCD method, identify the relevant component:

A, B, C, or D. Note that if there is a need to affect body function or impairment, the impairment must be clearly linked to function or focus on function.

Patient will be able to:

1. Stand with fixed front wheeled rolling walker with both feet flat, with minimal assist for foot positioning in order to obtain neutral dorsiflexion to facilitate functional standing for self-care

   A= B= C= D=

2. Achieve gait 50′ with front wheeled rolling walker, minimal assist for balance and walker placement with 90° directional change on even and uneven surfaces in order to get from bedroom safely to other rooms

   A= B= C= D=

3. Roll independently from supine to side-lying to initiate transfers and perform self-positioning to protect skin integrity and promote functional independence

   A= B= C= D=

4. Stand with posterior walker with feet flat, with minimal assist for foot positioning in order to obtain neutral dorsiflexion and facilitate functional standing in preparation for safe transfers and functional gait

   A= B= C= D=

5. Achieve gait 25′ with posterior walker, minimal assist for balance and walker placement without directional change in order to progress to functional gait at home or school

   A= B= C= D=

6. Roll independently from supine to prone to self-position in order to initiate creeping

   A= B= C= D=

7. Actively abduct the R shoulder 90°/180 without resistance to enable combing hair

   A= B= C= D=

8. Verbalize instructions to caretaker to assist with transition from sit to and from stand

   A= B= C= D=

9. Caretaker will be able to demonstrate car transfer with patient to and from WC into passenger seat in family sedan, using moderate assistance

   A= B= C= D=

10. Demonstrate gait with front wheeled rolling walker, large wheels, with heel/toe continuous pattern, erect posture with modified independence on grassy and pebble surface to safely get from car in driveway to front door 25′

    A = B= C= D=

11. Operate a sip and puff power chair on even surfaces with ability to turn R/L

    A = B= C= D=

Documentation and Clinical Reasoning Activity: ICF Model[4]

1. For each of the following sample medical diagnoses, complete the ICF Model chart, which will facilitate identification of the structural, functional, psychosocial, and environmental factors that will guide documentation of physical therapy goals, POC, intervention and overall patient management (indicate what the patient will need to do and achieve with physical therapy intervention).

APTA PT Evaluation Reference Table[11]

Activity limitations: Difficulties an individual may have in executing a task, action, or activities (e.g., inability to perform tasks due to abnormal vital sign response to increased movement or activity).

Body functions: The physiologic functions of body systems, including psychological functions.

Body regions: In reporting physical therapy evaluations, body regions are defined as head, neck, back, lower extremities, upper extremities, and trunk.

Body structures: The structural or anatomic parts of the body, such as organs, limbs, and their components, classified according to body systems.

Body systems: In reporting physical therapy evaluations, the systems review includes the following:

- For the cardiovascular/pulmonary system: the assessment of oxygen saturation (O_2), body temperature, heart rate heart rate, respiratory rate, blood pressure, and edema
- For the integumentary system: the assessment of pliability (texture), presence of scar formation, skin color, and skin integrity
- For the musculoskeletal system: the assessment of gross symmetry, gross ROM, gross strength, height, and weight
- For the neuromuscular system: a general assessment of gross coordinated movement (e.g., balance, gait, locomotion, transfers, and transitions) and motor function (motor control and motor learning)
- For communication ability: affect, cognition, language, processing, ability to follow simple versus complex commands/instruction and learning style: the assessment of the ability to make needs known, consciousness, orientation (person, place, and time), expected emotional/behavioral responses, and learning preferences (e.g., learning barriers, education needs)

Participation restrictions:

Problems an individual may experience in involvement in life situations (e.g., inability to engage in community social events due to exhaustion)

Personal factors:

Factors include sex, age, coping styles, social background, education, profession, past and current experience, overall behavior pattern, character, and other factors that influence how disability is experienced by the individual. Personal factors could exist but may or may not.

2. Once you have categorized the patient status, write one long-term goal for each identified category for the common diagnoses provided based on your knowledge of the pathology.

HEALTH CONDITION, DISEASE, OR DISORDER			
Body functions and structure	**Activities and activity limitations**	**Participation restrictions**	**Environmental factors that may facilitate recovery or present barriers**
Physiology	**Difficulty executing activities**	**Problems in life situations**	**Physical, social and attitudinal environment**
Goal 1:			
Goal 2:			
Goal 3:			
Goal 4:			

HEALTH CONDITION, DISEASE, OR DISORDER

UPPER QUARTER

- AC separation
- Amputation; above elbow, below elbow: dominant, nondominant
- Biceps tear
- Biceps tendinitis
- Brachial plexus injury
- Carpal tunnel syndrome
- Chronically subluxing shoulder
- Complex regional pain syndrome wrist; dominant hand
- Lateral epicondylitis
- Medial epicondylitis
- Pectoralis major tear; surgical repair
- Pectoralis major strain
- Post clavicular fracture; 8 weeks
- Post humeral fracture without surgical intervention
- Post olecranon fracture
- Post shoulder dislocation
- Post wrist fracture, external fixator removed
- Post wrist fracture; cast removed, no surgical intervention
- Status post biceps tendon repair
- Status post rotator cuff repair
- Status post rotator cuff tear without surgical repair
- Scaphoid fracture
- Shoulder bursitis
- Shoulder impingement syndrome
- Ulnar collateral ligament tear

LOWER QUARTER

- Achilles tendon rupture with surgical repair
- Achilles tendon tendonitis
- ACL rupture with surgical repair
- ACL rupture without surgical repair
- ACL tear
- Amputation: toe, foot, transtibial, transfemoral
- Ankle fracture s/p triple ankle arthrodesis
- Anterior approach
- Chondromalacia
- Compartment syndrome; lower leg surgical release
- Complex regional pain syndrome; ankle
- Greater trochanteric bursitis
- Hamstring rupture
- Hip fracture; ORIF, NWB
- Hip fracture; ORIF, PWB
- Iliopsoas syndrome
- Labral tear repair
- Meniscus tear
- Osteoarthritis of the knee
- Patella repair post fracture
- plantar fasciitis
- Post femoral shaft fracture with rod stabilization
- Posterolateral approach
- Status post bunion repair
- Status post triple ankle arthrodesis
- Total hip arthroplasty/replacement
- Total knee replacement: total, partial

TRUNK/SPINE

- Cervical
- Facet syndrome
- Lumbar
- Lumbar root syndrome
- Lumbar sprain
- Pelvic fracture
- Piriformis syndrome
- Scheuerman kyphosis
- Scoliosis
- SI joint misalignment
- Spinal stabilization; surgical
- Spinal stenosis: cervical, lumbar
- Spondylolisthesis
- Thoracic
- Torticollis
- Vertebral compression fracture
- Vertebral malalignment
- Whiplash

HEAD	UROGENITAL WOMEN'S HEALTH	NEUROMUSCULAR
Cephalgia/headaches	Anal sphincter incompetence	Amyotrophic lateral sclerosis
Facial nerve paralysis	Lymphedema: UE, LE	Cerebellar stroke
Labyrinthitis	Pelvic floor dysfunction	Cerebral palsy: consider varying levels of involvement
Post mandibular fracture	Post mastectomy	Cerebrovascular accident
Temporomandibular joint dysfunction	Urinary incontinence	Chronic fatigue syndrome
Vestibular neuritis	Vulvodynia	Developmental delay
		Duchenne muscular dystrophy, spinal muscular atrophy
		Dystonia
		Hemiplegia: R/L with varying limb involvement and communication disorders
		Low muscle tone
		Multiple sclerosis: progressive, remitting
		Muscular dystrophy; Duchenne
		Paraplegia
		Parkinson
		Quadriplegia
		Spinal cord injury; incomplete/complete:
		TBI: bilateral contusions, temporal lobe

ARTHRITIS/AUTOIMMUNE DISORDERS	SYSTEMS
Rheumatoid arthritis	Post myocardial infarct
Systemic lupus erythematosus	CABG; multiple
Scleroderma	Post organ transplant: kidney, lung, heart
Ankylosing spondylitis	LVAD placement
Multiple sclerosis; remitting and relapsing	COPD
	Cystic fibrosis

Rewrite Exercises

For each of the following, rewrite into objective and measurable goals.

Example:

Decrease swelling/edema:

In 2 weeks, L foot edema will be reduced from +4″ compared to R ankle/foot (size of R would be included) to +.5 – 1″ to enable patient to:

- wear required work shoes for safety on the job
- wear custom molded diabetic shoes to prevent skin breakdown
- wear foot wear to protect skin from objects on floor due to loss of protective sensation
- wear socks without undue compression causing circulatory compromise
- insert AFO into shoe to prevent foot drop during gait and falls secondary to same
- facilitate full weight bearing with normalized energy efficient gait pattern; initial contact with heel and effective toe off to prevent loss of balance

Rewrite Exercises: Gait, Bed, and Mobility

For each of the examples provided above, determine if the goal is complete (objective, measurable, and time defined) or needs revision.

INCREASE STRENGTH OF L ROTATOR CUFF	PATIENT WILL DEMONSTRATE INCREASED ROTATOR CUFF STRENGTH (R/L) FROM 3/5 TO 4/5 WITHOUT SUBSTITUTION	IN ORDER TO REACH BEHIND HER HEAD AND...	IN ______ DAYS/WEEKS
Decrease ankle swelling			
Bend over in standing			
Improve balance			
Prevent contracture			
Decrease contracture			
Improve transfers			
Increase knee strength			
Increase ankle ROM			
Propel wheelchair			
Independently ambulate			
Stabilize gait			
Will avoid objects			
Increase UE coordination			
Decrease spasm			
Stand on 1 leg			
Teach home program			
Maximize function			
Not fall			
Better head control			
Increase core strength			

With regard to gait, goals are multidimensional. Gait is used as an example, as it is a common intervention and includes multiple elements, all of which require inclusion.

All elements of gait are important, including a pattern as normal as possible based on patient presentation. Objective tests and measures, such as gait speed, the Six-Minute Walk Test, Functional Gait Assessment, Four Step, and 10-Meter Walk Test, and related measures such as the Dynamic Gait Index (DGI), Functional Gait Assessment (FGA), and others, including observational gait, should be used. The initial examination and results can then be readministered periodically or at discharge as objective measurement of progress. However, inclusion of only numeric results without explanation, such as the total numeric score or a measured outcome, will be problematic if not described. The element of a standardized measure that is a deviation from the norm should be integrated into the goals.

The following elements of gait should be included in the examination, progress over time, and response to treatment and goals:

- Gait pattern; observational
- Gait cycle
  - Stance and swing phases
    - Initial double stance, single limb, terminal stance
- Assistive device use or need
  - If a device is already being used, the height and type may need change ultimately, but the initial examination should be completed with the device currently being used
  - Specificity is needed with device description
    - Example:
      - Front wheeled rolling walker (FWRW) with large caster wheels and rear skis
      - Large based quad cane
      - Axillary crutches with rubber tips and ice pick tips (for winter)
      - Bilateral forearm crutches for forearm support
- Gait speed and quality of gait relative to functional gait speed step and stride length
  - Abnormally slow speed may prevent safe activities such as crossing a street or getting to the toilet in adequate time to prevent incontinence
  - Rapid speed without ability to moderate may indicate a balance problem
- Width; base of support (BOS)
  - A narrow base or wide base may indicate balance dysfunction
- Coordination
- Balance
- Ability to dual-task such as walk and talk; walk and be attentive to the environment; safely navigate obstacles, limited space, and other people; and carry items
- Adjust rapidly to a changing environment, stability on multiple surfaces (specified) indoor (smooth tile, irregular tile, low-pile carpet, high-pile carpet, other) and outdoor (i.e., dirt, grass, cement, sand, pavers/uneven brick or stones)
- Managing with or without an assistive device
- Directional changes: forward, backward, lateral/side stepping, turning R/L, 180°, 360°, other at normal pace, and rapid
- Postural control
- Visual compensation as indicated for sensory impairment, scanning of environment for safe movement if there is visual impairment strategies to negotiate with safe mobility
- Gait in environments of low light or with low vision
  - Compensatory strategies being used or vision deficits, sensory deficits that may require compensatory gait training strategies
- Vision screening
- Stability correction in response to sudden events during gait, such as crowd avoidance or navigation through a crowded environment, hanging branches, unexpected surface changes, and others

- Gait pattern: normal as possible
- Transition from one surface to another or surfaces at different heights
- Endurance, respiratory pattern/rate
- Coordination
- Muscle performance
- Need for orthoses or prosthesis or use of
- Vital sign stability or fluctuation
- Capillary glucose response in individuals with diabetes
- Distance

All of these factors and more should be included in gait-related goals.

Verbal instruction and tactile/manual facilitation and correction with stabilization are evidence of skilled gait training. Need for monitoring vital signs or using the Borg Rate of Perceived Exertion are also indicative of skill.

As an example of necessary gait speed, a few seconds could make the difference between incontinence and adequate time to make it to the toilet or to cross a street. In order to be accurate and appropriate in determining gait speed goals, determining outcomes are recommended at initial evaluation, assessment intervals, and discharge. Middleton et al[12] collated data from multiple sources to determine the range of walking or gait speed in meters/second (m/s). According to their study, 0.4 m/s and below indicates severe walking disability for household and hospital ambulation. Middleton et al[5] also found gait speeds of 0.4 to 0.8 m/s indicates limited community ambulation, 0.8 to 1.2 m/s community ambulation, 1.0 to 1.4 m/s indicates ability to carry light packages/groceries and perform light yard work, and 1.3 to 1.6 m/s ability to safely cross the street.

Example: Patient will be able to or demonstrate ______ gait speed with ___________ level of function/assistance in ______weeks or by date: (name device or indicate without an assistive device) in order to ______________________________

Determine if the goals stated here meet the criteria of a well-written goal. Indicate why or why not and rewrite as indicated.

1. Patient will demonstrate independent (or modified independent gait if using this term because of a walker or other assistive device) continuous gait with large front wheeled caster walker, posterior rubber tips, with directional changes: R/L turns; 90°, 180°, and 360° on even and uneven surfaces; flat tile, carpet, cement, grass, dirt in order to navigate all surfaces in his home and outside of home in community without hesitation, effectively navigating obstacles.
2. Patient will demonstrate supervised step to gait with fixed front wheel walker, PWB LLE on even surface with R/L 90° turns, and backwards stepping
3. Modified independent gait with straight cane R hand, for safe gait on tile and carpet indoors and cement and grass outside in order to safely navigate inside her home and through the parking lot of her condo development to safely get to a car
4. Modified independent gait with standard forearm crutches NWB LLE on indoor and outdoor surfaces
5. Patient will demonstrate modified (or) independent gait with forearm crutches NWB LLE up and down a flight of 12 stairs, with 6" to 10" rise, a ramp, and all curbs
6. Sustain NWB as required on LLE with standard walker in static standing for 2 minutes to prepare for functional NWB gait
7. Independent gait with single axillary crutch on all indoor and outdoor surfaces with ability to right self with intermittent balance loss to R or L in order to prevent falls
8. Using the straight cane for support, get up from floor independently in the event of a fall
9. With or without device, or using handrails R/L, independently navigate flight(s) of ___ stairs up and down, in order to get in out of her home on ____floor, or into basement of house to do her laundry

Bed mobility

1. Independently transition from supine to long sit in bed
2. Independently transition from long sit to short sit over side of bed
3. Independently transition from supine, to side lying to short sit over side of bed, without using bedrails
4. Independently transition from short sit to supine and self-position in bed
5. Demonstrate abdominal strength of at least 3/5 to lift head and shoulders off bed and stabilize on elbows to be able to reposition upper body in bed
6. Independently roll from supine to R side-lying, L side-lying, to relieve pressure on bony prominences, to reposition self, reach to bedside table/end tables for objects
7. Independently bridge to unweight and reposition buttocks for pressure relief, bedpan use, assist caretaker with position changes to facilitate dressing
8. Transition from supine to prone and assume elbow propping in preparation for quadruped
9. Transition from supine to prone and quadruped to facilitate the developmental sequence for rocking and progressing to creeping, or to facilitate shoulder girdle development for stabilization in upright
10. Independently transition from supine on floor, to quadruped, to chair or from supine to floor sit to WC

LE prosthetic independence

1. Improve balance backwards and forward, to prevent loss of balance and falls in all directions, with ability to self-correct.
2. Demonstrate ability to reach to floor in sitting to independently put on LE prosthesis, socks, stockings, slacks, shorts, shoes without loss of balance.
3. Demonstrate independent side stepping or lateral stepping in order to navigate at counters in the bathroom for personal hygiene, kitchen for cooking and meal preparation.
4. Demonstrate 180- and 360-degree turns L/R with/without a named device in small spaces, to safely navigate into position to demonstrate self-care, gait, shower adjustments, procuring clothing from walk in closet or any small spaces.
5. Demonstrate safe, independent gait without veering R or L and be able to dual-task by talking, to prevent loss of balance and falls by focusing on distant visual point.
6. Be able to remain upright during gait (with or without a device) when navigating through a crowd, around obstacles, if pushed unexpectedly from any direction.
7. Demonstrate safe step-ups 4", 6", and 8" in order to navigate curbs in community of varying heights without use of assistive device.

Independent Activities of Daily Living (ADLs)

1. Actively elevate both UEs to 100° of flexion bilaterally and externally rotate shoulders to 70° in order to wash and dry hair independently.
2. Actively flex her R elbow 125° with upper arm against her trunk in order to be able to brush her teeth independently, bring food to her mouth to eat.
3. Forward trunk flexion in unsupported sitting over side of bed to don and doff socks and shoes.

Exercise: Goal writing based on brief history and medical record entry

A 67-year-old slightly obese female admitted to hospital with acute pneumonia/SOB, history of HTN, and type 2 diabetes controlled with diet and oral medication. She is on 2L of supplemental O_2 since admission. Prior level of function (PLOF): Independent without assistive device, independent in all self-care and ADLs. Psychosocial: Lives with husband on second floor of condo building; although there is an elevator it is frequently out of service. Babysits part-time to supplement her Social Security, does cooking for self and husband and drives.

Based on the following entry, write a series of goals that will progress this patient over the course of 7 days in acute care with IV to antibiotics in R forearm, followed by 3 weeks in a

skilled nursing for short-term rehabilitation and then home with spouse and home health for the following functional activities.

1. Endurance
2. Bed mobility and transitional movement in bed
3. Transfers in and out of bed
4. Transitioning to and from sit
5. Gait/walking
6. Wheelchair mobility

HOSPITAL GOALS: TOTAL LOS 8 DAYS, PATIENT IS EVALUATED ON DAY 3 AFTER BEING IN BED, PAYMENT DRG MEDICARE A

SKILLED NURSING FACILITY (SNF) GOALS: 2 WEEKS TOTAL, PART A MEDICARE PATIENT-DRIVEN PAYMENT MODEL (PDPM)

MEDICARE HOME HEALTH PART A GOALS: 30 DAYS TOTAL, PDPM MEDICARE (30-DAY INTERVALS OF CARE)

Commonly used American Medical Association (AMA) CPT[6] codes for physical therapy (not a complete list, and with the exception of physical therapy evaluation, not exclusive to physical therapy)

Note:

1. Consider the intent of the activity to determine the correct coding when more than one may apply
2. Description of intervention/treatment should always be preceded CPT verbiage
3. Patient education for any intervention is included in the CPT code treatment and time for completion/training

Author's Note

Under the Health Insurance Portability and Accountability Act (HIPAA), the Department of Health and Human Services (DHHS) adopted specific code sets for diagnoses and procedures used in all transactions.

About Code Sets
Code sets classify medical:

- *Diagnoses*
- *Procedures*
- *Diagnostic tests*
- *Treatments*
- *Equipment and supplies*

They inform diverse healthcare functions, from billing to tracking public health.

HIPAA Code Sets
Code sets outlined in HIPAA regulations include:
ICD-10 International Classification of Diseases, 10th edition[5]
Health Care Common Procedure Coding System (HCPCS)
CPT Current Procedure Terminology[6]
CDT Code on Dental Procedures and Nomenclature
NDC National Drug Codes

As stated on the CMS website:[13]

The Healthcare Common procedure Coding System (HCPCS) is divided into two principal subsystems, referred to as level I and level II of the HCPCS. Level I of the HCPCS is comprised of Current Procedural Terminology (CPT), a numeric coding system maintained by the American Medical Association (AMA). The CPT is a uniform coding system consisting of descriptive terms and identifying codes that are used primarily to identify medical services and procedures furnished by physicians and other health care professionals. These health care professionals use the CPT to identify services and procedures for which they bill public or private health insurance programs. Level I of the HCPCS, the CPT codes, does not include codes needed to separately report medical items or services that are regularly billed by suppliers other than physicians.

Level II of the HCPCS is a standardized coding system that is used primarily to identify products, supplies, and services not included in the CPT codes, such as ambulance services and durable medical equipment, prosthetics, orthotics, and supplies (DMEPOS) when used outside a physician's office. Because Medicare and other insurers cover a variety of services, supplies, and equipment that are not identified by CPT codes, the level II HCPCS codes were established for submitting claims for these items (https://www.cms.gov/Medicare/Coding/MedHCPCSGenInfo/HCPCS_Coding_Questions)

CODE	VERBIAGE	DESCRIPTION
97001	Physical therapy evaluation (replaced by AMA CPT effective 1/1/2017) May be used for worker's compensation and auto insurance Physical therapy evaluation—based on complexity	Initial evaluation; untimed: see new codes for Medicare and commercial payers
97161	Low complexity	No personal factors (20 mins/average)
97162	Moderate complexity	1 to 2 personal factors (30 mins/average
97163	High complexity	3 or more personal and/or comorbidities (45 min/average)
97164	Physical therapy re-evaluation (replaced by AMA CPT effective 1/1/2017) revised	Subsequent re-evaluation
97110	Therapeutic exercise	Strengthening, AROM, PROM, stretching, endurance
97112	Neuromuscular re-education	Balance, coordination, proprioception, stabilization, inhibition, motor control, desensitization
97113	Aquatic therapy	Treatment and exercises that are performed in water
97116	Gait training	All elements
97140	Manual therapy	Soft tissue mobilization, joint mobilization, scar mobilization, manual traction, manual lymphatic drainage
97124	Massage therapy	Therapeutic massage
97150	Group therapy	Two or more patients treated simultaneously
97530	Therapeutic activity	Dynamic activity training: transfer training, transitional movement training, activities that are functionally oriented
97535	Self-care/home management training	ADLs: eating, dressing, hygiene, toileting, transferring, continence training; bowel and bladder training, teaching of wound care, TENS use, self-administered MLD, taping
97542	Wheelchair management	Fitting, assessment, mobility training
97760	Orthotic(s) management and training (including assessment and fitting when not otherwise reported), upper extremity(ies), lower extremity(ies) and/or trunk, initial orthotic(s) encounter, each 15 minutes	Intended to be reported only for initial encounter with patient
97761	Prosthetic training, upper and/or lower extremities, initial prosthetic encounter, each 15 minutes	Intended to be reported only for initial encounter with patient
97763	Orthotic(s)/prosthetic(s) management and/or training, upper extremity(ies), lower extremity(ies), and/or trunk, subsequent orthotic(s)/prosthetic(s) encounter, each 15 minutes	Subsequent encounter

90912	Biofeedback training, initial 15 minutes of 1 on 1 contact	Behavioral training using feedback
90913	Biofeedback training, each additional 15 minutes of 1-1 contact	
97750	Physical performance test or measurement	Functional capacity evaluations, sports specific, video analysis, exertional, functional testing, isokinetic testing
97305	Ultrasound	Deep heating provided by sound waves
20560	Needle insertion(s) without injection(s), 1 or 2 muscle(s)	Dry needling
20561	Needle insertion(s) without injection(s), 3 or more muscle(s)	Dry needling

Author's Note

Regarding CPT codes 20560 and 20561, CMS initially assigned 20560 and 20561 the status of "non-covered" services under Medicare, meaning they weren't eligible for payment when furnished by any provider. Subsequently, CMS changed the status of these codes to "active" but only in the context of the above NCD, meaning only the assigned providers could be paid for the service. CMS confirmed this in communications with APTA. Medicare Administrative Contractors cannot choose to cover dry needling services that don't conform with the guidance outlined in the acupuncture NCD. However, because these continue to be non-covered services when performed by a PT, PTs may bill a Medicare beneficiary directly for the services.[14] Because Medicare does not cover dry needling codes, CMS has not designated them as either "sometimes therapy" or "always therapy." "Always therapy" services must be furnished under the POC of a PT, occupational therapist (OT), or speech-language pathologist (SLP), regardless of who provides them. The codes always are accompanied by the appropriate GP (for PTs), GO (for OTs), or GN (for SLPs) modifier.

Author's Note

Based on the intent of an intervention, there may be more than one applicable code. The documentation should reflect the intent so that the best code can be selected.

Sample entry:

Day 4 acute care: In daily treatment/encounter note:

Therapeutic Activities: Transfer training: Patient required moderate assistance, 75% from wheelchair to mat table to facilitate manual unweighting/transition of buttocks to partial standing during stand pivot transfer, pivot and facilitate controlled descent to sit. Patient was able to demonstrate head control and assist with static stand prior to pivot with minimal weight shift ability. SOB on exertion; instructed in Rate of Perceived Exertion Scale (RPE)

Provide the CPT code,[6] CPT verbiage, and ICD-10 codes[5] in the content as indicated

For each of the following, indicate the ICD-10 code for the medical diagnosis; the expected treatment or physical therapy diagnostic codes; CPT codes for Medicare, commercial insurance, and workers' compensation; and correct verbiage for evaluation and POC elements

1. Total Hip Arthroplasty Posterior Approach: Evaluation
2. Total Hip Arthroplasty Anterior Approach: Evaluation
3. Total Hip Arthroplasty: Transfer training
4. Total Knee Arthroplasty: Strengthening, PROM
5. Total Knee Arthroplasty: Scar mobilization
6. Ankle Sprain, Grade III: Evaluation
7. Spinal Fusion, Diabetes Type 2, HTN: Evaluation
8. Acute Exacerbation of OA of the R Knee:
   a. Ultrasound
   b. Soft tissue mobilization
   c. Exercise
   d. Walking
9. Re-evaluation
10. Proprioceptive Loss Both Feet: Visual Compensation with Ambulation

Description of the following documentation elements

For each of the following, identify the content elements that are required, regardless of the payer.

1. Initial evaluation
2. Plan of care
3. Treatment/encounter daily note
4. Progress note
5. Progress report
6. Re-evaluation
7. Discharge summary

Flow Sheet Exercise

Identify the elements that are missing to justify the care included in the flow sheet and the errors over 2 weeks in outpatient (OP) physical therapy.

ACTIVITY	DATE 6/10/20	DATE 6/12/20	DATE 6/14/20	DATE 6/17/20	DATE 6/19/20	DATE 6/21/20	SKILLED COMPONENTS OF INTERVENTION:
Long arc quads	10 reps						
SLR	10 reps						
Bridging	10 reps						
Ankle pumps	20 reps						
Sit to from stand	10 reps CGA min A						
Stand pivot WC to from bed	5 reps CGA min A						
Nustep, no resistance	15 mins						

Exercises Activity:

1. Correct errors in the document; rewrite to comply with skilled documentation.
2. Rewrite the goals, justifying the skilled physical therapy needed and to reflect the ICF model for a 4-week course of physical therapy.
3. Rewrite the POC into reimbursable terminology that is CPT compatible.
4. Describe the justification for each intervention.
5. Write a practical home exercise plan (HEP) that progresses a patient over 4 weeks.
6. Intervention is expected to be initiated on the same visit. Write an encounter note that is consistent with brief, but appropriate, intervention using all relevant principles.

Documentation Initial Evaluation # 1: Colin Brooks

PT Evaluation

Name: Colin Brooks **Date:** 02/24/2020

DOB: 06/30/50

Time: 10:00 am

Case# 123456

Referring Physician: Dr. Jones

ICD-10

Diagnosis: Medical: Z96.641: R Total hip replacement posterior approach

PT treatment diagnosis R26 .2 (Difficulty in Walking), M62.81 (muscle weakness)

Subjective:

Patient is a 70-year-old male referred by Dr. Jones s/p 02/20/2020 R THA, posterior lateral approach, secondary to osteoarthritis. Home Health evaluation and treat 3 × week for 4 weeks by Dr. Jones. Per Dr. Jones patient needs to follow hip precautions and is WBAT R LE. Mr. Brooks reports that R hip pain level on a 0 to 10 scale is 5/10 at rest, 7/10 WB, and when ambulating 7/10. Patient reports that he is taking prescription Hydrocodone for pain as needed, but will switch to acetaminophen after 1 week. Patient's chief complaints are that he is dependent on walker for ambulation, unable to enjoy or participate in leisure activities, unable to drive, and unable to play with grandchildren. He is married, and lives in a single story home with threshold step. Per patient, he is independently using the bathroom with an elevated commode seat and receives assistance from spouse when showering and for donning on and off clothes. He states that he is retired, drives a car with an automatic transmission. Patient reports his leisure activities include cycling, gardening, and spending time with grandchildren. Patient goals are to become independent in ambulation without a device and driving, pain free.

Objective:

Barriers to learning: None

Cognition: Alert, orientated to time, orientated to place, accurate historian, and appropriate communication

PMH: OA of both hips

Medications: atenolol, indapamide

Vitals at rest: BP: 128/80 P: 80 RR: 14

Vitals post eval: BP: 131/81 P: 83 RR: 17

Height 5′11″

Weight 205 lb

Capillary refill test: normal, toes

Integument/Sensation: intact for right and left lower extremity

Girth measurement: (4 inches above apex of patella)	Right knee 21 inches Left knee 18 inches

Wound Observation: incision is healing without any signs of infection area around surgical area, ecchymosis noted in the periwound area

ROM: LLE no deficits noted

ROM: goniometer:

Hip abduction 33° passive 30° active
Hip external rotation 0° degrees post surgical limitation
Knee flexion 119° passive 125° active

Muscle performance: Because of precautions, RLE: no muscle performance testing of R hip flexion, IR or adduction. Active initiation of movements observed

RLE:
Hip abduction 2/5 (supine)
Hip extension 3/5 (side-lying tested)
Hip external rotation able to tolerate moderate resistance
Knee flexion 4+/5
Knee extension 4/5
Ankle dorsiflexion 5/5
Ankle plantar flexion 5/5
LLE:
Hip abduction 5/5
Hip flexion 5/5
Hip extension 5/5
Hip external rotation 5/5
Knee flexion 5/5
Knee extension 5/5
Ankle dorsiflexion 5/5
Ankle plantar flexion 5/5

Pain: R hip: at rest 5/10, with WB 7/10, when ambulating 7/10
DTRs: Normal
Timed Up and Go test (TUG): 30 seconds w/ AD, normal values (7.1 to 9.0) ages 60 to 69
Harris hip score: 53 (poor)
Ambulation: 300ft without directional changes even surface
Precautions: standard precautions; patient able to articulate
Assessment:

Patient has weak and decreased ROM in hip abduction. He is dependent on front wheeled rolling walker for ambulation on even surfaces in an abnormal step-through pattern with uneven step length and decreased WB on RLE. During ambulation pt. became fatigued after activity for 5 minutes and had pain of 7/10 on a scale of 0 to 10. He required verbal cues to take breaks after 5 minutes for 1 minute at a time. Surgical incision is normal with slight bruising and swelling. Bed mobility: rolling L/R: I, but cautious, with consistent application of hip precautions; transitional movement supine/side-lying to short sit is I, slow. Stable in unsupported short sit once up.

He is unable to dress and bathe independently. His home has all required modifications to assist with ADLs. Pt would benefit from ADL education using AD in donning clothes and self-care from OT. Pt would benefit from more strength and functional mobility training to progress toward his goals to be I.

STG: 2 Weeks

- Pt. will begin to ambulate 600 ft
- Pt. will decrease pain, resting to 3/10, ambulation to 5/10, and WB 5/10
- Pt. will reduce TUG test time by 10 seconds
- Pt. will increase Harris hip score by 15 points
- Pt. will increase hip abduction to 4/5
- Pt. will work towards I in ADLs of bathing and ambulating

LTG: 4 Weeks

- Pt. will be able to ambulate community distances using AD (cane)
- Pt. will be independent with HEP
- Pt. will decrease pain, resting to 0/10, ambulation 3/10, and WB 0/10

- Pt. will improve TUG test by 10s
- Pt. will increase Harris hip score by 15 points
- Pt. will increase hip abduction strength and ROM
- Pt. will gain I in ADLs of bathing, ambulating, and driving

Plan:

Initiate therapy home PT ×3/week for therapeutic exercise: strength, endurance, and gait training, therapeutic activities: functional mobility training. Cold pack following exercises for pain control. Plan to add resistance exercise by end of week 2.

- Ankle pumps to improve ambulation
- Short arc quads to increase leg strength
- Long arc quads to increase leg strength
- Bilateral sitting hip abduction to increase strength
- Prone hip extension exercises
- Standing walker hip abduction to increase strength
- Mini squats with walker to increase strength and endurance
- Gait training to increase strength, endurance and functional mobility
- Step training (1 step) to increase functional mobility

11:15 am
Michael Smith, PT 12345

Instructions: For the following initial examination and evaluation, complete the following

Documentation Activity:

1. Correct errors in the document; rewrite to comply with skilled documentation.
2. Rewrite the goals, justifying the need for skilled physical therapy and to reflect the ICF model for a 4-week course of physical therapy.
3. Rewrite the POC into reimbursable terminology that is CPT compatible.
4. Describe the justification for each intervention.
5. Write a practical HEP that progresses patient over 4 weeks.
6. Intervention is expected to be initiated on the same visit. Write an encounter note that is consistent with brief, but appropriate, intervention using all relevant principles.

Documentation Note 2: John Smith
PT Examination and Evaluation: SOAP format
Name: John Smith
DOB: 1/20/1953
#243230
ICD-10 Z96.649
Diagnosis: 81.51
Referring Physician: Dr. James Waler
Physical Therapist: John Doe
Visit 1 of 18
Date: March 27, 2020
Time: 8:03 AM
S:

The patient is a 65-year-old male who underwent an R THA from Dr. Waler using the posterior lateral cemented approach on 2/20/20 secondary to osteoarthritis. There were no complications during surgery and inpatient and home health rehab progressed as planned. He was discharged from home health on 3/24/20. He is currently WBAT and able to ambulate using a cane throughout the house with minimal fear of falling. He is confident in all ADLs except he feels some pain and difficulty when climbing the 7 stairs to his front door and the 6 stairs to the altar. He reports that he feels as if his R LE is weaker than the other one and he is unable to stand on it for more than an hour without resting. He also reports pain while standing for long periods of time as a 6/10. The patient is a priest who previously led Mass 5 days a week, but is currently only able to perform Mass 2 days a week because of pain and weakness. He hopes to return to full time with no pain. The patient is currently taking Advil for pain and 20 mg daily of lisinopril to control moderate hypertension. He has a medical history of hypertension and R hip osteoarthritis. He also enjoys golfing when he can and volunteering at the soup kitchen, which he has been unable to do. He drives a car with automatic transmission.

O:

Cognition

Intact, appropriate communication, accurate historian

Vitals: At Rest and Following Evaluation

BP 130/84 132/82

HR 74 bpm 78 bpm

RR 17 18

Pain

At rest 2/10

WB 3/10

WB over an hour 6/10

Posture/Gait Observation

Patient walks with a cane with decreased WB on RLE

Slight forward head posture

Wound Observation

Sutures removed and scar is closing with no indication of infection

Blue and yellow bruising on posterior gluteal and thigh regions

ROM

UEs
- No deficits noted

LLE
- No deficits noted

R Hip
- Fl not measured
- Ext 0 to 3° AROM, 0 to 7° PROM
- Abduction 0 to 25° AROM, 0 to 30° PROM
- Adduction not measured
- IR not measured
- ER 0 to 20° AROM, 0 to 23° PROM

R Knee
- Fl 105° AROM, 110° PROM
- Ext 0°

R Ankle
- Dorsiflexion 5° AROM, 10° PROM
- Plantarflexion 40° AROM, 40° PROM

Leg Length

R 100 cm

L 99.5 cm

Strength MMT

UEs:
- Gross strength 5/5

L Hip
- Flexion 4/5 (not past 90°)
- Extension 5/5
- Abduction 4/5
- Adduction 5/5 (not past midline)
- IR 5/5 (not past neutral)

- ER 4/5

R Hip
- Flex 3/5 (not past 90°)
- Ext 3/5
- Abduction 3/5
- Adduction 4/5 (not past midline)
- IR 3/5 (not past neutral)
- ER 3/5

L Knee
- Flex 5/5
- Ext 5/5

R Knee
- Flex 4/5
- Ext 4/5

Left Ankle
- Dorsiflexion 5/5
- Plantarflexion 5/5

Right Ankle
- Dorsiflexion 5/5
- Plantarflexion 4/5

Sensation Bilateral UE and LE

Light touch	Only impaired in the area of the incision
Sharp touch	Only impaired in the area of the incision
2 point discrimination	Only impaired in the area of the incision

Reflexes Bilateral

Patellar	2+
Achilles	2+

Circulation Bilateral

Femoral, popliteal, dorsal pedal, and posterior tibial pulses intact
Capillary refill in <1 second

Mobility

Drove himself to therapy
Able to sit to supine, sit to stand I, and stand pivot with and without cane
FWB on R LE
Able to negotiate stairs with cane and rail with minimal/moderate difficulty and pain

ADLs

Patient has an elevated toilet seat and utilizes a shower seat but is independent
He dresses while seated and uses a sock aid

Balance

Stable with cane
Without cane: Has balance loss with single leg stance on R LE

Education

Patient was able to recite the hip precautions with confidence

- No internal rotation past neutral, no adduction past neutral, and no hip flexion or trunk flexion past 90°

A:

Problem Summary:

The patient is progressing from surgery and has an excellent prognosis.

- Weakness in RLE, ROM deficits in RLE, balance deficit without an assistive device secondary to weakness, pain in RLE, dependent on the use of a cane.
- Difficulty with negotiating stairs to get into his house and on the altar.
- Increase in pain when weight bearing has led to a decrease in the amount of Masses he is able to perform and a decrease in his volunteer work. He has also been unable to golf.

Goals:

STGs: 4/11/20

- Patient will be able to ambulate 250 feet on even and carpeted surfaces without the use of a cane
- MMT RLE—Hip flexion 3+/5, Hip extension 4/5, Hip abduction 4/5, Hip IR 3+/5, Hip ER 3+/5
- ROM hip extension 0 to 10°AROM and 0 to 15° PROM
- Decrease pain to a 1/10 with WB and 0/10 NWB.

LTGs: 5/11/20

- Patient will be able to ambulate safely and confidently without the use of a cane
- Patient with regain strength and ROM in order to walk with a normal gait pattern
- Patient will have no pain in the R hip with weight bearing
- Patient will be able to return to performing Mass 5 days a week and volunteering as tolerated. The cane should be used if the patient begins experiencing fatigue.

P:

The patient will go to outpatient physical therapy 2 × week for 6 weeks to consist of gait training without an assistive device and progressive ther ex to help strengthen the muscles affected by the surgery. Balance exercises will be implemented as well, such as single leg standing and walking on uneven surfaces. Pain and swelling will be controlled with cryotherapy. Massage will be implemented over the area of the incision.

8:58 am

John Doe, RPT

For the following PT encounter note, rewrite the entry components so they are written with skilled verbiage.

Note 3: Hillary Hubbard

PT Encounter Note:

PINEWOOD SKILLED NURSING FACILITY

PHYSICAL THERAPY DEPARTMENT

Patient: Hillary Hubbard

Procedure: R Hip fracture; ORIF 3/14/2020

Diagnosis: sp R hip fracture

Patients ID: 2554

Physician: S. Shamus, MD

Physical Therapist: Colin Brooks, PT

Date: 3/30/2020, visit number: 6

PROBLEM STATEMENT/HISTORY:

Patient (Pt.) admitted to the Pinewood SNF 5 days following the right ORIF hip. Admitted for PT, NWB R

SUBJECTIVE:

Patient states that she is having R hip pain. She says that she is prescribed Vicodin every 8 hours, but trying to get off it and has been taking it twice a day. Patient describes her a pain as 7/10 with standing; has been unable to effectively NWB, and requires a lot of help to hold RLE up during transfers as well. 5/10 pain at rest. Pt. has difficulty doing "usual things such as moving easily in bed as well as self-care. Patient's goal is to go home and be independent "as soon as possible."

OBJECTIVE:

DOB: 10/21/1941
Height: 64 in, weight: 132 lb

BP at rest: 135/72	HR at rest: 74 bpm	RR at rest: 15
BP during ther exercise: 140/72	HR during tx: 79 bpm	RR during tx: 20
BP after: 135/70	HR after tx: 75 bpm	RR after tx: 16

Precautions: NWB RLE Patient (Pt.) presents with limited independence in performing activities of the daily living (ADL), weakness of the right lower extremity, overall soft tissue damage associated with the surgery.

20 minutes: 97116: Gait training: 3 trials with breaks after each trial using 2WW contact guard with gait belt assist ambulating on even ground 150 ft on carpet, and tile/linoleum, and patient instructed to avoid any throw rugs and move around set obstacles. Patient demonstrates slight antalgic gait with tendency to have a compensatory left lean and stoop during ambulation. Verbal cues given to correct gait pattern, patient is compliant and corrects posture with minimal verbal cues needed towards the end of the gait training

25 minutes: 97110: Therapeutic Exercise: In supine: patient performed active right hamstring stretch to 65 degrees ×3, 30-second holds. Patient also performed passive right calf stretch ×3, 30-second holds and passive rectus femoris stretch ×3/30-second holds. Quad sets and glut sets with strong contraction performs 20 times holding 5 seconds each. Strength: L Hip Flexion 4+/5, R Hip Flexion 3+/5. L Hip Abduction 5/5, R Hip Abduction 3+/5. In standing: active hip abduction strengthening using walker to stabilize balance and patient performed 3 sets of 10 repetitions with the right LE with light TheraBand around knee for resistance with rests in between sets. Active hip flexion to 85 degrees and extension were performed using walker to stabilize balance. Pt. performed 4 sets of 15 repetitions with no resistance with rests in between sets.

16 minutes: 97112: Neuromuscular re-education: balance training with parallel bars and walker, single leg balance on L LE, eyes open using fingertips on parallel bars and minimal assist of 20%; moderate assist to unweight RLE and sustain NWB. Patient is encouraged to remain on LLE for 10 seconds or longer. Verbal cueing and encouragement was given.

15 minutes: 97010: Cold pack placed on right hip, pt. side lying on a left side with a pillow in between knees (to avoid adduction) and a pillow under head of comfort. Checked skin each 5 minutes, sensation was intact.

ASSESSMENT:

Following treatment patient's pain level reported at 7/10, but was better 3/10 following application of ice. Pt. demonstrates good functional mobility, ambulates well with verbal cues. Following balance training fatigue level was high and rest was needed. The skin around incision area is healing well, incision looks pink with no abnormalities noted prior to and after the application of the ice pack. Pt. is instructed to use the walker when returning home until progressed by home health PT. Pt. was instructed to exercise twice a day and ice afterwards. Patient is progressing toward her goals being able to walk with standard walker upon discharge from Pinewood SNF.

PLAN:

Patient will be seen 1 more work for final gait training and neuromuscular re-education, and ice to prepare for D/C to home. Plan to instruct HEP with patient, hand out written copy, and answer any questions the patient may have regarding the HEP. Plan to perform D/C summary and assess Strength, integument, ROM, and prognosis. Plan to D/C to home health 3×/week for gait training, neuromuscular re-education, progressive therapeutic exercises, and functional training.

John Burke, PT 141466

Instructions: For the following initial examination and evaluation, complete the following:
Documentation Activity:

1. Correct errors in the document; rewrite to comply with skilled documentation.
2. Rewrite the goals, justifying the skilled physical therapy needed and to reflect the ICF model for a 4-week course of physical therapy.
3. Rewrite the POC into reimbursable terminology that is CPT compatible.
4. Describe the justification for each intervention.
5. Write a practical HEP that progresses the patient over 4 weeks.
6. Intervention is expected to be initiated on the same visit. Write an encounter note that is consistent with brief, but appropriate, intervention using all relevant principles.

Note 4: James Richards
Initial Examination and Evaluation
Patient Name: James Richards
Patient ID: 123484
Date: March 24, 2020
Time in: 11:00 am
Time out: 12:15 pm
Dx: L. TKA, Z96.65
Secondary: Osteoarthritis of the knee M17.11
Initial Evaluation

Subjective:

Pt is a 67 y.o. male referred to PT by Dr. Williams s/p LTKA performed on February 20, 2020. Pt reports pain as a 5 to 6/10 at worst and 1 to 2/10 at best. Pain is generally worse at night right before bed or in the middle of the day if he has a busy morning. Still has increased swelling and discomfort when standing for over 15 to 20 minutes and while driving for extended periods in the car. Pt denies any radiating pain down his LLE.

Reports that he is in good overall health and denies smoking and drug use. He occasionally has 1 to 2 alcoholic beverages on the weekend. Denies any history of cancer or diabetes. Has high blood pressure, osteoarthritis of the knee and low back. PMH: having a RTKA in July 2010. Reports taking OTC ibuprofen and Lopressor. Family hx of heart disease, colon cancer, and diabetes.

Prior to surgery, Pt reports being an avid golfer 3 × a week, walker; 40 minutes a day and a kayaker. Pt is right hand dominant. Swelling and pain are limiting his home responsibilities as well as his return to work. Has a hard time putting on his pants because he feels "off balance" as if he is going to fall over.

Personal goals are to cut the grass, assist his wife with household chores, cook a meal occasionally without needing to rest, be able to ambulate around the golf course and return to playing golf. Pt also reports he would like to be to drive in a car for a prolonged period of time to see his grandchildren in Central Florida.

Pt currently works part time at a golf course, but has taken the past month off and would like to return to work as soon as possible. Pt reports at work he cleans golf carts, caddies occasionally, and drives around the course tending to the course.

Pt lives in a single-story ranch-style home, with a small step in the garage with his wife and their golden retriever. Floors of the house are all tile and he has limited carpeting throughout.

Pt will return to see Ortho MD on 4/15/2020.

Objective

Vitals

Blood Pressure	130/80
Respiratory Rate	16 RR
O_2 Saturation	97%
Heart Rate	73 bpm

Deep Tendon Reflexes

	Right	Left
Achilles Reflex	2+	2+
Patella Tendon Reflex	2+	Not assessed due to incision site

AROM

	Right	Left
Hip Flexion	0 to 110°	0 to 108°
Hip Extension (standing leaning over a bolster)	0 to 25°	0 to 23°
Knee Extension	1 degree of hyperextension	Lacks 5 degrees to full extension
Knee Flexion	0 to 115°	0 to 110°
Ankle Dorsiflexion	0 to 10°	0 to 10°
Ankle Plantarflexion	0 to 35°	0 to 35°
Ankle EV	0 to 14°	0 to 15°
Ankle INV	0 to 20°	0 to 20°
Hamstring Flexibility	0 to 82°	0 to 75°

PROM

	Right	Left
Knee Extension (standing leaning over a bolster)	Did not assess, Pt is already hyperextended	Lacks 3 degrees to full extension
Knee Flexion	0 to 120°	0 to 113°

Muscle Performance

	Right	Left
Quadriceps	5/5	3+/5
Hamstring (standing leaning over a bolster)	5/5	4-/5
Hip adductors	4+/5	3+/5

Hip abductors	4+/5	3+/5
Calf Plantarflexion	25 single leg calf raises	5 single leg calf raises w/2 fingers on the table

30-Second Single Leg Stance (SLS) Test	Right	Left
Eyes Open	30 seconds	24 seconds
Eyes Closed	25 seconds	18 seconds

Girth	Right	Left
Center of Patella	40 cm	46 cm
5 cm proximal from center of patella	43 cm	48 cm
5 cm distal from center of patella	41 cm	45 cm

Berg Balance Score: 40/56

Cognition: Orientation × 3

Dermatome Sensation: Patient has decreased sensation around the L. knee on the anterior side over the incision. The rest of the LE has normal sensation throughout both limbs.

Assessment

Pt presents with limited AROM/PROM at L knee. Pt has impaired joint mobility, motor function, and muscular performance associated with L TKA. Pt did not present with an AD but during ambulation has an extension lag in his gait. Increased swelling and scar adhesions, with the scar healing well. Good-excellent candidate for PT.

Short-Term Goals

1. Pt will be able to stand for 15 minutes with pain at a 2 to 3/10 to increase endurance and decrease pain in L. LE for standing activities, functional ADLs, and personal responsibilities.
2. Pt will increase ROM to minus 3 degrees of full knee extension and 110 degrees of knee flexion to increase gait mobility.
3. Pt will increase strength of the knee to 4/5 to improve gait mobility and increase muscle endurance.
4. Pt will have decreased swelling by overall 4 cm to address stiffness and tightness of the joint which cause pain during driving.
5. Pt will increase single leg stance (SLS) on uneven surface with eyes open for 30 seconds to assist with balance and coordination deficits that limit Pt's ability to dress safely.

Long-Term Goals

1. Pt will be able to stand for 30 minutes at a 0 to 1/10 pain to cook meals, work, and cut the grass.
2. Pt will be able to ambulate with a full heel to toe strike without an extension lag to increase walking comfort and improve gait.
3. Pt will increase strength to 5/5 to increase muscle endurance with standing activities and work activities that require patient to ambulate frequently.
4. Pt will be able to drive for 40 minutes in the car without increased discomfort.
5. Pt will be able to perform SLS to don/off clothes.

Plan:

Patient will attend OP PT ×3/week for 4 to 6 weeks per protocol. Therapy to include: Ther ex (open chain and closed chain) to increase strength and mobility; Neuromuscular re-ed for balance, coordination and posture; modalities for pain reduction, circulations and muscle re-ed including ultrasound, E-STIM, thermal modalities; Manual therapy to include joint mobilizations grades I though III, traction, muscle stretching, PROM, functional massage and STM; Gait training on even/uneven surfaces; HEP education; functional ADL to condition Pt to return to work and attend to household chores.

Time out: 12:00 pm

John Burke, PT

Note 5

For the following entry, identify the correctly stated information and information that needs modification, and rewrite.

Name: Stuart Smith **Date:** 03/24/2020

DOB: 05/12/1935 **I.D. #:** 51245453

Referring Physician: Dr. Shamus

Diagnosis: Z96.651 Total Knee Arthroplasty

Treatment/PT diagnoses:

R26.89: gait dysfunction

R53.1: weakness RLE pain R knee

R60.0: edema

M2.60 Range of motion limiting gait and functional mobility

Visit #: 1–1:00 pm

Subjective

83 y.o. female presents to clinic four days post R total knee arthroplasty. Surgery was performed by referring physician. Surgery was performed at Lee Memorial hospital on 3/30/2013. Pt has history of osteoporosis, hypothyroidism, and high blood pressure. Medications include Levothyroxine, Levatol, and over-the-counter ibuprofen. Pt remained in hospital for three days post-surgery. Pt is a widow and resides alone in a one-bedroom apartment. There are no stairs in the apartment, nor does the patient have to climb any stairs to gain entry into the apartment. Has two grown children that do not reside in Florida. Pt is a retired teacher. Pt would like to return to driving and daily walks around the neighborhood. Patient states that prior to surgery she was able to walk a mile every day. When released from the SNF, Pt would like to return to living at home and being able to perform all ADLs independently. Pt has no precautions.

Objective

Vitals at rest: BP: 132/93 mmHg HR: 68 bpm RR: 16 breaths/min Temp: 98.6

Endurance: Sit to stand: 11 × in 30 seconds with CGA. Pt was short of breath after the completion of the test.

Cognition: Intact, aware of self, appropriate communication.

Integumentary/Sensation: Surgical incision on right knee, staples present, no sign of infection, swelling present in the area. No sensation loss. Cap refill: 3 seconds. Bruise present on left upper thigh.

Circumference/Girth (Taken two inches above superior pole of patella)

Left: 33 cm Right: 37 cm

ROM

LLE: No deficits seen

RLE	Active	Passive
Knee Flexion	93°	100°
Knee Extension	–5°	–3°

Strength

Left Knee Flexion	5/5
Left Knee Extension	5/5
Right Knee Flexion	3+/5
Right Knee Extension	4/5

Reflexes: Normal
Balance:

Normal balance seen on the LLE. Single leg stance on RLE × 3 seconds. Balance good when using wheeled walker. Educated patient in sit to stand transfer from bed with moderate assistance (50%). Pt was educated in gait training with the use of a walker. Pt was able to ambulate 10 ft to bathroom and required moderate assist in transferring to and from the toilet. Pt was educated in ther ex and asked to perform 3× daily. Exercises included 3 set of 20 repetitions of: ankle pumps, quad sets, heel slides with slide board, and short arc quads with bolster under the knees. Pt was able to demonstrate adequate quad contraction.

Assessment
General weakness seen in RLE.
Balance deficit in single leg stance on right side.
Walker dependent during gait.
Abnormal gait pattern seen with limp on the right side.
Endurance limitations.
Unable to return to independent living, unable to perform all ADLs independently, unable to function at prior level and participate in leisure activities.

Plan of Care
Goals:
STGs:

1. Patient will be able to ambulate for 50 feet while using a walker with minimal assistance at the end of 1 week.
2. Patient will be able to independently ambulate 150 feet while using a walker at the end of 2 weeks.
3. Patient will increase active ROM to 100 degrees and passive ROM to 110 degrees by the end of week one.
4. Patient will increase active range of motion to 105 degrees and passive ROM to 115 degrees by the end of week two.
5. Patient will be able to perform ADLs with minimal assistance and time to rest every 5 minutes by the end of the first week.
6. Patient will be able to perform all ADLs with minimal assistance and no rest time by the end of two weeks.

LTGs:

1. Patient will be able to ambulate 500 feet with the use of a walker on even surfaces before discharge from the SNF.
2. Among discharge, patient will increase active range of motion to 110° of flexion.
3. Among discharge, Patient will be able to perform ADLs independently with the assistance of a cane when needed.

P: SNF PT 5×/week for 3 weeks to consist of gait training with walker and progressive ther ex.
1:30 pm
Colin Brooks, PT 15154

Note 6

Instructions: For the following initial examination and evaluation, complete the following:

Documentation Activity:

1. Correct errors in the document; rewrite to comply with skilled documentation.
2. Rewrite the goals, justifying the skilled physical therapy needed and to reflect the ICF[4] model for a 4-week course of PT.
3. Rewrite the POC into reimbursable terminology that is CPT[6] compatible.
4. Describe the justification for each intervention.
5. Write a practical HEP that progresses the patient over 4 weeks.
6. Intervention is expected to be initiated on the same visit. Write an encounter note that is consistent with brief, but appropriate, intervention using all relevant principles.

Name: John Maple
Age: 25 M Date: 01/01/20
Referral: Dr. Knapp
Physician Orders: Eval and Treat L ankle pain
Medical Diagnosis: Left ankle pain
Rehab Diagnosis: Left hypomobile talocrural joint

Clinical Impression: Pt presents with a hypomobile talocrural joint as **evidenced by:** decreased A/PROM; DF with knee ext/flex, PF, inv/ev with abnormal capsule end-feel, hypomobile accessory mobility of A/P, P/A, med/lat glides and distraction of talus. **Causative factors** include 3 months self-immobilization secondary to swelling/effusion. Pt's ↓ A/PROM, swelling, hypomobility and deviated gait make **working** as a carpenter **difficult** and unsafe. **PT is necessary** to ↓ swelling, ↑ A/PROM, ↑accessory mobility, restore strength and gait so pt. can ambulate and work without pain/compensation and safely. **Stage of condition** is chronic 2° injury occurring 3 months ago even though condition is worse after working a full day but eases quickly if the pt. stays off his feet. **Tissue reactivity** of capsule is low 2° no pain with accessory mobility testing (high: pain with PROM). **Subject reactivity** is high as pt. works with pain and compensation.

1. *Swelling: Fig. 8 measurement around ankle R (42.0 cm), L (42.5 cm)*
2. A/PROM: *DF with knee ext/flex (10°/15°), PF (20°/25°), INV (25°/30°), EV (9°/12°),____ __with abnormal capsular end feel and 1/10 pain.*
3. *Accessory: ↑ A/P, P/A, med/lat glides and talus distraction by ½ grade.*
4. *Incomplete exams: Complete MLT and balance exams, set goals accordingly.*
5. *MMT: TA/TP, peroneus long/brev/tert (4+/5), gastroc R=L (4/5).*
6. *Function: (LEFI 60/80 = 75%) Pt able to ambulate*

Prognosis: Pt has a good prognosis of returning to framing houses pain-free secondary to his age, unremarkable PMH and no complicating factors that may impede his healing.

Impairments/Functional Limitations:

1. Swelling: ↑ swelling (+1.0 cm) with figure 8 measurement of ankle.
2. A/PROM: ↓ DF with knee ext/flex, PF, INV/EV, with abnormal capsular end feel and pain.
3. Accessory: Hypomobile A/P, P/A, Med/Lat glide of talus and talus distraction.
4. Incomplete exams: MLT deferred 2° inability to achieve test position/balance test incomplete 2° pain.
5. MMT: TA/TP, peroneus long/brev/tert (4/5), gastro (4–/5).
6. Function: (LEFI 43/80 = 53.75%) Pt unable to ambulate over level or unlevel surfaces, pick up items from floor *to waist or negotiate stairs without pain or compensation.*

LTG: Pt will achieve the following in 6 weeks in order to return to house framing pain free.

1. Swelling: Fig. 8 measurement around ankle R=L.
2. A/PROM: DF with knee ext/flex, PF, INV/EV R=L with N end feel and no pain.
3. Accessory: A/P, P/A, med/lat glides and talus distraction R=L.
4. Incomplete exams: Complete MLT and balance exams, set goals accordingly.
5. MMT: TA/TP, peroneus long/brev/tert and gastroc *R=L (5/5).*
6. Function: (LEFI 80/80 = 100%) Pt able to ambulate on treadmill for 30 minutes @ 2.2 mph with 3% incline and 0/10 pain

In 3 weeks, Pt will achieve the following
on treadmill for 15 minutes @ 2.2 mph____ __with 0% incline and 0/10 pain
Direct Interventions: Frequency: *3×/wk then 2×/wk* **Duration:** *4 weeks then 2* weeks

1. Swelling: Ice/HVPC → ankle pumps → alphabet → retrograde massage → wrap
2. A/PROM: PROM into DF/PF/INV/EV → AAROM → AROM → PROM with overpressure
3. Accessory: grade II A/P, P/A, med/lat glides→grade III→IV, talus distraction grade I, II, III
4. Incomplete exams: Complete MLT and balance exams, Tx accordingly.
5. MMT: AROM → MRE into DF/PF/INV/EV→ T-band → seated rocker board → standing_ __rocker board → weight shifts-
6. Function: Standing weight shifts → single leg stance → ambulate 5 minutes @ 1.6 mph @ 0% incline __→ 2.0 mph → 2.2 mph → 1% incline → 2% → 3% → 10 min → 20 min → 30 min.

Communication: Fax POC to MD
Patient related Instructions: Ice 5×/day, 10-15 minutes with elevation/ankle pumps. Rest/elevate 5 minutes every hr. Wear high boots and Aircast (ankle brace) for support.
Discharge Plan:
Pt (I) with ambulate over level/unlevel surface. Aircast (ankle brace) provided. No f/u necessary.
Matthew Daugh, DPT 01/01/20
Physical Therapist Signature
Physician's Signature

Note 7
Name: John Master
Age: 68
Gender: Male
Physician Orders: Eval and treat R leg pain
Medical Diagnosis: Multilevel lumbar facet joint arthrosis and stenosis
Rehab Diagnosis: Lateral foraminal stenosis with neuropathy

Clinical Impression: Pt presents with lateral foraminal stenosis with lumbar radiculopathy into RLE evidenced by: positive radiographic findings of lumbar facet joint arthrosis and stenosis, limited AROM with lumbar flexion, extension, and R side-bending with pain into R calf, diminished sensation in R lateral calf, 3–/5 strength in R extensor hallucis longus (EHL), tenderness between L4 and L5 spinous processes, and positive SLR test on the RLE. Causative factor includes facet joint degeneration secondary to abnormal stresses and aging. Pt presents with limited lumbar AROM with flexion, extension, and R side-bending with pain into R calf, limited R and L lumbar rotation with muscle guarding, diminished sensation in R lateral calf, 3–/5 strength in R EHL, limited R hip flexion and ER, positive lumbar distraction test and SLR on RLE, limited lumbar PIVMs in all directions, and tenderness over L4/5 interspinous space. These limitations have resulted in patient being unable to independently perform yardwork, housework, bowling, and shooting at the gun range. Pt was independent with all activities before s/s appeared. Pt will benefit from skilled PT to increase lumbar IV mobility, increase lumbar AROM, increase R hip ROM, and improve strength in R EHL. Pt's tissue reactivity of lumbar IV joints is low due to no pain at end-range. Pt's has the participation restriction of unable to perform his daily grandfather role due to the activity limitation of impaired sit to stand tasks due to pain. Pt's stage of condition is chronic due to the 4-month time frame duration of symptoms.

Prognosis: Pt has fair prognosis for a full recovery due to pt.'s age and decreased joint space in lumbar spine shown via x-ray.

Impairments:

- Posture: pt. presents with a forward flexed posture at the hips with excess lumbar lordosis
- A/PROM: pt. presents with decreased AROM with lumbar flexion, extension, and R side-bending that radiate pain into R calf. Pt also presents with decreased lumbar rotation bilaterally with muscle guarding
- Accessory: pt. presents with limited PIVM's in the lumbar spine in all directions
- Neurological: pt. presents with diminished sensation in R lateral calf and 3–/5 strength in R EHL
- Function: (OD I =62%) pt. ambulates with decreased weight-bearing through RLE and a forward flexed posture

Short-Term Goals:

- In 3 weeks, pt. will demo independence with HEP to improve postural deficits
- In 3 weeks, pt. will improve ODI score by 8% to improve overall functional mobility
- In 3 weeks, pt. will improve all lumbar AROM by at least 5 degrees to improve mobility

Long-Term Goals:

- In 6 weeks, pt. will improve ODI score by 15% to improve overall functional mobility.
- In 6 weeks, pt. will increase R EHL strength to at least a 4/5 to improve functional mobility
- In 6 weeks, pt. will improve all lumbar AROM by at least 10 degrees to improve functional mobility.

Interventions: **Frequency**: 3×/wk **Duration**: 4 weeks

- Posture: manual hip flexor stretch, self-stretch for hip flexors, STM to lumbar paraspinals and R piriformis, stretch ER rotators
- A/PROM: lumbar distraction, joint mobilizations to lumbar spine, double knees to chest, ball roll-outs
- MMT: AROM with EHL against gravity, MRE with EHL, abdominal strengthening

Delegation and/or Appropriate Referral

- PTA will continue with the following treatment sessions and continue the PT's POC.

Specific HEP/Pt. Education:

- Pt education on posture and importance of self-stretching in HEP
- Pt education on abdominal and multifidus strengthening and constant contractions to protect spine
- HEP will include self-stretching of hip flexors, PPT, double knee to chest, and lumbar rotations in supine

Discharge Summary:

- Pt independent with all ADLs, housework, yardwork, and return to bowling and shooting. Follow up with physician.

Matthew Daugherty, DPT *01/01/20*
Physical Therapist Signature
Physician's Signature

For each of the following entries, rewrite the content to emphasize skill, status, patient progress, skilled components of PT intervention, and appropriate verbiage or goals.

- Patient transfers have improved from max assist to mod assist; weakness persists in all extremities. Patient has difficulty sequencing components, preventing further progress at this time.

- Now able to go up four 6-inch steps holding on to rails, with minimal assist, needs a lot of help to descend.
- Patient is able to walk on even surface without directional changes × 1 rep, 50′, front wheeled rolling walker. Occasional verbal cues for attempts of step through pattern, flat footed.
- Gait in hallway, leans forward, bent at waist, short steps, CO SOB constantly, hemiwalker R, min asst to move hemiwalker, 25′.
- Able to extend and flex L knee with 2# weight 3 sets of 10 reps with assistance counting, resting as needed.
- Patient now able to don long pants with dressing stick with min to mod asst LLE; but unable to don L sock or shoe. With min asst able to don button shirt using RUE, 2° L neglect. Poor follow-through.
- Patient able to lean forward in unsupported sitting but unable to reach to floor without losing balance.
- Can now rotate neck 25° and 10° to the left from midline with pain at end range.
- Patient goes from supine to side-lying using bedrail and mod asst. Mod asst to assume short sitting; minimal improvement.
- IV L forearm, indwelling catheter, NG tube; ambulation training bedside chair to door of room and back, FWRW, shuffled, mod asst to move walker forward, constant instructions.
- Child is able to roll R, using LUE and R head turning, no LE use; LE extensor tone.
- Ambulation with posterior walker, bilateral AFOs, flexed in standing, drags legs forward laboriously, moderate asst for balance.
- Exercise in prone to decrease extension and facilitate reaching.

SUMMARY

Chapter 16 focuses on documentation activities that reinforce appropriate content. PTs and PTAs should remember that entries should reflect the following:

1. Where the patient was functionally and medically prior to the current episode
   a. PLOF; components of history
2. Where the patient is functionally and medically at the start of care
   a. Initial examinations; tests and measures, objective and standardized (if possible)
   b. Initial evaluation
3. Where the patient is going
   a. Initial evaluation: Goals; objective and measurable
4. How the patient will get there
   a. Initial evaluation: Interventions; POC
5. How the patient is doing at any point in time
   a. Daily notes, progress notes/summaries, and reports; documentation of progress over time; patient response
6. How the physical therapy intervention affected the patient and discharge instructions
   a. Discharge summary and plan

All medical record documentation must be complete, in total and individual entries. It must include the patient's legal name, full legal signature of the treating professional, time or total minutes, adequate and appropriate details, legible (if manual), and all other required elements.

Anyone needing access to a physical therapy record should be able to review the initial evaluation and discharge summary to determine the effectiveness of care. The same standardized tests and measures should be administered for measurable, objective results for comparison. Progress and justification of skill should be reflected. If they match, the overall content should also provide evidence of the effectiveness of care. If they do not match, payment and patient satisfaction may be at risk; in addition, there may be liability issues.

It is incumbent upon the treating therapist to know the coding, billing, and documentation requirements of all third-party payers. Therapists also should verify that they or their employer are approved providers for the payer and determine if preauthorization is required or if there is a limit on the number of visits. It is also incumbent on the PT/PTA to ensure appropriate skilled documentation, whether electronic or manual, to reflect medical necessity and to justify care, effectiveness, and delivery of skilled services.

REFERENCES

1. *Documentation Overview. Alexandria,* VA: American Physical Therapy Association. Available at https://www.apta.org/your-practice/documentation/overview. Accessed August 20, 2020.
2. *Sample Checklist for Documentation.* Alexandria, VA: American Physical Therapy Association. Available at http://www.apta.org/DefensibleDocumentation/SampleChecklist/. Accessed August 20, 2020.
3. *Defensible Documentation.* Alexandria, VA: American Physical Therapy Association. Available at http://www.apta.org/DefensibleDocumentation/Tips/#General. Accessed August 20, 2020.
4. *International Classification of Functioning, Disability and Health (ICF).* World Health Organization, WHO. Available at https://www.who.int/classifications/icf/en/. Accessed August 20, 2020.
5. *ICD-10 update.* American Medial Association. Available at https://www.ama-assn.org/practice-management/claims-processing/icd-10-overview. Accessed August 20, 2020.
6. *CPT.* American Medical Association. https://www.ama-assn.org/practice-management/cpt. Accessed August 20, 2020.
7. *National Provider Identifier Standard (NPI).* Centers for Medicare & Medicaid Services. Available at https://www.cms.gov/Regulations-and-Guidance/Administrative-Simplification/NationalProvIdentStand#:~:text=The%20NPI%20is%20a%2010,live%20or%20their%20medical%20specialty. Accessed August 20, 2020.
8. *Medicare Benefit Policy Manual Chapter 15 – Covered Medical and Other Health Services.* Centers for Medicare & Medicaid Services. Available at https://www.cms.gov/Regulations-and-Guidance/Guidance/Manuals/downloads/bp102c15 pdf. Accessed August 20, 2020.
9. *Medicare Claims Processing Manual Chapter 5 – Part B Outpatient Rehabilitation and CORF/OPT Services.* Centers for Medicare & Medicaid Services. Available at https://www.cms.gov/Regulations-and-guidance/Guidance/Manuals/downloads/clm104c05.pdf. Accessed August 20, 2020.
10. *Functional Independence Measure (FIM).* Alexandria, VA: American Physical Therapy Association. Available at https://www.apta.org/patient-care/evidence-based-practice-resources/test-measures/functional-independence-measure-fim. Accessed August 20, 2020.
11. *Quick Guide to the Three Levels of Physical Therapy Evaluation.* Alexandria, VA: American Physical Therapy Association. Available at https://www.apta.org/your-practice/payment/coding-billing/tiered-evaluation-codes/tiered-codes-evaluation-table. Accessed August 20, 2020.
12. Middleton A, Fritz SL, Lusardi M. Walking speed: The functional vital sign. *J Aging Phys Act.* 2015;23(2):314-322. doi:10.1123/japa.2013-0236.
13. *HCPCS Coding Questions.* Centers for Medicare & Medicaid Services. Available at https://www.cms.gov/Medicare/Coding/MedHCPCSGenInfo/HCPCS_Coding_Questions. Accessed August 20, 2020.
14. *Busting Payment Myths (and Regulating Your Expectations) Part 4.* Alexandria, VA: American Physical Therapy Association. Available at https://www.apta.org/article/2020/07/29/busting-medicare-part-b-myths-and-regulating-your-expectations-part-4. Accessed August 20, 2020.

Appendices

Appendix A

ABBREVIATIONS

Δ change
↓ decrease
↑ increase
↔ to/from, in/out of
~ approximate
= equals
< less than
> greater than
number
- minus
+ plus
& and
etc. etcetera
% percentage
| parallel bars
@ each, at, before
’ foot
" inch
° degree
p̄ after
c̄ with
s̄ without
♀ female
♂ male
¶ paragraph

a artery
ā ante (L)
A assistance
AA atlantoaxial; adjusted age; active assist, alcoholics anonymous
AAA abdominal aortic aneurysm
AAO ×3 alert, awake, and oriented to date, person, place
AAROM active assisted range of motion
AARP American Association of Retired Persons
Abd abduction
ABG arterial blood gases
AC alternating current; acromioclavicular
a.c. before a meal
ACA anterior communicating artery; anterior cerebral artery
ACCE academic coordinator of clinical education
ACL anterior cruciate ligament
ACM Arnold–Chiari malformation
ACO Accountable Care Organization
ACSM American College of Sports Medicine

AD	advanced directive
ADA	American Dental Association; American Dietetics Association
ad lib	ad libitum (Latin), at pleasure
ADD	attention deficit disorder; adduction
ADHD	attention deficit hyperactivity disorder
ADL	activities of daily living
Adm	admitted; admission
ADR	additional development required
AE(A)	above elbow amputation; preferred term is transhumeral amputation
AF	atrial fibrillation, Arthritis Foundation
AFB	acid-fast bacillus
AFO	ankle foot orthosis
AFP	alpha-fetoprotein
AGA	appropriate for gestational age
AHA	American Heart Association; American Hospital Association
AHIMA	American Health Information Management Association
AI	aortic incompetence
AIDS	acquired immune deficiency syndrome
AIMS	Alberta Infant Motor Scale
AK(A)	above knee amputation; preferred term is transfemoral amputation
ALJ	administrative law judge
ALL	acute lymphocytic leukemia; anterior longitudinal ligament
ALS	amyotrophic lateral sclerosis; advanced life support
AM	morning
AMA	against medical advice; American Medical Association
amb	ambulate; ambulation
AML	acute myelogenous leukemia; acute myelocytic leukemia
ANA	American Nursing Association
ANS	autonomic nervous system
ant	anterior
AOTA	American Occupational Therapy Association
AP	anteroposterior; before dinner
APGAR	appearance, pulse, grimace, activity, respiration
APM	Alternative Payment Method
APTA	American Physical Therapy Association
ARC	Association for Retarded Citizens
ARD	assessment reference dates
ARDS	adult respiratory distress syndrome; acute respiratory distress syndrome
ARF	acute renal failure; acute respiratory failure
AROM	active range of motion
AS	aortic stenosis; ankylosing spondylitis
As & Bs	apnea and bradycardia
ASA	aspirin
ASAP	as soon as possible
ASD	atrial septal defect
ASHA	American Speech and Hearing Association
ASIS	anterior superior iliac spine
Asst, assist	assistance; assist
ATC	athletic trainer, certified
ATNR	asymmetric tonic neck reflex
AV	arteriovenous; atrioventricular; aortic valve
AVM	arteriovenous malformation
B	bilateral; both
BAER	brainstem auditory evoked response (hearing screening)
BBA	Balanced Budget Act

BBB	blood–brain barrier; bundle-branch block
BCBS	Blue Cross and Blue Shield
BE	barium enema
BE(A)	below elbow amputation; preferred term is transradial amputation
BFR	blood flow rate; blood flow restriction
BIB	drink
BICU	burn intensive care unit
BID	bis in die (Latin); twice a day
bil, bilat	bilateral
BIN	twice at night
BK(A)	below knee amputation; preferred term is transtibial amputation
bl	blood; bleeding
BM	bowel movement
BMI	body mass index
BMR	basal metabolic rate
BMT	bone marrow transplant
BOS	base of support
BP	blood pressure; bed pan
BPCI	Bundled Payment for Care Improvements
BPD	bronchopulmonary disease/dysplasia
BPH	benign prostatic hyperplasia/hypertrophy
bpm	beats per minute; breaths per minute
BPPV	benign paroxysmal positional vertigo
BR	bathroom
BRP	bathroom privileges
BS	breath sounds; blood sugar; bowel sounds
B/S	bedside
BSA	body surface area
BT	Blalock–Taussig (shunt)
BUN	blood urea nitrogen
bw	body weight, birth weight
bx	biopsy
$\bar{c}$	with, calorie
C	centigrade scale
C & S	culture and sensitivity
Ca	calcium; about
CA	cancer; chronological age
Cal	calories
CABG	coronary artery bypass graft
CAD	coronary artery disease
CARF	Commission on Accreditation of Rehabilitation Facilities
cath.	catheter
CBC	complete blood count
CC, C/C	chief complaint; carbon copy
cc	cubic centimeter
CCCE	clinical coordinator of clinical education
CCI	Correct Coding Initiative
CCU	cardiac care unit; coronary care unit
CDC	Centers for Disease Control and Prevention
CDM	Clinical decision making
CDMM	Clinical Decision-Making Model
CF	cystic fibrosis
CFS	chronic fatigue syndrome
CG	contact guard
CHAMPUS	Civilian Health and Medical Program-Uniformed Services

CHD	congenital heart disease
CHF	congestive heart failure
CI	clinical instructor; curie
CICU	coronary intensive care unit; cardiac intensive care unit
CK	creatine kinase
CLD	chronic liver disease; chronic lung disease
CLL	chronic lymphocytic leukemia
cm	centimeter
CMC	carpometacarpal (joint)
CME	continuing medical education
CML	chronic myelogenous leukemia
CMR	computerized medical record
CMS	Centers for Medicare & Medicaid Services
CMV	cytomegalovirus
CNA	certified nursing assistant
CN	cranial nerve; tomorrow night
CN I	olfactory nerve
CN II	optic nerve
CN III	oculomotor nerve
CN IV	trochlear nerve
CN V	trigeminal nerve
CN VI	abducens nerve
CN VII	facial nerve
CN VIII	vestibulocochlear nerve
CN IX	glossopharyngeal nerve
CN X	vagus nerve
CN XI	accessory nerve
CN XII	hypoglossal nerve
CNS	central nervous system
c/o	complains of
CO	cardiac output; carbon monoxide; complains of
CO_2	carbon dioxide
COG	center of gravity
cont.	continued
COPD	chronic obstructive pulmonary disease/disorder
CORF	Comprehensive Outpatient Rehabilitation Facility
COTA	certified occupational therapist assistant
COVID	corona virus disease
CP	cerebral palsy; chest pain; cold pack
CPAP	continuous positive airway pressure
CPI	clinical performance instrument
CPK	creatine phosphokinase
CPM	continuous passive motion machine
CPR	cardiopulmonary resuscitation; computerized-based patient record
CPT	Current Procedural Terminology
CPS	Clinical problem solving
CR	Clinical reasoning
CRPS	complex regional pain syndrome
CS	cesarean section; cervical spine
CSF	cerebrospinal fluid
CT	chest tube; computed axial tomography (CAT)
CV	cardiovascular
CVA	cerebrovascular accident
CVL	central venous line
CWI	crutch walking instructions
CXR	chest x-ray

D & C	dilation and curettage
DAFO	dynamic foot ankle orthosis
DC	direct current
D/C, DC, d/c	discharge; discontinue
DDD	degenerative disc disease
DDE	direct data entry
DDH	developmental dysplasia of hip
DDS	doctor of dental science
Dept.	department
DF	dorsiflexion
DHT	Dobhoff (feeding) tube
DIP	distal interphalangeal (joint)
DJD	degenerative joint disease
DLE	discoid lupus erythematosus; disseminated lupus erythematosus
DLT	double lung transplant
DM	diabetes mellitus
DMD	Duchenne muscular dystrophy; doctor of medical dentistry
DME	durable medical equipment
DNA	deoxyribonucleic acid
DNR	do not resuscitate
DO	disorder; doctor of osteopathy
DOA	dead on arrival; date of admission
DOB	date of birth
DOE	dyspnea on exertion
DOI	date of injury
DPT	diphtheria-pertussis-tetanus vaccine; doctor of physical therapy
DRGs	diagnostic-related groups
DT	delirium tremens; diptheria tetanus
DTR	deep tendon reflexes
DVT	deep vein thrombosis
Dx	diagnosis
EBP	evidence-based practice
EBV	Epstein–Barr virus
ECF	extended care facility; extracellular fluid
ECG	electrocardiogram
ECMO	extracorporeal membrane oxygenation
EEG	electroencephalogram
EENT	eye, ear, nose, and throat
EF	ejection fraction
EFA	essential functional activities
EHR	electronic health record
EIA	exercise-induced asthma
EID	easily identified depression
EIP	early intervention program
ELBW	extremely low birth weight
ELISA	enzyme-linked immunosorbent assay
ELS	Eaton–Lambert syndrome
EMG	electromyography
EMR	electronic medical record
EMS	emergency medical services
EMT	emergency medical technician
ENT	ear, nose, and throat
EOB	edge of bed
ER	emergency room; external rotation
ERT	estrogen replacement therapy

ES	electrical stimulation
ESR	erythrocyte sedimentation rate
ESRD	end-stage renal disease
ETOH	alcohol (use/abuse)
ETT	endotracheal tube
Eval	evaluation
EX	exercise
EXT	extension; extensive
F	♀ fair; female
f/u	follow-up
FAQ	frequently asked questions
FAS	fetal alcohol syndrome
FBG	fasting blood glucose
FBS	fasting blood sugar
FES	functional electrical stimulation
FEV1	forced expiratory volume in 1 second
FFS	Fee for Service
FI	fiscal intermediary
FIM	Functional Independence Measure
FIN	federal identification number
FL	functional limitation; Florida
Flex	flexion
FOB	father of baby
FOIA	Freedom of Information Act
FOR	functional outcome reporting
FOTO	Focus on Therapeutic Outcomes, Inc.
FSH	fascioscapulohumeral dystrophy
FSP	family service plan
Ft.	feet
FT	feeding tube; full term
FTT	failure to thrive
Funct	functional
FUO	fever of unknown origin
FVC	forced vital capacity
FWB	full weight bearing
FWW	four-wheeled walker or front-wheeled rolling walker
Fx	fracture
G	good
G tube	gastrostomy tube
G#P#A#	number of births, pregnancies, and abortions
GA	gestational age
GAO	Governmental Accounting Agency
GB	gallbladder
GBS	Guillain–Barré syndrome
GCS	Glasgow Coma Scale
GERD	gastroesophageal reflux disease
GI	gastrointestinal
gm	gram
GMFM	Gross Motor Function Measure
GPCI	geographic practice cost indices
grava	gravida = number of births
GSW	gunshot wound
gt	gait training
GU	genitourinary
GVHD	graft-versus-host disease
GYN	gynecology

H	Haemophilus influenza B; hydrogen; hour
H & P	history and physical
h/o	history of
HA	headache
Hams, hs	hamstrings
Hb	hemoglobin
HBP	high blood pressure
HC	heelcords
HCFA	Healthcare Finance Administration (now CMS)
hct	hematocrit
HCPCS	Healthcare Common Procedure Coding Systems
HCVD	hypertensive cardiovascular disease
HDL	high-density lipoprotein
HEENT	head, ears, eyes, nose, and throat
HEP	home exercise program
Hg, Hgb	hemoglobin
HH	home health; handheld
HHA	home health aide; handheld assist; home health agency
HHS	Department of Health and Human Services
HIB	Haemophilus influenza B (vaccine)
HICN	health insurance claim number
HIE	hypoxic-ischemic encephalopathy
HIM	Health Information Management
HIPAA	Health Information and Portability Accountability Act
HIV	human immunodeficiency virus
HKAFO	hip knee ankle foot orthosis
HLA	human leukocyte antigen; homologous leukocytic antibodies
HLT	heart, lung transplant
HMD	hyaline membrane disease
HMO	health maintenance organization
HNP	herniated nucleus pulposus
HO	heterotopic ossification; house officer
HOB	head of bed
HOH	hard of hearing
HOOS	Hip Disability Osteoarthritis and Outcome Score
HP	hot pack
HPI	history of present illness
hr.	hour
HR	heart rate
HRT	hormone replacement therapy
HS	at bedtime
HSV	herpes simplex virus
Ht	height
HT	heart transplant
HTN	hypertension
HVGS	high volt galvanic stimulation
HX	history
I	independent
I & D	incision and drainage
I & O	input and output
IADL	independent/instrumental activities of daily living
IBS	irritable bowel syndrome
ICA	internal carotid artery
ICD	International Classification of Diseases
ICH	intracranial hemorrhage; intracerebral hemorrhage

ICF	International Classification of Functioning, Disability and Health
ICP	intracranial pressure
ICU	intensive care unit
ID	infectious disease
IDDM	insulin-dependent diabetes mellitus
IDEA	Individuals with Disabilities Education Act
IEP	individualized exercise program; individualized education plan
IFC	interferential current
IFSP	Individual Family Support Plan
Ig	immunoglobulin
IM	intramuscular
Indep	independent
inf.	inferior
instr	instructions
Imp	impression
IPA	independent practice association
IPPB	intermittent positive pressure breathing
IPO	independent practice organization
IQ	intelligence quotient
IR	internal rotation
IRB	institutional review board
ITB	intrathecal baclofen
IUD	intrauterine device
IUGR	intrauterine growth retardation
IV	intravenous
IVC	inferior vena cava
IVH	intraventricular hemorrhage
IVP	intravenous pyelogram
J tube	jejunostomy tube
JCAHO	Joint Commission on Accreditation of Healthcare Organizations
JP	Jackson–Pratt (drain)
JRA	juvenile rheumatoid arthritis
jt	joint
KAFO	knee ankle foot orthosis
kcal	kilocalories
kg	kilogram
KUB	kidney, ureter, bladder; kidney and upper bladder
L	left; lower
L, l	liter
l/min	liters per minute
LAP	laparoscopy; laparotomy
LAQ	long arc quad
LBP	low back pain
LBQC	large-based quad cane
LBW	low birth weight
LCL	lateral collateral ligament
LD	learning disability
LDL	low-density lipoprotein
LE	lower extremity
LFT	liver function test
LG	limb girdle dystrophy
LGA	large for gestational age
Lim	limited
LLC	long leg cast
LLE	left lower extremity

LLL	left lower lobe
LLQ	left lower quadrant
LMN	lower motor neuron
LMRP	local medical review policies
LOB	loss of balance
LOC	loss of consciousness
LOS	length of stay
LP	lumbar puncture
LPN	licensed practical nurse
LS, L/S	lumbar spine
LT	lung transplant; light
LTACH	Long-Term Acute Care Hospital
LTCF	long-term care facility
LTD	limited
LTG	long-term goal
LTM	long-term memory
LUE	left upper extremity
LUL	left upper lobe
LUQ	left upper quadrant
M	male, ♂
MAO	monoamine oxidase
max	maximum; maximal
MCA	middle cerebral artery
MCL	medial collateral ligament
MCO	managed care organization
MCP	metacarpophalangeal (joint)
MD	muscular dystrophy; medical doctor
MDA	Muscular Dystrophy Association
MDS	medical data sheet; material data safety sheets; minimum data set
MED	minimal erythemal dose
MENS	microcurrent electrical stimulation
mets	metastasis
MET	metabolic equivalent of task
MFT	muscle function test
MFR	myofascial release
MH	moist heat
MHP	moist hot pack
MI	myocardial infarction
MICU	medical intensive care unit
min	minimal; minute
MIPS	Merit-based Incentive Payment System
mL	milliliter
mm	millimeter
mm Hg	millimeters of mercury
MMPI	Minnesota Multiphasic Personality Inventory
MMR	measles, mumps, rubella (vaccine)
MMT	manual muscle test
mo	month; months old
mob	mobilization; mobility
mod	moderate
MOI	mechanism of injury
MOM	milk of magnesia
mph	miles per hour
MRE	manual resistive exercise
MRI	magnetic resonance imaging
MS	multiple sclerosis; mitral stenosis, musculoskeletal

MSDS	Material Safety Data Sheet
MT	medical technologist; metatarsal
MTBI	minimal traumatic brain injury
MTP	metatarsophalangeal joint
MV	mitral valve; movement
MVA	motor vehicle accident
MVP	mitral valve prolapse
MWD	microwave diathermy
N	normal; nausea
N & V	nausea and vomiting
N/A	not applicable
NAD	no appreciable disease; nothing abnormal detected; no acute distress
NCQA	National Committee on Quality Assurance
NCV	nerve conduction velocity
NDT	neurodevelopmental treatment
neb	nebulizer
NEC	necrotizing enterocolitis
Neg	negative (–)
neuro-ICU	neurological intensive care unit
NG	nasogastric
NGT	nasogastric tube
NICU	neonatal intensive care unit; newborn intensive care unit
NIDDM	noninsulin-dependent diabetes mellitus
NIH	National Institutes of Health
NIOSH	National Institute for Occupational Safety and Health
NKA	no known allergies
nl	normal
NMES	neuromuscular electrical stimulation
NPP	Non physician practitioner
NPO	non per os (Latin); nothing by mouth
NSAID	nonsteroidal anti-inflammatory drug
NSR	normal sinus rhythm
NWB	non-weight bearing
O	objective; oral
O_2, O2	oxygen
OA	osteoarthritis
OASIS	Outcome and Assessment Information Set
OB	obstetrics
Obj	objective
OBRA	Omnibus Budget Reconciliation Act
OBS	organic brain syndrome
OD	overdose; doctor of optometry
OHTx	orthotopic heart transplant
OI	osteogenesis imperfecta
OIG	Office of the Inspector General
OLD	obstructive lung disease
OLT	orthotopic lung transplant
OM	otitis media
OMRA	Other Medicare Required Assessment
OOB	out-of-bed
OP	outpatient
OPV	oral polio vaccine
OR	operating room
ORIF	open reduction internal fixation
OSHA	Occupational Safety and Health Administration

OT	occupational therapy; occupational therapist
OTA	Occupational therapy assisstant
OTC	over-the-counter
OTR	occupational therapist, registered
oz	ounce
p̄	after
P	poor; plan
PA	pulmonary artery; posterior-anterior; physician's assistant
PAC	premature atrial contraction
para	number of births, paraplegic
Path	pathology
PCA	patient-controlled analgesic; posterior cerebral artery; posterior communicating artery
PCL	posterior cruciate ligament
PCP	primary care physician
PD	Parkinson disease; peritoneal dialysis
PDA	patent ductus arteriosus; personal data application
PDD	pervasive developmental delay
PDGM	Patient Driven Grouping Model
PDPM	Patient Driven Payment Model
PE	pulmonary embolus; pulmonary edema
PEDI	Pediatric Evaluation of Disability Inventory
PEEP	positive end-expiratory pressure
PEG	percutaneous endoscopic gastrostomy
per	by, through
PERRLA	pupils equal, round, react to light, accommodate
PET	positron emission tomography
PF	plantarflexion
PFS	Physician fee schedule
PharmD	doctor of pharmacy
PH	past history
PI	present illness
PICA	posterior inferior cerebellar artery; posterior inferior communicating artery
PICC	peripherally inserted central catheter
PICU	pediatric intensive care unit
PID	pelvic inflammatory disease
PIP	proximal interphalangeal (joint); personal injury protection
PKU	phenylketonuria
PLF/PLOF	prior level of function
PLL	posterior longitudinal ligament, postero-lateral left
PM	afternoon
PM & R	physical medicine and rehabilitation
PMH	past medical history
PMS	premenstrual syndrome
PNF	proprioceptive neuromuscular facilitation
PNI	peripheral nerve injury
PNS	peripheral nervous system
PO	per os (Latin); by mouth
POC	plan of care
POD	post-operative day (followed by number)
POMR	problem-oriented medical record
Pos	positive (+)
POS	point-of-service plan
Poss	possible
post	posterior, after
post-op	postoperative

PPE	personal protective equiptment
PPH	primary pulmonary hypertension
PPO	preferred provider organization
PPS	prospective payment system
PRE	progressive resistance exercises
pre-op	preoperative
Pron	pronation
PRN	pro re nata (Latin); as needed
PRO	peer review organization; patient-reported outcome
PROM	passive range of motion; premature rupture of membranes
PROMIS	patient-reported outcome measurement information system
PRSO	professional standards review organization
PSIS	posterior superior iliac spine
Psych	psychology, psychiatric
Pt., pt	patient; point; pint
PT	physical therapy; physical therapist prothrombin time
PTA	physical therapist assistant; prior to admission; post-traumatic amnesia
PTB	patellar tendon bearing (prosthesis)
PTIP	physical therapist in independent practice
PTPP	physical therapist in private practice (per CMS)
PVC	premature ventricular contraction
PVD	peripheral vascular disease
PVH	periventricular hemorrhage
PVL	periventricular leukomalacia
PWB	partial weight bearing
q	every
QA	quality assurance
QC	quad
qd	once daily
qh	every hour
QI	quality improvement; quality indicator
qid	quater in die (Latin); four times a day
qiw	four times per week
qod	every other day
QOL	quality of life
QPP	quality payment program
qt	quart
quad	quadriplegic; quadriceps
R	right
R/O, RO	rule out
RA	rheumatoid arthritis; right atrium; rehabilitation agency (certified)
RAM	random access memory, rapid alternating movements
RAD	reactive airway disease
RAI	resident assessment instrument
RAP	resident assessment protocol
RAS	reticular activating system
RBBB	right bundle branch block
RBC	red blood cell
RBRVS	Resource-Based Relative Value Scale
RCA	right carotid artery, right coronary artery
RD	registered dietician
RDS	respiratory distress syndrome
Re	regarding
Rehab	rehabilitation
REM	rapid eye movement

Reps	repetitions
RF	radio frequency; rectus femoris
RGO	reciprocating gait orthosis
RLE	right lower extremity
RLL	right lower lobe
RLQ	right lower quadrant
RML	right middle lobe
RN	registered nurse
ROM	range of motion; read-only memory
ROP	retinopathy of prematurity
ROS	review of systems
RPE	rate of perceived exertion
RR	respiratory rate
RRR	regular rate and rhythm; relative risk ratio
RSD	reflex sympathetic dystrophy
RSV	respiratory syncytial virus
RT	respiratory therapist; recreational therapy; renal transplabt, radiation therapy
RTx	radiation therapy; renal transplant
RUE	right upper extremity
RUG	resource utilization group
RUL	right upper lobe
RUQ	right upper quadrant
RV	right ventricle
RVRBS	relative value resource-based systems
RVU	relative value component
RW	rolling walker
Rx	drug; treatment; therapy; prescription
$\bar{s}$	without
S	sine (Latin); subjective; supervision
S & S	signs and symptoms
S/P	status post
SA	sinoatrial
SACH	solid ankle, cushion heel
SBA	stand-by assistance
SBQC	small-based quad cane
SC	sternoclavicular
SCC	sickle cell crisis
SCD	sickle cell disease; sequential compression device
SCFE	slipped capital femoral epiphysis
SCI	spinal cord injury
SCID	severe combined immunodeficiency disorder
SCM	sternocleidomastoid
SD	seizure disorder; standard deviation
SDAT	senile dementia, Alzheimer type
SDR	selective dorsal rhizotomy
sec	second
sed	sedimentation
SED	suberythemal dose
SGA	small for gestational age
SI	sacroiliac; sensory integration
SICU	surgical intensive care unit
SIDS	sudden infant death syndrome
SLC	short leg cast
SLE	systemic lupus erythematosus
SLP	speech-language pathology
SLR	straight leg raise

SMA	spinal muscular atrophy
SNF	skilled nursing facility
SOAP	subjective, objective, assessment, plan
SOB	short of breath
SOC	start of care
SOMR	source-oriented medical record
SPL	subjective pain level
SR	sinus rhythm
SSN	Social Security number
ST	speech therapy; speech therapist; straight
Stat	immediately
Stats	statistics
STD	sexually transmitted disease
STG	short-term goal
STM	soft tissue massage; short-term memory
Str	strength
STNR	symmetric tonic neck reflex
STSG	split-thickness skin graft
sup	superior; supination; supervision
SV	stroke volume
SVC	superior vena cava
SVD	spontaneous vaginal delivery
SWD	shortwave diathermy
Sx	symptoms
Sz	seizure
T	trace; temperature
T & A	tonsillectomy and adenoidectomy
TA	tricuspid atresia
TAH	total abdominal hysterectomy
TAR	total ankle replacement
TB	tuberculosis
TBA	to be announced
TBI	traumatic brain injury
TBSA	total body surface area
Tbsp	tablespoon
TCU	transitional care unit
TD	tardive dyskinesia
TEF	tracheoesophageal fistula
TENS	transcutaneous electrical nerve stimulation
TER	total elbow replacement
TES	threshold electrical stimulation
TGA	transposition of great arteries
THA	total hip arthroplasty
Ther ex	therapeutic exercise
THR	total hip replacement
TIA	transient ischemic attack
tid	three times a day
tin	three times a night
tiw	three times a week
TKA	total knee arthroplasty
TKE	terminal knee extension
TKR	total knee replacement
TLSO	thoracic lumbar spine orthosis
TMJ	temporomandibular joint
TO	telephone order
TOF	tetralogy of Fallot
TOS	thoracic outlet syndrome

TPN	total parenteral nutrition
TPR	temperature, pulse, and respiration
Trng	training
TS, T/S	thoracic spine
TSA	total shoulder arthroplasty
tsp	teaspoon
TTWB	toe-touch weight bearing
TUR	transurethral resection
Tx	treatment; traction; therapy; transplant
U	upper
UA	urinalysis
UE	upper extremity
UM	utilization management
UMN	upper motor neuron
UQ	upper quadrant
UR	utilization review
URI	upper respiratory infection
URO	utilization review organization
URQA	utilization review quality assurance
US	ultrasound
UTI	urinary tract infection
UV	ultraviolet
VA	Veterans Administration; visual acuity
VAD	ventricular assistive device; vertebral axial decompression
VAS	Visual Analogue Scale
VC	vital capacity
VD	venereal disease
vent	ventilator; ventilate
VLBW	very low birth weight
VO	verbal order
Vol	volume
VPA	valproic acid
VS	vital signs
VSD	ventricular septal defect
VT	ventricular tachycardia
W	walker; white
W/C, WC	wheelchair
W/O	without
WB	weight bearing
WBAT	weight bearing as tolerated
WBC	white blood cell; white blood count
WFL	within functional limits; within full limits
WHO	World Health Organization
WIC	women, infants, children
wk	week
WNL	within normal limits
wp, wpl	whirlpool
wt	weight
$\bar{x}$	except, times
XRT	radiation therapy
Yd	yard
y.o.	years old
yr	year

Appendix B

OASIS-D All Items. Center for Medicare & Medicaid Services; Baltimore, MD.

OMB #0938-1279 Expiration date 12/31/2021

Home Health Patient Tracking Sheet

(M0010) CMS Certification Number: ☐☐☐☐☐☐

(M0014) Branch State: ☐☐

(M0016) Branch ID Number: ☐☐☐☐☐☐☐☐☐☐

(M0018) National Provider Identifier (NPI) for the attending physician who has signed the plan of care:

☐☐☐☐☐☐☐☐☐☐ ☐ **UK – Unknown or Not Available**

(M0020) Patient ID Number: ☐☐☐☐☐☐☐☐☐☐☐☐☐☐☐☐☐☐☐☐

(M0030) Start of Care Date: ☐☐ / ☐☐ / ☐☐☐☐
month day year

(M0032) Resumption of Care Date: ☐☐ / ☐☐ / ☐☐☐☐ ☐ **NA – Not Applicable**
month day year

(M0040) Patient Name:

☐☐☐☐☐☐☐☐☐☐☐☐ ☐ ☐☐☐☐☐☐☐☐☐☐☐☐☐☐☐☐☐☐ ☐☐☐
(First) (M I) (Last) (Suffix)

(M0050) Patient State of Residence: ☐☐

(M0060) Patient ZIP Code: ☐☐☐☐☐ – ☐☐☐☐

(M0063) Medicare Number: ☐☐☐☐☐☐☐☐☐☐☐☐ ☐ **NA – No Medicare**
(including suffix)

(M0064) Social Security Number: ☐☐☐ - ☐☐ - ☐☐☐☐ ☐ **UK – Unknown or Not Available**

(M0065) Medicaid Number: ☐☐☐☐☐☐☐☐☐☐☐☐☐ ☐ **NA – No Medicaid**

(M0066) Birth Date: ☐☐ / ☐☐ / ☐☐☐☐
month day year

Outcome and Assessment Information Set OASIS-D Guidance Manual Effective January 1, 2019. Centers for Medicare & Medicaid Services; Baltimore, MD. Available at https://www.cms.gov/Medicare/Quality-Initiatives-Patient-Assessment-Instruments/HomeHealthQualityInits/Downloads/OASIS-D-Guidance-Manual-final.pdf. Accessed August 25, 2020.

(M0069) Gender	
Enter Code ☐	1 Male 2 Female

(M0140) Race/Ethnicity: (Mark all that apply.)

- ☐ 1 - American Indian or Alaska Native
- ☐ 2 - Asian
- ☐ 3 - Black or African-American
- ☐ 4 - Hispanic or Latino
- ☐ 5 - Native Hawaiian or Pacific Islander
- ☐ 6 - White

(M0150) Current Payment Sources for Home Care: (Mark all that apply.)

- ☐ 0 - None; no charge for current services
- ☐ 1 - Medicare (traditional fee-for-service)
- ☐ 2 - Medicare (HMO/managed care/Advantage plan)
- ☐ 3 - Medicaid (traditional fee-for-service)
- ☐ 4 - Medicaid (HMO/managed care)
- ☐ 5 - Workers' compensation
- ☐ 6 - Title programs (for example, Title III, V, or XX)
- ☐ 7 - Other government (for example, TriCare, VA)
- ☐ 8 - Private insurance
- ☐ 9 - Private HMO/managed care
- ☐ 10 - Self-pay
- ☐ 11 - Other (specify) ____________________
- ☐ UK - Unknown

Outcome and Assessment Information Set
Items to be Used at Specific Time Points

Time Point	Items Used
Start of Care	M0010-M0030, M0040-M0150, M1000-M1033, M1060-M1306, M1311-M2003, M2010, M2020-M2200, GG0100-GG0170
Start of care – further visits planned	
Resumption of Care	M0032, M0080-M0110, M1000-M1033, M1060-M1306, M1311-M2003, M2010, M2020-M2200, GG0100-GG0170
Resumption of care (after inpatient stay)	
Follow-Up	M0080-M0100, M0110, M1021- M1023, M1030, M1200-M1306, M1311-M1400, M1610-M1630, M1810-M1840, M1850-M1860, M2030, M2200, GG0130-GG0170
Recertification (follow-up) assessment Other follow-up assessment	
Transfer to an Inpatient Facility	M0080-M0100, M1041-M1056, M2005, M2016, M2301-M2410, M0906, J1800-J1900
Transferred to an inpatient facility – patient not discharged from an agency Transferred to an inpatient facility – patient discharged from agency	
Discharge from Agency – Not to an Inpatient Facility	
Death at home	M0080-M0100, M2005, M0906, J1800-J1900
Discharge from agency	M0080-M0100, M1041-M1056, M1242-M1311, M1324-M1330, M1334-M1600, M1620, M1700-M1720, M1740-M1870, M2005, M2016-M2020, M2102, M2301-M2420, M0906, GG0130-J1900

CLINICAL RECORD ITEMS

(M0080)	Discipline of Person Completing Assessment
Enter Code ☐	1 RN 2 PT 3 SLP/ST 4 OT

(M0090) Date Assessment Completed:

☐☐ / ☐☐ / ☐☐☐☐
month day year

(M0100)	This Assessment is Currently Being Completed for the Following Reason:
Enter Code ☐	**Start/Resumption of Care** 1 Start of care – further visits planned 3 Resumption of care (after inpatient stay) **Follow-Up** 4 Recertification (follow-up) reassessment ***[Go to M0110]*** 5 Other follow-up ***[Go to M0110]*** **Transfer to an Inpatient Facility** 6 Transferred to an inpatient facility – patient not discharged from agency ***[Go to M1041]*** 7 Transferred to an inpatient facility – patient discharged from agency ***[Go to M1041]*** **Discharge from Agency – Not to an Inpatient Facility** 8 Death at home ***[Go to M2005]*** 9 Discharge from agency ***[Go to M1041]***

CLINICAL RECORD ITEMS, continued

(M0102) Date of Physician-ordered Start of Care (Resumption of Care): If the physician indicated a specific start of care (resumption of care) date when the patient was referred for home health services, record the date specified.

☐☐ / ☐☐ / ☐☐☐☐ [*Go to M0110, if date entered*]
month day year

☐ NA - No specific SOC date ordered by physician

(M0104) Date of Referral: Indicate the date that the written or verbal referral for initiation or resumption of care was received by the HHA.

☐☐ / ☐☐ / ☐☐☐☐
month day year

(M0110)	**Episode Timing:** Is the Medicare home health payment episode for which this assessment will define a case mix group an "early" episode or a "later" episode in the patient's current sequence of adjacent Medicare home health payment episodes?
Enter Code ☐	1 Early 2 Later UK Unknown NA Not Applicable: No Medicare case mix group to be defined by this assessment.

PATIENT HISTORY AND DIAGNOSES

(M1000) From which of the following **Inpatient Facilities** was the patient discharged within the past 14 days? **(Mark all that apply.)**

☐ 1 - Long-term nursing facility (NF)

☐ 2 - Skilled nursing facility (SNF/TCU)

☐ 3 - Short-stay acute hospital (IPPS)

☐ 4 - Long-term care hospital (LTCH)

☐ 5 - Inpatient rehabilitation hospital or unit (IRF)

☐ 6 - Psychiatric hospital or unit

☐ 7 - Other (specify) ______________________

☐ NA - Patient was not discharged from an inpatient facility [*Go to M1021*]

(M1005) Inpatient Discharge Date (most recent):

☐☐ / ☐☐ / ☐☐☐☐
month day year

☐ UK - Unknown

PATIENT HISTORY AND DIAGNOSES, continued

(M1021/1023) Diagnoses and Symptom Control: List each diagnosis for which the patient is receiving home care in Column 1, and enter its ICD-10-CM code at the level of highest specificity in Column 2 (diagnosis codes only – no surgical or procedure codes allowed). Diagnoses are listed in the order that best reflects the seriousness of each condition and supports the disciplines and services provided. Rate the degree of symptom control for each condition in Column 2. ICD-10-CM sequencing requirements must be followed if multiple coding is indicated for any diagnoses.

Code each row according to the following directions for each column:

Column 1: Enter the description of the diagnosis. Sequencing of diagnoses should reflect the seriousness of each condition and support the disciplines and services provided.

Column 2: Enter the ICD-10-CM code for the condition described in Column 1 – no surgical or procedure codes allowed. Codes must be entered at the level of highest specificity and ICD-10-CM coding rules and sequencing requirements must be followed. Note that external cause codes (ICD-10-CM codes beginning with V, W, X, or Y) may not be reported in M1021 (Primary Diagnosis) but may be reported in M1023 (Secondary Diagnoses). Also note that when a Z-code is reported in Column 2, the code for the underlying condition can often be entered in Column 2, as long as it is an active on-going condition impacting home health care.

Rate the degree of symptom control for the condition listed in Column 1. Do not assign a symptom control rating if the diagnosis code is a V, W, X, Y or Z-code. Choose one value that represents the degree of symptom control appropriate for each diagnosis using the following scale:

0 - Asymptomatic, no treatment needed at this time
1 - Symptoms well controlled with current therapy
2 - Symptoms controlled with difficulty, affecting daily functioning; patient needs ongoing monitoring
3 - Symptoms poorly controlled; patient needs frequent adjustment in treatment and dose monitoring
4 - Symptoms poorly controlled; history of re-hospitalizations

Note that the rating for symptom control in Column 2 should not be used to determine the sequencing of the diagnoses listed in Column 1. These are separate items and sequencing may not coincide.

(Form on next page)

(M1021) Primary Diagnosis & (M1023) Other Diagnoses	
Column 1	**Column 2**
Diagnoses (Sequencing of diagnoses should reflect the seriousness of each condition and support the disciplines and services provided)	ICD-10-CM and symptom control rating for each condition. Note that the sequencing of these ratings may not match the sequencing of the diagnoses
Description	ICD-10-CM / Symptom Control Rating
(M1021) Primary Diagnosis a. ____________	**V, W, X, Y codes NOT allowed** a. ☐☐☐ ☐☐☐☐ ☐0 ☐1 ☐2 ☐3 ☐4
(M1023) Other Diagnoses b. ____________	**All ICD-10–CM codes allowed** b. ☐☐☐ ☐☐☐☐ ☐0 ☐1 ☐2 ☐3 ☐4
c. ____________	c. ☐☐☐ ☐☐☐☐ ☐0 ☐1 ☐2 ☐3 ☐4
d. ____________	d. ☐☐☐ ☐☐☐☐ ☐0 ☐1 ☐2 ☐3 ☐4
e. ____________	e. ☐☐☐ ☐☐☐☐ ☐0 ☐1 ☐2 ☐3 ☐4
f. ____________	f. ☐☐☐ ☐☐☐☐ ☐0 ☐1 ☐2 ☐3 ☐4

(M1028) Active Diagnoses – Comorbidities and Co-existing Conditions – Check all that apply
See OASIS Guidance Manual for a complete list of relevant ICD-10 codes.

- ☐ 1 - Peripheral Vascular Disease (PVD) or Peripheral Arterial Disease (PAD)
- ☐ 2 - Diabetes Mellitus (DM)
- ☐ 3 - None of the above

(M1030) Therapies the patient receives at home: **(Mark all that apply.)**

- ☐ 1 - Intravenous or infusion therapy (excludes TPN)
- ☐ 2 - Parenteral nutrition (TPN or lipids)
- ☐ 3 - Enteral nutrition (nasogastric, gastrostomy, jejunostomy, or any other artificial entry into the alimentary canal)
- ☐ 4 - None of the above

PATIENT HISTORY AND DIAGNOSES, continued

(M1033) Risk for Hospitalization: Which of the following signs or symptoms characterize this patient as at risk for hospitalization? **(Mark all that apply.)**

- ☐ 1 - History of falls (2 or more falls – or any fall with an injury – in the past 12 months)
- ☐ 2 - Unintentional weight loss of a total of 10 pounds or more in the past 12 months
- ☐ 3 - Multiple hospitalizations (2 or more) in the past 6 months
- ☐ 4 - Multiple emergency department visits (2 or more) in the past 6 months
- ☐ 5 - Decline in mental, emotional, or behavioral status in the past 3 months
- ☐ 6 - Reported or observed history of difficulty complying with any medical instructions (for example, medications, diet, exercise) in the past 3 months
- ☐ 7 - Currently taking 5 or more medications
- ☐ 8 - Currently reports exhaustion
- ☐ 9 - Other risk(s) not listed in 1 - 8
- ☐ 10 - None of the above

(M1041)	**Influenza Vaccine Data Collection Period:** Does this episode of care (SOC/ROC to Transfer/Discharge) include any dates on or between October 1 and March 31?
Enter Code ☐	0 No ***[Go to M1051]*** 1 Yes
(M1046)	**Influenza Vaccine Received:** Did the patient receive the influenza vaccine for this year's flu season?
Enter Code ☐	1 Yes; received from your agency during this episode of care (SOC/ROC to Transfer/Discharge) 2 Yes; received from your agency during a prior episode of care (SOC/ROC to Transfer/Discharge) 3 Yes; received from another health care provider (for example, physician, pharmacist) 4 No; patient offered and declined 5 No; patient assessed and determined to have medical contraindication(s) 6 No; not indicated – patient does not meet age/condition guidelines for influenza vaccine 7 No; inability to obtain vaccine due to declared shortage 8 No; patient did not receive the vaccine due to reasons other than those listed in responses 4-7.
(M1051)	**Pneumococcal Vaccine:** Has the patient ever received the pneumococcal vaccination (for example, pneumovax)?
Enter Code ☐	0 No 1 Yes ***[Go to M2005 at TRN; Go to M1242 at DC]***
(M1056)	**Reason Pneumococcal Vaccine not received:** If patient has never received the pneumococcal vaccination (for example, pneumovax), state reason:
Enter Code ☐	1 Offered and declined 2 Assessed and determined to have medical contraindication(s) 3 Not indicated; patient does not meet age/condition guidelines for Pneumococcal Vaccine 4 None of the above

(M1060) Height and Weight – While measuring, if the number is X.1-X.4 round down; X.5 or greater round up

☐☐ inches — a. Height (in inches). Record most recent height measure since the most recent SOC/ROC

☐☐☐ pounds — b. Weight (in pounds). Base weight on most recent measure in last 30 days; measure weight consistently, according to standard agency practice (for example, in a.m. after voiding, before meal, with shoes off, etc.)

LIVING ARRANGEMENTS

(M1100) Patient Living Situation: Which of the following best describes the patient's residential circumstance and availability of assistance? **(Check one box only.)**

	Availability of Assistance				
Living Arrangement	Around the clock	Regular daytime	Regular nighttime	Occasional / short-term assistance	No assistance available
a. Patient lives alone	☐ 01	☐ 02	☐ 03	☐ 04	☐ 05
b. Patient lives with other person(s) in the home	☐ 06	☐ 07	☐ 08	☐ 09	☐ 10
c. Patient lives in congregate situation (for example, assisted living, residential care home)	☐ 11	☐ 12	☐ 13	☐ 14	☐ 15

SENSORY STATUS

(M1200)	**Vision** (with corrective lenses if the patient usually wears them):
Enter Code ☐	0 Normal vision: sees adequately in most situations; can see medication labels, newsprint. 1 Partially impaired: cannot see medication labels or newsprint, but <u>can</u> see obstacles in path, and the surrounding layout; can count fingers at arm's length. 2 Severely impaired: cannot locate objects without hearing or touching them, or patient nonresponsive.
(M1242)	**Frequency of Pain Interfering** with patient's activity or movement:
Enter Code ☐	0 Patient has no pain 1 Patient has pain that does not interfere with activity or movement 2 Less often than daily 3 Daily, but not constantly 4 All of the time

INTEGUMENTARY STATUS

(M1306)	Does this patient have at least one **Unhealed Pressure Ulcer/Injury at Stage 2 or Higher** or designated as Unstageable? (Excludes Stage 1 pressure injuries and all healed pressure ulcers/injuries)
Enter Code ☐	0 No ***[Go to M1322 at SOC/ROC/FU; Go to M1324 at DC]*** 1 Yes
(M1307)	The **Oldest Stage 2 Pressure Ulcer** that is present at discharge: (Excludes healed Stage 2 pressure ulcers)
Enter Code ☐	1 Was present at the most recent SOC/ROC assessment 2 Developed since the most recent SOC/ROC assessment. Record date pressure ulcer first identified: ☐☐ / ☐☐ / ☐☐☐☐ month day year NA No Stage 2 pressure ulcers are present at discharge

SOC/ROC

(M1311) Current Number of Unhealed Pressure Ulcers/Injuries at Each Stage	Enter Number
A1. Stage 2: Partial thickness loss of dermis presenting as a shallow open ulcer with a red or pink wound bed, without slough. May also present as an intact or open/ruptured blister. **Number of Stage 2 pressure ulcers**	☐
B1. Stage 3: Full thickness tissue loss. Subcutaneous fat may be visible but bone, tendon, or muscle is not exposed. Slough may be present but does not obscure the depth of tissue loss. May include undermining and tunneling. **Number of Stage 3 pressure ulcers**	☐
C1. Stage 4: Full thickness tissue loss with exposed bone, tendon, or muscle. Slough or eschar may be present on some parts of the wound bed. Often includes undermining and tunneling. **Number of Stage 4 pressure ulcers**	☐
D1. Unstageable: Non-removable dressing/device: Known but not stageable due to non-removable dressing/device **Number of unstageable pressure ulcers/injuries due to non-removable dressing/device**	☐
E1. Unstageable: Slough and/or eschar: Known but not stageable due to coverage of wound bed by slough and/or eschar **Number of unstageable pressure ulcers due to coverage of wound bed by slough and/or eschar**	☐
F1. Unstageable: Deep tissue injury **Number of unstageable pressure injuries presenting as deep tissue injury**	☐

Follow-Up

(M1311) Current Number of Unhealed Pressure Ulcers/Injuries at Each Stage	Enter Number
A1. **Stage 2:** Partial thickness loss of dermis presenting as a shallow open ulcer with a red or pink wound bed, without slough. May also present as an intact or open/ruptured blister. **Number of Stage 2 pressure ulcers**	☐
B1. **Stage 3:** Full thickness tissue loss. Subcutaneous fat may be visible but bone, tendon, or muscle is not exposed. Slough may be present but does not obscure the depth of tissue loss. May include undermining and tunneling. **Number of Stage 3 pressure ulcers**	☐
C1. **Stage 4:** Full thickness tissue loss with exposed bone, tendon, or muscle. Slough or eschar may be present on some parts of the wound bed. Often includes undermining and tunneling. **Number of Stage 4 pressure ulcers**	☐
D1. **Unstageable: Non-removable dressing/device**: Known but not stageable due to non-removable dressing/device **Number of unstageable pressure ulcers/injuries due to non-removable dressing/device**	☐
E1. **Unstageable: Slough and/or eschar:** Known but not stageable due to coverage of wound bed by slough and/or eschar **Number of unstageable pressure ulcers due to coverage of wound bed by slough and/or eschar**	☐
F1. **Unstageable: Deep tissue injury** **Number of unstageable pressure injuries presenting as deep tissue injury**	☐

INTEGUMENTARY STATUS, continued

Discharge

(M1311) Current Number of Unhealed Pressure Ulcers/Injuries at Each Stage	Enter Number
A1. Stage 2: Partial thickness loss of dermis presenting as a shallow open ulcer with a red or pink wound bed, without slough. May also present as an intact or open/ruptured blister. **Number of Stage 2 pressure ulcers** [If 0 – Go to M1311B1, Stage 3]	☐
A2. Number of <u>these</u> Stage 2 pressure ulcers that were present at most recent SOC/ROC – enter how many were noted at the time of most recent SOC/ROC	☐
B1. Stage 3: Full thickness tissue loss. Subcutaneous fat may be visible but bone, tendon, or muscle is not exposed. Slough may be present but does not obscure the depth of tissue loss. May include undermining and tunneling. **Number of Stage 3 pressure ulcers** [If 0 – Go to M1311C1, Stage 4]	☐
B2. Number of <u>these</u> Stage 3 pressure ulcers that were present at most recent SOC/ROC – enter how many were noted at the time of most recent SOC/ROC	☐
C1. Stage 4: Full thickness tissue loss with exposed bone, tendon, or muscle. Slough or eschar may be present on some parts of the wound bed. Often includes undermining and tunneling. **Number of Stage 4 pressure ulcers** [If 0 – Go to M1311D1, Unstageable: Non-removable dressing/device]	☐
C2. Number of <u>these</u> Stage 4 pressure ulcers that were present at most recent SOC/ROC – enter how many were noted at the time of most recent SOC/ROC	☐
D1. Unstageable: Non-removable dressing/device: Known but not stageable due to non-removable dressing/device **Number of unstageable pressure ulcers/injuries due to non-removable dressing/device** [If 0 – Go to M1311E1, Unstageable: Slough and/or eschar]	☐
D2. Number of <u>these</u> unstageable pressure ulcers/injuries that were present at most recent SOC/ROC – enter how many were noted at the time of most recent SOC/ROC	☐
E1. Unstageable: Slough and/or eschar: Known but not stageable due to coverage of wound bed by slough and/or eschar **Number of unstageable pressure ulcers due to coverage of wound bed by slough and/or eschar** [If 0 – Go to M1311F1, Unstageable: Deep tissue injury]	☐
E2. Number of <u>these</u> unstageable pressure ulcers that were present at most recent SOC/ROC – enter how many were noted at the time of most recent SOC/ROC	☐
F1. Unstageable: Deep tissue injury **Number of unstageable pressure injuries presenting as deep tissue injury** [If 0 – Go to M1324]	☐
F2. Number of <u>these</u> unstageable pressure injuries that were present at most recent SOC/ROC – enter how many were noted at the time of most recent SOC/ROC	☐

(M1322)	**Current Number of Stage 1 Pressure Injuries:** Intact skin with non-blanchable redness of a localized area usually over a bony prominence. Darkly pigmented skin may not have a visible blanching; in dark skin tones only it may appear with persistent blue or purple hues.
Enter Code ☐	0 1 2 3 4 or more
(M1324)	**Stage of Most Problematic Unhealed Pressure Ulcer/Injury that is Stageable:** (Excludes pressure ulcer/injury that cannot be staged due to a non-removable dressing/device, coverage of wound bed by slough and/or eschar, or deep tissue injury.)
Enter Code ☐	1 Stage 1 2 Stage 2 3 Stage 3 4 Stage 4 NA Patient has no pressure ulcers/injuries or no stageable pressure ulcers/injuries
(M1330)	Does this patient have a **Stasis Ulcer**?
Enter Code ☐	0 No ***[Go to M1340]*** 1 Yes, patient has BOTH observable and unobservable stasis ulcers 2 Yes, patient has observable stasis ulcers ONLY 3 Yes, patient has unobservable stasis ulcers ONLY (known but not observable due to non-removable dressing/device) ***[Go to M1340]***
(M1332)	**Current Number of Stasis Ulcer(s) that are Observable:**
Enter Code ☐	1 One 2 Two 3 Three 4 Four or more
(M1334)	**Status of Most Problematic Stasis Ulcer that is Observable:**
Enter Code ☐	1 Fully granulating 2 Early/partial granulation 3 Not healing
(M1340)	Does this patient have a **Surgical Wound?**
Enter Code ☐	0 No ***[Go to M1400]*** 1 Yes, patient has at least one observable surgical wound 2 Surgical wound known but not observable due to non-removable dressing/device ***[Go to M1400]***
(M1342)	**Status of Most Problematic Surgical Wound that is Observable**
Enter Code ☐	0 Newly epithelialized 1 Fully granulating 2 Early/partial granulation 3 Not healing

RESPIRATORY STATUS

(M1400)	When is the patient dyspneic or noticeably **Short of Breath**?
Enter Code ☐	0 Patient is not short of breath 1 When walking more than 20 feet, climbing stairs 2 With moderate exertion (for example, while dressing, using commode or bedpan, walking distances less than 20 feet) 3 With minimal exertion (for example, while eating, talking, or performing other ADLs) or with agitation 4 At rest (during day or night)

ELIMINATION STATUS

(M1600)	Has this patient been treated for a **Urinary Tract Infection** in the past 14 days?
Enter Code ☐	0 No 1 Yes NA Patient on prophylactic treatment UK Unknown **[*Omit "UK" option on DC*]**
(M1610)	**Urinary Incontinence or Urinary Catheter Presence:**
Enter Code ☐	0 No incontinence or catheter (includes anuria or ostomy for urinary drainage) 1 Patient is incontinent 2 Patient requires a urinary catheter (specifically: external, indwelling, intermittent, or suprapubic)
(M1620)	**Bowel Incontinence Frequency:**
Enter Code ☐	0 Very rarely or never has bowel incontinence 1 Less than once weekly 2 One to three times weekly 3 Four to six times weekly 4 On a daily basis 5 More often than once daily NA Patient has ostomy for bowel elimination UK Unknown **[*Omit "UK" option on FU, DC*]**
(M1630)	**Ostomy for Bowel Elimination:** Does this patient have an ostomy for bowel elimination that (within the last 14 days): a) was related to an inpatient facility stay; <u>or</u> b) necessitated a change in medical or treatment regimen?
Enter Code ☐	0 Patient does <u>not</u> have an ostomy for bowel elimination. 1 Patient's ostomy was <u>not</u> related to an inpatient stay and did <u>not</u> necessitate change in medical or treatment regimen. 2 The ostomy <u>was</u> related to an inpatient stay or <u>did</u> necessitate change in medical or treatment regimen.

NEURO/EMOTIONAL/BEHAVIORAL STATUS

(M1700)	**Cognitive Functioning:** Patient's current (day of assessment) level of alertness, orientation, comprehension, concentration, and immediate memory for simple commands.
Enter Code ☐	0 Alert/oriented, able to focus and shift attention, comprehends and recalls task directions independently. 1 Requires prompting (cuing, repetition, reminders) only under stressful or unfamiliar conditions. 2 Requires assistance and some direction in specific situations (for example, on all tasks involving shifting of attention) or consistently requires low stimulus environment due to distractibility. 3 Requires considerable assistance in routine situations. Is not alert and oriented or is unable to shift attention and recall directions more than half the time. 4 Totally dependent due to disturbances such as constant disorientation, coma, persistent vegetative state, or delirium.
(M1710)	**When Confused (Reported or Observed Within the Last 14 Days):**
Enter Code ☐	0 Never 1 In new or complex situations only 2 On awakening or at night only 3 During the day and evening, but not constantly 4 Constantly NA Patient nonresponsive
(M1720)	**When Anxious (Reported or Observed Within the Last 14 Days):**
Enter Code ☐	0 None of the time 1 Less often than daily 2 Daily, but not constantly 3 All of the time NA Patient nonresponsive
(M1730)	**Depression Screening:** Has the patient been screened for depression, using a standardized, validated depression screening tool?
Enter Code ☐	0 No 1 Yes, patient was screened using the PHQ-2©* scale.

Instructions for this two-question tool: Ask patient: "Over the last two weeks, how often have you been bothered by any of the following problems?"

PHQ-2©*	Not at all 0-1 day	Several days 2-6 days	More than half of the days 7-11 days	Nearly every day 12-14 days	NA Unable to respond
a) Little interest or pleasure in doing things	☐0	☐1	☐2	☐3	☐NA
b) Feeling down, depressed, or hopeless?	☐0	☐1	☐2	☐3	☐NA

2 Yes, patient was screened with a different standardized, validated assessment and the patient meets criteria for further evaluation for depression.
3 Yes, patient was screened with a different standardized, validated assessment and the patient does not meet criteria for further evaluation for depression.

(M1740) **Cognitive, behavioral, and psychiatric symptoms** that are demonstrated <u>at least once a week</u> **(Reported or Observed): (Mark all that apply.)**

- ☐ 1 - Memory deficit: failure to recognize familiar persons/places, inability to recall events of past 24 hours, significant memory loss so that supervision is required
- ☐ 2 - Impaired decision-making: failure to perform usual ADLs or ADLs inability to appropriately stop activities, jeopardizes safety through actions
- ☐ 3 - Verbal disruption: yelling, threatening, excessive profanity, sexual references, etc.
- ☐ 4 - Physical aggression: aggressive or combative to self and others (for example, hits self, throws objects, punches, dangerous maneuvers with wheelchair or other objects)
- ☐ 5 - Disruptive, infantile, or socially inappropriate behavior (**excludes** verbal actions)
- ☐ 6 - Delusional, hallucinatory, or paranoid behavior
- ☐ 7 - None of the above behaviors demonstrated

(M1745)	**Frequency of Disruptive Behavior Symptoms (Reported or Observed):** Any physical, verbal, or other disruptive/dangerous symptoms that are injurious to self or others or jeopardize personal safety.
Enter Code ☐	0 Never 1 Less than once a month 2 Once a month 3 Several times each month 4 Several times a week 5 At least daily

<u>ADL/IADLs</u>

(M1800)	**Grooming:** Current ability to tend safely to personal hygiene needs (specifically: washing face and hands, hair care, shaving or make up, teeth or denture care, or fingernail care).
Enter Code ☐	0 Able to groom self unaided, with or without the use of assistive devices or adapted methods. 1 Grooming utensils must be placed within reach before able to complete grooming activities. 2 Someone must assist the patient to groom self. 3 Patient depends entirely upon someone else for grooming needs.
(M1810)	Current **Ability to Dress <u>Upper</u> Body** safely (with or without dressing aids) including undergarments, pullovers, front-opening shirts and blouses, managing zippers, buttons, and snaps:
Enter Code ☐	0 Able to get clothes out of closets and drawers, put them on and remove them from the upper body without assistance. 1 Able to dress upper body without assistance if clothing is laid out or handed to the patient. 2 Someone must help the patient put on upper body clothing. 3 Patient depends entirely upon another person to dress the upper body.
(M1820)	Current **Ability to Dress <u>Lower</u> Body** safely (with or without dressing aids) including undergarments, slacks, socks or nylons, shoes:
Enter Code ☐	0 Able to obtain, put on, and remove clothing and shoes without assistance. 1 Able to dress lower body without assistance if clothing and shoes are laid out or handed to the patient. 2 Someone must help the patient put on undergarments, slacks, socks or nylons, and shoes. 3 Patient depends entirely upon another person to dress lower body.

ADL/IADLs, continued

(M1830)	**Bathing:** Current ability to wash entire body safely. **Excludes grooming (washing face, washing hands, and shampooing hair).**
Enter Code ☐	0 Able to bathe self in shower or tub independently, including getting in and out of tub/shower. 1 With the use of devices, is able to bathe self in shower or tub independently, including getting in and out of the tub/shower. 2 Able to bathe in shower or tub with the intermittent assistance of another person: (a) for intermittent supervision or encouragement or reminders, OR (b) to get in and out of the shower or tub, OR (c) for washing difficult to reach areas. 3 Able to participate in bathing self in shower or tub, but requires presence of another person throughout the bath for assistance or supervision. 4 Unable to use the shower or tub, but able to bathe self independently with or without the use of devices at the sink, in chair, or on commode. 5 Unable to use the shower or tub, but able to participate in bathing self in bed, at the sink, in bedside chair, or on commode, with the assistance or supervision of another person. 6 Unable to participate effectively in bathing and is bathed totally by another person.
(M1840)	**Toilet Transferring:** Current ability to get to and from the toilet or bedside commode safely and transfer on and off toilet/commode.
Enter Code ☐	0 Able to get to and from the toilet and transfer independently with or without a device. 1 When reminded, assisted, or supervised by another person, able to get to and from the toilet and transfer. 2 Unable to get to and from the toilet but is able to use a bedside commode (with or without assistance). 3 Unable to get to and from the toilet or bedside commode but is able to use a bedpan/urinal independently. 4 Is totally dependent in toileting.
(M1845)	**Toileting Hygiene:** Current ability to maintain perineal hygiene safely, adjust clothes and/or incontinence pads before and after using toilet, commode, bedpan, urinal. If managing ostomy, includes cleaning area around stoma, but not managing equipment.
Enter Code ☐	0 Able to manage toileting hygiene and clothing management without assistance. 1 Able to manage toileting hygiene and clothing management without assistance if supplies/implements are laid out for the patient. 2 Someone must help the patient to maintain toileting hygiene and/or adjust clothing. 3 Patient depends entirely upon another person to maintain toileting hygiene.
(M1850)	**Transferring:** Current ability to move safely from bed to chair, or ability to turn and position self in bed if patient is bedfast.
Enter Code ☐	0 Able to independently transfer. 1 Able to transfer with minimal human assistance or with use of an assistive device. 2 Able to bear weight and pivot during the transfer process but unable to transfer self. 3 Unable to transfer self and is unable to bear weight or pivot when transferred by another person. 4 Bedfast, unable to transfer but is able to turn and position self in bed. 5 Bedfast, unable to transfer and is unable to turn and position self.

ADL/IADLs, continued

(M1860)	**Ambulation/Locomotion:** Current ability to walk safely, once in a standing position, or use a wheelchair, once in a seated position, on a variety of surfaces.
Enter Code ☐	0 Able to independently walk on even and uneven surfaces and negotiate stairs with or without railings (specifically: needs no human assistance or assistive device). 1 With the use of a one-handed device (for example, cane, single crutch, hemi-walker), able to independently walk on even and uneven surfaces and negotiate stairs with or without railings. 2 Requires use of a two-handed device (for example, walker or crutches) to walk alone on a level surface and/or requires human supervision or assistance to negotiate stairs or steps or uneven surfaces. 3 Able to walk only with the supervision or assistance of another person at all times. 4 Chairfast, unable to ambulate but is able to wheel self independently. 5 Chairfast, unable to ambulate and is unable to wheel self. 6 Bedfast, unable to ambulate or be up in a chair.
(M1870)	**Feeding or Eating:** Current ability to feed self meals and snacks safely. Note: This refers only to the process of eating, chewing, and swallowing, not preparing the food to be eaten.
Enter Code ☐	0 Able to independently feed self. 1 Able to feed self independently but requires: (a) meal set-up; OR (b) intermittent assistance or supervision from another person; OR (c) a liquid, pureed or ground meat diet. 2 Unable to feed self and must be assisted or supervised throughout the meal/snack. 3 Able to take in nutrients orally and receives supplemental nutrients through a nasogastric tube or gastrostomy. 4 Unable to take in nutrients orally and is fed nutrients through a nasogastric tube or gastrostomy. 5 Unable to take in nutrients orally or by tube feeding.
(M1910)	Has this patient had a multi-factor **Falls Risk Assessment** using a standardized, validated assessment tool?
Enter Code ☐	0 No. 1 Yes, and it does not indicate a risk for falls. 2 Yes, and it does indicate a risk for falls.

MEDICATIONS

(M2001)	**Drug Regimen Review:** Did a complete drug regimen review identify potential clinically significant medication issues?
Enter Code ☐	0 No – No issues found during review ***[Go to M2010]*** 1 Yes – Issues found during review 9 NA – Patient is not taking any medications ***[Go to M2102]***
(M2003)	**Medication Follow-up:** Did the agency contact a physician (or physician-designee) by midnight of the next calendar day and complete prescribed/recommended actions in response to the identified potential clinically significant medication issues?
Enter Code ☐	0 No 1 Yes
(M2005)	**Medication Intervention:** Did the agency contact and complete physician (or physician-designee) prescribed/recommended actions by midnight of the next calendar day each time potential clinically significant medication issues were identified since the SOC/ROC?
Enter Code ☐	0 No 1 Yes 9 NA – There were no potential clinically significant medication issues identified since SOC/ROC or patient is not taking any medications
(M2010)	**Patient/Caregiver High-Risk Drug Education:** Has the patient/caregiver received instruction on special precautions for all high-risk medications (such as hypoglycemics, anticoagulants, etc.) and how and when to report problems that may occur?
Enter Code ☐	0 No 1 Yes NA Patient not taking any high-risk drugs OR patient/caregiver fully knowledgeable about special precautions associated with all high-risk medications
(M2016)	**Patient/Caregiver Drug Education Intervention**: At the time of, or at any time since the most recent SOC/ROC assessment, was the patient/caregiver instructed by agency staff or other health care provider to monitor the effectiveness of drug therapy, adverse drug reactions, and significant side effects, and how and when to report problems that may occur?
Enter Code ☐	0 No 1 Yes NA Patient not taking any drugs
(M2020)	**Management of Oral Medications:** Patient's current ability to prepare and take all oral medications reliably and safely, including administration of the correct dosage at the appropriate times/intervals. **Excludes injectable and IV medications. (NOTE: This refers to ability, not compliance or willingness.)**
Enter Code ☐	0 Able to independently take the correct oral medication(s) and proper dosage(s) at the correct times. 1 Able to take medication(s) at the correct times if: (a) individual dosages are prepared in advance by another person; OR (b) another person develops a drug diary or chart. 2 Able to take medication(s) at the correct times if given reminders by another person at the appropriate times 3 Unable to take medication unless administered by another person. NA No oral medications prescribed.

(M2030)	**Management of Injectable Medications:** Patient's current ability to prepare and take all prescribed injectable medications reliably and safely, including administration of correct dosage at the appropriate times/intervals. **Excludes IV medications.**
Enter Code ☐	0 Able to independently take the correct medication(s) and proper dosage(s) at the correct times. 1 Able to take injectable medication(s) at the correct times if: (a) individual syringes are prepared in advance by another person; OR (b) another person develops a drug diary or chart. 2 Able to take medication(s) at the correct times if given reminders by another person based on the frequency of the injection 3 Unable to take injectable medication unless administered by another person. NA No injectable medications prescribed.

CARE MANAGEMENT

SOC/ROC

(M2102)	**Types and Sources of Assistance:** Determine the ability and willingness of non-agency caregivers (such as family members, friends, or privately paid caregivers) to provide assistance for the following activities, if assistance is needed. Excludes all care by your agency staff.
Enter Code ☐	f. **Supervision and safety** (for example, due to cognitive impairment) 0 No assistance needed –patient is independent or does not have needs in this area 1 Non-agency caregiver(s) currently provide assistance 2 Non-agency caregiver(s) need training/ supportive services to provide assistance 3 Non-agency caregiver(s) are not likely to provide assistance OR it is unclear if they will provide assistance 4 Assistance needed, but no non-agency caregiver(s) available

Discharge

(M2102)	**Types and Sources of Assistance:** Determine the ability and willingness of non-agency caregivers (such as family members, friends, or privately paid caregivers) to provide assistance for the following activities, if assistance is needed. Excludes all care by your agency staff.
Enter Code ☐	a. **ADL assistance** (for example, transfer/ ambulation, bathing, dressing, toileting, eating/feeding) 0 No assistance needed –patient is independent or does not have needs in this area 1 Non-agency caregiver(s) currently provide assistance 2 Non-agency caregiver(s) need training/ supportive services to provide assistance 3 Non-agency caregiver(s) are not likely to provide assistance OR it is unclear if they will provide assistance 4 Assistance needed, but no non-agency caregiver(s) available
Enter Code ☐	c. **Medication administration** (for example, oral, inhaled or injectable) 0 No assistance needed –patient is independent or does not have needs in this area 1 Non-agency caregiver(s) currently provide assistance 2 Non-agency caregiver(s) need training/ supportive services to provide assistance 3 Non-agency caregiver(s) are not likely to provide assistance OR it is unclear if they will provide assistance 4 Assistance needed, but no non-agency caregiver(s) available
Enter Code ☐	d. **Medical procedures/ treatments** (for example, changing wound dressing, home exercise program) 0 No assistance needed –patient is independent or does not have needs in this area 1 Non-agency caregiver(s) currently provide assistance 2 Non-agency caregiver(s) need training/ supportive services to provide assistance 3 Non-agency caregiver(s) are not likely to provide assistance OR it is unclear if they will provide assistance 4 Assistance needed, but no non-agency caregiver(s) available
Enter Code ☐	f. **Supervision and safety** (for example, due to cognitive impairment) 0 No assistance needed –patient is independent or does not have needs in this area 1 Non-agency caregiver(s) currently provide assistance 2 Non-agency caregiver(s) need training/ supportive services to provide assistance 3 Non-agency caregiver(s) are not likely to provide assistance OR it is unclear if they will provide assistance 4 Assistance needed, but no non-agency caregiver(s) available

THERAPY NEED AND PLAN OF CARE

(M2200) Therapy Need: In the home health plan of care for the Medicare payment episode for which this assessment will define a case mix group, what is the indicated need for therapy visits (total of reasonable and necessary physical, occupational, and speech-language pathology visits combined)? **(Enter zero ["000"] if no therapy visits indicated.)**

(☐☐☐) Number of therapy visits indicated (total of physical, occupational and speech-language pathology combined).

☐ NA - Not Applicable: No case mix group defined by this assessment.

EMERGENT CARE

(M2301)	**Emergent Care:** At the time of or at any time since the most recent SOC/ROC assessment has the patient utilized a hospital emergency department (includes holding/observation status)?
Enter Code ☐	0 No ***[Go to M2401]*** 1 Yes, used hospital emergency department WITHOUT hospital admission 2 Yes, used hospital emergency department WITH hospital admission UK Unknown ***[Go to M2401]***

(M2310) Reason for Emergent Care: For what reason(s) did the patient seek and/or receive emergent care (with or without hospitalization)? **(Mark all that apply.)**

☐ 1 - Improper medication administration, adverse drug reactions, medication side effects, toxicity, anaphylaxis

☐ 10 - Hypo/Hyperglycemia, diabetes out of control

☐ 19 - Other than above reasons

☐ UK - Reason unknown

DATA ITEMS COLLECTED AT INPATIENT FACILITY ADMISSION OR AGENCY DISCHARGE ONLY

(M2401) Intervention Synopsis: (Check only **one** box in each row.) At the time of or at any time since the most recent SOC/ROC assessment, were the following interventions BOTH included in the physician-ordered plan of care AND implemented?

Plan / Intervention	No	Yes	Not Applicable	
a. Diabetic foot care including monitoring for the presence of skin lesions on the lower extremities and patient/caregiver education on proper foot care	☐0	☐1	☐NA	Patient is not diabetic or is missing lower legs due to congenital or acquired condition (bilateral amputee).
b. Falls prevention interventions	☐0	☐1	☐NA	Every standardized, validated multi-factor fall risk assessment conducted at or since the most recent SOC/ROC assessment indicates the patient has no risk for falls.
c. Depression intervention(s) such as medication, referral for other treatment, or a monitoring plan for current treatment	☐0	☐1	☐NA	Patient has no diagnosis of depression AND every standardized validated depression screening conducted at or since the most recent SOC/ROC assessment indicates the patient has: 1) no symptoms of depression; or 2) has some symptoms of depression but does not meet criteria for further evaluation of depression based on screening tool used.
d. Intervention(s) to monitor and mitigate pain	☐0	☐1	☐NA	Every standardized, validated pain assessment conducted at or since the most recent SOC/ROC assessment indicates the patient has no pain.
e. Intervention(s) to prevent pressure ulcers	☐0	☐1	☐NA	Every standardized, validated pressure ulcer risk assessment conducted at or since the most recent SOC/ROC assessment indicates the patient is not at risk of developing pressure ulcers.
f. Pressure ulcer treatment based on principles of moist wound healing	☐0	☐1	☐NA	Patient has no pressure ulcers OR has no pressure ulcers for which moist wound healing is indicated.

(M2410)	To which **Inpatient Facility** has the patient been admitted?
Enter Code ☐	1 Hospital 2 Rehabilitation facility 3 Nursing home 4 Hospice NA No inpatient facility admission **[*Omit "NA" option on TRN*]**
(M2420)	**Discharge Disposition:** Where is the patient after discharge from your agency? **(Choose only one answer.)**
Enter Code ☐	1 Patient remained in the community (without formal assistive services) 2 Patient remained in the community (with formal assistive services) 3 Patient transferred to a non-institutional hospice 4 Unknown because patient moved to a geographic location not served by this agency UK Other unknown

(M0906) Discharge/Transfer/Death Date: Enter the date of the discharge, transfer, or death (at home) of the patient.

☐☐ / ☐☐ / ☐☐☐☐
month day year

Section GG	Functional Abilities and Goals

GG0100. Prior Functioning: Everyday Activities: Indicate the patient's usual ability with everyday activities prior to the current illness, exacerbation, or injury.

Coding:	↓ Enter Codes in Boxes	
3. Independent – Patient completed the activities by him/herself, with or without an assistive device, with no assistance from a helper. **2. Needed Some Help** – Patient needed partial assistance from another person to complete activities. **1. Dependent** – A helper completed the activities for the patient. **8. Unknown** **9. Not Applicable**	☐	**A. Self Care:** Code the patient's need for assistance with bathing, dressing, using the toilet, or eating prior to the current illness, exacerbation, or injury.
	☐	**B. Indoor Mobility (Ambulation):** Code the patient's need for assistance with walking from room to room (with or without a device such as cane, crutch or walker) prior to the current illness, exacerbation, or injury.
	☐	**C. Stairs:** Code the patient's need for assistance with internal or external stairs (with or without a device such as cane, crutch, or walker) prior to the current illness, exacerbation or injury.
	☐	**D. Functional Cognition:** Code the patient's need for assistance with planning regular tasks, such as shopping or remembering to take medication prior to the current illness, exacerbation, or injury.

GG0110. Prior Device Use. Indicate devices and aids used by the patient prior to the current illness, exacerbation, or injury.

↓ Check all that apply	
☐	**A. Manual wheelchair**
☐	**B. Motorized wheelchair and/or scooter**
☐	**C. Mechanical lift**
☐	**D. Walker**
☐	**E. Orthotics/Prosthetics**
☐	**Z. None of the above**

Section GG: Self-Care

SOC/ROC

GG0130. Self-Care

Code the patient's usual performance at SOC/ROC for each activity using the 6-point scale. If activity was not attempted at SOC/ROC, code the reason. Code the patient's discharge goal(s) using the 6-point scale. Use of codes 07, 09, 10 or 88 is permissible to code discharge goal(s).

Coding:

Safety and **Quality of Performance** – If helper assistance is required because patient's performance is unsafe or of poor quality, score according to amount of assistance provided.

Activities may be completed with or without assistive devices.

06. **Independent** – Patient completes the activity by him/herself with no assistance from a helper
05. **Setup or clean-up assistance** – Helper sets up or cleans up; patient completes activity. Helper assists only prior to or following the activity.
04. **Supervision or touching assistance** – Helper provides verbal cues and/or touching/steadying and/or contact guard assistance as patient completes activity. Assistance may be provided throughout the activity or intermittently.
03. **Partial/moderate assistance** – Helper does LESS THAN HALF the effort. Helper lifts, holds or supports trunk or limbs, but provides less than half the effort.
02. **Substantial/maximal assistance** – Helper does MORE THAN HALF the effort. Helper lifts or holds trunk or limbs and provides more than half the effort.
01. **Dependent** – Helper does ALL of the effort. Patient does none of the effort to complete the activity. Or, the assistance of 2 or more helpers is required for the patient to complete the activity.

If activity was not attempted, code reason:

07. **Patient refused**
09. **Not applicable** – Not attempted and the patient did not perform this activity prior to the current illness, exacerbation or injury.
10. **Not attempted due to environmental limitations** (e.g., lack of equipment, weather constraints)
88. **Not attempted due to medical conditions or safety concerns**

1. SOC/ROC Performance	2. Discharge Goal	
↓ Enter Codes in Boxes ↓		
☐☐	☐☐	**A. Eating:** The ability to use suitable utensils to bring food and/or liquid to the mouth and swallow food and/or liquid once the meal is placed before the patient.
☐☐	☐☐	**B. Oral Hygiene:** The ability to use suitable items to clean teeth. Dentures (if applicable): The ability to remove and replace dentures from and to the mouth, and manage equipment for soaking and rinsing them.
☐☐	☐☐	**C. Toileting Hygiene:** The ability to maintain perineal hygiene, adjust clothes before and after voiding or having a bowel movement. If managing an ostomy, include wiping the opening but not managing equipment.
☐☐	☐☐	**E. Shower/bathe self:** The ability to bathe self, including washing, rinsing, and drying self (excludes washing of back and hair). Does not include transferring in/out of tub/shower
☐☐	☐☐	**F. Upper body dressing:** The ability to dress and undress above the waist; including fasteners, if applicable.
☐☐	☐☐	**G. Lower body dressing:** The ability to dress and undress below the waist, including fasteners; does not include footwear.
☐☐	☐☐	**H. Putting on/taking off footwear:** The ability to put on and take off socks and shoes or other footwear that is appropriate for safe mobility; including fasteners, if applicable.

Follow-Up

GG0130. Self-Care

Code the patient's usual performance at Follow-Up for each activity using the 6-point scale. If activity was not attempted at Follow-Up, code the reason.

Coding:

Safety and **Quality of Performance –** If helper assistance is required because patient's performance is unsafe or of poor quality, score according to amount of assistance provided.

Activities may be completed with or without assistive devices.

06. **Independent** – Patient completes the activity by him/herself with no assistance from a helper.
05. **Setup or clean-up assistance –** Helper sets up or cleans up; patient completes activity. Helper assists only prior to or following the activity.
04. **Supervision or touching assistance –** Helper provides verbal cues and/or touching/steadying and/or contact guard assistance as patient completes activity. Assistance may be provided throughout the activity or intermittently.
03. **Partial/moderate assistance –** Helper does LESS THAN HALF the effort. Helper lifts, holds or supports trunk or limbs, but provides less than half the effort.
02. **Substantial/maximal assistance –** Helper does MORE THAN HALF the effort. Helper lifts or holds trunk or limbs and provides more than half the effort.
01. **Dependent –** Helper does ALL of the effort. Patient does none of the effort to complete the activity. Or, the assistance of 2 or more helpers is required for the patient to complete the activity.

If activity was not attempted, code reason:

07. **Patient refused**
09. **Not applicable** – Not attempted and the patient did not perform this activity prior to the current illness, exacerbation or injury.
10. **Not attempted due to environmental limitations** (e.g., lack of equipment, weather constraints)
88. **Not attempted due to medical conditions or safety concerns**

4. Follow-Up Performance	
Enter Codes in Boxes ↓	
☐☐	**A. Eating:** The ability to use suitable utensils to bring food and/or liquid to the mouth and swallow food and/or liquid once the meal is placed before the patient.
☐☐	**B. Oral Hygiene:** The ability to use suitable items to clean teeth. Dentures (if applicable): The ability to insert and remove dentures into and from the mouth, and manage denture soaking and rinsing with use of equipment.
☐☐	**C. Toileting Hygiene:** The ability to maintain perineal hygiene, adjust clothes before and after voiding or having a bowel movement. If managing an ostomy, include wiping the opening but not managing equipment.

Discharge

GG0130. Self-Care	
Code the patient's usual performance at Discharge for each activity using the 6-point scale. If activity was not attempted at Discharge, code the reason.	

Coding:

Safety and **Quality of Performance –** If helper assistance is required because patient's performance is unsafe or of poor quality, score according to amount of assistance provided.

Activities may be completed with or without assistive devices.

06. **Independent** – Patient completes the activity by him/herself with no assistance from a helper.
05. **Setup or clean-up assistance –** Helper sets up or cleans up; patient completes activity. Helper assists only prior to or following the activity.
04. **Supervision or touching assistance –** Helper provides verbal cues and/or touching/steadying and/or contact guard assistance as patient completes activity. Assistance may be provided throughout the activity or intermittently.
03. **Partial/moderate assistance** – Helper does LESS THAN HALF the effort. Helper lifts, holds or supports trunk or limbs, but provides less than half the effort.
02. **Substantial/maximal assistance –** Helper does MORE THAN HALF the effort. Helper lifts or holds trunk or limbs and provides more than half the effort.
01. **Dependent –** Helper does ALL of the effort. Patient does none of the effort to complete the activity. Or, the assistance of 2 or more helpers is required for the patient to complete the activity.

If activity was not attempted, code reason:

07. **Patient refused**
09. **Not applicable** – Not attempted and the patient did not perform this activity prior to the current illness, exacerbation or injury.
10. **Not attempted due to environmental limitations** (e.g., lack of equipment, weather constraints)
88. **Not attempted due to medical conditions or safety concerns**

3. Discharge Performance ↓ **Enter Codes in Boxes**	
☐☐	**A. Eating:** The ability to use suitable utensils to bring food and/or liquid to the mouth and swallow food and/or liquid once the meal placed before the patient.
☐☐	**B. Oral Hygiene:** The ability to use suitable items to clean teeth. Dentures (if applicable): The ability to insert and remove dentures into and from the mouth, and manage denture soaking and rinsing with use of equipment.
☐☐	**C. Toileting Hygiene:** The ability to maintain perineal hygiene, adjust clothes before and after voiding or having a bowel movement. If managing an ostomy, include wiping the opening but not managing equipment.
☐☐	**E. Shower/bathe self:** The ability to bathe self, including washing, rinsing, and drying self (excludes washing of back and hair). Does not include transferring in/out of tub/shower.
☐☐	**F. Upper body dressing:** The ability to dress and undress above the waist; including fasteners, if applicable.
☐☐	**G. Lower body dressing:** The ability to dress and undress below the waist, including fasteners; does not include footwear.
☐☐	**H. Putting on/taking off footwear:** The ability to put on and take off socks and shoes or other footwear that is appropriate for safe mobility; including fasteners, if applicable.

Section GG: Mobility

SOC/ROC

GG0170. Mobility		
Code the patient's usual performance at SOC/ROC for each activity using the 6-point scale. If activity was not attempted at SOC/ROC, code the reason. Code the patient's discharge goal(s) using the 6-point scale. Use of codes 07, 09, 10 or 88 is permissible to code discharge goal(s).		
Coding: **Safety** and **Quality of Performance** – If helper assistance is required because patient's performance is unsafe or of poor quality, score according to amount of assistance provided. *Activities may be completed with or without assistive devices.* 06. **Independent** – Patient completes the activity by him/herself with no assistance from a helper. 05. **Setup or clean-up assistance** – Helper sets up or cleans up; patient completes activity. Helper assists only prior to or following the activity. 04. **Supervision or touching assistance** – Helper provides verbal cues and/or touching/steadying and/or contact guard assistance as patient completes activity. Assistance may be provided throughout the activity or intermittently. 03. **Partial/moderate assistance** – Helper does LESS THAN HALF the effort. Helper lifts, holds or supports trunk or limbs, but provides less than half the effort. 02. **Substantial/maximal assistance** – Helper does MORE THAN HALF the effort. Helper lifts or holds trunk or limbs and provides more than half the effort. 01. **Dependent** – Helper does ALL of the effort. Patient does none of the effort to complete the activity. Or, the assistance of 2 or more helpers is required for the patient to complete the activity. **If activity was not attempted, code reason:** 07. **Patient refused** 09. **Not applicable** – Not attempted and the patient did not perform this activity prior to the current illness, exacerbation or injury. 10. **Not attempted due to environmental limitations** (e.g., lack of equipment, weather constraints) 88. **Not attempted due to medical conditions or safety concerns**		
1. SOC/ROC Performance	**2. Discharge Goal**	
↓ Enter Codes in Boxes ↓		
☐☐	☐☐	**A. Roll left and right:** The ability to roll from lying on back to left and right side, and return to lying on back on the bed.
☐☐	☐☐	**B. Sit to lying:** The ability to move from sitting on side of bed to lying flat on the bed.
☐☐	☐☐	**C. Lying to sitting on side of bed:** The ability to move from lying on the back to sitting on the side of the bed with feet flat on the floor, and with no back support.
☐☐	☐☐	**D. Sit to stand:** The ability to come to a standing position from sitting in a chair, wheelchair, or on the side of the bed.
☐☐	☐☐	**E. Chair/bed-to-chair transfer:** The ability to transfer to and from a bed to a chair (or wheelchair).
☐☐	☐☐	**F. Toilet transfer:** The ability to get on and off a toilet or commode.
☐☐	☐☐	**G. Car Transfer:** The ability to transfer in and out of a car or van on the passenger side. Does not include the ability to open/close door or fasten seat belt.
☐☐	☐☐	**I. Walk 10 feet:** Once standing, the ability to walk at least 10 feet in a room, corridor, or similar space. *If SOC/ROC performance is coded 07, 09, 10 or 88, skip to GG0170M, 1 step (curb)*
☐☐	☐☐	**J. Walk 50 feet with two turns:** Once standing, the ability to walk 50 feet and make two turns.

		K. Walk 150 feet: Once standing, the ability to walk at least 150 feet in a corridor or similar space.
		L. Walking 10 feet on uneven surfaces: The ability to walk 10 feet on uneven or sloping surfaces (indoor or outdoor), such as turf or gravel.
		M. 1 step (curb): The ability to go up and down a curb and/or up and down one step. *If SOC/ROC performance is coded 07, 09, 10 or 88, skip to GG0170P, Picking up object.*
		N. 4 steps: The ability to go up and down four steps with or without a rail. *If SOC/ROC performance is coded 07, 09, 10 or 88, skip to GG0170P, Picking up object.*
		O. 12 steps: The ability to go up and down 12 steps with or without a rail.
		P. Picking up object: The ability to bend/stoop from a standing position to pick up a small object, such as a spoon, from the floor.
		Q. Does patient use wheelchair and/or scooter? **0. No** → Skip GG0170R, GG0170RR1, GG0170S, and GG0170SS1. **1. Yes** → Continue to GG0170R, Wheel 50 feet with two turns.
		R. Wheel 50 feet with two turns: Once seated in wheelchair/scooter, the ability to wheel at least 50 feet and make two turns.
		RR1. Indicate the type of wheelchair or scooter used. **1. Manual** **2. Motorized**
		S. Wheel 150 feet: Once seated in wheelchair/scooter, the ability to wheel at least 150 feet in a corridor or similar space.
		SS1. Indicate the type of wheelchair or scooter used. **1. Manual** **2. Motorized**

Follow-Up

GG0170. Mobility

Code the patient's usual performance at Follow-Up for each activity using the 6-point scale. If activity was not attempted at Follow-Up code the reason.

Coding:

Safety and **Quality of Performance** – If helper assistance is required because patient's performance is unsafe or of poor quality, score according to amount of assistance provided.

Activities may be completed with or without assistive devices.

06. **Independent** – Patient completes the activity by him/herself with no assistance from a helper.
05. **Setup or clean-up assistance** – Helper sets up or cleans up; patient completes activity. Helper assists only prior to or following the activity.
04. **Supervision or touching assistance** – Helper provides verbal cues and/or touching/steadying and/or contact guard assistance as patient completes activity. Assistance may be provided throughout the activity or intermittently.
03. **Partial/moderate assistance** – Helper does LESS THAN HALF the effort. Helper lifts, holds or supports trunk or limbs, but provides less than half the effort.
02. **Substantial/maximal assistance** – Helper does MORE THAN HALF the effort. Helper lifts or holds trunk or limbs and provides more than half the effort.
01. **Dependent** – Helper does ALL of the effort. Patient does none of the effort to complete the activity. Or, the assistance of 2 or more helpers is required for the patient to complete the activity.

If activity was not attempted, code reason:

07. **Patient refused**
09. **Not applicable** – Not attempted and the patient did not perform this activity prior to the current illness, exacerbation or injury.
10. **Not attempted due to environmental limitations** (e.g., lack of equipment, weather constraints)
88. **Not attempted due to medical conditions or safety concerns**

4. Follow-Up Performance	
Enter Codes in Boxes	
☐☐	A. **Roll left and right:** The ability to roll from lying on back to left and right side, and return to lying on back on the bed.
☐☐	B. **Sit to lying:** The ability to move from sitting on side of bed to lying flat on the bed.
☐☐	C. **Lying to sitting on side of bed:** The ability to move from lying on the back to sitting on the side of the bed with feet flat on the floor, and with no back support.
☐☐	D. **Sit to stand:** The ability to come to a standing position from sitting in a chair, wheelchair, or on the side of the bed.
☐☐	E. **Chair/bed-to-chair transfer:** The ability to transfer to and from a bed to a chair (or wheelchair).
☐☐	F. **Toilet transfer:** The ability to get on and off a toilet or commode.
☐☐	I. **Walk 10 feet:** Once standing, the ability to walk at least 10 feet in a room, corridor, or similar space. *If Follow-Up performance is coded 07, 09, 10 or 88 → skip to GG0170M, 1 step (curb).*
☐☐	J. **Walk 50 feet with two turns:** Once standing, the ability to walk 50 feet and make two turns.
☐☐	L. **Walking 10 feet on uneven surfaces:** The ability to walk 10 feet on uneven or sloping surfaces (indoor or outdoor), such as turf or gravel.
☐☐	*M.* **1 step (curb):** The ability to go up and down a curb and/or up and down one step. *If Follow-up performance is coded 07, 09, 10 or 88, skip to GG0170Q, Does patient use wheelchair and/or scooter?*
☐☐	N. **4 steps:** The ability to go up and down four steps with or without a rail.
	☐ **Q. Does patient use wheelchair and/or scooter?** **0. No** →Skip GG0170R **1. Yes** → Continue to GG0170R, Wheel 50 feet with two turns.
☐☐	R. **Wheel 50 feet with two turns:** Once seated in wheelchair/scooter, the ability to wheel at least 50 feet and make two turns.

Discharge

GG0170. Mobility	
Code the patient's usual performance at Discharge for each activity using the 6-point scale. If activity was not attempted at Discharge, code the reason.	
Coding: **Safety** and **Quality of Performance** – If helper assistance is required because patient's performance is unsafe or of poor quality, score according to amount of assistance provided. *Activities may be completed with or without assistive devices.* 06. **Independent** – Patient completes the activity by him/herself with no assistance from a helper. 05. **Setup or clean-up assistance** – Helper sets up or cleans up; patient completes activity. Helper assists only prior to or following the activity. 04. **Supervision or touching assistance** – Helper provides verbal cues and/or touching/steadying and/or contact guard assistance as patient completes activity. Assistance may be provided throughout the activity or intermittently. 03. **Partial/moderate assistance** – Helper does LESS THAN HALF the effort. Helper lifts, holds or supports trunk or limbs, but provides less than half the effort. 02. **Substantial/maximal assistance** – Helper does MORE THAN HALF the effort. Helper lifts or holds trunk or limbs and provides more than half the effort. 01. **Dependent** – Helper does ALL of the effort. Patient does none of the effort to complete the activity. Or, the assistance of 2 or more helpers is required for the patient to complete the activity. **If activity was not attempted, code reason:** 07. **Patient refused** 09. **Not applicable** – Not attempted and the patient did not perform this activity prior to the current illness, exacerbation or injury. 10. **Not attempted due to environmental limitations** (e.g., lack of equipment, weather constraints) 88. **Not attempted due to medical conditions or safety concerns**	
3. Discharge Performance	
Enter Codes in Boxes	
☐☐	**A. Roll left and right:** The ability to roll from lying on back to left and right side, and return to lying on back on the bed.
☐☐	**B. Sit to lying:** The ability to move from sitting on side of bed to lying flat on the bed.
☐☐	**C. Lying to sitting on side of bed:** The ability to move from lying on the back to sitting on the side of the bed with feet flat on the floor, and with no back support.
☐☐	**D. Sit to stand:** The ability to come to a standing position from sitting in a chair, wheelchair, or on the side of the bed.
☐☐	**E. Chair/bed-to-chair transfer:** The ability to transfer to and from a bed to a chair (or wheelchair).
☐☐	**F. Toilet transfer:** The ability to get on and off a toilet or commode.
☐☐	**G. Car Transfer:** The ability to transfer in and out of a car or van on the passenger side. Does not include the ability to open/close door or fasten seat belt.
☐☐	**I. Walk 10 feet:** Once standing, the ability to walk at least 10 feet in a room, corridor, or similar space. *If Discharge performance is coded 07, 09, 10 or 88, skip to GG0170M, 1 step (curb).*
☐☐	**J. Walk 50 feet with two turns:** Once standing, the ability to walk 50 feet and make two turns.
☐☐	**K. Walk 150 feet:** Once standing, the ability to walk at least 150 feet in a corridor or similar space.
☐☐	**L. Walking 10 feet on uneven surfaces:** The ability to walk 10 feet on uneven or sloping surfaces (indoor or outdoor), such as turf or gravel.
☐☐	**M. 1 step (curb):** The ability to go up and down a curb and/or up and down one step. *If Discharge performance is coded 07, 09, 10 or 88, skip to GG0170P, Picking up object.*

☐☐	**N.** **4 steps:** The ability to go up and down four steps with or without a rail. *If Discharge performance is coded 07, 09, 10 or 88, skip to GG0170P, Picking up object.*	
☐☐	**O.** **12 steps:** The ability to go up and down 12 steps with or without a rail.	
☐☐	**P.** **Picking up object**: The ability to bend/stoop from a standing position to pick up a small object, such as a spoon, from the floor.	
	☐	**Q. Does patient use wheelchair and/or scooter?** **0. No →** Skip to J1800 Any falls since SOC/ROC, whichever is more recent. **1. Yes →** Continue to GG0170R, Wheel 50 feet with two turns.
☐☐	**R.** **Wheel 50 feet with two turns:** Once seated in wheelchair/scooter, the ability to wheel at least 50 feet and make two turns.	
	☐	**RR3. Indicate the type of wheelchair or scooter used.** **1. Manual** **2. Motorized**
☐☐	**S.** **Wheel 150 feet:** Once seated in wheelchair/scooter, the ability to wheel at least 150 feet in a corridor or similar space.	
	☐	**SS3. Indicate the type of wheelchair or scooter used.** **1. Manual** **2. Motorized**

Section J: Health Conditions

J1800.	**Any Falls Since SOC/ROC,** whichever is more recent	
Enter Code ☐	Has the patient **had any falls since SOC/ROC,** whichever is more recent? 0. **No** → Skip J1900 1. **Yes** → Continue to J1900, Number of Falls Since SOC/ROC, whichever is more recent	
J1900.	**Number of Falls Since SOC/ROC,** whichever is more recent	
CODING: 0. None 1. One 2. Two or more	↓ **Enter Codes in Boxes**	
	☐	**A. No injury:** No evidence of any injury is noted on physical assessment by the nurse or primary care clinician; no complaints of pain or injury by the patient; no change in the patient's behavior is noted after the fall
	☐	**B. Injury (except major):** Skin tears, abrasions, lacerations, superficial bruises, hematomas and sprains; or any fall-related injury that causes the patient to complain of pain
	☐	**C. Major injury:** Bone **fractures**, joint dislocations, closed head injuries with altered consciousness, subdural hematoma

Appendix C

CMS FORM 1500 WITH INSTRUCTIONS

CMS-1500 Instructions

The following table identifies the fields that are required and provides a description of the field.

FORM FIELD	REQUIRED	DESCRIPTION
Element 01-Program Block/Claim Sort Indicator	YES	
Element 01a–Insured's I.D. Number	YES	All claims require one of the following recipient numbers in order for processing. Enter the recipient's Alien Identification Number. If not available, enter recipient's Fingerprint ID Number. If not available, enter recipient's Event Number. Do not enter any other numbers or letters. It is the referring custodial facility's responsibility to provide this information to the provider.
Element 02 – Patient's Name	YES	Enter the recipient's last name, first name, and middle initial.
Element 03 – Patient's Birth Date, Patient's Sex	YES	Enter the recipient's birth date in MM/DD/YY format (e.g., February 3, 1955, would be 02/03/55) or in MM/DD/YYYY format (e.g., February 3, 1955, would be 02/03/1955). Specify whether the recipient is male or female by placing an "X" in the appropriate box.
Element 04 – Insured's Name	YES	
Element 05 – Patient's Address	YES	Enter the detention facility's address where the recipient resides. If recipient in custody of Border Patrol, enter the Border Patrol Station of the Border Patrol Officer(s). Do not use the detainee's home address.
Element 06 - Patient Relationship to Insured		
Element 07 – Insured's Address	YES	Enter the detention facility's address where the recipient resides. If recipient in custody of Border Patrol, enter the Border Patrol Station of the custodial Border Patrol Officers.
Element 08 - Patient Status		
Element 09 -Other Insured's Name		
Element 10 - Is Patient's Condition Related to	YES	
Element 11 – Insured's Policy, Group, or FECA Number	YES	

FORM FIELD	REQUIRED	DESCRIPTION
Element 11a – Insured's Date of Birth and Sex	YES	
Element 11b - Employer's Name or School Name		
Element 11c - Insurance Plan Name or Program Name	YES	Enter "Immigration Health Services."
Elements 12 and 13 - Authorized Person's Signature	YES	
Element 14 -Date of Current Illness, Injury, or Pregnancy		
Element 15 - If Patient Has Had Same or Similar Illness		
Element 16 -Dates Patient Unable to Work in Current Occupation (not required)		
Elements 17 and 17a - Name and I.D. Number of Referring Physician or Other Source	YES WHEN APPLICABLE	
Element 18 -Hospitalization Dates Related to Current Services	YES WHEN APPLICABLE	
Element 19 - Reserved for Local Use		
Element 20 -Outside Lab?		
Element 21 -Diagnosis or Nature of Illness or Injury	YES	Enter the most current International Classification of Diseases, Clinical Modification (ICD-9-CM) diagnosis code for each symptom or condition related to the services provided. List the primary diagnosis first.
Element 22 - Medicaid Resubmission		
Element 23 - Prior Authorization Number	YES	Enter the Authorization # for service. All Claims require an Authorization # for processing. It is the referring custodial facility's responsibility to provide this information to the provider.
Element 24A - Date(s) of Service	YES	Enter the month, day, and year for each service using the following guidelines.
Element 24A - Date(s) of Service		When billing for one date of service (DOS), enter the date in MM/DD/YY or MM/DD/YYYY format in the "From" field.

FORM FIELD	REQUIRED	DESCRIPTION
Element 24A - Date(s) of Service	YES	When billing for one date of service (DOS), enter the date in MM/DD/YY or MM/DD/YYYY format in the "From" field. When billing for two, three, or four DOS on the same detail line, enter the first DOS in MM/DD/YY or MM/DD/YYYY format in the "From" field and enter subsequent DOS in the "To" field by listing only the date(s) of the month. For example, for DOS December 1, 8, 15, and 22, 2003, indicate 12/01/03 or 12/01/2003 in the "From" field and indicate 08/15/22 in the "To" field. It is allowable to enter up to four DOS per line if: All DOS are in the same calendar month. All services are billed using the same procedure code and modifier(s), if applicable. All services have the same place of service (POS) code. All services were performed by the same provider. The same diagnosis is applicable for each service. The charge for all services is identical. (Enter the total charge per detail line in Element 24F.) The number of services performed on each DOS is identical. All services have the same family planning indicator, if applicable. All services have the same emergency indicator, if applicable.
Element 24B - Place of Service	YES	Enter the appropriate two-digit POS code for each service.
Element 24C - Type of Service	YES	
Element 24D - Procedures, Services, or Supplies	YES	Enter the single most appropriate five-character procedure code. Claims received without an appropriate procedure code may be denied. Modifiers: Enter the appropriate modifier(s) in the "Modifier" column of Element 24D.
Element 24E - Diagnosis Code	YES	Enter the number (1, 2, 3, or 4) that corresponds to the appropriate ICD-9-CM diagnosis code listed in Element 21.
Element 24F - $ Charges	YES	Enter the total charge for each line item.
Element 24G - Days or Units	YES	Enter the appropriate number of units billed for each line item. Always use a decimal (e.g., 30 minutes equals 2.0 units).
Element 24H - EPSDT/ Family Plan	YES WHEN APPLICABLE	
Element 24I - EMG		Enter an "E" for each procedure performed as an emergency. If the procedure is not an emergency, leave this element blank.
Element 24J - COB		
Element 24K - Reserved for Local Use		
Element 24K - Reserved for Local Use		
Element 25 - Federal Tax I.D. Number	YES	Enter tax ID information.
Element 26 – Patient's Account No.		
Element 27 - Accept Assignment		
Element 28 - Total Charge	YES	Enter the total charges for the claim.

FORM FIELD	REQUIRED	DESCRIPTION
Element 29 -Amount Paid	YES WHEN APPLICABLE	
Element 30 - Balance Due	YES	
Element 31 - Signature of Physician or Supplier	YES	The provider or the authorized representative must sign in Element 31. The month, day, and year the form is signed must also be entered in MM/DD/YY or MM/DD/YYYY format. Note: The signature may be a computer-printed or typed name and date, or a signature stamp with the date.
Element 32 -Name and Address of Facility Where Services Were Rendered	YES	
Element 33 – Physician's, Supplier's Billing Name, Address, ZIP Code, and Phone #	YES	Enter the provider's name (exactly as indicated on the provider's notification of certification letter) and address of the billing provider. At the bottom of Element 33, enter the billing provider's eight-digit Medicaid provider number.

PLEASE
DO NOT
STAPLE
IN THIS
AREA

PICA **HEALTH INSURANCE CLAIM FORM** PICA

CARRIER

1. MEDICARE (Medicare #) MEDICAID (Medicaid #) CHAMPUS (Sponsor's SSN) CHAMPVA (VA File #) GROUP HEALTH PLAN (SSN or ID) FECA BLK LUNG (SSN) OTHER (ID)

1a. INSURED'S I.D. NUMBER (FOR PROGRAM IN ITEM 1)

2. PATIENT'S NAME (Last Name, First Name, Middle Initial)

3. PATIENT'S BIRTH DATE MM DD YY SEX M F

4. INSURED'S NAME (Last Name, First Name, Middle Initial)

5. PATIENT'S ADDRESS (No., Street)

6. PATIENT RELATIONSHIP TO INSURED Self Spouse Child Other

7. INSURED'S ADDRESS (No., Street)

CITY STATE

8. PATIENT STATUS Single Married Other

CITY STATE

ZIP CODE TELEPHONE (Include Area Code) ( )

Employed Full-Time Student Part-Time Student

ZIP CODE TELEPHONE (INCLUDE AREA CODE) ( )

9. OTHER INSURED'S NAME (Last Name, First Name, Middle Initial)

10. IS PATIENT'S CONDITION RELATED TO:

11. INSURED'S POLICY GROUP OR FECA NUMBER

a. OTHER INSURED'S POLICY OR GROUP NUMBER

a. EMPLOYMENT? (CURRENT OR PREVIOUS) YES NO

a. INSURED'S DATE OF BIRTH MM DD YY SEX M F

b. OTHER INSURED'S DATE OF BIRTH MM DD YY SEX M F

b. AUTO ACCIDENT? YES NO PLACE (State)

b. EMPLOYER'S NAME OR SCHOOL NAME

c. EMPLOYER'S NAME OR SCHOOL NAME

c. OTHER ACCIDENT? YES NO

c. INSURANCE PLAN NAME OR PROGRAM NAME

d. INSURANCE PLAN NAME OR PROGRAM NAME

10d. RESERVED FOR LOCAL USE

d. IS THERE ANOTHER HEALTH BENEFIT PLAN? YES NO *If yes, return to and complete item 9 a-d.*

READ BACK OF FORM BEFORE COMPLETING & SIGNING THIS FORM.

12. PATIENT'S OR AUTHORIZED PERSON'S SIGNATURE I authorize the release of any medical or other information necessary to process this claim. I also request payment of government benefits either to myself or to the party who accepts assignment below.

SIGNED ______ DATE ______

13. INSURED'S OR AUTHORIZED PERSON'S SIGNATURE I authorize payment of medical benefits to the undersigned physician or supplier for services described below.

SIGNED ______

PATIENT AND INSURED INFORMATION

14. DATE OF CURRENT: MM DD YY ILLNESS (First symptom) OR INJURY (Accident) OR PREGNANCY(LMP)

15. IF PATIENT HAS HAD SAME OR SIMILAR ILLNESS. GIVE FIRST DATE MM DD YY

16. DATES PATIENT UNABLE TO WORK IN CURRENT OCCUPATION MM DD YY FROM MM DD YY TO

17. NAME OF REFERRING PHYSICIAN OR OTHER SOURCE

17a. I.D. NUMBER OF REFERRING PHYSICIAN

18. HOSPITALIZATION DATES RELATED TO CURRENT SERVICES MM DD YY FROM MM DD YY TO

19. RESERVED FOR LOCAL USE

20. OUTSIDE LAB? YES NO $ CHARGES

21. DIAGNOSIS OR NATURE OF ILLNESS OR INJURY. (RELATE ITEMS 1,2,3 OR 4 TO ITEM 24E BY LINE)

1. ___ . ___ 3. ___ . ___

2. ___ . ___ 4. ___ . ___

22. MEDICAID RESUBMISSION CODE ORIGINAL REF. NO.

23. PRIOR AUTHORIZATION NUMBER

24. A DATE(S) OF SERVICE From MM DD YY To MM DD YY	B Place of Service	C Type of Service	D PROCEDURES, SERVICES, OR SUPPLIES (Explain Unusual Circumstances) CPT/HCPCS MODIFIER	E DIAGNOSIS CODE	F $ CHARGES	G DAYS OR UNITS	H EPSDT Family Plan	I EMG	J COB	K RESERVED FOR LOCAL USE
1										
2										
3										
4										
5										
6										

25. FEDERAL TAX I.D. NUMBER SSN EIN

26. PATIENT'S ACCOUNT NO.

27. ACCEPT ASSIGNMENT? (For govt. claims, see back) YES NO

28. TOTAL CHARGE $

29. AMOUNT PAID $

30. BALANCE DUE $

31. SIGNATURE OF PHYSICIAN OR SUPPLIER INCLUDING DEGREES OR CREDENTIALS (I certify that the statements on the reverse apply to this bill and are made a part thereof.)

SIGNED DATE

32. NAME AND ADDRESS OF FACILITY WHERE SERVICES WERE RENDERED (If other than home or office)

33. PHYSICIAN'S, SUPPLIER'S BILLING NAME, ADDRESS, ZIP CODE & PHONE #

PIN# GRP#

PHYSICIAN OR SUPPLIER INFORMATION

(APPROVED BY AMA COUNCIL ON MEDICAL SERVICE 8/88) *PLEASE PRINT OR TYPE* APPROVED OMB-0938-0008 FORM CMS-1500 (12-90), FORM RRB-1500, APPROVED OMB-1215-0055 FORM OWCP-1500 APPROVED OMB-0720-0001 (CHAMPUS)

REFERENCE

Medicare Claims Processing Manual. Centers for Medicare & Medicaid Services. Available at https://www.cms.gov/Regulations-and-Guidance/Guidance/Manuals/downloads/clm104c26.pdf. Accessed August 20, 2020.

Appendix D

ICD-10 GUIDELINES

ICD-10-CM Official Guidelines for Coding and Reporting
FY 2021
(October 1, 2020 - September 30, 2021)

Narrative changes appear in bold text
Items underlined have been moved within the guidelines since the FY 2020 version
***Italics* are used to indicate revisions to heading changes**

The Centers for Medicare and Medicaid Services (CMS) and the National Center for Health Statistics (NCHS), two departments within the U.S. Federal Government's Department of Health and Human Services (DHHS) provide the following guidelines for coding and reporting using the International Classification of Diseases, 10th Revision, Clinical Modification (ICD-10-CM). These guidelines should be used as a companion document to the official version of the ICD-10-CM as published on the NCHS website. The ICD-10-CM is a morbidity classification published by the United States for classifying diagnoses and reason for visits in all health care settings. The ICD-10-CM is based on the ICD-10, the statistical classification of disease published by the World Health Organization (WHO).

These guidelines have been approved by the four organizations that make up the Cooperating Parties for the ICD-10-CM: the American Hospital Association (AHA), the American Health Information Management Association (AHIMA), CMS, and NCHS.

These guidelines are a set of rules that have been developed to accompany and complement the official conventions and instructions provided within the ICD-10-CM itself. The instructions and conventions of the classification take precedence over guidelines. These guidelines are based on the coding and sequencing instructions in the Tabular List and Alphabetic Index of ICD-10-CM, but provide additional instruction. Adherence to these guidelines when assigning ICD-10-CM diagnosis codes is required under the Health Insurance Portability and Accountability Act (HIPAA). The diagnosis codes (Tabular List and Alphabetic Index) have been adopted under HIPAA for all healthcare settings. A joint effort between the healthcare provider and the coder is essential to achieve complete and accurate documentation, code assignment, and reporting of diagnoses and procedures. These guidelines have been developed to assist both the healthcare provider and the coder in identifying those diagnoses that are to be reported. The importance of consistent, complete documentation in the medical record cannot be overemphasized. Without such documentation accurate coding cannot be achieved. The entire record should be reviewed to determine the specific reason for the encounter and the conditions treated.

The term encounter is used for all settings, including hospital admissions. In the context of these guidelines, the term provider is used throughout the guidelines to mean physician or any qualified health care practitioner who is legally accountable for establishing the patient's diagnosis. Only this set of guidelines, approved by the Cooperating Parties, is official.

The guidelines are organized into sections. Section I includes the structure and conventions of the classification and general guidelines that apply to the entire classification, and chapter-specific guidelines that correspond to the chapters as they are arranged in the classification. Section II includes guidelines for selection of principal diagnosis for non-outpatient settings. Section III includes guidelines for reporting additional diagnoses in non-outpatient settings. Section IV is for outpatient coding and reporting. It is necessary to review all sections of the guidelines to fully understand all of the rules and instructions needed to code properly.

Section I. Conventions, general coding guidelines and chapter specific guidelines

The conventions, general guidelines and chapter-specific guidelines are applicable to all health care settings unless otherwise indicated. The conventions and instructions of the classification take precedence over guidelines.

A. Conventions for the ICD-10-CM

The conventions for the ICD-10-CM are the general rules for use of the classification independent of the guidelines. These conventions are incorporated within the Alphabetic Index and Tabular List of the ICD-10-CM as instructional notes.

1. The Alphabetic Index and Tabular List

The ICD-10-CM is divided into the Alphabetic Index, an alphabetical list of terms and their corresponding code, and the Tabular List, a structured list of codes divided into chapters based on body system or condition. The Alphabetic Index consists of the following parts: the Index of Diseases and Injury, the Index of External Causes of Injury, the Table of Neoplasms and the Table of Drugs and Chemicals.

See Section I.C2. General guidelines
See Section I.C.19. Adverse effects, poisoning, underdosing and toxic effects

2. Format and Structure:

The ICD-10-CM Tabular List contains categories, subcategories and codes. Characters for categories, subcategories and codes may be either a letter or a number. All categories are 3 characters. A three-character category that has no further subdivision is equivalent to a code. Subcategories are either 4 or 5 characters. Codes may be 3, 4, 5, 6 or 7 characters. That is, each level of subdivision after a category is a subcategory. The final level of subdivision is a code. Codes that have applicable 7th characters are still referred to as codes, not subcategories. A code that has an applicable 7th character is considered invalid without the 7th character.

The ICD-10-CM uses an indented format for ease in reference.

3. Use of codes for reporting purposes

For reporting purposes only codes are permissible, not categories or subcategories, and any applicable 7th character is required.

4. Placeholder character

The ICD-10-CM utilizes a placeholder character "X". The "X" is used as a placeholder at certain codes to allow for future expansion. An example of this is at the poisoning, adverse effect and underdosing codes, categories T36-T50.

Where a placeholder exists, the X must be used in order for the code to be considered a valid code.

5. 7th Characters

Certain ICD-10-CM categories have applicable 7th characters. The applicable 7th character is required for all codes within the category, or as the notes in the Tabular List instruct. The 7th character must always be the 7th character in the data field. If a code that requires a 7th character is not 6 characters, a placeholder X must be used to fill in the empty characters.

6. Abbreviations

a. Alphabetic Index abbreviations

NEC "Not elsewhere classifiable"
This abbreviation in the Alphabetic Index represents "other specified." When a specific code is not available for a condition, the Alphabetic Index directs the coder to the "other specified" code in the Tabular List.

NOS "Not otherwise specified"
This abbreviation is the equivalent of unspecified.

b. Tabular List abbreviations

NEC "Not elsewhere classifiable"
This abbreviation in the Tabular List represents "other specified". When a specific code is not available for a condition, the Tabular List includes an NEC entry under a code to identify the code as the "other specified" code.

NOS "Not otherwise specified"
This abbreviation is the equivalent of unspecified.

7. Punctuation

[ ] Brackets are used in the Tabular List to enclose synonyms, alternative wording or explanatory phrases. Brackets are used in the Alphabetic Index to identify manifestation codes.

( ) Parentheses are used in both the Alphabetic Index and Tabular List to enclose supplementary words that may be present or absent in the statement of a disease or procedure without affecting the code number to which it is assigned. The terms within the parentheses are referred to as nonessential modifiers. The nonessential modifiers in the Alphabetic Index to Diseases apply to subterms following a main term except when a nonessential modifier and a subentry are mutually exclusive, the subentry takes precedence. For example, in the ICD-10-CM Alphabetic Index under the main term Enteritis, "acute" is a nonessential modifier and "chronic" is a subentry. In this case, the nonessential modifier "acute" does not apply to the subentry "chronic".

: Colons are used in the Tabular List after an incomplete term which needs one or more of the modifiers following the colon to make it assignable to a given category.

8. Use of "and".

See Section I.A.14. Use of the term "And"

9. Other and Unspecified codes

a. "Other" codes

Codes titled "other" or "other specified" are for use when the information in the medical record provides detail for which a specific code does not exist. Alphabetic Index entries with NEC in the line designate "other" codes in the Tabular List. These Alphabetic Index entries represent specific disease entities for which no specific code exists, so the term is included within an "other" code.

b. "Unspecified" codes

Codes titled "unspecified" are for use when the information in the medical record is insufficient to assign a more specific code. For those categories for which an unspecified code is not provided, the "other specified" code may represent both other and unspecified.

See Section I.B.18 Use of Signs/Symptom/Unspecified Codes

10. Includes Notes

This note appears immediately under a three-character code title to further define, or give examples of, the content of the category.

11. Inclusion terms

List of terms is included under some codes. These terms are the conditions for which that code is to be used. The terms may be synonyms of the code title, or, in the case of "other specified" codes, the terms are a list of the various conditions assigned to that code. The inclusion terms are not necessarily exhaustive. Additional terms found only in the Alphabetic Index may also be assigned to a code.

12. Excludes Notes

The ICD-10-CM has two types of excludes notes. Each type of note has a different definition for use but they are all similar in that they indicate that codes excluded from each other are independent of each other.

a. Excludes1

A type 1 Excludes note is a pure excludes note. It means "NOT CODED HERE!" An Excludes1 note indicates that the code excluded should never be used at the same time as the code above the Excludes1 note. An Excludes1 is used when two conditions cannot occur together, such as a congenital form versus an acquired form of the same condition.

An exception to the Excludes1 definition is the circumstance when the two conditions are unrelated to each other. If it is not clear whether the two conditions involving an Excludes1 note are related or not, query the provider. For example, code F45.8, Other somatoform disorders, has an Excludes1 note for "sleep related teeth grinding (G47.63)," because "teeth grinding" is an inclusion term under F45.8. Only one of these two codes should be assigned for teeth grinding. However psychogenic dysmenorrhea is also an inclusion term under F45.8, and a patient could have both this condition and sleep related teeth grinding. In this case, the two conditions are clearly unrelated to each other, and so it would be appropriate to report F45.8 and G47.63 together.

b. Excludes2

A type 2 Excludes note represents "Not included here." An excludes2 note indicates that the condition excluded is not part of the condition represented by the code, but a patient may have both conditions at the same time. When an Excludes2 note appears under a code, it is acceptable to use both the code and the excluded code together, when appropriate.

13. Etiology/manifestation convention ("code first", "use additional code" and "in diseases classified elsewhere" notes)

Certain conditions have both an underlying etiology and multiple body system manifestations due to the underlying etiology. For such conditions, the ICD-10-CM has a coding convention that requires the underlying condition be sequenced first, if applicable, followed by the manifestation. Wherever such a combination exists, there is a "use additional code" note at the etiology code, and a "code first" note at the manifestation code. These instructional notes indicate the proper sequencing order of the codes, etiology followed by manifestation.

In most cases the manifestation codes will have in the code title, "in diseases classified elsewhere." Codes with this title are a component of the etiology/ manifestation convention. The code title indicates that it is a manifestation code. "In diseases classified elsewhere" codes are never permitted to be used as first listed or principal diagnosis codes. They must be used in conjunction with an underlying condition code and they must be listed following the underlying condition. See category F02, Dementia in other diseases classified elsewhere, for an example of this convention.

There are manifestation codes that do not have "in diseases classified elsewhere" in the title. For such codes, there is a "use additional code" note at the etiology code and a "code first" note at the manifestation code, and the rules for sequencing apply.

In addition to the notes in the Tabular List, these conditions also have a specific Alphabetic Index entry structure. In the Alphabetic Index both conditions are listed together with the etiology code first followed by the manifestation codes in brackets. The code in brackets is always to be sequenced second.

An example of the etiology/manifestation convention is dementia in Parkinson's disease. In the Alphabetic Index, code G20 is listed first, followed by code F02.80 or F02.81 in brackets. Code G20 represents the underlying etiology, Parkinson's disease, and must be sequenced first, whereas code F02.80 and F02.81 represent the manifestation of dementia in diseases classified elsewhere, with or without behavioral disturbance.

"Code first" and "Use additional code" notes are also used as sequencing rules in the classification for certain codes that are not part of an etiology/ manifestation combination.

See Section I.B.7. Multiple coding for a single condition.

14. "And"

The word "and" should be interpreted to mean either "and" or "or" when it appears in a title.

For example, cases of "tuberculosis of bones", "tuberculosis of joints" and "tuberculosis of bones and joints" are classified to subcategory A18.0, Tuberculosis of bones and joints.

15. "With"

The word "with" or "in" should be interpreted to mean "associated with" or "due to" when it appears in a code title, the Alphabetic Index (either under a main term or subterm), or an instructional note in the Tabular List. The classification presumes a causal relationship between the two conditions linked by these terms in the Alphabetic Index or Tabular List. These conditions should be coded as related even in the absence of provider documentation explicitly linking them, unless the documentation clearly states the conditions are unrelated or when another guideline exists that specifically requires a documented linkage between two conditions (e.g., sepsis guideline for "acute organ dysfunction that is not clearly associated with the sepsis").

For conditions not specifically linked by these relational terms in the classification or when a guideline requires that a linkage between two conditions be explicitly documented, provider documentation must link the conditions in order to code them as related.

The word "with" in the Alphabetic Index is sequenced immediately following the main term or subterm, not in alphabetical order.

16. "See" and "See Also"

The "see" instruction following a main term in the Alphabetic Index indicates that another term should be referenced. It is necessary to go to the main term referenced with the "see" note to locate the correct code.

A "see also" instruction following a main term in the Alphabetic Index instructs that there is another main term that may also be referenced that may provide additional Alphabetic Index entries that may be useful. It is not necessary to follow the "see also" note when the original main term provides the necessary code.

17. "Code also" note

A "code also" note instructs that two codes may be required to fully describe a condition, but this note does not provide sequencing direction. The sequencing depends on the circumstances of the encounter.

18. Default codes

A code listed next to a main term in the ICD-10-CM Alphabetic Index is referred to as a default code. The default code represents that condition that is most commonly associated with the main term or is the unspecified code for the condition. If a condition is documented in a medical record (for example, appendicitis) without any additional information, such as acute or chronic, the default code should be assigned.

19. Code assignment and Clinical Criteria

The assignment of a diagnosis code is based on the provider's diagnostic statement that the condition exists. The provider's statement that the patient has a particular condition is sufficient. Code assignment is not based on clinical criteria used by the provider to establish the diagnosis.

B. General Coding Guidelines

1. Locating a code in the ICD-10-CM

To select a code in the classification that corresponds to a diagnosis or reason for visit documented in a medical record, first locate the term in the Alphabetic Index, and then verify the code in the Tabular List. Read and be guided by instructional notations that appear in both the Alphabetic Index and the Tabular List.

It is essential to use both the Alphabetic Index and Tabular List when locating and assigning a code. The Alphabetic Index does not always provide the full code. Selection of the full code, including laterality and any applicable 7th character can only be done in the Tabular List. A dash (-) at the end of an Alphabetic Index entry indicates that additional characters are required. Even if a dash is not included at the Alphabetic Index entry, it is necessary to refer to the Tabular List to verify that no 7th character is required.

2. Level of Detail in Coding

Diagnosis codes are to be used and reported at their highest number of characters available.

ICD-10-CM diagnosis codes are composed of codes with 3, 4, 5, 6 or 7 characters. Codes with three characters are included in ICD-10-CM as the heading of a category of codes that may be further subdivided by the use of fourth and/or fifth characters and/or sixth characters, which provide greater detail.

A three-character code is to be used only if it is not further subdivided. A code is invalid if it has not been coded to the full number of characters required for that code, including the 7th character, if applicable.

3. Code or codes from A00.0 through T88.9, Z00-Z99.8

The appropriate code or codes from A00.0 through T88.9, Z00-Z99.8 must be used to identify diagnoses, symptoms, conditions, problems, complaints or other reason(s) for the encounter/visit.

4. Signs and symptoms

Codes that describe symptoms and signs, as opposed to diagnoses, are acceptable for reporting purposes when a related definitive diagnosis has not been established (confirmed) by the provider. Chapter 18 of ICD-10-CM, Symptoms, Signs, and Abnormal Clinical and Laboratory Findings, Not Elsewhere Classified (codes R00.0 - R99) contains many, but not all, codes for symptoms.

See Section I.B.18 Use of Signs/Symptom/Unspecified Codes

5. Conditions that are an integral part of a disease process

Signs and symptoms that are associated routinely with a disease process should not be assigned as additional codes, unless otherwise instructed by the classification.

6. Conditions that are not an integral part of a disease process

Additional signs and symptoms that may not be associated routinely with a disease process should be coded when present.

7. Multiple coding for a single condition

In addition to the etiology/manifestation convention that requires two codes to fully describe a single condition that affects multiple body systems, there are other single conditions that also require more than one code. "Use additional code" notes are found in the Tabular List at codes that are not part of an etiology/manifestation pair where a secondary code is useful to fully describe a condition. The sequencing rule is the same as the etiology/manifestation pair, "use additional code" indicates that a secondary code should be added, if known.

For example, for bacterial infections that are not included in chapter 1, a secondary code from category B95, Streptococcus, Staphylococcus, and Enterococcus, as the cause of diseases classified elsewhere, or B96, Other bacterial agents as the cause of diseases classified elsewhere, may be required to identify the bacterial organism causing the infection. A "use additional code" note will normally be found at the infectious disease code, indicating a need for the organism code to be added as a secondary code.

"Code first" notes are also under certain codes that are not specifically manifestation codes but may be due to an underlying cause. When there is a "code first" note and an underlying condition is present, the underlying condition should be sequenced first, if known.

"Code, if applicable, any causal condition first" notes indicate that this code may be assigned as a principal diagnosis when the causal condition is unknown or not applicable. If a causal condition is known, then the code for that condition should be sequenced as the principal or first-listed diagnosis.

Multiple codes may be needed for sequela, complication codes and obstetric codes to more fully describe a condition. See the specific guidelines for these conditions for further instruction.

8. Acute and Chronic Conditions

If the same condition is described as both acute (subacute) and chronic, and separate subentries exist in the Alphabetic Index at the same indentation level, code both and sequence the acute (subacute) code first.

9. Combination Code

A combination code is a single code used to classify:
Two diagnoses, or
A diagnosis with an associated secondary process (manifestation)
A diagnosis with an associated complication

Combination codes are identified by referring to subterm entries in the Alphabetic Index and by reading the inclusion and exclusion notes in the Tabular List.

Assign only the combination code when that code fully identifies the diagnostic conditions involved or when the Alphabetic Index so directs. Multiple coding should not be used when the classification provides a combination code that clearly identifies all of the elements documented in the diagnosis. When the combination code lacks necessary specificity in describing the manifestation or complication, an additional code should be used as a secondary code.

10. Sequela (Late Effects)

A sequela is the residual effect (condition produced) after the acute phase of an illness or injury has terminated. There is no time limit on when a sequela code can be used. The residual may be apparent early, such as in cerebral infarction, or it may occur months or years later, such as that due to a previous injury. Examples of sequela include: scar formation resulting from a burn, deviated septum due to a nasal fracture, and infertility due to tubal occlusion from old tuberculosis. Coding of sequela generally requires two codes sequenced in the following order: the condition or nature of the sequela is sequenced first. The sequela code is sequenced second.

An exception to the above guidelines are those instances where the code for the sequela is followed by a manifestation code identified in the Tabular List and title, or the sequela code has been expanded (at the fourth, fifth or sixth character levels) to include the manifestation(s). The code for the acute phase of an illness or injury that led to the sequela is never used with a code for the late effect.

See Section I.C.9. Sequelae of cerebrovascular disease
See Section I.C.15. Sequelae of complication of pregnancy, childbirth and the puerperium
See Section I.C.19. Application of 7th characters for Chapter 19

11. Impending or Threatened Condition

Code any condition described at the time of discharge as "impending" or "threatened" as follows:

If it did occur, code as confirmed diagnosis.
If it did not occur, reference the Alphabetic Index to determine if the condition has a subentry term for "impending" or "threatened" and also reference main term entries for "Impending" and for "Threatened."
If the subterms are listed, assign the given code.
If the subterms are not listed, code the existing underlying condition(s) and not the condition described as impending or threatened.

12. Reporting Same Diagnosis Code More than Once

Each unique ICD-10-CM diagnosis code may be reported only once for an encounter. This applies to bilateral conditions when there are no distinct codes identifying laterality or two different conditions classified to the same ICD-10-CM diagnosis code.

13. Laterality

Some ICD-10-CM codes indicate laterality, specifying whether the condition occurs on the left, right or is bilateral. If no bilateral code is provided and the condition is bilateral, assign separate codes for both the left and right side. If the side is not identified in the medical record, assign the code for the unspecified side.

When a patient has a bilateral condition and each side is treated during separate encounters, assign the "bilateral" code (as the condition still exists on both sides), including for the encounter to treat the first side. For the second encounter for treatment after one side has previously been treated and the condition no longer exists on that side, assign the appropriate unilateral code for the side where the condition still exists (e.g., cataract surgery performed on each eye in separate encounters). The bilateral code would not be assigned for the subsequent encounter, as the patient no longer has the condition in the previously-treated site. If the treatment on the first side did not completely resolve the condition, then the bilateral code would still be appropriate.

14. Documentation *by Clinicians Other than the Patient's Provider*

Code assignment is based on the documentation by patient's provider (i.e., physician or other qualified healthcare practitioner legally accountable for establishing the patient's diagnosis). There are a few exceptions, such as codes for the Body Mass Index (BMI), depth of non-pressure chronic ulcers, pressure ulcer stage, coma scale, and NIH stroke scale (NIHSS) codes, code assignment may be based on medical record documentation from clinicians who are not the patient's provider (i.e., physician or other qualified healthcare practitioner legally accountable for establishing the patient's diagnosis), since this information is typically documented by other clinicians involved in the care of the patient (e.g., a dietitian often documents the BMI, a nurse often documents the pressure ulcer stages, and an emergency medical technician often documents the coma scale). However, the associated diagnosis (such as overweight, obesity, acute stroke, or pressure ulcer) must be documented by the patient's provider. If there is conflicting medical record documentation, either from the same clinician or different clinicians, the patient's attending provider should be queried for clarification.

For social determinants of health, such as information found in categories Z55-Z65, Persons with potential health hazards related to socioeconomic and psychosocial circumstances, code assignment may be based on medical record documentation from clinicians involved in the care of the patient who are not the patient's provider since this information represents social information, rather than medical diagnoses. **Patient self-reported documentation may also be used to assign codes for social determinants of health, as long as the**

patient self-reported information is signed-off by and incorporated into the health record by either a clinician or provider.

The BMI, coma scale, NIHSS codes and categories Z55-Z65 should only be reported as secondary diagnoses.

15. Syndromes

Follow the Alphabetic Index guidance when coding syndromes. In the absence of Alphabetic Index guidance, assign codes for the documented manifestations of the syndrome. Additional codes for manifestations that are not an integral part of the disease process may also be assigned when the condition does not have a unique code.

16. Documentation of Complications of Care

Code assignment is based on the provider's documentation of the relationship between the condition and the care or procedure, unless otherwise instructed by the classification. The guideline extends to any complications of care, regardless of the chapter the code is located in. It is important to note that not all conditions that occur during or following medical care or surgery are classified as complications. There must be a cause-and-effect relationship between the care provided and the condition, and an indication in the documentation that it is a complication. Query the provider for clarification, if the complication is not clearly documented.

17. Borderline Diagnosis

If the provider documents a "borderline" diagnosis at the time of discharge, the diagnosis is coded as confirmed, unless the classification provides a specific entry (e.g., borderline diabetes). If a borderline condition has a specific index entry in ICD-10-CM, it should be coded as such. Since borderline conditions are not uncertain diagnoses, no distinction is made between the care setting (inpatient versus outpatient). Whenever the documentation is unclear regarding a borderline condition, coders are encouraged to query for clarification.

18. Use of Sign/Symptom/Unspecified Codes

Sign/symptom and "unspecified" codes have acceptable, even necessary, uses. While specific diagnosis codes should be reported when they are supported by the available medical record documentation and clinical knowledge of the patient's health condition, there are instances when signs/symptoms or unspecified codes are the best choices for accurately reflecting the healthcare encounter. Each healthcare encounter should be coded to the level of certainty known for that encounter.

If a definitive diagnosis has not been established by the end of the encounter, it is appropriate to report codes for sign(s) and/or symptom(s) in lieu of a definitive diagnosis. When sufficient clinical information isn't known or available about a particular health condition to assign a more specific code, it is acceptable to report the appropriate "unspecified" code (e.g., a diagnosis of pneumonia has been determined, but not the specific type). Unspecified codes should be reported when they are the codes that most accurately reflect what is known about the patient's condition at the time of that particular encounter. It would be inappropriate to select a specific code that is not supported by the medical record documentation or conduct medically unnecessary diagnostic testing in order to determine a more specific code.

19. Coding for Healthcare Encounters in Hurricane Aftermath

a. Use of External Cause of Morbidity Codes

An external cause of morbidity code should be assigned to identify the cause of the injury(ies) incurred as a result of the hurricane. The use of external cause of morbidity codes is supplemental to the application of ICD-10-CM codes. External cause of morbidity codes are never to be recorded as a principal diagnosis (first-listed in non-inpatient settings). The appropriate injury code should be sequenced before any external cause codes. The external cause of morbidity codes capture how the injury or health condition happened (cause), the intent (unintentional or accidental; or intentional, such as suicide or assault), the place where the event occurred, the activity of the patient at the time of the event, and the person's status (e.g., civilian, military). They should not be assigned for encounters to treat hurricane victims' medical conditions when no injury, adverse effect or poisoning is involved. External cause of morbidity codes should be assigned for each encounter for care and treatment of the injury. External cause of morbidity codes may be assigned in all health care settings. For the purpose of capturing complete and accurate ICD-10-CM data in the aftermath of the hurricane, a healthcare setting should be considered as any location where medical care is provided by licensed healthcare professionals.

b. Sequencing of External Causes of Morbidity Codes

Codes for cataclysmic events, such as a hurricane, take priority over all other external cause codes except child and adult abuse and terrorism and should be sequenced before other external cause of injury codes. Assign as many external cause of morbidity codes as necessary to fully explain each cause. For example, if an injury occurs as a result of a building collapse during the hurricane, external cause codes for both the hurricane and the building collapse should be assigned, with the external causes code for hurricane being sequenced as the first external cause code. For injuries incurred as a direct result of the hurricane, assign the appropriate code(s) for the injuries, followed by the code X37.0-, Hurricane (with the appropriate 7th character), and any other applicable external cause of injury codes. Code X37.0- also should be assigned when an injury is incurred as a result of flooding caused by a levee breaking related to the hurricane. Code X38.-, Flood (with the appropriate 7th character), should be assigned when an injury is from flooding resulting directly from the storm. Code X36.0.-, Collapse of dam or man-made structure, should not be assigned when the cause of the collapse is due to the hurricane. Use of code X36.0- is limited to collapses of man-made structures due to earth surface movements, not due to storm surges directly from a hurricane.

c. Other External Causes of Morbidity Code Issues

For injuries that are not a direct result of the hurricane, such as an evacuee that has incurred an injury as a result of a motor vehicle accident, assign the appropriate external cause of morbidity code(s) to describe the cause of the injury, but do not assign code X37.0-, Hurricane. If it is not clear whether the injury was a direct result of the hurricane, assume the injury is due to the hurricane and assign code X37.0-, Hurricane, as well as any other applicable external cause of morbidity codes. In addition to code X37.0-, Hurricane, other possible applicable external cause of morbidity codes include:

W54.0-, Bitten by dog
X30-, Exposure to excessive natural heat
X31-, Exposure to excessive natural cold
X38-, Flood

d. Use of Z codes

Z codes (other reasons for healthcare encounters) may be assigned as appropriate to further explain the reasons for presenting for healthcare services, including transfers between healthcare facilities. The ICD-10-CM Official Guidelines for Coding and Reporting identify which codes maybe assigned as principal or first-listed diagnosis only secondary diagnosis only, or principal/first-listed or secondary (depending on the circumstances). Possible applicable Z codes include:

Z59.0, Homelessness
Z59.1, Inadequate housing
Z59.5, Extreme poverty
Z75.1, Person awaiting admission to adequate facility elsewhere
Z75.3, Unavailability and inaccessibility of health-care facilities
Z75.4, Unavailability and inaccessibility of other helping agencies
Z76.2, Encounter for health supervision and care of other healthy infant and child
Z99.12, Encounter for respirator [ventilator] dependence during power failure

REFERENCE

ICD-10-CM Official Guidelines for Coding and Reporting FY 2021. Centers for Disease Control and Prevention. Available at https://www.cdc.gov/nchs/data/icd/10cmguidelines-FY2021.pdf. Accessed August 20, 2020.

Appendix E

APTA GUIDELINES: PHYSICAL THERAPY DOCUMENTATION OF PATIENT/CLIENT MANAGEMENT

APTA
American Physical Therapy Association

Last Updated: 05/19/14
Contact: nationalgovernance@apta.org

GUIDELINES: PHYSICAL THERAPY DOCUMENTATION OF PATIENT/CLIENT MANAGEMENT BOD G03-05-16-41
[Amended BOD 02-02-16-20; BOD 11-01-06-10; BOD 03-01-16-51; BOD 03-00-22-54; BOD 03-99-14-41; BOD 11-98-19-69; BOD 03-97-27-69; BOD 03-95-23-61; BOD 11-94-33-107; BOD 06-93-09-13; Initial BOD 03-93-21-55] [Guideline]

PREAMBLE

The American Physical Therapy Association (APTA) is committed to meeting the physical therapy needs of society, to meeting the needs and interests of its members, and to developing and improving the art and science of physical therapy, including practice, education and research. To help meet these responsibilities, APTA's Board of Directors has approved the following guidelines for physical therapy documentation. It is recognized that these guidelines do not reflect all of the unique documentation requirements associated with the many specialty areas within the physical therapy profession. Applicable for both hand written and electronic documentation systems, these guidelines are intended to be used as a foundation for the development of more specific documentation guidelines in clinical areas, while at the same time providing guidance for the physical therapy profession across all practice settings. Documentation may also need to address additional regulatory or payer requirements.

Finally, be aware that these guidelines are intended to address *documentation* of patient/client management, not to describe the provision of physical therapy services. Other APTA documents, including APTA Standards of Practice for Physical Therapy, Code of Ethics and Guide for Professional Conduct, and the Guide to Physical Therapist Practice, address provision of physical therapy services and patient/client management.

APTA POSITION ON DOCUMENTATION

Documentation Authority For Physical Therapy Services

Physical therapy examination, evaluation, diagnosis, prognosis, and plan of care (including interventions) shall be documented, dated, and authenticated by the physical therapist who performs the service. Interventions provided by the physical therapist or selected interventions provided by the physical therapist assistant under the direction and supervision of the physical therapist are documented, dated, and authenticated by the physical therapist or, when permissible by law, the physical therapist assistant.

Other notations or flow charts are considered a component of the documented record but do not meet the requirements of documentation in or of themselves.

Students in physical therapist or physical therapist assistant programs may document when the record is additionally authenticated by the physical therapist or, when permissible by law, documentation by physical therapist assistant students may be authenticated by a physical therapist assistant.

OPERATIONAL DEFINITIONS

Guidelines
APTA defines a "guideline" as a statement of advice.

Authentication
The process used to verify that an entry is complete, accurate and final. Indications of authentication can include original written signatures and computer "signatures" on secured electronic record systems only.
The following describes the main documentation elements of patient/client management: 1) initial examination/evaluation, 2) visit/encounter, 3) reexamination, and 4) discharge or discontinuation summary.

Initial Examination/Evaluation
Documentation of the initial encounter is typically called the "initial examination," "initial evaluation," or "initial examination/evaluation." Completion of the initial examination/ evaluation is typically completed in one visit, but may occur over more than one visit. Documentation elements for the initial examination/evaluation include the following:

Examination: Includes data obtained from the history, systems review, and tests and measures.

Evaluation: Evaluation is a thought process that may not include formal documentation. It may include documentation of the assessment of the data collected in the examination and identification of problems pertinent to patient/client management.

Diagnosis: Indicates level of impairment, activity limitation and participation restriction determined by the physical therapist. May be indicated by selecting one or more preferred practice patterns from the Guide to Physical Therapist Practice.

Prognosis: Provides documentation of the predicted level of improvement that might be attained through intervention and the amount of time required to reach that level. Prognosis is typically not a separate documentation elements, but the components are included as part of the plan of care.

Plan of care: Typically stated in general terms, includes goals, interventions planned, proposed frequency and duration, and discharge plans.

<u>Visit/Encounter</u>
Documentation of a visit or encounter, often called a progress note or daily note, documents sequential implementation of the plan of care established by the physical therapist, including changes in patient/client status and variations and progressions of specific interventions used. Also may include specific plans for the next visit or visits.

<u>Reexamination</u>
Documentation of reexamination includes data from repeated or new examination elements and is provided to evaluate progress and to modify or redirect intervention.

<u>Discharge or Discontinuation Summary</u>
Documentation is required following conclusion of the current episode in the physical therapy intervention sequence, to summarize progression toward goals and discharge plans.

GENERAL GUIDELINES

- Documentation is required for every visit/encounter.
- All documentation must comply with the applicable jurisdictional/regulatory requirements.
- All handwritten entries shall be made in ink and will include original signatures. Electronic entries are made with appropriate security and confidentiality provisions.
- Charting errors should be corrected by drawing a single line through the error and initialing and dating the chart or through the appropriate mechanism for electronic documentation that clearly indicates that a change was made without deletion of the original record.
- All documentation must include adequate identification of the patient/client and the physical therapist or physical therapist assistant:
    - The patient's/client's full name and identification number, if applicable, must be included on all official documents.
    - All entries must be dated and authenticated with the provider's full name and appropriate designation:
        - Documentation of examination, evaluation, diagnosis, prognosis, plan of care, and discharge summary must be authenticated by the physical therapist who provided the service.
        - Documentation of intervention in visit/encounter notes must be authenticated by the physical therapist or physical therapist assistant who provided the service.
        - Documentation by physical therapist or physical therapist assistant graduates or other physical therapists and physical therapist assistants pending receipt of an unrestricted license shall be authenticated by a licensed physical therapist, or, when permissible by law, documentation by physical therapist assistant graduates may be authenticated by a physical therapist assistant.
        - Documentation by students (SPT/SPTA) in physical therapist or physical therapist assistant programs must be additionally authenticated by the physical therapist or, when permissible by law, documentation by physical therapist assistant students may be authenticated by a physical therapist assistant.
- Documentation should include the referral mechanism by which physical therapy services are initiated. Examples include:

  - Self-referral/direct access
  - Request for consultation from another practitioner
- Documentation should include indication of no shows and cancellations.

INITIAL EXAMINATION/EVALUATION

Examination (History, Systems Review, and Tests and Measures)

History:

Documentation of history may include the following:

- General demographics
- Social history
- Employment/work (Job/School/Play)
- Growth and development
- Living environment
- General health status (self-report, family report, caregiver report)
- Social/health habits (past and current)
- Family history
- Medical/surgical history
- Current condition(s)/Chief complaint(s)
- Functional status and activity level
- Medications
- Other clinical tests

Systems Review:

Documentation of systems review may include gathering data for the following systems:

- Cardiovascular/pulmonary
  - Blood Pressure
  - Edema
  - Heart Rate
  - Respiratory Rate
- Integumentary
  - Pliability (texture)
  - Presence of scar formation
  - Skin color
  - Skin integrity
- Musculoskeletal
  - Gross range of motion
  - Gross strength
  - Gross symmetry
  - Height
  - Weight
- Neuromuscular
  - Gross coordinated movement (e.g., balance, locomotion, transfers,) and transitions)
  - Motor function (motor control, motor learning)

Documentation of systems review may also address communication ability, affect, cognition, language, and learning style:

- Ability to make needs known
- Consciousness
- Expected emotional/behavioral responses
- Learning preferences (e.g., education needs, learning barriers)
- Orientation (person, place, time)

Tests and Measures:

Documentation of tests and measures may include findings for the following categories:

- Aerobic Capacity/Endurance

Examples of examination findings include:
- Aerobic capacity during functional activities
- Aerobic capacity during standardized exercise test protocols
- Cardiovascular signs and symptoms in response to increased oxygen demand with exercise or activity
- Pulmonary signs and symptoms in response to increased oxygen demand with exercise or activity

- Anthropometric Characteristics
  Examples of examination findings include:
  - Body composition
  - Body dimensions
  - Edema

- Arousal, attention, and cognition
  Examples of examination findings include:
  - Arousal and attention
  - Cognition
  - Communication
  - Consciousness
  - Motivation
  - Orientation to time, person, place, and situation
  - Recall

- Assistive and adaptive devices
  Examples of examination findings include:
  - Assistive or adaptive devices and equipment use during functional activities
  - Components, alignment, fit, and ability to care for the assistive or adaptive devices and equipment
  - Remediation of impairments, activity limitations and participation restrictions with use of assistive or adaptive devices and equipment
  - Safety during use of assistive or adaptive devices and equipment

- Circulation (Arterial, Venous, Lymphatic)
  Examples of examination findings include:
  - Cardiovascular signs
  - Cardiovascular symptoms
  - Physiological responses to position change

- Cranial and Peripheral Nerve Integrity
  Examples of examination findings include:
  - Electrophysiological integrity
  - Motor distribution of the cranial nerves
  - Motor distribution of the peripheral nerves
  - Response to neural provocation
  - Response to stimuli, including auditory, gustatory, olfactory, pharyngeal, vestibular, and visual
  - Sensory distribution of the cranial nerves
  - Sensory distribution of the peripheral nerves

- Environmental, Home, and Work (Job/School/Play) Barriers
  Examples of examination findings include:
  - Current and potential barriers
  - Physical space and environment

- Ergonomics and Body mechanics
  Examples of examination findings for *ergonomics* include:
  - Dexterity and coordination during work
  - Functional capacity and performance during work actions, tasks, or activities
  - Safety in work environments

  - Specific work conditions or activities
  - Tools, devices, equipment, and work-stations related to work actions, tasks, or activities

  Examples of examination findings for *body mechanics* include:
  - Body mechanics during self-care, home management, work, community, or leisure actions, tasks, or activities

- Gait, locomotion, and balance
  Examples of examination findings include:
  - Balance during functional activities with or without the use of assistive, adaptive, orthotic, protection, supportive, or prosthetic devices or equipment
  - Balance (dynamic and static) with or without the use of assistive, adaptive, orthotic, protective, supportive, or prosthetic devices or equipment
  - Gait and locomotion during functional activities with or without the use of assistive, adaptive, orthotic, protective, supportive, or prosthetic devices or equipment
  - Gait and locomotion with or without the use of assistive, adaptive, orthotic, protective, supportive, or prosthetic devices or equipment
  - Safety during gait, locomotion, and balance

- Integumentary Integrity
  Examples of examination findings include:
  Associated skin:
  - Activities, positioning, and postures that produce or relieve trauma to the skin
  - Assistive, adaptive, orthotic, protective, supportive, or prosthetic devices and equipment that may produce or relieve trauma to the skin
  - Skin characteristics

- Wound
  - Activities, positioning, and postures that aggravate the wound or scar or that produce or relieve trauma
  - Burn
  - Signs of infection
  - Wound characteristics
  - Wound scar tissue characteristics

- Joint Integrity and Mobility
  Examples of examination findings include:
  - Joint integrity and mobility
  - Joint play movements
  - Specific body parts

- Motor Function
  Examples of examination findings include:
  - Dexterity, coordination, and agility
  - Electrophysiological integrity
  - Hand function
  - Initiation, modification, and control of movement patterns and voluntary postures

- Muscle Performance
  Examples of examination findings include:
  - Electrophysiological integrity
  - Muscle strength, power, and endurance
  - Muscle strength, power, and endurance during functional activities
  - Muscle tension

- Neuromotor development and sensory integration
  Examples of examination findings include:
  - Acquisition and evolution of motor skills
  - Oral motor function, phonation, and speech production
  - Sensorimotor integration

- Orthotic, protective, and supportive devices
  Examples of examination findings include:
  - Components, alignment, fit, and ability to care for the orthotic, protective, and supportive devices and equipment
  - Orthotic, protective, and supportive devices and equipment use during functional activities
  - Remediation of impairments, activity limitations, and participation restrictions with use of orthotic, protective, and supportive devices and equipment
  - Safety during use of orthotic, protective, and supportive devices and equipment

- Pain
  Examples of examination findings include:
  - Pain, soreness, and nocioception
  - Pain in specific body parts

- Posture
  Examples of examination findings include:
  - Postural alignment and position (dynamic)
  - Postural alignment and position (static)
  - Specific body parts

- Prosthetic requirements
  Examples of examination findings include:
  - Components, alignment, fit, and ability to care for prosthetic device
  - Prosthetic device use during functional activities
  - Remediation of impairments, activity limitations, and participation restrictions with use of the prosthetic device
  - Residual limb or adjacent segment
  - Safety during use of the prosthetic device

- Range of motion (including muscle length)
  Examples of examination findings include:
  - Functional ROM
  - Joint active and passive movement
  - Muscle length, soft tissue extensibility, and flexibility

- Reflex integrity
  Examples of examination findings include:
  - Deep reflexes
  - Electrophysiological integrity
  - Postural reflexes and reactions, including righting, equilibrium, and protective reactions
  - Primitive reflexes and reactions
  - Resistance to passive stretch
  - Superficial reflexes and reactions

- Self-care and home management (including activities of daily living and instrumental activities of daily living)
  Examples of examination findings include:
  - Ability to gain access to home environments
  - Ability to perform self-care and home management activities with or without assistive, adaptive, orthotic, protective, supportive, or prosthetic devices and equipment
  - Safety in self-care and home management activities and environments

- Sensory integrity
  Examples of examination findings include:
  - Combined/cortical sensations
  - Deep sensations
  - Electrophysiological integrity

- Ventilation and respiration
  Examples of examination findings include:
  - Pulmonary signs of respiration/gas exchange
  - Pulmonary signs of ventilatory function
  - Pulmonary symptoms

- Work (job/school/play), community, and leisure integration or reintegration (including instrumental activities of daily living)
  Examples of examination findings include:
  - Ability to assume or resume work (job/school/play), community, and leisure activities with or without assistive, adaptive, orthotic, protective, supportive, or prosthetic devices and equipment
  - Ability to gain access to work (job/school/play), community, and leisure environments
  - Safety in work (job/school/play), community, and leisure activities and environments

Evaluation

- Evaluation is a thought process that may not include formal documentation. However, the evaluation process may lead to documentation of impairments, activity limitations, and participation restrictions using formats such as:
  - A problem list
  - A statement of assessment of key factors (e.g., cognitive factors, co-morbidities, social support) influencing the patient/client status.

Diagnosis

- Documentation of a diagnosis determined by the physical therapist may include impairment, activity limitation, and participation restrictions. Examples include:
  - Impaired Joint Mobility, Motor Function, Muscle Performance, and Range of Motion Associated With Localized Inflammation (4E)
  - Impaired Motor Function and Sensory Integrity Associated With Progressive Disorders of the Central Nervous System (5E)
  - Impaired Aerobic Capacity/Endurance Associated With Cardiovascular Pump Dysfunction or Failure (6D)
  - Impaired Integumentary Integrity Associated With Partial-Thickness Skin Involvement and Scar Formation (7C)

Prognosis

- Documentation of the prognosis is typically included in the plan of care. See below

Plan of Care

- Documentation of the plan of care includes the following:
  - Overall goals stated in measurable terms that indicate the predicted level of improvement in functioning
  - A general statement of interventions to be used
  - Proposed duration and frequency of service required to reach the goals
  - Anticipated discharge plans

VISIT/ENCOUNTER

- Documentation of each visit/encounter shall include the following elements:
  - Patient/client self-report (as appropriate).
  - Identification of specific interventions provided, including frequency, intensity, and duration as appropriate. Examples include:
    - Knee extension, three sets, ten repetitions, 10# weight
    - Transfer training bed to chair with sliding board
    - Equipment provided
  - Changes in patient/client impairment, activity limitation, and participation restriction status as they relate to the plan of care.
  - Response to interventions, including adverse reactions, if any.
  - Factors that modify frequency or intensity of intervention and progression goals, including patient/client adherence to patient/client-related instructions.
  - Communication/consultation with providers/patient/client/family/significant other.

- Documentation to plan for ongoing provision of services for the next visit(s), which is suggested to include, but not be limited to:
  - The interventions with objectives
  - Progression parameters
  - Precautions, if indicated

REEXAMINATION

- Documentation of reexamination shall include the following elements:
  - Documentation of selected components of examination to update patient's/client's functioning, and/or disability status.
  - Interpretation of findings and, when indicated, revision of goals.
  - When indicated, revision of plan of care, as directly correlated with goals as documented.

DISCHARGE/DISCONTINUATION SUMMARY

- Documentation of discharge or discontinuation shall include the following elements:
  - Current physical/functional status.
  - Degree of goals achieved and reasons for goals not being achieved.
  - Discharge/discontinuation plan related to the patient/client's continuing care. Examples include:
    - Home program.
    - Referrals for additional services.
    - Recommendations for follow-up physical therapy care.
    - Family and caregiver training.
    - Equipment provided.

Relationship to Vision 2020: Professionalism; (Practice Department, ext 3176)

Explanation of Reference Numbers:
<u>BOD P00-00-00-00</u> stands for Board of Directors/month/year/page/vote in the Board of Directors Minutes; the "P" indicates that it is a position (see below). For example, BOD P11-97-06-18 means that this position can be found in the November 1997 Board of Directors minutes on Page 6 and that it was Vote 18.

P: Position | S: Standard | G: Guideline | Y: Policy | R: Procedure

REFERENCE

Guidelines: Physical Therapy Documentation of Patient/Client Management. Alexandria, Va: American Physical Therapy Association. Available at https://www.apta.org/siteassets/pdfs/policies/guidelines-documentation-patient-client-management.pdf. Accessed August 25, 2020.

Appendix F

This is a *sample* documentation review checklist only. Check with the payer, state law and the applicable accreditation organization, such as The Joint Commission and Commission on Accreditation of Rehabilitation Facilities (CARF), for specific compliance requirements.

Therapist reviewed: **Date:**

REVIEW OF MEDICAL RECORDS DOCUMENTATION FOR PHYSICAL THERAPY			
PHYSICAL THERAPIST INITIAL VISIT ELEMENTS FOR DOCUMENTATION			
Examination	**YES**	**NO**	**N/A**
1. Date/time			
2. Legibility			
3. Referral mechanism by which physical therapy services are initiated			
4. History: medical/surgical history, past physical therapy, social history, growth order and development, living environment, work status, cultural preferences, current condition(s)/chief complaint(s), onset, previous functional status and activity level, medications, allergies Review of systems: cardiovascular and pulmonary; endocrine; eyes, ears, nose, throat; gastrointestinal; genitourinary and reproductive; hematologic and lymphatic; integumentary, musculoskeletal, neuromuscular			
5. Patient's or client's rating of health status, current complaints			
6. Systems Review: brief, limited exam of musculoskeletal, neuromuscular, cardiovascular/pulmonary, and integumentary systems that may or may not be related to chief complaint, and may require outside consultation or referral; also may include patient's or client's communication ability, cognition, factors that might influence care, language, learning style			
7. Tests and Measures: specific tests and measures used, with emphasis on standardized tests (such as OPTIMAL and Oswestry); associated findings or outcomes			
Evaluation	**YES**	**NO**	**N/A**
1. Synthesis of the data and findings gathered from the examination, highlighting pertinent factors; level of severity; should guide the diagnosis and prognosis; formats could include a problem list or statement of assessment of key factors that influence patient or client status (such as cognitive factors, comorbidities, social support, additional services)			
Diagnosis	**YES**	**NO**	**N/A**
1. Made at the levels of impairment of body function and structure, activities and participations, and health conditions; uses common terminology such as ICD-10-CM diagnostic coding system; includes impact of condition on movement			

(continued)

Prognosis	**YES**	**NO**	**N/A**
1. Conveys the PT's professional judgment on the predicted functional outcome and estimated duration and intensity of services to achieve the desired outcome			
Plan of Care	**YES**	**NO**	**N/A**
1. Overall goals stated in measurable terms that indicate the predicted level of improvement in function over the entire episode of care			
2. Statement of interventions to be used; whether a PTA will provide some interventions; physical therapist of record			
3. Proposed duration and frequency of services to reach desired goals (such as number of visits per week, number of weeks)			
4. Anticipated discharge plans			
Authentication	**YES**	**NO**	**N/A**
1. Signature, title, and license number (if required by state law)			
Physical Therapist Daily Visit Note Elements for Documentation	**YES**	**NO**	**N/A**
1. Date			
2. Cancellations and no-shows			
3. Patient or client, or caregiver self-report (as appropriate) and subjective response to previous treatment			
4. Identification of specific interventions and/or equipment provided, including frequency, intensity, and duration as appropriate			
5. Changes in patient or client status in terms of impairment, functional limitation, and disability status as they relate to the plan of care			
6. Patient or client response to interventions, including adverse reactions, if any			
7. Variations and progressions of specific interventions used			
8. Factors that modify frequency or intensity of intervention and progression toward anticipated goals, including patient or client adherence to patient- or client-related instructions			
9. Communication/consultation with other providers/patient or client/family/significant other			
10. Plan for ongoing provision of services for the next visit(s), which may include: • Interventions with objectives • Progression parameters • Precautions, if indicated			
11. Continuation of or modifications in plan of care			
12. Signature, title, and license number (if required by state law)			
PT Progress Report Elements for Documentation*	**YES**	**NO**	**N/A**
1. Labeled as a Progress Report/Note or Summary of Progress			
2. Date			
3. Cancellations and no-shows			
4. Treatment information regarding the current status of the patient or client			

5. Update of the baseline information provided at the initial evaluation and any needed re-evaluation(s)
6. Extent of progress (or lack thereof) between the patient's or client's current functional abilities/limitations and that of the previous progress report or at the initial evaluation
7. Factors that modify frequency or intensity of intervention and progression toward anticipated goals, including patient or client adherence to patient- or client-related instructions
8. Communication/consultation with providers/patient or client/family/significant other
9. Any modifications in the plan of care (such as goals, interventions, prognosis)
10. Signature, title, and license number (if required by state law)

**The physical therapist may be required by state law or by a payer, such as Medicare, to write a progress report. The daily note is not sufficient for this purpose unless it includes the elements listed earlier.*

PT Re-examination Elements for Documentation	**YES**	**NO**	**N/A**
1. Date			
2. Reason for re-examination, such as:			
• Unanticipated change in patient's or client's status			
• Failure for patient or client to respond to physical therapy intervention as expected			
• Need for new plan of care and/or time factors based on state practice act or other requirements			
3. Selected components of examination to update patient's or client's impairment, function, or disability status			
4. Interpretation of findings and, when indicated, revision of goals			
5. Changes from previous objective findings			
6. Interpretation of results			
7. When indicated, modification of plan of care, as directly correlated with documented goals			
8. Signature, title, and license number (if required by state law)			

PT Discharge/Discontinuation/Conclusion of Episode of Care/Final Visit Elements for Documentation*	**YES**	**NO**	**N/A**
1. Date			
2. Criteria for termination of services			
3. Patient's or client's current physical/functional status			
4. Degree of goals and outcomes achieved (patient's or client's progress or lack thereof) and reasons for goals and outcomes not being achieved			
5. Discharge/discontinuation plan that includes written and verbal communication related to the patient's or client's continuing care			
6. Justification of the medical necessity for the episode of care			
7. Signature, title, and license number (if required by state law)			

**Note: Discharge summary must be written by the PT and may be combined with the final visit note if seen by the PT on final visit.*

PTA Visit Note Elements for Documentation	YES	NO	N/A
1. Date			
2. Cancellations and no-shows			
3. Patient or client, or caregiver self-report (as appropriate) and subjective response to previous treatment			
4. Identification of specific interventions and/or equipment provided, including frequency, intensity, and duration as appropriate			
5. Changes in patient or client status in terms of impairment, functional limitation, and disability as they relate to the interventions provided			
6. Patient or client response to interventions, including adverse reactions, if any			
7. Continuation of intervention(s) as established by the PT or change of intervention(s) as authorized by PT			
8. Signature, title, and license number (if required by state law)			

Index

Page numbers followed by the letters "*f*" and "*t*" indicate figures and tables, respectively.